A B   REVISION GUIDE ?

MCQs and EMQs in Surgery

SECOND EDITION

Pradip K Datta MBE, MS, FRCS (Ed, Eng, Irel, Glasg), Honorary Consultant Surgeon, Caithness General Hospital, Wick, Member of Council and College Tutor, Royal College of Surgeons of Edinburgh

Christopher J K Bulstrode MCh, FRCS (Orth), Professor and Honorary Consultant Trauma and Orthopaedic Surgeon, University of Oxford, Member of Council, Royal College of Surgeons of Edinburgh

Iain J Nixon MBChB, FRCS (ORL-HNS), PhD, Consultant Head and Neck Oncological Surgeon, East Kent University Hospitals NHS Foundation Trust, Canterbury, United Kingdom

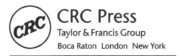

CRC Press
Taylor & Francis Group
Boca Raton London New York

CRC Press is an imprint of the
Taylor & Francis Group, an **informa** business

Contents

First published in 1932, *Bailey & Love's Short Practice of Surgery* has stood the test of time. Perhaps this is an understatement, considering all three of us have used the book as medical students. This book has been the result of good foresight on the part of Hodder Arnold to keep up with the changing trends in the pattern of surgical examinations, at both undergraduate and postgraduate levels. The publishers should be congratulated on bringing out this book—converting the original Silver Jubilee (25th) edition—all 77 chapters of it—as Multiple Choice Questions (MCQs) and Extended Matching Questions (EMQs).

The book is aptly titled as a companion to *Bailey & Love*. We would therefore hope that the reader, specifically preparing for a written examination, would use this book as the major reading material and refer to the original for detailed elucidation of a particular point or operative detail.

Most of the contributors are different from *Bailey & Love's Short Practice of Surgery* except for chapters 5, 25, the section on orthopaedics, and part of trauma. Thus while retaining the essence of the original material, this book has been seasoned by different authors, giving it a fresh flavour without losing any of its original ingredients. We are grateful to all the contributors for their prompt response in spite of the pressures of work in the National Health Service.

The images and pictures are mostly different than those in the original book, giving this tome an added attraction. While the MCQs test knowledge, the EMQs with the illustrations give a good format for a self-assessment exercise. The chapters are specifically geared toward helping the reader with preparation for the written papers of the MRCS and FRCS(Gen) examinations. The undergraduate will also find this book equally stimulating for the same reasons. In surgical examinations in the English-speaking world, where essays have been replaced by short answer questions (short notes of yesteryear), the reader will find the EMQs ideal preparation.

Any book must be dynamic, much more so a new venture such as this. It was said in the preface of the parent book, 'Whereas the past informs the present, it must never enslave the future.' As authors of this very exciting project, we can stay true to the spirit of this statement only with help from you—our readers. Therefore, we look forward to your suggestions and constructive criticisms for the next edition.

Pradip K Datta
Christopher JK Bulstrode
BV Praveen

November 2009

Preface to Second Edition

This is the Second Edition of the book which initially published in 2010, and mirrored the 25th Edition of *Bailey & Love* in the form of MCQs and EMQs. The success of *Bailey & Love* as an international surgical tome continues unabated, with the 26th Edition published in 2013. In keeping with the prestige of such a publication, we are now bringing out the Second Edition.

There has been a change both in authorship and in contributors. While the basic tenet of the book remains much the same, we have asked the contributors to give the answers in much greater detail, which has resulted in some changes to the set-up. This has enhanced some of the chapters to such an extent that we feel that in parts it is a new book.

The book is ideally suited for the first part (section A) of the FRCS in General Surgery; this is the theory paper which deals with MCQs and EMQs. Since 2013, a new Intercollegiate FRCS (International) examination has started. We hope that the readership will include this new group of international senior surgical trainees wishing to appear in this examination. Most surgical examinations, postgraduate and undergraduate, now have an EMQ and MCQ component. We have catered to their needs.

In keeping with the parent book, there are 81 chapters and an appendix, which is a chapter on surgical instruments. Images and pictures of clinical cases and pathological specimens help the reader to cement the knowledge gleaned from the text. Readers' suggestions would be most welcome.

Pradip K Datta
Christopher JK Bulstrode
Iain J Nixon

Acknowledgments

We would like to thank Henry Spilberg for initiating the process of publishing the Second Edition and his team for seeing it through to completion. All the contributors have done a tremendous job of producing comprehensive chapters—and this in spite of the pressures of the present-day National Health Service. To them we record our grateful thanks. We thank Julia Molloy and Rachael Russell from the Editorial Department for liaising with the authors and contributors on a regular basis, a task carried out with infinite patience. We would like to thank Laurie Schlags for her most diligent work toward the book, which has helped in its on-time publication. Finally, to CRC Press of Taylor & Francis Group we owe a debt of immeasurable gratitude for bringing out a Second Edition.

PKD
CJKB
IJN

Contributors

Christopher JK Bulstrode MCh, FRCS (Orth)
Emeritus Professor
University of Oxford
Oxford, United Kingdom

Harry Bulstrode MA (Cantab), BM BCh, MRCS (Eng)
Scottish Centre for Regenerative Medicine
Edinburgh, United Kingdom

Pradip K Datta MBE, MS, FRCS(Ed), FRCS (Eng), FRCS (Ire), FRCS (Glas)
Honorary Consultant Surgeon
Caithness General Hospital
Wick, United Kingdom

Sanjay De Bakshi MS, FRCS (Eng), FRCS(Ed)
Consultant Surgeon
Calcutta Medical Research Institute
Kolkata, India

Andrew D Duckworth MSc, MRCS(Ed)
Specialist Registrar and Clinical
Research Fellow
Edinburgh Orthopaedic Trauma Unit
Edinburgh, United Kingdom

Stuart Enoch PhD, MRCS (Eng), MRCS(Ed)
Director for Education and Research
Doctors Academy Group
Cardiff, United Kingdom

Brian W Fleck MD, FRCOphth, FRCS(Ed)
Consultant Ophthalmic Surgeon
Princess Alexandra Eye Pavilion and Royal
Hospital for Sick Children
Edinburgh, United Kingdom

Andrew Hobkirk FDSRCS, MRCS
Specialist Registrar
Oral and Maxillofacial Surgery
University Hospital Aintree
Liverpool, United Kingdom

Tessa Housden MBBS, FRCA
ST 6 Anaesthetist
Royal Infirmary of Edinburgh
Edinburgh, United Kingdom

KS Krishna Kumar MBBS, MS(Gen Surg), FRCS(Ed), FRCS(Glasg), MCh(Plast Surg), FRCS(Plast Surg), CCT in Plastic Surgery (UK)
Fellowship in Hand and Microsurgery
Christine M Kleinert Institute
Louisville, Kentucky

and

Examiner and Trainer MRCS
(RCSEd)
Head of Department and Senior
Consultant, Plastic, Reconstructive and
Microsurgery
Baby Memorial Hospital
Calicut, Kerala, India

Pawanindra Lal MS, DNB, FIMSA, FRCS(Ed), FRCS(Eng), FRCS(Glas), FACS
Professor of Surgery
Maulana Azad Medical College
and
Associated Lok Nayak Hospital
New Delhi, India

Ian Leeuwenberg MB ChB, FRCA
Trainee in Anaesthesia
South East Scotland
Edinburgh, United Kingdom

Sarah M Lloyd FRCA, FFPMRCA
Member of Council and Former Honorary
Secretary
British Association of Day Surgery
Consultant Anaesthetist
Leeds Teaching Hospitals NHS Trust
Leeds, United Kingdom

CONTRIBUTORS

Pratap Nadar MBBS, MS (Gen Surg), MCh (Plast Surg)
Plastic Surgeon
Baby Memorial Hospital
Calicut, Kerala, India

Dumbor L Ngaage MBBS, FRCS(Ed), FWACS, FRCS(C-Th), FETCS (Cardiovascular), FETCS (Thoracic), MS
Consultant Cardiothoracic Surgeon
The Cardiothoracic Centre
Basildon University Hospital
Basildon, United Kingdom

Iain J Nixon MBChB, FRCS (ORL-HNS), PhD
Consultant Head and Neck Oncological Surgeon
East Kent University Hospitals NHS Foundation Trust
Canterbury, United Kingdom

Stephen J Nixon FRCS(Ed), FRCP (Edin)
Consultant Surgeon
Royal Infirmary of Edinburgh
Edinburgh, United Kingdom

Ajit Kumar Pati MBBS, MS(Gen Surg), MCh(Plast Surg)
Plastic Surgeon
Baby Memorial Hospital
Calicut, Kerala, India

BV Praveen MS, FRCS(Ed, Eng, Glas, Ire), FRCS(Gen)
Consultant Surgeon
Southend University Hospital
Southend, United Kingdom

Selvi Radhakrishna, FRCS(Ed), DNB, PGDip Clin Oncol (Univ of Birmingham)
Consultant Oncoplastic Breast Surgeon
Chennai Breast Centre and Apollo Specialty Hospitals
Chennai, India

P Raghu Ram MS, FRCS(Ed), FRCS(Eng), FRCS (Glasg), FRCS(Ire)
Director and Consultant Oncoplastic Breast Surgeon
KIMS-Ushalakshmi Centre for Breast Diseases
Krishna Institute of Medical Sciences
Hyderabad, India

Nandini Rao MRCP, MSc
Specialist Registrar in Chemical Pathology/ Metabolic Medicine
Royal Free Hampstead NHS Trust
London, United Kingdom

Pranathi Reddy MD, DGO, DNB, FRCOG (UK)
Clinical Director
Department of Obstetrics and Gynaecology
Rainbow Hospital
Hyderabad, India

CR Selvasekar MD, FRCS(Ed), FRCS(Gen), PGCert (Med Ed), PGCert (Health Executive)
Consultant General
Colorectal and Laparoscopic Surgeon
The Christie NHS Foundation Trust, Manchester
and
Honorary Senior Lecturer
University of Manchester
Manchester, United Kingdom

Benjamin M Stutchfield MBChB, BSc, MSc, MRCS
Registrar in General Surgery
Department of Surgery
Royal Infirmary of Edinburgh
Edinburgh, United Kingdom

Shamim Toma FRCS(ORL-HNS)
ENT Registrar
East Kent Hospitals
Canterbury, United Kingdom

S Vyjayanthi MD, DNB, MRCOG
Consultant in Reproductive Medicine
Krishna Institute of Medical Sciences
Hyderabad, India

Metabolic response to trauma

Pradip K Datta

Multiple choice questions

Homeostasis

1. Which one of the following statements about homeostasis is false?

A It is defined as a stable state of the normal body.

B The central nervous system, heart, lungs, kidneys and spleen are the essential organs that maintain normal homeostasis.

C Elective surgery should cause little disturbance to homeostasis.

D Emergency surgery should cause little disturbance to homeostasis.

E Return to normal homeostasis after an insult (operation, injury, infection) would depend upon the presence of comorbid conditions.

Stress response

2. Neuroendocrine pathways of the stress response consist of the following except:

A Spinal cord

B Thalamus

C Hypothalamus

D Pituitary

E Thyroid

Body metabolism

3. Changes in body metabolism that occur in response to trauma are the following except:

A Lipolysis

B Gluconeogenesis

C Protein breakdown

D Hypoglycaemia

E Hypermetabolism

Mediators

4. Which of the following statements about mediators are true?

A They consist of neural, endocrine and inflammatory.

B Every endocrine gland plays a part.

C They play an important role in the flow phase.

D These mediators are released over several days.

E They play an important role in the recovery process.

Optimal perioperative care

5. Which of the following statements are true of optimal perioperative care?

A Surgery should be carried out by the use of adequate large incisions to give good exposure.

B Adequate pain relief is essential.

C Early mobilisation.

D Avoid ongoing insults and secondary trauma.

E Maintain good fluid load with several litres of normal saline.

6. The following statements are true regarding Enhanced Recovery After Surgery (ERAS) programmes except:

A It optimises rehabilitation following major surgery.

B It reduces hospital stay.

C Patient engagement is an integral part.

D It is only used in colorectal surgery.

E Blocking afferent painful stimuli is important in reducing stress response.

Answers to multiple choice questions

→ ## Homeostasis

1. D

Emergency surgery causes a marked disturbance in homeostasis. This disturbance is directly proportional to the degree of injury and inversely proportional to the fitness of the patient prior to the event. The greater the injury the more pronounced is the physiological, metabolic and immunological changes, all of which are graded according to the magnitude of the initial insult. Elective surgery causes minimal disturbance because the patient is optimised and precautions taken against comorbid conditions prior to an operation.

Homeostasis is the normal physiological state of the human body – *the milieu intérieur,* a term coined by Claude Bernard. The vital organs – the brain, heart, lungs and kidneys, and, to a lesser extent, the spleen – play an essential part in its maintenance. The brain, heart and kidneys by their specific ability of autoregulation play an added role in response to trauma. Fluid and electrolyte conservation is the vital first stage **(Figure 1.1)**. A return to normal physiology is always affected by the presence of ongoing complications or secondary insults, such as ischaemia from hypotension, inadequate oxygenation from hypoxia, or infection and complications such as compartment syndrome or deep venous thrombosis **(see Figure 1.2)**.

→ ## Stress response

2. E

The thyroid does not form a part of the neuroendocrine pathway to the stress response. Following any form of injury, the afferent nociceptive pathways consist of the spinal cord, thalamus, hypothalamus and the pituitary. The hypothalamus secretes corticotrophin-releasing factor (CRF), which acts on the anterior pituitary to secrete adrenocorticotrophic hormone (ACTH), which, in turn, acts on the adrenal glands to release cortisol **(Figure 1.3)**. Classically it has been described as the 'fight or flight' response. This occurs as a result of a concerted interplay between neural, endocrine and inflammatory factors **(Figure 1.4)**.

The stress response is graded. For instance, a 30-year-old fit woman undergoing an elective laparoscopic cholecystectomy will elicit a minor transient stress response compared to a 70-year-old involved in a road traffic accident who has to undergo major orthopaedic

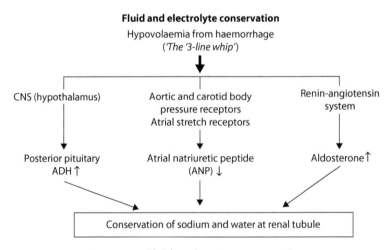

Fluid and electrolyte conservation

Hypovolaemia from haemorrhage
(*'The '3-line whip'*)

| CNS (hypothalamus) | Aortic and carotid body pressure receptors Atrial stretch receptors | Renin-angiotensin system |

| Posterior pituitary ADH ↑ | Atrial natriuretic peptide (ANP) ↓ | Aldosterone ↑ |

Conservation of sodium and water at renal tubule

Figure 1.1 Fluid and water conservation.

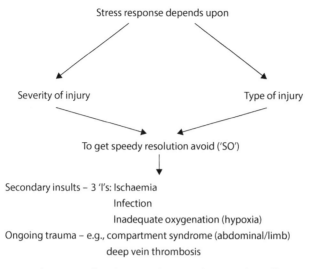

Figure 1.2 Ongoing complications and secondary insults affecting recovery.

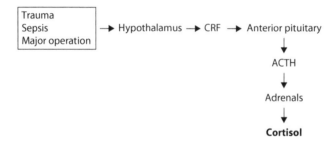

Figure 1.3 The release of cortisol.

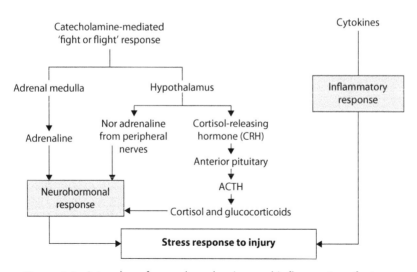

Figure 1.4 Interplay of neural, endocrine and inflammatory factors.

surgery. In the latter case, there is increase in metabolism and nitrogen excretion with immunological and metabolic changes reflected in the altered physiology – pyrexia, tachycardia and tachypnoea. In such a patient, the stress response can be modified by anticipating and preventing complications by management in an intensive care unit (ICU) and by attention to nutrition and organ support.

Body metabolism

3. D

It is hypergylcaemia and not hypolglycaemia that occurs in stress response. There is an increase in glucagon and reduction of insulin producing the 'diabetes of stress'. Marked changes occur in the body metabolism – lipolysis, hepatic gluconeogenesis, skeletal muscle protein breakdown, hypergylcaemia and hypermetabolism.

The changes that occur in body metabolism in the stress response have been divided into the 'ebb and flow' phases, a term that Sir David Cuthbertson first used in 1932. The initial ebb phase (a holding pattern), which lasts for a few hours, is characterized by the classical features of shock – hypovolaemia, hypothermia, reduced cardiac output and lactic acidosis (**Figure 1.5a** and **1.5b**). The hormones responsible for the ebb phase are catecholamines, cortisol and aldosterone, the latter activated by the renin–angiotensin–aldosterone system (RAAS) (**Figure 1.6**).

The ebb phase, following resuscitation, gives way to the flow phase (**Figure 1.7**). This phase concentrates on recovery and repair. There is increased basal metabolic rate, increased cardiac output, increased body temperature, leukocytosis and gluconeogenesis. The flow phase initially consists of the catabolic phase, which lasts up to 10 days, followed by the anabolic phase, which lasts for weeks. Obviously the duration of these phases will depend upon the severity of injury,

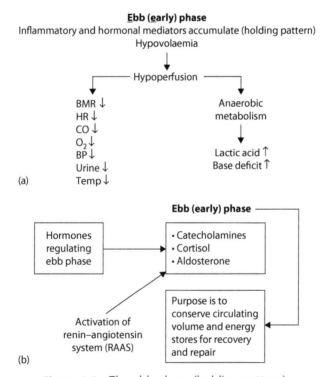

Figure 1.5   The ebb phase (holding pattern).

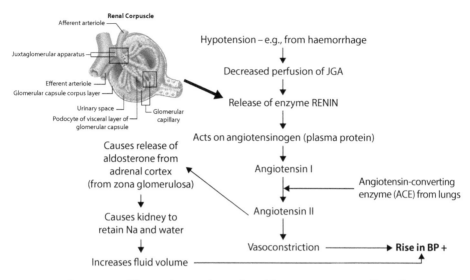

Figure 1.6 The renin–angiotensin–aldosterone system (RAAS).

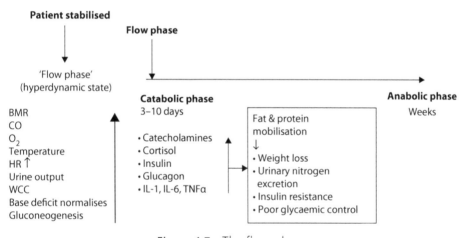

Figure 1.7 The flow phase.

effectiveness of management, presence of any comorbidities and any complications that might occur.

Mediators

4. D

The mediators are released immediately within the first few hours. The two immune systems are the innate (mainly macrophages) and the adaptive (T cells and B cells) systems. These produce the mediators – interleukin -1(IL-1), IL-6, IL-8 and tumour necrosis factor alpha (TNFα) **(Figure 1.8)**. They act on the hypothalamus to cause pyrexia. The pituitary, adrenal and pancreas play an integral role in this response; the thyroid and gonads play a minor role.

Proinflammatory cytokines thus released result in systemic inflammatory response syndrome (SIRS). At this stage, endogenous cytokine antagonists appear to control the proinflammatory cytokines, thus keeping in check the SIRS. If the response to SIRS is

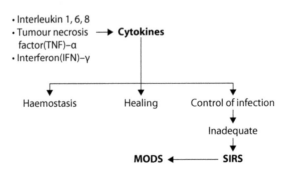

Figure 1.8 The mediators.

inadequate, multiple organ dysfunction syndrome (MODS) occurs, which is a step away from death.

Optimal perioperative care

5. B, C, D

Adequate pain relief is essential to reduce the stress response following surgical trauma. Blocking afferent painful stimuli by epidural analgesia is an efficient method of postoperative pain relief after major abdominal and thoracic surgery. It has the advantage of continuous analgesia by infusion (or with patient-controlled analgesia, PCA) through a catheter in the epidural space. A weak local anaesthetic with opioids (e.g., fentanyl) is used. This allows early mobilisation, thus reducing the incidence of deep vein thrombosis and chest complications.

Minimal access surgery instead of open surgical incisions is well known to reduce the stress response and return the patient to an early postoperative normal homeostasis. Steps should be taken to prevent any postoperative ongoing insults such as infection, ischaemia, inadequate oxygenation and secondary trauma such as acute compartment syndromes (limb and abdominal). It is important to avoid excessive administration of intravenous fluids (saline) and prolonged preoperative starvation to hasten recovery.

ERAS

6. D

Although the concept of ERAS was originally started in colorectal surgery it is now used across all surgical specialties. Enhanced recovery, also known as Rapid or Accelerated Recovery or Fast Track surgery, is an evidence-based innovative approach to the preoperative, intraoperative and postoperative care of patients undergoing elective surgery. It improves patient outcomes by speeding postoperative recovery, thus reducing the stress response following surgery.

First developed in Copenhagen by Professor Henrik Kehlet in 1997, it has been used in the United Kingdom since 2002. The concept optimises rehabilitation following major surgery with better outcomes and reduced hospital stay enabling faster postoperative recovery. This is achieved through patient engagement by shared decision making. This results in improved clinical outcomes and a better patient experience from a shorter hospital stay. As a final outcome, more patients are treated in the system, which is thus more streamlined.

Shock and blood transfusion

Pradip K Datta

→ ## Pathophysiology of shock

1. Which of the following statements are true in the pathophysiology of shock?

A In shock, cells switch from aerobic to anaerobic metabolism.

B The product of anaerobic respiration is carbon dioxide, resulting in respiratory acidosis.

C Hypoxia and acidosis generate oxygen free radicals and cytokine release.

D Renal ischaemia leads to decreased glomerular filtration (GFR), thus activating the renin-aldosterone-angiotensin system (RAAS).

E Once shock has been treated and circulation restored, the physiological disturbances return to normal.

→ ## Severity of shock

2. Which of the following statement/s are false?

A In compensated shock, blood flow is maintained to the brain, lungs and kidneys.

B Loss of 15% of circulating blood volume will overload the body's compensatory mechanisms.

C Capillary refill time is an accurate clinical parameter in all types of shock.

D Hypotension is an early sign of shock.

E Prolonged systemic ischaemia and reperfusion injury contribute to multi-organ failure.

→ ## Resuscitation

3. Which of the following statements are true?

A In a patient who is shocked from a leaking abdominal aortic aneurysm or a bleeding peptic ulcer, time should not be wasted in instituting high-volume fluid resuscitation.

B In a patient with intestinal obstruction with hypovolaemic shock, time should be spent in optimising with adequate fluid resuscitation.

C In hypovolaemia, inotropes must be started as soon as possible as first-line therapy.

D The ideal fluid is colloid in hypovolaemia.

E The shock status is best determined by an initial fluid challenge.

→ ## Monitoring

4. Which of the following statements are true?

A CVP monitoring is a dynamic reflection on fluid challenge.

B Measurement of cardiac output (CO) helps in distinguishing the type of shock.

C Mixed venous oxygen saturation is an indicator of systemic perfusion.

D Pulmonary artery wedge pressure (PAWP) measurement should be instituted in all shocked patients in the ICU.

E It is mandatory to perform Allen's test prior to insertion of an arterial line.

→ ## Haemorrhage

5. The following statements are true except:

A Haemorrhage with hypovolaemic shock results in a state of coagulopathy.

B Haemoglobin level is an accurate indicator of the degree of haemorrhage.

C The acid-base disturbance is metabolic acidosis.

D Permissive hypotension is a strategy to be followed until haemorrhage is controlled.

E Haemorrhagic shock can be classified into three groups – mild, moderate and severe.

→ Blood transfusion

6. Which of the following statements are true?

A Blood group 'O' is regarded as universal donor.

B Blood group 'AB' is regarded as universal recipient.

C The vast majority of the population is Rhesus negative.

D In coagulopathy packed red blood cells should be transfused.

E Fresh frozen plasma (FFP) has a shelf life of 2 years.

Extended matching questions

→ Diagnoses

1 Anaphylactic shock
2 Autologous blood transfusion
3 Cardiogenic shock
4 Hypovolaemic shock
5 Mismatched blood transfusion
6 Neurogenic shock
7 Septic shock

Match the diagnoses with the clinical scenarios that follow:

→ Clinical scenarios

A A 50-year-old man is undergoing partial hepatectomy for secondary metastasis. The operation proceeded smoothly for the first couple of hours, after which the surgical team noticed unusual bleeding in the form of oozing from all the wound sites. The patient has two intravenous cannula sites through one of which he is on his first unit of blood.

B A fit 30-year-old woman while gardening suddenly became very short of breath, had intense itching with rash and complained of a painful red spot on her arm. She has been brought to the A&E department and is hypotensive, hypoxic with warm peripheries.

C A fit 25-year-old man fell from a height of 40 feet at a building site. He has been brought in unconscious with a GCS of 13 and flaccid limbs. He has been immobilised in a spinal frame and has an intravenous line.

D A 70-year-old man of ASA anaesthetic category 3, underwent an emergency closure of a perforated duodenal ulcer. The anaesthetic and operation were uneventful. On the first postoperative day, he complained of feeling very unwell with a systolic blood pressure of 80 mm Hg with no unusual signs in his abdomen; there was impaired conscious level and peripheral vasoconstriction.

E A 60-year-old man of ASA 1 anaesthetic risk underwent a total gastrectomy for stomach cancer. While in the ITU, 12 hours postoperatively, his BP has fallen to 80 mm Hg systolic, he has not put out any urine over the past 3 hours and he is hypoxic with oxygen saturation of 92%.

F A 60-year-old woman has been admitted as an emergency with a 4-day history of severe right upper quadrant pain, vomiting, jaundice and intense pruritus and is very toxic – high temperature with rigors and hyperdynamic circulation.

G A 35-year-old woman is due for a bilateral mastectomy. She has requested a bilateral breast reconstruction at the same time. However, she is a strict Jehovah's Witness and would under no circumstances have a heterologous blood transfusion.

Pathophysiology of shock

1. A, C, D

Shock is a clinical state of inadequate tissue perfusion where there is reduced delivery of oxygen and glucose. The former leads to anaerobic metabolism. As glucose is reduced, anaerobic respiration stops with failure of the sodium/potassium pump in the cell membrane thus causing release of cell contents and potassium into the blood stream. Hypoxia and metabolic acidosis produces oxygen free radicals and cytokine release, causing damage to the capillary endothelium and resulting in tissue oedema, which worsens cellular hypoxia. At the same time the stress response is activated, causing renal ischaemia. This triggers the RAAS, helping sodium and water reabsorption by the kidney.

The product of anaerobic respiration is lactic acid and not carbon dioxide. This causes lactic acidosis, resulting in metabolic and not respiratory acidosis. The metabolic acidosis and increased sympathetic activity results in tachypnoea and increased excretion of carbon dioxide, thus producing a compensatory respiratory alkalosis. Once circulation is restored, further injury can occur from the stagnant potassium and lactic acid being flushed back into the circulation. This leads to myocardial depression, vascular dilatation and endothelial injury to lungs and kidneys. The process is called ischaemia-reperfusion injury, a classical example being compartment syndrome.

Severity of shock

2. B, C, D

With loss of 15% of blood volume, the body will compensate with its normal mechanisms by reducing the blood flow to the skin (hence, cold skin in shock), muscles and gastrointestinal tract. Capillary refill time is not an accurate clinical finding in shock as this may not be affected in the early stages; moreover, in septic shock the peripheries are warm with a brisk capillary refill. Similarly, hypotension is the last sign to be affected in shock. Fit and young patients maintain their blood pressure by increasing the stroke volume and peripheral vasoconstriction. Elderly hypertensive patients may show a misleading 'normal blood pressure' in the presence of shock just as patients on beta blockers may fail to show tachycardia.

In compensated shock, adequate preload is maintained to the vital organs such as the brain, lungs, heart and kidneys. This perfusion in the presence of adversity is also helped by the phenomenon of autoregulation in the brain, heart and kidneys. Prolonged ischaemia from profound shock leads to cell death, resulting in myocardial depression that is unresponsive to volume expansion or inotropes. This, coupled with reperfusion injury, contributes to multiple organ dysfunction syndrome, a condition defined by the failure of two or more organs.

Resuscitation

3. A, B, E

For a patient who is losing blood from a leaking abdominal aortic aneurysm (AAA) or upper gastrointestinal haemorrhage, trying to resuscitate with large amounts of fluid would be counterproductive and a waste of valuable time. Increasing the preload would make the patient lose all the infused fluid. Moreover, it would be dangerous, because it would cause hypothermia and dilute coagulation factors increasing the chances of disseminated intravascular coagulation (DIC). The 'leaking tap must be turned off' as soon as possible by surgery.

On the other hand, a patient with intestinal obstruction will have lost a large amount of fluid as a result of sequestration into the third space. Time should be spent in optimising this patient with intravenous fluids, the adequacy of resuscitation being monitored by an indwelling urinary catheter and central venous pressure (CVP) line. A good method of assessing the shock status is a 'fluid challenge' where the response of the patient is gauged by infusing 300–500 ml of crystalloid over 15–30 minutes. The response is gauged by the patient's blood pressure, heart rate, CVP and urinary output.

Inotrope administration is not the first-line treatment in hypovolaemia. It should never be used until confirming the presence of an adequate preload. An inotrope in the presence of inadequate preload will reduce diastolic filling and coronary perfusion with disastrous consequences. Although controversy continues with regard to the ideal intravenous fluid, it is customary to use crystalloids and not colloids. There is less benefit from the use of colloids, which are more expensive and have worse side effects.

Monitoring

4. A, B, C, E

Monitoring is an integral part of resuscitation. With CVP, one reading should never be relied upon. It is a dynamic measurement that assesses response to fluid resuscitation. The normal response will be a rise in CVP of 2–5 cm H_2O, indicating a positive response to a fluid challenge. Absence of response indicates need for more fluid, whereas a sustained rise denotes fluid overload or cardiac failure. Measurement of CO helps in distinguishing hypovolaemic, cardiogenic and distributive shock, particularly when they co-exist. This information is obtained by real-time monitoring by Doppler ultrasound and pulse waveform analysis without resorting to PAWP.

Mixed venous oxygen saturation is obtained from blood from the right atrium with an accurately placed CVP line. Normal levels are 50% to 70% and are an indicator of oxygen delivery and extraction by the tissues. Levels below 50% are a reflection of insufficient oxygen delivery or increased oxygen extraction by the cells – a situation that occurs in hypovolaemic or cardiogenic shock. High venous saturation is seen in distributive shock, as in sepsis.

When aggressive invasive monitoring is necessary, an arterial line for continuous blood pressure monitoring is advisable. Before inserting such a line, Allen's test is mandatory to make sure that the collateral circulation in the palm between the radial and ulnar arteries is efficient. PAWP measurement need not be instituted in all shocked patients. It has largely been superseded by more sophisticated and less invasive methods (see previous section), because insertion of a Swan-Ganz catheter can produce serious complications. Besides the monitoring tools previously mentioned, use of routine clinical parameters of pulse, blood pressure, urine output and pulse oximetry should be routine.

Haemorrhage

5. B, E

The level of haemoglobin is not an accurate indicator of the degree of haemorrhage, as it represents a concentration and not an absolute amount. Immediately after blood loss and in the presence of continued blood loss, the haemoglobin level is unchanged as whole blood is lost. The haemoglobin level will fall after some time when there is a fluid shift from the intracellular and interstitial spaces into the vascular compartment. Haemorrhagic shock is classified into four groups: 1 to 4 depending upon the estimated percentage of the total blood volume lost: 1 = <15%, 2 = 5%–30%, 3 = 30%–40% and 4 = >40%.

Hypovolaemic shock from haemorrhage results in acute traumatic coagulopathy (ATC) along with acidosis and hypothermia. A quarter of the patients develop ATC, which is associated with a four-fold increase in mortality. A multitude of factors cause this problem, which is explained in **Figure 2.1**. The acid-base disturbance is metabolic acidosis. This is because ischaemia results in anaerobic metabolism with resultant lactic acidosis reflected in the base deficit.

Patients who are actively bleeding, such as a leaking abdominal aortic aneurysm or acute upper or lower gastrointestinal tract haemorrhage, need immediate arrest of their haemorrhage and not fluid resuscitation and blood transfusion. Permissive hypotension is the

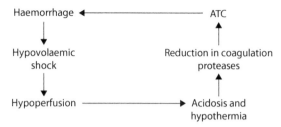

Figure 2.1 Acute traumatic coagulopathy (ATC) in haemorrhage.

key, as volume expansion will only result in further haemorrhage or dilutional coagulopathy, thus worsening the situation. Arrest of haemorrhage should be the immediate goal.

Blood transfusion

6. A, B, E

The red blood cells have agglutinogen (a sugar) on the outer coat. Blood group 'O' (46% of the population) is regarded as the universal donor because it has neither 'A' nor 'B' agglutinogen to provoke a reaction. Blood group A (42%) has agglutinogen A, group B (9%) has agglutinogen B and group AB (3%) has both agglutinogen A and B. Those belonging to blood group AB are universal recipients because they do not develop any agglutinins. The other sub-group in blood grouping is the Rhesus factor (rhesus D). The rhesus D is strongly antigenic and is present in 85% of the U.K. population, whilst the rest are rhesus negative.

In coagulopathy, packed red blood cells have no role. Fresh frozen plasma (FFP) is used in prolonged prothrombin or partial thromboplastin time, cryoprecipitate is used when there is reduced fibrinogen and platelets are transfused in thrombocytopenia. The shelf life of FFP is 2 years.

Answers to extended matching questions

1. B Anaphylactic shock

Anaphylactic shock, more common in patients with asthma and eczema, is an acute medical emergency that can follow insect bites, administration of drugs or vaccines and consumption of shellfish and many other foodstuffs (e.g., nuts). The patient presents with apprehension, urticaria, bronchospasm, respiratory distress, nausea, vomiting, diarrhea and signs such as laryngeal oedema, hypoxia, hypotension, shock and vasodilatation.

In this type of shock the antigen combines with immunoglobulin E (Ig E) on the mast cells and basophils, releasing large amounts of histamine and SRS-A (slow-release-substance–anaphylaxis). These compounds cause the symptoms. The mortality is about 10%.

In the acute stage, the patient should be made to lie down with elevation of the lower limbs. The airway should be free; the patient is given oxygen and venous access established with full monitoring; in severe hypoxia ventilation may be necessary. The patient is given the following:

- 0.5 ml of 1 in 1000 adrenaline intramuscular (0.5 mg) to be repeated after 5 minutes if shock persists
- Antihistamine (chlorphenamine/chlorpheniramine)10 mg by slow intravenous injection to be continued for 48 hours
- Intravenous hydrocortisone 100 mg

2. G Autologous blood transfusion

Autologous blood transfusion in elective surgery is ideal for prevention of transfusion reactions and in those who refuse to receive heterologous transfusion. This can be achieved in one of the following three ways:

- Preoperative Donation: A patient with a preoperative Hb of 11g/dL can donate once weekly for three weeks before operation; the patient is put on iron and recombinant human erythropoietin.
- Acute Normovolaemic Haemodilution: In the anaesthetic room under anaesthesia, three to four units of blood are withdrawn and replaced with crystalloid or colloid. The whole blood is reinfused at the end of the operation.
- Perioperative Blood Salvage: At the time of surgery lost blood is collected in a cell-saver that washes and collects red blood cells, which are then reinfused during or after the operation. Transfusion trigger: This is the threshold at which blood transfusion is indicated. A haemoglobin level of less than 10 g/dL used to be the reason for transfusion; this is no longer the case. A level of 6 to 7 g/dL is regarded as acceptable in patients who are not actively bleeding and in the absence of risk factors. In the young, healthy patient undergoing elective surgery, moderate haemodilution is tolerated. A balance has to be struck between the risks of transfusion, such as transmission of infection and immunosuppression against the lower oxygen-carrying capacity of the blood interfering with adequate tissue oxygenation. It is accepted when haemoglobin level (g/dL) is the following:

  - 8 or more, there is no indication for transfusion
  - 6–8, transfusion is unlikely to be beneficial in the absence of bleeding
  - < 6, will benefit from transfusion

3. D Cardiogenic shock

Cardiogenic shock indicates a state of inadequate circulatory perfusion caused by cardiac dysfunction. The causes are the following:

- Myocardial infarction (MI)
- Cardiac arrhythmias
- Tension pneumothorax
- Cardiac tamponade
- Vena caval obstruction
- Dissecting aneurysm

This patient will have ECG changes: ST elevation in precordial leads, new wide or deep Q waves and T wave inversion. Blood investigations such as creatine kinase (CK), alanine aminotransferase (ALT), aspartate aminotransferase (AST), lactic dehydrogenase and troponin T assay are carried out and the patient transferred to the coronary care unit (CCU). In the CCU, oxygen therapy will be started along with aspirin, nitrates, ACE inhibitors, opiates and intravenous beta blockers. Depending upon the unit's protocol, reperfusion strategy would be considered and the patient closely monitored with a CVP and sometimes with a pulmonary artery flotation catheter (PAFC). The complications are the following:

- Cardiac arrest (ventricular fibrillation, VF)
- Pump failure
- Arrhythmias
- Ventricular septal defect (VSD)
- Cardiac rupture

- Pericardial tamponade
- Ventricular aneurysm
- Mitral regurgitation

The risk factors in postoperative myocardial infarction are the following:

- Previous MI
- Unstable angina
- Disabling angina
- Silent ischaemia
- Hypertension

The risk of perioperative MI in the general surgical population is 0.07%, whereas if surgery is performed within 3 months of a MI, the risk rises to 25%.

4. E Hypovolaemic shock

Hypovolaemic shock arises from a reduction in the volume of circulating fluid. This can be due to inadequate preload or decreased contractility of the heart.

Inadequate preload can be the result of the following:

- Absolute reduction of fluid as in haemorrhage
- Severe vomiting and diarrhoea where fluid lass has not been adequately replaced
- Relative reduction of fluid from vasodilatation as in spinal shock
- Mechanical interference as in tension pneumothorax and pulmonary embolism

Decreased contractility can be the result of the following:

- Ischaemia
- Hypoxia
- Acidosis
- Sepsis
- Electrolyte imbalance
- Fluid overload
- Cardiac tamponade

In the management, careful monitoring is essential, particularly in the over-60s, to prevent overload. A close watch is maintained on the CVP, urinary output and clinical parameters such as oxygen saturation, capillary filling, blood pressure and heart rate.

The pathophysiology of hypovolaemic shock is shown in **Figure 2.2**. In the immediate postoperative period, hypovolaemic shock should be presumed to be from postoperative bleeding unless otherwise proved. The treatment is surgical exploration to stop the bleeding. When the cause may be due to traumatic rupture of a solid intra-abdominal organ, such as the liver, kidney or spleen, and the patient is stable, a CT scan should be performed. If the diagnosis is confirmed, an angiogram may be carried out if arterial embolization is considered.

5. A Mismatched blood transfusion

Although rare, the complication of ABO-incompatibility is always due to human error. It arises from mistakes that can occur at various levels, such as in taking the blood, labelling the sample, collecting the wrong blood from the blood bank refrigerator and, finally, inadequate or hurried checking prior to transfusion. As soon as this serious error is suspected, transfusion should be stopped at once, all clerical checks made, the blood bank informed and surgery halted.

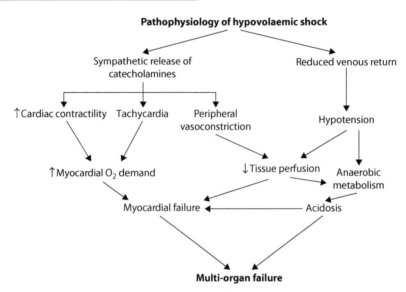

Pathophysiology of hypovolaemic shock

Figure 2.2   Pathophysiology of hypovolaemic shock.

Table 2.1   Complications of blood transfusion

General	Massive transfusion
• Disease transmission	• Hypothermia
– Bacterial	• Dilutional coagulopathy
– Parasitic	• DIC
– Viral	• Acid-base disturbance
• Transfusion reactions	• Hypocalcaemia
• Mismatched transfusion	• Hypomagnesaemia
• TRALI	• Hyperkalaemia
• Immunosuppression	

Incompatible red blood cells react with the patient's own anti-A and anti-B antibodies. This results in complement activation, acute intravascular haemolysis and disseminated intravascular coagulation (DIC). Ultimately, acute renal failure will result. Therefore, preparation for renal support such as dialysis should be made as soon as possible. The complications of blood transfusion are in **Table 2.1**.

6. C Neurogenic shock
In neurogenic shock (head or spinal injury) the cardiovascular response is sometimes referred to as distributive shock. Interruption of the thoracolumbar sympathetic outflow results in loss of the sympathetic drive to the heart. This causes hypotension from loss of vasomotor tone with warm extremities, bradycardia, flaccidity and loss of reflexes. The sympathetic tone takes 3 to 7 days to return to normal.

Fractures of the atlas (C1) account for 5% of all cervical spine (c-spine) injuries, and 40% of these are associated with a concomitant injury of the axis (C2). Because of the nature of the vertebra, which is very thin (because it is devoid of a body that is incorporated into the axis as the odontoid process), the most common fracture is a burst fracture (Jefferson fracture) caused by axial loading. Fractures of the axis account for 18% of all C-spine injuries, and 60% of these involve the odontoid process. Fracture occurs in the posterior element called hangman's fracture and is the most dangerous, occurring in 20%. Confirmation is by open-mouth lateral x-ray followed by CT scan. The mechanism of injury is hyperextension. The treatment of C1 injury is a halo jacket for 3 months; in C2 injury the treatment is sterno-occipito-mandibular immobiliser (SOMI) with surgical fixation when indicated.

The immediate management is to identify and exclude life-threatening problems. Whilst intravenous access is obtained, temptation for overzealous administration of intravenous fluids in view of hypotension should be resisted to prevent causing pulmonary oedema; vasopressors may be indicated. Methylprednisolone is administered for 24 hours. Once resuscitated and stabilised, the patient is referred to the spinal injuries centre.

7. F Septic shock

In septic shock, a source of sepsis is the primary cause. This may be postoperative or from a septic focus in the body – gastrointestinal, biliary, or genitourinary tracts. This may follow on from systemic inflammatory response syndrome (SIRS). The systemic changes in SIRS are loss of microvascular integrity, increased vascular permeability, systemic vasodilatation, depressed myocardial contractility, poor oxygen delivery and increased microvascular clotting.

This is also a distributive type of shock with vascular dilatation, hypotension, low systemic vascular resistance, inadequate afterload and a high cardiac output – hyperdynamic circulation. These features are the result of the release of endotoxins with activation of the cellular and humoral components of the immune system. If not promptly treated, the patient deteriorates due to hypovolaemia from fluid leaking into the interstitial spaces; this causes myocardial ischaemia.

The management is resuscitation, identification of the source of sepsis and definitive treatment. The patient is given oxygen, intravenous access is obtained, blood samples are taken for culture, haematological and biochemical investigations are performed and the patient is started on broad-spectrum antibiotics. The distributive nature of shock requires a CVP line besides other methods of monitoring, and the patient is cared for in the high-dependency unit. A CT scan identifies the source of sepsis. The definitive treatment of removing the cause is carried out either surgically or by the interventional radiologist depending upon the cause.

Wounds, tissue repair and scars

Pradip K Datta

Multiple choice questions

→ ### Normal wound healing

1. The following statements are true except:

A The inflammatory phase of wound healing lasts for 5 to 7 days.

B Platelet-rich blood clot and dilated vessels are typical of the inflammatory phase.

C Fibroblastic activity is the main feature of the proliferative phase.

D In a tendon injury, fibrous adhesion between the tendon and its sheath is an important mechanism of healing.

E In a fractured bone cortical structure and medullary cavity are restored in the remodelling phase.

→ ### Abnormal healing

2. Which of the following statements are true?

A The aim in treatment of a wound is to reduce the inflammatory and proliferative responses.

B The mechanism of wounding influences the healing of a wound.

C There is no role for tests for hepatitis and HIV when managing wounds.

D Primary repair of all damaged structures should be attempted in all wounds.

E Healing by tertiary intention should be the choice in certain situations.

→ ### Managing the acute wound

3. Which one of the following statements is false?

A In case of severe uncontrollable bleeding, a soft clamp must be applied immediately across the vessel in the wound.

B Wounds should be classified as tidy and untidy before deciding upon intervention.

C Repair of all damaged structures can be attempted under certain situations.

D Pulsed jet lavage for saline irrigation is not always ideal for saline irrigation.

E A large haematoma should be actively treated.

Extended matching questions

→ ### Diagnoses

1 Compartment syndrome
2 Contracture
3 Hypertrophic scar
4 Keloid
5 Leg ulcer
6 Necrotising soft-tissue infection
7 Pressure sore

Match the diagnoses with the clinical scenarios that follow:

Clinical scenarios

A A 72-year-old man, recovering from a stroke, has developed an ulcer over his sacrum over a week. There is also a patch of necrotic skin over his heel.

B A 54-year-old woman who is undergoing chemotherapy for breast carcinoma underwent an emergency appendectomy for acute perforated appendicitis 4 days ago. She complains of severe pain in the wound, which shows erythema, oedema, skin blistering and crepitus.

C A 76-year-old woman complains of an ulcer in the region of her medial malleolus for 6 months. She has had a swollen leg for many years following a deep vein thrombosis, which she suffered after childbirth.

D A 28-year-old man while working on a building site sustained a fracture of his tibia and fibula having fallen from a ladder. This was promptly treated by open reduction and internal fixation. On the second postoperative day, he developed severe pain in his leg exacerbated by passive movement and sensory loss.

E A 62-year-old man underwent a coronary artery bypass grafting 8 months ago. The longitudinal scar on his sternum has increased in width, is itchy and is cosmetically unsightly.

F An 18-year-old man sustained an assault injury to his face and neck with a broken glass bottle. This was sutured as an emergency and healed primarily. The scar is unsightly and he wishes further surgery.

G A 26-year-old woman sustained a burn to her upper limb, which straddled her cubital fossa. This has healed, leaving her with a flexion deformity.

Answers to multiple choice questions

Normal wound healing

1. A

The inflammatory phase of wound healing lasts for 2 to 3 days. Normal wound healing occurs in three phases – the inflammatory phase lasts for the first 2 to 3 days, the proliferative phase lasts for 3 days to 3 weeks and, finally, the remodelling (maturation) phase lasts from the end of the third week to years.

The inflammatory phase, also called the exudative phase, has no tensile strength to the wound. It consists of vascular, cellular and enzymatic processes. As a result of the wound, bleeding, vasoconstriction and thrombus formation occurs. Platelets stick to the damaged vessel endothelium, releasing adenosine diphosphate (ADP), cytokines, serotonin, prostaglandins and histamine. This causes vascular permeability, resulting in the migration of inflammatory cells and macrophages, the latter removing devitalised tissue and microorganisms. Fibrinogen produces fibrin, which forms the framework for the fibroblastic activity, which is the second phase.

The proliferative phase lasts from 3 days to the end of the third week. The principal feature of this is fibroblastic activity with the production of collagen and new capillaries (angiogenesis) and re-epithelialisation; this is called granulation tissue. This increased collagen gives the wound almost one-third of its original tensile strength. The third phase of remodelling constitutes re-arrangement and cross-linking of collagen fibres, which can go on for years while the wound regains 80% of its original tensile strength.

Wound healing in special situations such as tendon, consists of intrinsic and extrinsic mechanisms, the latter depending upon fibrous adhesions between the tendon and its sheath. In fractured bones, in the final phase of remodelling, restoration of cortical bone and the medullary cavity occurs.

→ Abnormal healing

2. A, B, E

The aim should always be to achieve healing by primary intention. This can occur by reducing the inflammatory and proliferative responses. By doing so, healing occurs by first or primary intention when the wound edges are accurately apposed, leaving minimal scarring. The mechanism of a wound has a profound bearing on the healing. For example, a clean-cut incision in an elective operation will heal well with the least prominent scar. On the other hand, a crush injury or one following burns will take a long time to heal and do so by secondary intention with ugly scarring.

In certain situations, such as emergency abdominal surgery in faecal peritonitis where the wound would be inevitably contaminated, it is prudent to leave the abdominal wall open after closing the peritoneum. Delayed closure of the wound is carried out when the inflammatory and proliferative phases of wound healing are well established. This is referred to as closure by tertiary or delayed primary intention.

There is a role for testing hepatitis and HIV viruses when multiple victims from the same site (terrorist-related injuries or bus crashes) have been brought in because these will carry the risk of tissue and viral contamination. Primary repair of structures such as bone, tendon, soft tissue, nerve and vessels should not be attempted in all wounds. Such repair should be carried out only in a tidy wound. Staged procedures should be attempted in untidy wounds such as explosions.

→ Managing the acute wound

3. A

In severe uncontrollable bleeding, a clamp should never be applied because nerves may be irreparably damaged. The bleeding wound should be elevated and a pressure pad applied until the wound can be properly examined under adequate analgesia or anaesthesia (local, regional, or general). When appropriate, this examination is carried out under the use of a tourniquet. Wounds are classified as 'tidy' and 'untidy' to help in their management. Tidy wounds are those with a clean incision on healthy tissue without any tissue loss. Untidy wounds are caused by crush or avulsion injuries and contaminated where there is tissue loss with ischaemia.

Repair of all damaged structures may be attempted in a tidy wound. Vessels, nerves and tendons are repaired, magnification being used whenever necessary. Wound irrigation with large amounts of saline is carried out as a part of debridement. Irrigation by pulsed jet lavage is not always advisable, because the procedure can push the dirt further deep into tissue planes. A large haematoma can cause pressure on nerves and therefore should be evacuated by incision or aspiration, but the latter is not always successful because the clot may be semi-solid.

Answers to extended matching questions

1. D Compartment syndrome

Compartment syndrome usually occurs in the lower limb, following closed injuries, circumferential burns and revascularisation procedures. The patient complains of severe pain out of proportion to the injury or operation; the pain is exacerbated by passive movement and associated with sensory disturbance and loss of two-point discrimination. The calf muscles feel tense and tender and in late stages peripheral pulses may not be palpable.

In vulnerable patients, compartment pressures may be measured by a catheter placed in the muscle compartment or through use of a pressure monitor. Normal pressure in the calf is up to 10 mm Hg. Pain and paraesthesia starts at 20–30 mm Hg when fasciotomy has to be undertaken. Decompression of the lower limbs is carried out by two incisions lateral to the subcutaneous border of the tibia, thus gaining access to the two posterior compartments, the peroneal and anterior compartments.

In crush injuries when the presentation may be late, delayed fasciotomy may be dangerous. This is because myoglobin released from the dead muscles may result in myoglobinuria, causing acute renal failure. Under such circumstances, amputation may be the safer alternative once the dead tissue has demarcated.

2. G Contracture
Contracture occurs when scars cross joints, causing deformity resulting in compromise of mobility. It most often occurs following burns or assault, causes disability and may require complex plastic surgery followed by intensive postoperative physiotherapy.

3. F Hypertrophic scar
This is the outcome of a prolonged inflammatory phase of wound healing, particularly when the site of the scar is in an unfavourable area such as across the lines of Langer. It results in excessive scar tissue that is confined within the boundary of the original cut (unplanned wound) or incision. This may require expert plastic surgery for cosmetic purpose.

4. E Keloid
A keloid is an exuberant scar, which is the result of excessive scar tissue that extends well beyond the boundaries of the original incision or wound. It is associated with raised levels of growth factor, occurs more commonly in pigmented skin and has an inherited tendency. Certain areas of the body are more susceptible, such as ear lobe and the area bounded by the two shoulder tips and the xiphisternum. Histologically, the dermis is markedly thickened with broad and irregular hyalinised collagen bundles and an excess of capillaries and fibroblasts than seen in normal scar tissue.

Several methods of treatment are available, a sure indication that it is a difficult condition to treat as recurrence is common. Steroid injection into the lesion and excision with postoperative radiation or steroid injection has been tried with limited success.

5. C Leg ulcer
An ulcer is defined as a break in epithelial continuity. Leg ulcers can be caused by vascular disease (arterial or venous, or a combination of both) and autoimmune diseases such as rheumatoid arthritis causing arteritis, trauma, chronic infection, inflammatory bowel disease, haematological disorders and skin cancers (**Figure 3.1**). One of the most common causes is post-phlebitic syndrome with venous hypertension (**Figure 3.2**), the mechanism of which is explained in **Figure 3.3**. An indolent ulcer unresponsive to the usual methods of conservative treatment should be biopsied to exclude a Marjolin's ulcer, which is a squamous carcinomatous change in a venous ulcer.

An arterial component (ischaemia) should always be excluded by Doppler ultrasound. The mainstay of management is to treat the underlying cause. Locally conservative regime of hygiene, rest, elevation and compression bandaging under the supervision of a district nurse is the key.

6. B Necrotising soft tissue infection
Necrotising soft tissue infection most often occurs in an immunosuppressed patient following trauma or surgery in the presence of wound contamination. The causative organisms are multiple with Gram-positive aerobes (*S. aureus* and pyogenes) and Gram-negative anaerobes (*E. coli,* pseudomonas, clostridia, bacteroides) and β-haemolytic streptococcus. The two main types are clostridial (gas gangrene) and non-clostridial (streptococcal origin). The latter type

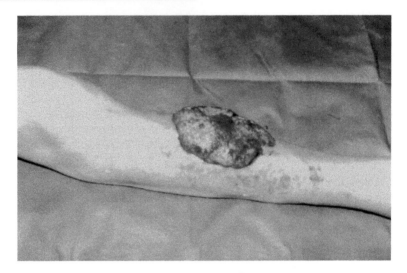

Figure 3.1 Squamous cell carcinoma.

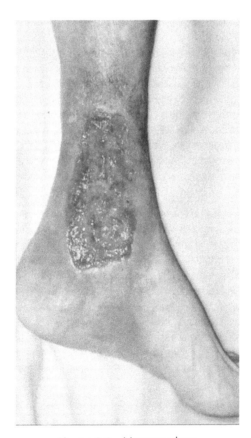

Figure 3.2 Venous ulcer.

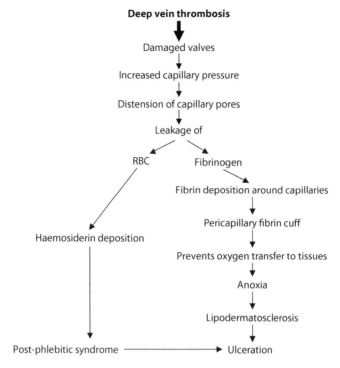

Deep vein thrombosis

Damaged valves

Increased capillary pressure

Distension of capillary pores

Leakage of

RBC   Fibrinogen

Fibrin deposition around capillaries

Pericapillary fibrin cuff

Haemosiderin deposition

Prevents oxygen transfer to tissues

Anoxia

Lipodermatosclerosis

Post-phlebitic syndrome ⟶ Ulceration

Figure 3.3   Formulation of venous ulcer.

is called necrotising fasciitis, which may lead to toxic shock syndrome from *S. pyogenes*. In lay parlance, it is called the 'flesh eating bug'.

Patients present with severe pain out of proportion to the signs, oedema beyond the erythema, crepitus and greyish discharge ('dishwater pus') with focal skin gangrene being a late sign. Unrecognised and hence when the diagnosis is made late, shock, coagulopathy and multiple organ dysfunction syndrome can be followed by death. Treatment is wide surgical excision, which may have to be repeated. Delayed skin grafting will be needed.

7. A Pressure sore

Also called bed sores, decubitus ulcers and pressure ulcers, pressure sores are chronic wounds that result in tissue necrosis due to prolonged pressure. Although preventable, such sores occur in 5% of hospitalised patients. The most susceptible are paraplegic patients, those with peripheral vascular disease, unconscious and bed-bound patients. The sites are any bony prominences such as sacrum, ischium, greater trochanter, heel and malleoli.

The mechanism of formation of a pressure sore is shown in **Figure 3.4**. Prevention is the most important. This is achieved by good skin care, special pressure dispersion cushions, foams and beds; meticulous nursing of the bed-bound patient who should be turned at regular intervals is essential. Overall management should be a multi-disciplinary approach

Prolonged weight bearing

Mechanical shear forces on soft tissue over bony prominences

↓

Increase in pressure across small vessels

↓

Reduced tissue perfusion

↓

Ischaemic necrosis

↓

Ulcer formation

Figure 3.4 Formation of pressure sores.

and surgery should be contemplated only after very careful and detailed assessment. A well-motivated clinically stable patient with good nutrition should be considered for surgery by graft or flap cover. This should be preceded by optimum preparation of the wound by debridement and vacuum-assisted closure (VAC) also called negative pressure wound closure.

 *4*

Basic surgical skills and anastomoses

Pradip K Datta

Multiple choice questions

⇀ Incisions

1. Which of the following statements are true about skin incisions?

A Skin incisions are best made along tension lines.

B Incisions should avoid bony prominences and skin creases.

C The 22-blade scalpel is ideal for all incisions.

D Incisions should be made bearing in mind cosmesis.

E Transverse abdominal incisions have fewer respiratory complications.

⇀ Wound closure

2. The following statements are true except:

A Mass closure technique is the usual method used for abdominal wall.

B Sutures lose 50% of their tensile strength at the knot.

C Non-absorbable suture material should be used in the biliary and urinary tract.

D Synthetic suture materials elicit minimal tissue reaction.

E Round-bodies needles are used in intestinal surgery.

⇀ Principles of anastomosis

3. Which of the following statements are true?

A The current favoured technique of bowel anastomosis is the one-layer extramucosal interrupted method.

B The bowel must be prepared prior to any anastomosis.

C It is essential that in end-to-end anastomosis the bowel ends should match the diameter.

D In vascular anastomosis, polypropylene is the suture material to be used.

E A transverse arteriotomy should always be used to prevent stenosis after closure.

⇀ Drains

4. Which of the following statements are false?

A A drain is best inserted through the end of a wound so as not to have another scar.

B 'When in doubt drain' should be the motto.

C Drains are mandatory after a thoracotomy.

D Drains are usually used following exploration of the common bile duct.

E During removal of a chest drain, the patient should be asked to do a Valsalva manoeuvre.

⇀ Principles of diathermy

5. Which of the following statements are true?

A The two types of diathermy in use are monopolar and bipolar.

B Monopolar diathermy is ideal for microsurgery and delicate procedures.

C Bipolar diathermy is ideal for patients who have pacemakers.

D Accidental burns are more common when monopolar diathermy is used.

E Capacitance coupling can occur when a metal port is used in laparoscopic surgery.

Answers to multiple choice questions

→ Incisions

1. A, B, D, E

Skin incisions are best made along Langers' lines (tension lines), which represent the direction of dermal collagen fibres. Therefore, incisions made parallel to these lines result in a good scar, the surgeon's signature, which is the only part of the operation the patient actually sees. They should avoid bony prominences and skin creases and should take into account the final cosmetic result. The latter factor should not however be of paramount importance, as any incision should provide adequate access to make the operation safe and functionally effective. Transverse abdominal incisions cut through fewer dermatomes and hence produce less postoperative pain. Therefore, the patient coughs much better producing less respiratory complications.

The 22-blade scalpel is not ideal for all incisions. It is best reserved for making an abdominal incision; the 15-blade is for minor procedures and an 11-blade is for arteriotomy.

→ Wound closure

2. C

Non-absorbable suture material should not be used in the biliary tract and urinary tract, as they would act as a nidus for a stone. Absorbable sutures should always be used when closing the common bile duct or placing sutures anywhere from the renal pelvis down to the urinary bladder.

In closure of the abdominal wall, mass closure technique is the usual method. In this large bites are taken in short steps using nylon or polypropylene (non-absorbable) or polydiaxanone (PDS, slowly absorbable) sutures. The length of suture material used should be at least four times the length of the incision to be closed; this is to minimise the risk of wound dehiscence or incisional hernia. Knot tying, one of the most basic of surgical techniques, should be thoroughly mastered as sutures lose 50% of their strength at the knot. Suture materials are generally classified as synthetic (non-absorbable) and natural (absorbable). Synthetic suture materials produce minimal tissue reaction. Sutures from biological or natural material elicit tissue reaction and hence are unpredictable in their behaviour.

The bodies of needles are round, triangular, or flat. Round-bodied needles gradually taper to a point and are designed to separate tissue fibres, as in intestinal and cardiovascular surgery. Triangular needles have cutting edges and are used when tough or dense tissue such as skin and fascia are to be sutured.

→ Principles of anastomosis

3. A, C, D

The current favoured technique of bowel anastomosis is one-layer extramucosal closure, because it causes the least tissue necrosis and luminal narrowing. The suture must include the submucosa, which, by virtue of its high collagen content, is the most stable suture layer. Several studies have shown that there are very little differences between the single-layer and two-layer anastomoses as long as the basic surgical principles are followed, which include ensuring a good blood supply, tension-free anastomosis and use of atraumatic bowel clamps to minimise contamination.

In end-to-end anastomosis, the bowel ends must be of similar diameter. Following resection for intestinal obstruction when the bowel ends to be anastomosed are unequal, a side-to-side or end-to-side anastomosis is done. In case the discrepancy is minimal, end-to-end anastomosis can be carried out by making a cut into the anti-mesenteric border (Cheatle split) of the distal collapsed lumen to bring the diameter into line with that of the proximal bowel.

In vascular anastomosis when prosthetic material or graft is used, the anastomosis will never be integrated into the graft tissues. Therefore, the suture line needs to be permanent. Hence, polypropylene, as it is not biodegradable, is the ideal suture to be used. When making an arteriotomy, particularly for a femoral embolectomy, a transverse arteriotomy, although it will not stenose on closure, is not suitable as it may not give adequate access. A longitudinal arteriotomy is preferable and is closed with a vein patch. In arterial anastomosis the needle should always go from within to without on the downstream edge of the vessel to prevent creating a dissection and fix any plaque.

Bowel preparation prior to anastomosis is a principle of the past. Conventional bowel preparation provides little benefit and may be harmful. However, meticulous prevention of spillage of bowel contents must be followed.

Drains

4. A, B

Drains are best placed through a separate incision. They should not be brought out through the end of an incision, because this leads to an increased chance of wound infection. It was Lawson Tait in 1887 who said 'When in doubt drain'. This dictum, however, is no longer true. The use of drains depends upon a surgeon's individual preference and type of surgery. Again, after the same operation one surgeon might drain whilst another might not. Protagonists believe that drains remove collections within a wound or peritoneal cavity and might indicate postoperative haemorrhage; those not in favour of drains claim that they increase the incidence of wound infections, abdominal pain and hospital stays, and that they reduce pulmonary function.

Following a thoracotomy, drains are always inserted to remove air and blood; they are connected to an underwater seal to which sometimes a suction pressure of 10 to 20 mm Hg is applied. After exploration of the common bile duct most surgeons insert a T-tube to remain in place for 10 days. This is to allow free postoperative bile drainage whilst there is spasm at the sphincter of Oddi; additionally, when a postoperative T-tube cholangiogram is done after 10 days, it helps to show up any residual stones that might have been left inadvertently. T-tubes are left for 10 days to prevent intraperitoneal bile leakage after removal. When removing a chest drain, the patient is always asked to take a deep breath and hold it (Valsalva manoeuvre) to prevent air being sucked into the pleural cavity during removal of the tube.

Principles of diathermy

5. A, C, D, E

There are two types of diathermy, monopolar and bipolar. The principle is used to coagulate, cut and fulgurate. The most common type is monopolar diathermy where normal electric current is converted into high-frequency alternating current (HFAC). In this, HFAC is passed through the patient's body tissues and returned to the machine by a large surface plate (70 cm²) called the indifferent electrode. The surface area of contact of the active electrode is small compared with the indifferent electrode; this concentrated powerful current produces heat at the operation site, thus exercising the desired effect.

In bipolar diathermy, the HFAC passes from the diathermy machine down one prong of the forceps through to the tissue being held and returned to the machine via the second prong thus concentrating the desired effect on the small piece of tissue held by the forceps. Therefore, bipolar diathermy is ideal for patients who have a pacemaker because current does not flow through other tissues of the body.

Accidental burns is more common in monopolar diathermy for the following reasons: the indifferent electrode may be incorrectly applied with inadequate contact, the patient being earthed by metal contact on the operating table, there may be faulty insulation of the diathermy leads and accidental contact of the active electrode may occur with other metal instruments in use.

Capacitance coupling is the cause of an accidental burn injury to intraperitoneal structures during laparoscopic surgery. For example, when an insulated diathermy hook is passed through a metal laparoscopic port, HFAC is transferred from the insulated instrument to the metal port, which, if in contact with an intra-abdominal organ, results in burning the organ, say a part of the bowel. This danger is avoided by using entirely plastic ports.

Monopolar diathermy is never to be used for microsurgery and delicate procedures. Bipolar diathermy should be the choice.

5 Surgical infection

Pradip K Datta

Multiple choice questions

Physiology

1. Which of the following statements are true?

A Microorganisms are prevented from causing infection by intact skin, chemical, humoral and cellular factors.

B Reduced resistance to infection may result from metabolic problems, disseminated disease and iatrogenic causes.

C Colonisation and translocation in the gastrointestinal tract is a risk factor for SIRS, MODS and wound infection (surgical site infections, or SSIs).

D When closing a skin incision, silk has the least chance of causing infection.

E In reduced host resistance, non-pathogenic microorganisms may behave as pathogens.

Presentation

2. The following statements are true except:

A Whether a wound becomes infected depends upon the host response.

B All SSIs are secondary and due to HAI (health-care–associated infection).

C Presence of antibiotics during the 'decisive period' is crucial to the prevention of SSIs.

D Poor surgical technique is a recipe for SSIs.

E Primary infection occurs when the source of the pathogen is endogenous.

Treatment of surgical infection

3. Which of the following statements is not true?

A Surgical incision through infected tissue is best managed by delayed primary or secondary closure.

B SSIs are usually missed by the surgical team and picked up by the primary care doctors.

C Antibiotics should be started only once sensitivities are available.

D Extensive debridement is necessary in Meleney's synergistic gangrene.

E An infected wound is ideally treated by opening it up.

Prophylaxis

4. The following statements are true except:

A The blood and tissue levels of antibiotics should be maximal before contamination occurs.

B In a long operation, under certain conditions, antibiotics should be repeated at 4-hourly intervals.

C Further doses of antibiotics postoperatively helps in reducing infection.

D Patients with cardiac valve disease or a prosthesis should have prophylaxis.

E Ideally, preoperative shaving should be done in the operating theatre just before the operation.

Bacteria involved in surgical infection

5. Which of the following statements are true?

A Streptococci are most often responsible for cellulitis.

B The most common organism in an abscess is Staphylococci.

C Bacteroides are aerobic spore-bearing organisms.

D *Clostridium difficile* causes *pseudomembranous enterocolitis*.

E *Staphylococcus epidermidis* is a cause of HAI.

→ **Principles of antimicrobial treatment**

6. Which of the following statements is not true?

A A broad-spectrum antibiotic should be used to treat a known sensitive infection.

B Combination of broad-spectrum antibiotics is to be used while awaiting sensitivities.

C Under certain circumstances it may be necessary to rotate antibiotics.

D Antibiotics should not be used instead of surgical drainage.

E In SIRS and MODS when there is no response within 3 to 4 days, one should revisit the clinical situation.

→ **Antibiotics used in treatment and prophylaxis of surgical infection**

7. Which of the following statements are true?

A Benzylpenicillin is the treatment of choice against Gram-positive organisms.

B Ampicillin and amoxicillin are the antibiotics of choice against *Pseudomonas* and *Klebsiella*.

C Aminoglycosides may have ototoxicity and nephrotoxicity.

D Carbapenems are effective against Gram-positive and anaerobic organisms.

E Quinolones have a limited role in treating surgical infections.

→ **Human immunodeficiency virus, AIDS and the surgeon**

8. The following statements are true except:

A In surgical practice, the risk of transmission of the HIV virus is through needlestick injury.

B Those with the virus have an increased risk of neoplasms and opportunistic infections.

C Untreated HIV infection proceeds to AIDS within 2 years in 25%–35% of patients.

D In the early phases of infection, drug treatment is not required.

E Treatment after exposure should be dictated by local policies.

Extended matching questions

→ Diagnoses

1 Abscess
2 Bacteraemia and sepsis
3 Cellulitis and lymphangitis
4 Clostridium tetani
5 Gas gangrene
6 Synergistic spreading gangrene

Match the diagnoses with the clinical scenarios that follow:

→ Clinical scenarios

A A 58-year-old cattle farmer normally a resident in the subcontinent, on a short visit to the United Kingdom, was brought into the A&E department with convulsions. The episode started with lassitude, irritability, dysphagia and spasm of facial muscles. He showed generalised tonic and clonic spasm.

B A 68-year-old woman underwent an amputation of her right leg following severe crush injury. Three days postoperatively she has pyrexia and tachycardia and looks toxic. The amputation site looks red and brawny with the limb swollen with crepitus in the intermuscular planes.

C A 75-year-old man underwent a low anterior resection. Five days postoperatively he became toxic. A contrast CT scan showed an anastomotic leak.

D A 38-year-old woman sustained a superficial wound of her thumb from a puncture while gardening. Twenty-four hours later, her thumb became swollen and very painful, with red inflamed streaks all along the skin up to the axilla.

E A 42-year-old woman underwent an emergency appendectomy for perforated suppurative appendicitis. Three days postoperatively, her wound became red and tender with gross oedema; on removal of the sutures, the wound showed slough and ulceration.

F A 25-year-old man presented with a tender lump in the right supraclavicular area of 3 days' duration. The lump is red and fluctuant. He looks unwell with pyrexia. A week before the onset of this episode he had his right ear pierced, which became infected.

Answers to multiple choice questions

→ Physiology

1. A, B, C, E

Infection by microorganisms is normally prevented by intact epithelial surfaces, such as skin, chemical factors such as the low pH of gastric acid, humoral factors such as antibodies, and cellular factors such as phagocytic cells, macrophages, polymorphonuclear cells and killer lymphocytes. The organism gains the upper hand when resistance to infection is compromised in situations such as metabolic – diabetes, malnutrition and obesity, jaundice, chronic renal failure; disseminated disease – malignancy, AIDS; iatrogenic – radiotherapy, steroids, chemotherapy.

When a patient's immunity is depressed as in cancer, sepsis and shock, bacteria, particularly aerobic Gram-negative bacilli, tend to colonise the upper gastrointestinal tract. They then translocate to the mesenteric lymph nodes causing release of endotoxins, which may then go on to produce SIRS, MODS and SSIs. In a situation of compromised host resistance, harmless microorganisms such as fungi become pathogenic, producing opportunistic infections much more so when prolonged, and changing antibiotic regimes have been in place.

Silk as a suture material acts as a nidus for infection and encourages the invasion of bacteria, causing suture abscesses. Hence, it should not be used.

→ Presentation

2. B

Not all SSIs are secondary and of health-care–associated origin. The origin of an SSI can be primary when it is endogenous in origin and present in the host, such as in faecal peritonitis from perforated diverticulitis or acute perforated appendicitis, and secondary or exogenous when it is health-care–associated or nosocomial infection.

Host response is a very important factor that will determine whether a wound becomes infected. After trauma or surgery it takes at least 4 hours for the host's inflammatory, humoral and cellular defence mechanisms to be in place. This is referred to as the 'decisive period' during which time the causative organisms become established in the host. Therefore, the concentration of antibiotics must reach its peak during this period so that the antibiotic level in the tissue should reach above the minimum inhibitory concentration for the likely pathogens. Poor surgical technique, such as leaving a dead space, or ischaemic and necrotic tissue and a haematoma are potent causes for SSIs and no attempt should ever be made to counterbalance this by using antibiotics.

→ Treatment of surgical infection

3. C

Antibiotics should be started on clinical grounds in surgical infections. One should not wait for culture and sensitivities, because it takes two to three days for the answer to be available. Empirical treatment should be started when there is swinging pyrexia, spreading infection, cellulitis and bacteraemia. A triple-therapy combination of broad-spectrum penicillin (ampicillin), with aminoglycoside (gentamicin) and metronidazole is started; this is obviously modified once the results are available.

As most patients have a short hospital stay after surgery and wound infections take up to 10 days to develop, surgical teams miss most SSIs; they are managed in primary care. In necrotising fasciitis of the abdominal wall (Meleney's synergistic gangrene), extensive debridement should be carried out; all necrotic tissue is excised and affected areas laid open, which will require skin grafting later. When there is infected postoperative wound with evidence of underlying pus, the wound should be laid open by removal of the sutures and wound curettage to drain the pus. In severely contaminated wounds, such as a laparotomy for faecal peritonitis, it is prudent to leave the wound open to be closed by delayed primary or secondary closure.

→ Prophylaxis

4. C

There is no evidence that extra doses of antibiotics postoperatively are of any value in the prevention of infection. Such extra doses can actually be harmful as the process can cause antibiotic resistance. Prophylactic antibiotics are ideally given in the 'decisive period' when local wound defences are minimal and before contamination occurs. In long operations or in the presence of excessive blood loss as in vascular surgery, or in unexpected contamination, antibiotics are repeated at 4-hourly intervals during operation as tissue levels fall faster than serum levels.

Patients with valvular disease of the heart and those with prosthesis should have prophylactic antibiotics to prevent bacteraemia when undergoing any form of surgical intervention, such as dental work or urethral instrumentation. In preoperative preparation, shaving of the skin should be done just before the operation in the theatre, as SSI rate after clean wound surgery doubles if it is done the night before.

→ Bacteria involved in surgical infection

5. A, B, D, E

Streptococci are Gram-positive organisms, the most important of which is the β-haemolytic Streptococcus, which is the normal inhabitant of the pharynx in up to 10% of the population. Group A Streptococcus (*S. pyogenes*) is the most pathogenic, with the ability to spread, and causes cellulitis and tissue destruction by releasing the streptolysin, streptokinase and streptodornase enzymes. The organism is sensitive to penicillin and erythromycin. Staphylococci are Gram-positive organisms normally present in the nasopharynx of up to 15% of the population. *Staphylococcus aureus* is the most important pathogen that causes an abscess. Most of these strains are β-lactamase producers resistant to penicillin (MRSA) but sensitive to flucloxacillin, vancomycin, aminoglycosides, some cephalosporins and fusidic acid.

Bacteroides are non-spore-bearing anaerobes found in the large bowel, vagina and oropharynx. *Bacteroides fragilis* is the main organism that acts in concert with aerobic Gram-negative bacilli to cause SSIs after colorectal and gynaecological surgery. Such organisms are sensitive to metronidazole and cefotaxime.

The Clostridia are Gram-positive anaerobes that produce resistant spores. *C. difficile* is the cause of the HAI, *pseudomembranous enterocolitis*. This is caused by the injudicious use of several antibiotics sequentially, and the elderly and immunocompromised are particularly vulnerable. *Staphylococcus epidermidis* (*S. albus*) is a coagulase-negative staphylococcus that is an important cause of HAI and a major threat in operations where prostheses are used (vascular and orthopaedic surgery).

Principles of antimicrobial treatment

6. A

A broad-spectrum antibiotic should not be used to treat an infection when the sensitivities are known. The specific antibiotic should be used. For instance when MRSA is isolated, it should be treated by specific antibiotics such as vancomycin and teicoplanin. Antibiotics should not be withheld when clinically indicated. A combination of broad-spectrum antibiotics such as ampicillin or mezlocillin (penicillins), gentamicin (aminoglycoside) and metronidazole is used whilst awaiting sensitivities.

In situations where commensals such as Pseudomonas and Klebsiella (Gram-negative species) become resident opportunist pathogens, it may be prudent to rotate anti-pseudomonal and anti-Gram-negative therapy. Antibiotics should never be used as a substitute for good surgical technique and surgical drainage; wherever pus is present, it needs to be let out. In SIRS and MODS with antibiotic treatment if the patient has not improved, the surgical team should revisit the diagnosis and methods of imaging to identify the source. Adherence to local hospital protocols and consultation with the infection-control team and microbiologist are essential in difficult situations.

Antibiotics used in treatment and prophylaxis of surgical infection

7. A, C, D, E

Benzylpenicillin is the antibiotic of choice against Gram-positive organisms such as streptococci, clostridia and staphylococci that do not produce lactamase. It is effective against *Actinomyces*, a pathogen causing chronic wound infection in developing countries and very potent in gas gangrene. It is effective against spreading streptococcal infections and also used as a component of multiple therapy.

Aminoglycosides (gentamicin and tobramycin), effective against Gram-negative *Enterobacteriaceae* and *Pseudomonas*, may cause ototoxicity and nephrotoxicity at sustained high levels. Therefore, serum levels should be monitored 48 hours after commencing treatment and the dosage modified to satisfy peak and trough levels. Sometimes single large doses may be effective, and the dose may be reduced in the presence of raised urea and creatinine. Carbapenems (meropenem, ertapenem, imipenem) are stable to β-lactamase and have an useful broad-spectrum effect against anaerobic and Gram-positive organisms causing urinary tract and abdominal infections. Quinolones (ciprofloxacin) have a limited role in surgical infections because of the development of resistant strains.

Ampicillin and amoxicillin are not effective against *Pseudomonas* and *Klebsiella*. These are β-lactam penicillins that can be used orally and parenterally but are rarely used now as there are more effective alternatives.

Human immunodeficiency virus, AIDS and the surgeon

8. D

In the early phases of treatment, drug treatment is most effective. Highly active anti-retroviral therapy (HAART) acts by inhibiting reverse-transcriptase and protease synthesis, which are the main mechanisms through which HIV progresses.

Needlestick injury during operations is the most common risk of transmission of the disease. In general this retrovirus virus is transmitted by body fluids, especially blood. On exposure, the virus binds to CD4 receptors with loss of CD4+ cells, T-helper cells and other cells involved in cell-mediated immunity and antibody production. Therefore, the chances of opportunistic infections (*Pneumocystis carinii* pneumonia, tuberculosis and cytomegalovirus) and neoplasms (Kaposi's sarcoma and lymphoma) are enhanced. Untreated HIV infection leads to AIDS in 25% to 35% of patients within 2 years.

Surgeons may be involved with HIV patients who suffer from surgical conditions or need surgical intervention related to their illness. Guidelines for universal precautions in the NHS are available to be followed. Contamination most often occurs due to needlestick injury on the nondominant index finger during an operation. Active management, and whether highly active anti-retroviral therapy (HAART) is instituted, is determined according to local policies.

Answers to extended matching questions

1. F Abscess
This patient has developed an abscess secondary to infection of his pierced ear. The infection has spread to the cervical lymph nodes where liquefaction necrosis has resulted in an abscess. An abscess is a cavity lined by granulation tissue containing pus, which is the cause of his local signs. The organism is most likely to be *Staphylococcus aureus*.

This is a clinical diagnosis. Because the patient is toxic, the patient is started on antibiotics and the abscess is drained and left open to heal by granulation. Abscesses in certain situations can be treated by aspiration and appropriate antibiotic therapy.

2. C Bacteraemia and sepsis
This patient has bacteraemia and sepsis from anastomotic breakdown (deep space SSI). Aerobic Gram-negative bacilli are usually responsible. This patient needs vigorous resuscitation followed by laparotomy. The procedure should be to dismantle the anastomosis, bring the proximal end out as an end colostomy and close off the distal rectum. This should be followed by copious warm saline washouts. The abdominal wall may be left open to be closed by delayed primary closure.

If on imaging the leak looks small and contained, a decision may be made to drain the leak by interventional radiology.

3. D Cellulitis and lymphangitis
This patient has spreading infection from her injured thumb to her axilla along the lymphatic channels. This is an invasive non-suppurative, poorly localised infection caused by β-haemolytic streptococci, staphylococci and *Clostridium perfringens*. Cellulitis is localised to site of injury, whilst lymphangitis is the vehicle of spread of the infection to the regional lymph nodes. The release of proteases results in tissue destruction, gangrene and ulceration with systemic signs of chills, fever and rigors (toxaemia).

Blood cultures are sent and the patient started on empirical broad-spectrum antibiotics. Blood cultures are often negative, as the patient's clinical features are from a cytokine-mediated systemic inflammatory response that causes release of toxins. The arm should be elevated and rested with close watch kept for the development of systemic inflammatory response syndrome (SIRS).

4. A *Clostridium tetani*
Clostridium tetani is rare in Western countries because of the strict prophylactic regimen in place of 5-yearly booster doses of tetanus toxoid. The condition is tetanus caused

by the anaerobic, spore-bearing Gram-positive bacterium that has entered the tissues through a wound that is often trivial, unrecognised, or forgotten. The spores are abundant in soil or manure and hence the condition is more common in traumatic civilian or military injuries. The clinical features arise from the release of the exotoxin tetanospasmin, which affects the myoneural junctions, motor neurons and the anterior horn cells of the spinal cord.

The treatment consists of benzylpenicillin with debridement of the wound. In established infection, antitoxin using human immunoglobulin should be considered. In severe cases, the patient needs ventilation with muscle relaxants. Prolonged ventilation will require a tracheostomy. However, prevention is the most important.

5. B Gas gangrene

This is caused by *Clostridium perfringens*, a Gram-positive anaerobic, spore-bearing bacillus abundantly found in soil and faeces. The condition is more common in military and traumatic surgery and in colorectal operations. Also, the immunocompromised patient is more susceptible. The patient complains about severe wound pain out of proportion to the size of the wound, with local crepitus from gas, which may be seen on a plain x-ray **(Figure 5.1)**. The wound exudes a thin, brown, sweet-smelling fluid, which soon gives way to gangrene. Unless promptly and aggressively treated, this may lead to multiple organ dysfunction syndrome (MODS).

Prophylaxis is the key in the form of benzylpenicillin in patients undergoing amputation for peripheral vascular disease. In established disease, large doses of antibiotics and wide debridement of tissue is carried out.

6. E Synergistic spreading gangrene

This is caused by a group of organisms acting in concert. The group includes coliforms, staphylococci, Bacteroides species and anaerobic streptococci. When it occurs on the abdominal wall it is called Meleney's synergistic hospital gangrene; when it affects the

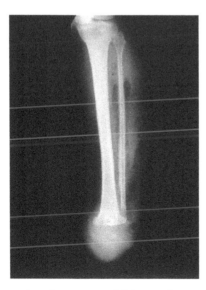

Figure 5.1   Local crepitus from gas, which may be seen on a plain x-ray.

scrotum it is referred to as Fournier's gangrene. Contaminated wounds are more likely to be affected, causing severe wound pain and signs of spreading inflammation with crepitus and foul-smelling discharge.

The patient is treated with broad-spectrum antibiotics with circulatory support. This is combined with aggressive excision of local necrotic tissue, which may need to be repeated. The patient once recovered will require extensive skin grafting.

6 Surgery in the tropics

Pawanindra Lal and Sanjay De Bakshi

Multiple choice questions

→ Amoebiasis

1. Which of the following are true of amoebiasis?
A The disease is common in the Indian subcontinent, Africa and parts of Central and South America.
B The majority of sufferers are symptomatic.
C Amoebic liver abscess, the most common extraintestinal manifestation, occur in more than 50%.
D The mode of infection is via the faeco-oral route due to poor hygiene and sanitation.
E The organism enters the gut via contaminated food and water.

2. *Entamoeba histolytica*, the causative organism, enters the body as cysts contaminating water or food. Which of the following occurs?
A The cysts hatch in the large bowel and colonise the colon.
B The cysts cause flask-shaped ulcers in the colon.
C The trophozoites may invade the wall of the colon and pass to liver via the portal circulation, causing focal infarction and liquefactive necrosis in the liver.
D Cysts are passed in the faeces in an infective form.
E The right lobe of the liver is affected in 10% of cases, the left in 80% and the rest are multiple.

3. A middle-aged man presents with pain in the right upper quadrant of the abdomen. He has had fever, night sweats, anorexia, malaise, cough and weight loss. He is found to be toxic, anaemic and mildly jaundiced. He has a tender hepatomegaly with tenderness over the right lower intercostal spaces. An ultrasound scan had shown a hypoechoic lesion in the right lobe of the liver and his CT scan is shown in Figure 6.1. Which of the following statements are true?
A While the clinical features are suggestive of amoebiasis, travel to an endemic area and a history of bloody diarrhoea may also be present.
B The CT scan is compatible with an amoebic liver abscess.
C The abscess cavity contains blackcurrant jelly-like fluid.
D The collection is normally odourless and sterile but becomes smelly if secondarily infected.
E Trophozoites may be found in the wall of the abscess cavity in a minority of cases.

4. Which of the following are presenting features of amoebiasis?
A Chronic diarrhoea, often blood-stained, with colicky abdominal pain.
B Pain in the upper right abdomen and right shoulder-tip with hiccoughs and a painful dry cough.
C An apple-core lesion on barium enema due to the formation of a chronic granuloma, most common in the caecum.
D Features of peritonitis with shock.
E All of the above.

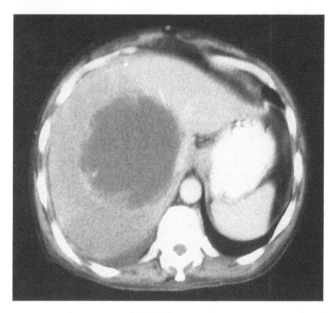

Figure 6.1 Computed tomographic (CT) scan showing an amoebic liver abscess in the right lobe.

5. **What is the treatment for an amoebic abscess?**

A Urgent laparotomy upon diagnosis.

B Medical treatment with metronidazole or tinidazole.

C Medical treatment with diloxanide furoate is sufficient.

D Aspiration may be carried out for abscesses that present with features of imminent rupture.

E Surgical treatment for amoebiasis is indicated for a ruptured liver abscess, for patients with severe haemorrhage and toxic megacolon and for a suspected amoeboma, which is not responding to treatment or where carcinoma cannot be excluded.

Ascariasis (roundworms)

6. **Which of the following are caused by *Ascaris lumbricoides*?**

A Intestinal symptoms as a larva.

B Pulmonary symptoms as a larva.

C Intestinal symptoms as an adult worm.

D Pulmonary symptoms primarily as an adult worm.

E Biliary disease as a larva.

7. **What percentage of the world's population is affected by roundworms (*Ascaris lumbricoides*)?**

A 2%

B 10%

C 25%

D 50%

E 75%

8. **How is roundworm disease transmitted?**

A Inadvertent ingestion of the larva in soil.

B Inadvertent ingestion of the fertilised egg in soil.

C The larva penetrates unbroken skin.

D Inadvertent ingestion of fertilised eggs in contaminated meat.

E The larva is transmitted to the lung as a droplet infection.

9. **Which of the following are true of the life cycle of the *Ascaris lumbricoides*?**

A Eggs release larvae in the lumen of the intestine, which then develop into adult worms.

B Eggs release larvae into the portal blood and thereafter into the liver and then the lungs.

C Eggs penetrate the intestinal wall and travel to the liver where they develop into adult worms and are released into the intestinal lumen via the biliary tract.

D The larvae are released in the lungs. The developing larvae are swallowed in sputum and complete their maturation in the intestine.

E Eggs are released into the environment in stool as cysts, which survive.

10. How is Loeffler's syndrome characterised?

A Chest pain with productive cough, friction rub and a chest x-ray showing pleural effusion.

B Retrosternal burning, discomfort on ingestion of food, fever and mediastinal widening on chest x-ray.

C Epigastric pain radiating to the right, a tender palpable liver and an elevated right dome of the diaphragm.

D Chest pain, dry cough, dyspnoea and fever with fluffy exudates on chest x-ray.

E Haemoptysis.

11. Which of the following are caused by roundworm infestation?

A Malnutrition and failure to thrive.

B Mechanical obstruction of the intestine.

C Perforation of the intestine.

D Ascending cholangitis, obstructive jaundice and acute pancreatitis.

E Chest symptoms.

12. Which of the following may be found in roundworm infestations?

A A high eosinophil count.

B Charcot–Leyden crystals in stool.

C Larvae in sputum or bronchoscopic lavage.

D Fluffy exudates on chest x-rays.

E Barium meal may show the worm lying freely in the lumen.

13. Which of the following are recognised treatments in uncomplicated roundworm intestinal obstruction?

A Urgent laparotomy.

B Nasogastric suction, intravenous (IV) saline and hypertonic saline enemas.

C Kneaded a worm bolus into the large intestine at laparotomy, to be subsequently treated with hypertonic saline enemas.

D Gastrojejunostomy.

E A long-standing small intestinal perforation may require exteriorisation in the presence of a heavy worm load.

14. A patient presents with sudden severe upper abdominal pain with chills and rigors. He has icterus and is diffusedly tender over the right upper abdomen. His blood tests show an elevated white cell count (WCC) with high polymorphs and obstructive jaundice. The ultrasound scan (Figure 6.2) shows stones in the gall bladder and a linear shadow in a dilated common bile duct (CBD). The magnetic resonance cholangiopancreatograpm (MRCP) shows a linear shadow in the CBD, which in real time is found to change its position. Which of the following statements are true?

A The most likely diagnosis is a line of stones in the CBD.

B The condition is likely to be due to a live worm in the CBD.

C The condition should be treated with pyrantel palmoate.

D The condition should be treated with albendazole.

E Following an anthelmintic, the condition may be treated by endoscopic removal of the roundworm followed by cholecystectomy.

→ Asiatic cholangiohepatitis

15. Asiatic cholangiohepatitis, also called 'Oriental cholangiohepatitis', results from infestation of the hepatobiliary system by *Clonorchis sinensis*, a liver fluke. Which of the following pertain to the disease?

A The human acts as the intermediate host, by the ingestion of infected fish and snails, which are the definitive host.

B The parasite matures into an adult worm in the intrahepatic biliary channel, causing epithelial hyperplasia and periductal fibrosis.

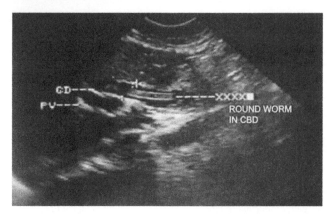

Figure 6.2 Ultrasound scan showing a roundworm in the common bile duct (CBD). The patient presented with obstructive jaundice and had asymptomatic gallstones. On endoscopic retrograde cholangiopancreatography (ERCP), part of the worm was seen outside the ampulla in the duodenum and was removed through the endoscope. Subsequent laparoscopic cholecystectomy was uneventful.

C The eggs or dead worms may form the nidus for stone formation in the biliary system.

D Changes around the intrahepatic biliary channels often cause dysplasia, which may lead to cholangiocarcinoma.

E Ultrasound scan characteristically shows uniform dilatation of small peripheral intrahepatic ducts with only minimal dilatation of the common duct system.

16. What is the treatment of Asiatic cholangiohepatitis?

A Praziquantel and albendazole are the drugs of choice.

B Cholecystectomy, exploration of the common bile duct and choledochoduodenostomy.

C A Roux-en-Y choledochojejunostomy with or without an access loop.

D The disease should ideally be diagnosed and treated in its subclinical form.

E All of the above.

→ Filariasis

17. Which of the following statements about filariasis are true?

A It is mainly caused by the parasite *Brugia malayi* and *Brugia timori*. In 10% of sufferers, the parasite *Wuchereria bancrofti* also causes the disease.

B Once inoculated by a mosquito bite, the matured eggs enter the circulation to hatch and grow into adult worms.

C The adult worms cause lymphatic blockage, resulting in massive limb oedema. This is often compounded by streptococcal secondary infection, leading to additional fibrosis of the lymphatic channels and further leading to elephantiasis.

D Chyluria and chylous ascites seen in cancers blocking lymphatics are never seen in filariasis.

E A mild form of the disease, which affects the respiratory tract and presents with dry cough is called tropical pulmonary eosinophilia.

18. Which of the following statements about filariasis are true?

A Blood tests often reveal an elevated lymphocyte count.

B Immature worms can be seen in nocturnal peripheral blood smear.

C Medical treatment with diethylcarbamazepine is effective even when huge elephantiasis occurs.

D Hydroceles are treated in the usual way, but excess skin may need trimming.

E Elephantiasis can be treated easily with operations to reduce the size of the limb.

→ Hydatid disease

19. Which of the following are true with regard to hydatid disease caused by *Echinococcus granulosus*?

A   Man is the definitive host.

B   Dog is the definitive host.

C   Sheep and cattle are intermediate hosts.

D   The disease causes cystic lesions mainly in the liver but may affect any organ.

E   The disease causes an infiltration of the liver without any definite margin.

20. How is hydatid disease transmitted?

A   By eating infected meat and therefore affects only non-vegetarians.

B   By the faeco-oral route through ingestion of eggs.

C   Through penetration of the skin of the bare-footed by larvae.

D   It may be vector-borne.

E   It spreads by droplet infection.

21. Which of the following statements regarding cystic hydatid disease are true?

A   It contains an outer pericyst made up of spreading living parasites.

B   It contains an intermediate ectocyst, which is non-infective.

C   It contains an inner endocyst, which has a germinal membrane containing viable parasites.

D   The germinal envelope may give rise to daughter cysts.

E   It spreads to the liver by travelling along the intestinal lymphatics.

22. Which of the following features are the presentations of hydatid disease?

A   Chest symptoms of a dry cough with fluffy exudates called Loeffler's syndrome.

B   A dull aching pain in the upper right abdomen.

C   Abdominal pain, anaphylactic shock and collapse after trivial trauma.

D   Patients often complain of passing live worms in stool.

E   Features of obstructive jaundice.

23. Which ultrasound scan features characterise a hepatic hydatid cyst?

A   A cyst with multiple septations.

B   A cyst wall with shaggy and irregular outlines.

C   A cyst wall with calcifications.

D   A solid lesion with a surrounding rim of oedema.

E   A cyst with split walls.

24. A young girl was dancing in school and felt a dull pain in the abdomen. In the evening the mother noticed a diffuse skin rash and started her on a course of antihistamines to which she responded and the pain reduced in intensity. A week later she underwent an ultrasound scan, which showed a cystic lesion with a split wall. Blood tests showed a high eosinophil count and a CT scan is shown (Figure 6.3). Which of the following are true of this clinical scenario?

A   The feature is compatible with a ruptured simple cyst of the liver.

B   The feature suggests a ruptured hydatid cyst.

C   Treatment is expectant.

D   Treatment is exploratory laparotomy under cover of albendazole.

E   Anaphylaxis can occur during laparotomy.

25. A young woman presented with pain in her upper abdomen with chills and rigors followed by high-coloured urine. She is jaundiced and tender over the upper abdomen. An ultrasound scan shows gall bladder calculi, a dilated CBD with echogenic material and a septated cyst in the left lobe of the liver. A CT scan shows a septated cyst of the left lobe of the liver (Figure 6.4). At endoscopic retrograde cholangiopancreatography (ERCP), multiple membranous structures were delivered after sphincterotomy. Which of the following are true of this condition?

A   The likely diagnosis is cholecystitis and choledocholithiasis with an incidental liver cyst.

B   The likely diagnosis is a multiseptated hydatid cyst with biliary communication, causing daughter cysts in the CBD and gall bladder calculi, due to hydatid sand.

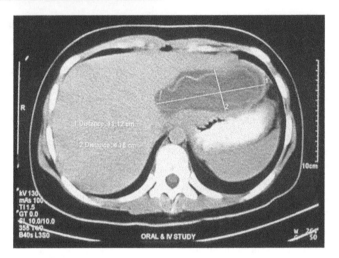

Figure 6.3 CT scan of the upper abdomen showing a hypodense lesion of the left lobe of the liver; the periphery of the lesion shows a double edge. This is the lamellar membrane of the hydatid cyst that separated after trivial injury. The patient was a 14-year-old girl who developed a rash and pain in the upper abdomen after dancing. The rash settled down after a course of antihistamines. The CT scan was done 2 weeks later for persisting upper abdominal pain.

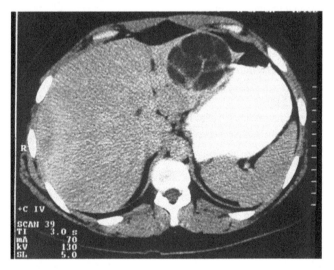

Figure 6.4 CT scan showing a hydatid cyst with septa in the left lobe of the liver.

C Treatment following endoscopic clearance of the CBD should only require a cholecystectomy.

D Treatment following endoscopic clearance of the CBD should be with a cholecystectomy followed by injection of sclerosants into the cyst.

E Treatment of the cyst by injection of scolicidal solutions has a risk of causing sclerosing cholangitis because of the presence of biliary communications.

26. Which of the following statements are true of hydatid cysts?

A Anaphylactic shock is more common in the treatment of unilocular hydatid cysts than in the treatment of multiloculated cysts.

B Sclerosing cholangitis is more common following injection of scolicidal solutions into multiloculated hydatid cysts.

C Small deep cysts that show calcification in their walls may be watched and treated with albendazole.

D Surgical curettage of the cyst wall is mandatory.

E Rupture of a cyst may cause dissemination of the disease.

27. Which of the following is true of thoracic hydatid disease?

A The lung is the most common organ affected.

B The right lower lobe is affected slightly more than any other site.

C The cysts are usually multiple.

D Silent cysts may sometimes present with an allergic reaction.

E Pulmonary hydatid disease characteristically presents with a silent pleural effusion.

28. A fit active young man presents suddenly with cough, expectoration of clear fluid, fever, chest pain and occasional haemoptysis. His chest x-ray shows a rounded cystic lesion and another rounded lesion with air in it (Figure 6.5). Which of the following are true of this condition.

A Air is introduced as the lesion erodes into the bronchiole, giving rise to a fine radiolucent shadow.

B This x-ray finding is called the 'meniscus sign or crescent sign'.

C Pulmonary hydatid disease never presents with pleural effusion.

D The 'water-lily sign' on CT scan of the chest indicates inactive disease (Figure 6.6).

E Surgery is the mainstay of hydatid disease of the lungs.

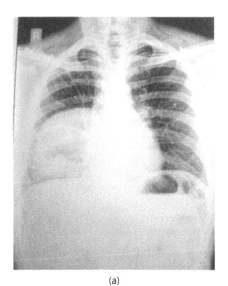
(a)

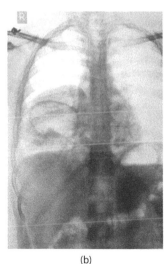
(b)

Figure 6.5   Chest x-ray: (a) a smooth rounded cystic lesion in the right lower lobe; (b) 'meniscus or crescent' sign. (Courtesy of Professor Saibal Gupta, Professor of Cardiovascular Surgery, Kolkata, India and Dr Rupak Bhattacharya, Kolkata, India.)

→ Leprosy

29. A 33-year-old woman presents with loss of eyebrows, collapse of the nasal bridge and lifting of the tip of the nose, paralysis of the left orbicularis oculi causing exposure keratitis and blindness (Figures 6.7 and 6.8). A diagnosis of leprosy is made. Which of the following features are relevant to the disease?

A The disease is caused by the acid-fast bacillus, *Mycobacterium tuberculosis*.

B The disease is transmitted by sexual contact.

C The disease is classified into two groups, lepromatous and tuberculoid, depending on the immune response of the patient to the disease.

D The disease is slowly progressive and affects the skin, upper respiratory tract and peripheral nerves.

E The deformities produced are primary, which are caused by leprosy or its reactions, and secondary from the effects such as anaesthesia of the hands and feet.

30. Which of the following statements about leprosy (Hansen's disease) are true?

A Patients have neural involvement characterised by thickening of the nerves, which are tender.

B Patients may present with 'leprids', which are asymmetrical, well-defined, anaesthetic, hypopigmented, or erythematous macules with elevated edges and a dry rough surface.

C There are often nodular lesions on the patient's face in the acute phase of the lepromatous type. The characteristic facies thus produced is known as 'leonine facies' (resembling a lion).

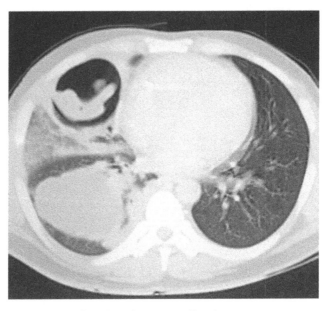

Figure 6.6 CT scan showing the 'water-lily' sign. A young mountaineer, while on a high-altitude trip, complained of sudden shortness of breath, cough and copious expectoration consisting of clear fluid and flaky material. At first thought to be due to pulmonary oedema, it turned out to be a ruptured hydatid cyst, which was successfully treated by surgery. (Courtesy of Professor Saibal Gupta, Professor of Cardiovascular Surgery, Kolkata, India and Dr Rupak Bhattacharya, Kolkata, India.)

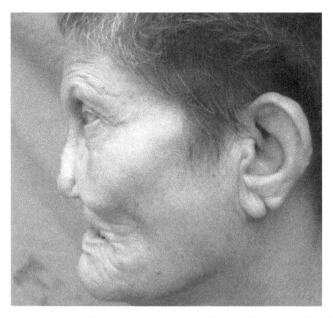

Figure 6.7 Lateral view of the face showing collapse of the nasal bridge due to destruction of nasal cartilage by leprosy.

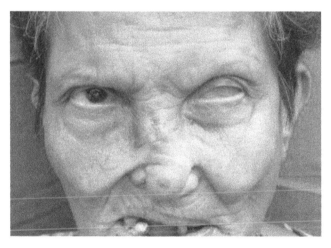

Figure 6.8 Frontal view of the face showing eye changes in leprosy – paralysis of orbicularis oculi and loss of eyebrows.

D The condition is diagnosed by demonstrating the bacilli in urine.

E The patient is treated by a multidisciplinary team of infectious disease specialist, plastic surgeon, ophthalmologist and hand and orthopaedic surgeon.

→ Mycetoma

31. Which of the following statements are true?

A It is a chronic, progressive, destructive granulomatous disease.

B The causative organism could be a fungus or bacteria.

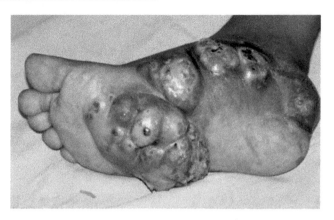

Figure 6.9 Mycetoma of the foot.

C Patients present with painful nodules, multiple sinuses and mucus discharge **(Figure 6.9)**.

D The condition occurs in Sudan, Somalia, Senegal, India, Yemen and Mexico.

E The route of infection is through direct transmission from another patient.

32. **Which of the following is/are true regarding the diagnosis?**

A Ultrasound cannot differentiate between eumycetoma and actinomycetoma.

B A deep biopsy should be obtained from the nodule, under general or regional anesthesia to identify one of the three types of host tissue reactions.

C Type III reaction is characterised by formation of epitheloid granulomas and Langhan's type giant cells.

D FNAC is not useful in yielding an accurate diagnosis and not used in distinguishing between eumycetoma and actinomycetoma.

E Culture and immunoelectrophoresis are diagnostic of Mycetoma.

33. **Which of the following is/are true regarding the management?**

A In actinomycetoma, combined drug therapy with amikacin sulphate and co-trimoxazole in the form of cycles is the treatment of choice.

B There is no definitive drug therapy for Eumycetoma.

C Surgery is indicated for widespread lesions, after medical treatment.

D Amputation, used as a life-saving procedure, is indicated in advanced mycetoma refractory to medical treatment with severe secondary bacterial infection.

E Recurrence can be prevented with radiotherapy.

→ Poliomyelitis

34. **Which of the following are true of poliomyelitis?**

A It is an enteroviral infection that spreads by inhalation or ingestion.

B It is a rotavirus that spreads by the faeco-oral route.

C It targets the anterior horn cells of the spinal cord.

D It causes sensory loss, which spreads cranially.

E It causes a lower motor neuron type of flaccid paralysis.

→ Tropical chronic pancreatitis

35. **Tropical chronic pancreatitis affects the younger age group from poor socioeconomic strata in developing countries. Which of the following statements about the condition are true?**

A It is caused by ingestion of cassava (tapioca), a root vegetable, which contains derivatives of cyanide. The concurrent absence of sulphur-containing amino acid in the diet prevents the cyanide from being detoxified in the liver, leading to cyanogen toxicity and the disease.

B It is caused by alcoholism.

C Patients present with extensive pancreatic periductal fibrosis, intraductal calcium carbonate stones and type I diabetes mellitus.

D Patients show pancreatic calcification in the form of discrete stones on straight abdominal X-ray. Ultrasound and CT scans of the pancreas confirm the disease.

E Patients need medical support for exocrine and endocrine pancreatic insufficiency and treatment for pain. Some require surgery.

→ ## Tuberculosis of the small intestine

36. Which of the following types of infection may be caused by intestinal infection with *Mycobacterium tuberculosis*?

A Transverse ulcers with undermined edges in the ileum.

B Tubercles on the serosa of the intestine.

C Apple-core lesions of the colon.

D Hyperplasia and thickening of the terminal ileum.

E Transmural inflammation with a propensity for fistula formation.

37. What presenting features do patients with tuberculosis of the small intestine show?

A Weight loss, vague abdominal pain and evening rise of temperature.

B A doughy feel of the abdomen from area of localised ascites.

C A mass in the right iliac fossa.

D A water-can perineum with undermined edges and watery discharge.

E Characteristically, a non-caseating granuloma on histology.

38. A 24-year-old woman presents with repeated attacks of abdominal pain with abdominal distension. A barium meal X-ray is carried out (Figure 6.10). Which of the following should make you consider a diagnosis of tuberculosis?

A A resident of a developing country from a poor socioeconomic background.

B Presence of active tuberculosis of the lungs.

C Skip lesions of the intestine.

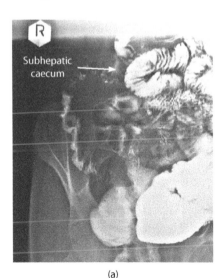
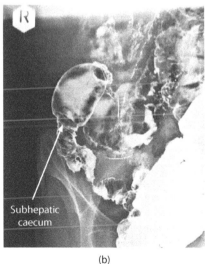

(a) (b)

Figure 6.10 (a and b) Series of a barium meal and follow-through showing strictures in the ileum with the caecum pulled up into a subhepatic position.

D The barium meal x-ray shows a narrowing of the terminal ileum with a normally placed caecum.

E The barium meal x-ray shows a narrowing of the terminal ileum with a pulled-up subhepatic caecum.

39. Which of the following surgical procedures can be carried out for ileal and ileocaecal tuberculosis:

A Strictureplasty.

B Limited ileocolic resection.

C Right hemicolectomy.

D Ileo-transverse anastomosis.

E All of the above.

40. Which of the following are true in tuberculous perforation?

A Free gas under the diaphragm is always present.

B It is treated by resuscitation followed by resection of the affected segment.

C It may be treated by resuscitation, followed by strictureplasty through the perforation.

D It may be treated by resection and exteriorisation as a first step, followed by restoration of bowel continuity after completion of antituberculous chemotherapy.

E It should always be treated conservatively.

→ Typhoid

41.Typhoid fever is caused by *Salmonella typhi*, which is a Gram-negative bacillus. Which of the following are true of the disease?

A The bacteria enter the body through infected blood or contaminated needles.

B The organism colonises the Peter's patches in the terminal ileum, initially causing hyperplasia and later necrosis and ulceration.

C If left untreated or inadequately treated, the ulcers may bleed or perforate.

D A typical patient may present with high fever for 2 to 3 weeks after a visit to an endemic area, with abdominal distension due to paralytic ileus.

E Patients may present as an emergency due to melaena and hypovolaemia or with features of peritonitis and shock.

42. Which of the following statements are true?

A It is diagnosed by positive blood and stool cultures.

B The Widal test, although obsolete, looks for the presence of bacteria in red blood cells.

C In the presence of inadequate treatment when blood cultures are often negative, special kits such as Multi-Test Dip-S-Ticks to detect immunoglobulin G, Tubex to detect immunoglobulin M and TyphiDot to detect IgG and IgM may be used.

D In the second or third week, any patient who shows signs of deterioration accompanied by abdominal pain should be considered to have a perforation unless otherwise proved.

E Abdominal distension in typhoid disease in the second or third week of the fever should be treated by high-bowel washout to get rid of the toxins.

43. Which of the following statements are true with regard to the treatment of typhoid perforation?

A Treatment involves vigorous resuscitation with IV fluids and antibiotics in an intensive care unit.

B Chloramphenicol is the drug of choice.

C Several surgical options are available, depending on the condition of the patient, site and number of perforations and amount of peritoneal soiling.

D After operation the skin and subcutaneous tissue are often kept open for delayed closure, as wound infection inevitably occurs, leading to wound dehiscence.

E Perforation occurring in the first week of typhoid fever has a better prognosis, as the patient's nutritional and immunological status is better.

Extended matching questions

→ ## Diagnoses

1 Actinomycetoma
2 Amoebic liver abscess
3 Ascariasis
4 Filariasis
5 Hydatid disease
6 Hyperplastic ileocaecal tuberculosis
7 Leprosy
8 Poliomyelitis
9 Psoas abscess
10 Tropical chronic pancreatitis
11 Tubercular peritonitis
12 Typhoid perforation

Match the diagnoses with the clinical scenarios that follow:

A   A 35-year-old man presents with episodic severe upper abdominal pain radiating to back for 5 months. He has increased thirst with polyuria and passage of bulky pale stools. He consumes tapioca as a staple diet. On examination, there is no abnormality. His fasting blood sugar level is 18 mmol/L; plain abdominal x-ray shows linear calcification in the upper abdomen across the spine.

B   A 45-year-old man presents with anorexia with pain in the upper abdomen associated with high-grade fever, night sweats and general malaise for 5 days. The pain has been constant in the right upper abdomen and is exacerbated by movement and coughing. He had bloody diarrhoea over the preceding 3 to 4 weeks. On examination there is tender hepatomegaly 5 cm below the right costal margin with intercostal tenderness in the right 5th, 6th and 7th spaces.

C   A 45-year-old sheep farmer complains about a gradually enlarging painful lump in the right upper abdomen for 3 months. He is otherwise healthy. Physical examination reveals firm tender hepatomegaly. He has a total leucocyte count (TLC) of 8600 with a differential leucocyte count (DLC) showing 12% eosinophils.

D   A 19-year-old woman presents with a history of intermittent colicky central abdominal pain for the past 6 months. She has diarrhoea alternating with constipation over this period. Her father died 2 years ago of a prolonged respiratory illness. On examination she is pale, with slight fullness in the right iliac fossa and a firm lump in the same region that is tender. The rest of her abdomen is unremarkable. A barium meal and follow-through reveals irregular narrowing of the terminal ileum.

E   A 25-year-old woman patient gives a history of high-grade fever with chills over the past 3 weeks, and diarrhoea 10 days previously, which lasted for about 1 week. She also gives a history of abdominal pain for the past 4 to 5 days that started in the lower abdomen and later became severe as well as generalized. On examination, she is severely dehydrated and febrile. Abdominal examination reveals a board-like rigidity with absent bowel sounds. There is free gas under the diaphragm on erect abdominal radiograph.

F   A 40-year-old man complains of progressive swelling of his right leg over the past 6 months. He has had episodes of high-grade fever for 4 months, during which the leg becomes red and painful with increase in the size of the swelling. On examination, the girth of the affected limb is found to be increased, and the skin is very thick and rough. The swelling of the limb does not pit with pressure. Blood examination reveals the presence of marked eosinophilia.

G A 40-year-old female resident of Myanmar complains of progressive deformity affecting both of her hands over the past 3 to 4 years. She also complains of numbness of the tips of her fingers and non-healing ulcers involving several of them. There is no history of any trauma. On examination, there is bilaterally symmetrical clawing of all the digits of both the hands with non-healing ulcers over the tips of several of the digits. There are multiple hypoaesthetic and anaesthetic areas involving both the forearms and hands. Incidentally, she is also found to have lost her eyebrows.

H A 6-year-old boy is brought by his parents with complaints of sudden-onset fever, with severe headache and weakness and deformities of both the upper limbs. On examination, the boy is malnourished, with no neck rigidity. There is weakness of the muscles of shoulders, elbows and wrist, more on the left side. There is also accompanying flattening of the thenar eminence with weakness of flexion of the fingers and apposition of the thumb. The sensory examination is normal.

I A 30-year-old woman presents with an inability to straighten her left lower limb at the hip joint for the past 2 weeks. The deformity was preceded by a history of backache for 6 months for which she took some analgesics. She also has history of low-grade evening fever over the past 4 to 5 months. On examination there is flexion deformity of the left hip joint with evidence of fullness in the abdomen over the left iliac fossa. There is also a gibbus deformity of the upper lumbar spine, which is tender with fullness along the left paravertebral region.

J A 36-year-old man presents with irregular swelling in the inguinal region with multiple purulent discharging sinuses involving the anterior abdominal wall and perineum, a swollen knee and a previous history of a swelling in the foot with similar discharging sinuses.

K A 30-year-old woman presents with intermittent colicky central abdominal pain for 10 months with weight loss and amenorrhoea over the past 3 months. She has had alternating constipation and diarrhoea during this period. In the past week the pain has been continuous and is increasing in severity. Over the past 2 days, she has had absolute constipation. Her husband was treated for pulmonary tuberculosis in the recent past. On examination the patient is pale and dehydrated with a distended rigid abdomen with rebound tenderness and absent bowel sounds. An erect x-ray of the abdomen reveals free gas under the diaphragm.

L A 10-year-old boy is brought to the hospital by his mother with complaints of sudden onset of severe colicky abdominal pain associated with several episodes of vomiting. There is a history of failure to thrive and also of the passage of worms per rectum in the past. On examination, he is pale and underweight for his age. The abdomen is distended with palpable bowel loops. The bowel sounds are exaggerated. His haemoglobin is 10.2 g/dL and 12% eosinophils.

Answers to multiple choice questions

→ Amoebiasis

1. A, D, E
The disease is common in the Indian subcontinent, Africa and parts of Central and South America. The majority produce no symptoms and amoebic liver abscess occurs in less than 10% of patients affected with amoebiasis. The mode of infection is via the faeco-oral route through contaminated food or water.

2. B, C, D
The cysts hatch in the small intestine and large numbers of trophozoites are released and carried to the colon. Here they attach themselves to the mucosa and may penetrate to cause flask-shaped ulcers, or invade the portal vein to be carried to the liver. They affect the right

lobe in 80% of cases, the left lobe in 10% of the cases and the rest are multiple. A large number in the intestine form cysts, which are passed in stool that can infect other humans as well.

3. A, B, D, E

The clinical features are those of an amoebic liver abscess. The CT scan features of a hypodense lesion with irregular walls showing peripheral enhancement are characteristic of an abscess. The fluid is chocolate-coloured, odourless and 'anchovy sauce'-like, a mixture of blood and necrotic liver tissue. This fluid becomes smelly when secondarily infected. The abscess is usually high in the diaphragmatic surface of the right lobe. This may cause pulmonary symptoms. Untreated abscesses are likely to rupture.

4. E

A large majority of patients will present with bloody diarrhoea due to colonic infestation. A liver abscess often presents with upper abdominal and chest symptoms. Rupture of the abscess causes peritonitis and shock. A chronic granuloma, called an amoeboma, may form, commonly on the right side of the colon, where the patient has had a long history of repeated indiscriminate and inadequate self-medication. This condition may mimic a carcinoma. When a patient is from an endemic background with a history of altered bowel habit and a right-sided lesion, an amoeboma should be suspected; it is imperative to exclude a carcinoma. The two conditions often co-exist; therefore, it is mandatory to take repeat biopsies on colonoscopy after adequate treatment.

5. B, D, E

The primary treatment for an amoebic liver abscess is medical. Metronidazole and tinidazole are the effective drugs. After treatment with metronidazole or tinidazole, diloxanide furoate, which is not effective against hepatic infestation, is used for 10 days to destroy any residual intestinal infestation. Aspiration not only prevents rupture, but also promotes the penetration of amoebicidal drugs. Surgery is carried out for complications of amoebiasis. However, the general principles of vigorous resuscitation must be applied to these very sick patients.

→ *Ascaris lumbricoides* (roundworm)

6. B, C

The life cycle of the roundworm is as follows: The ingested eggs release larva, which penetrate the intestinal wall and get carried via the bloodstream to the lungs. In the lung, the larvae penetrate the bronchioles. This causes inflammation with a dry cough, chest pain and fluffy exudates on chest X-ray called Loeffler's syndrome. The larvae are swallowed in sputum and complete their maturation in the intestine. In the intestine, they mature and cause intestinal symptoms.

7. C

Almost 25% of the world's population, principally in the developing world, harbour the roundworm in their intestines. The vast majority are asymptomatic or have transient ill-defined symptoms.

8. B

The egg of *Ascaris lumbricoides* survives in the external environment even under hostile conditions. Hot and humid conditions are ideally suited for the eggs to turn into embryos. The fertilised eggs are present in the soil contaminated with infected faeces. Faeco-oral contamination causes human infection.

9. B, D

Having been swallowed in the sputum (see Number 6 previously), they mature in the intestines where they cause their symptoms. Larvae are released into the portal circulation.

They then travel to the liver and via the hepatic veins to the lungs. The larvae are present in the sputum. The swallowed sputum enables the larvae to enter the gut and repeat the cycle again.

10. D
The release of larvae causes an inflammation of the lung characterised by dry cough, chest pain, dyspnoea and fever with fluffy exudates on chest x-ray. This combination of symptoms, combined with characteristic features on chest x-ray, is called Loeffler's syndrome.

11. A, B, C, D, E
Roundworms cause problems in the lungs when larvae are released into the bronchioles from the circulation. Additionally, roundworms colonise the intestine and if the infestation is very heavy, compete for nutrients. This may lead to malnutrition and failure to thrive. A worm bolus may cause intestinal obstruction and perforation. The worms may travel up the papilla of Vater, causing ascending cholangitis, obstructive jaundice and acute pancreatitis.

12. A, C, D, E
Worm infestation is often associated with a high eosinophil count, as in most parasitic infestations. Bronchoscopic lavage may show larvae or Charcot–Leyden crystals. In Loeffler's syndrome, chest x-ray shows fluffy exudates. A barium meal often demonstrates roundworms in the intestine either by a negative shadow or linear streak lying parallel to the intestine. This represents barium ingested by the worm.

13. B, C, E
An uncomplicated roundworm obstruction of the intestine should always be treated conservatively with nasogastric suction, IV fluids and hypertonic saline enemas. When laparotomy is indicated, there is never a situation of an actual pyloric narrowing, and therefore a gastrojejunostomy is not indicated. Kneading the bolus of worms into the large bowel and subsequent treatment with hypertonic saline enemas is a way of treating the condition. A long-standing perforation in a malnourished patient ideally requires exteriorisation of the bowel.

14. B, D, E
The imaging in real time is found to change its position. Therefore, it is more likely to be due to a roundworm in the common bile duct. Following the use of albendazole, an anthelmintic, the worm may be extricated by an endoscope followed by cholecystectomy.

→ Asiatic cholangiohepatitis
15. B, C, D, E
Clonorchis sinensis infects snails and fish, which act as the intermediate host. Ingestion of infected fish and snails when eaten raw or partly cooked causes infection in humans and other fish-eating mammals. The disease may remain dormant for years. It often presents with non-specific symptoms but can also present with features of ascending cholangitis, obstructive jaundice and acute pancreatitis.

16. E
Patients from endemic areas should be offered screening by ultrasonography of the biliary system. Stool examination for eggs or worms is diagnostic. The disease can be cured when treated in its subclinical form. Therefore, the risk of developing cholangiocarcinoma is eliminated.

Filariasis

17. B, C, E

The disease is mainly caused by *Wuchereria bancrofti* and in 10% of cases is caused by the parasite *Brugia malayi* and *Brugia timori*. Chyluria and chylous ascites may be seen in filariasis.

18. B, D

Blood tests reveal eosinophilia. Treatment with diethylcarbamazepine is very effective but only in the early stages before the gross deformity of elephantiasis sets in. Once elephantiasis sets in, the condition is rarely treated with surgery, as none of the operations described are universally successful.

Hydatid disease

19. B, C, D

Echinococcus granulose, the parasite that causes cystic echinococcal disease, infects dogs and grows in their intestine. They are the definitive host. The eggs infect sheep, cattle and humans. The worms spread into the bloodstream via the portal system. Therefore, the liver is the most common site of infection but any organ may be infected. The lesions are cystic and spread by expanding rather than by direct invasion.

20. B

In the dog, the adult worm reaches the small intestine, and the eggs are passed in the faeces. The ovum gains access to humans by being ingested. On excystation, the parasite penetrates the intestine to reach and spread through the portal system.

21. B, C, D

The cyst is characterised by three layers, an outer pericyst derived from compressed host organ tissues, an intermediate hyaline ectocyst that is non-infective and an inner endocyst that is the germinal membrane and contains viable parasites, which can separate forming daughter cysts.

22. B, C, E

Hydatid disease commonly affects the liver. Hence, patients present with a dull ache in the upper right abdomen from hepatomegaly. Exposure to the hydatid antigen means that patients often present with anaphylactic shock and collapse in addition to pain, because trivial trauma sometimes causes a rupture of the cyst. A large cyst may exert pressure on the CBD, and additionally daughter cysts may communicate with the biliary tract, causing obstructive jaundice.

23. A, C, E

Hydatid cysts are characterised by the presence of multiple septations, and calcification in the wall and periphery of the lesion may show a double edge. In addition, the presence of multiple daughter cysts sometimes gives rise to the characteristic 'cartwheel' appearance.

24. B, D, E

The clinical scenario of abdominal pain after a trivial trauma, followed by skin rash that responds to antihistamines is suggestive of a ruptured hydatid cyst. The blood tests reveal an elevated eosinophil count and imaging shows a cyst with a split wall. The cyst, having already ruptured, needs immediate treatment with albendazole followed by laparotomy. As the patient is already exposed to the hydatid antigen, a repeat exposure during exploration of the cyst could initiate a violent anaphylactic attack. This needs to be anticipated and appropriate prophylactic measures initiated.

25. B, E
ERCP reveals multiple membranous structures in the CBD with a septated hydatid cyst. A septated cyst, often caused by trivial trauma, is more likely to communicate with the biliary channel. Therefore, the likely diagnosis is that the entire biliary system has become colonised by hydatid disease. Injecting scolicidal solutions into this patient runs a real risk of the solution escaping into the biliary channel and causing sclerosing cholangitis.

26. B, C, E
Multiloculated cysts often occur after insignificant trauma. They are more likely to communicate with the biliary channels, and thus injection of scolicidal solutions is more likely to cause sclerosing cholangitis. Moreover, the host is more likely to have been exposed to hydatid antigen, and anaphylactic reactions are more common in multiloculated hydatid cysts. Some of these cysts are large, and the ectocyst often has a thin layer of compressed tissue spread over vital structures such as the intrahepatic inferior vena cava. Surgical curettage of the cyst wall is often fraught with danger. Deep cysts that show calcification signify that the parasite may be dying or dead and need only be treated with albendazole.

27. B, D
The lung is the second most common organ affected after the liver. Cysts can vary in size from very small to very large. Usually single, the disease is slightly more common in the lower lobe of the right lung. The cysts may also be multiple and affect other organs at the same time. The disease may be silent but may also present with cough, expectoration, fever, chest pain and haemoptysis, and may sometimes rupture and present with an allergic reaction or anaphylaxis.

28. A, B, E
Uncomplicated cysts present with a rounded or oval opacity on a chest x-ray. Air is often introduced by erosions into the bronchioles. This air collects in between the pericyst and the laminated membrane, giving a fine radiological crescent (**Figure 6.5**) called the 'meniscus or crescent sign'. Rupture causes the membrane to collapse, the crumpled-up endocyst floats on the residual fluid giving the 'water-lily' sign on a CT scan (**Figure 6.6**). Rupture into the pleural cavity is usually symptomatic and leads to pleural effusion. The mainstay of treatment is surgery. Medical treatment is less successful and reserved for patients with very poor general condition or with diffuse, recurrent, or ruptured pulmonary hydatidosis. The principle of surgery is to maintain as much viable lung tissue as possible. The exact procedure can be cystotomy, capittonage (suturing the walls together), pericystectomy, segmentectomy, or, rarely, pneumonectomy.

→ ## Leprosy

29. C, D, E
The disease is caused by a *Mycobacterium leprae*, which is weakly acid-fast compared with *Mycobacterium tuberculosis*. The disease is transmitted by the nasal secretions of a patient, the infection being contracted in childhood or early adolescence. After an incubation period of several years, the disease presents with skin and upper respiratory or neurological manifestations. The deformities are therefore a direct cause of the disease or its reactions referred to as 'primary deformities', and secondary, resulting from effects such as anaesthesia of hands and feet causing repeated unrecognised trauma. The tissue damage is proportional to the host's immune response, with a plethora of grades between tuberculoid, where there is a strong immune response with scanty bacteria and epithelioid granuloma formation to lepromatous, where there is a poor immune response, with widespread dissemination of abundant bacilli in the tissues with macrophages and few lymphocytes.

30. A, B, C, E

The disease is diagnosed by obtaining a skin smear, which often demonstrates the acid-fast bacillus, and by a skin biopsy, which shows the characteristic histology. Treatment is carried out according to WHO guidelines with rifampicin, dapsone and clofazimine. Deformities need a multidisciplinary team approach with the involvement of the physician, hand surgeon, orthopaedic surgeon, physiotherapist, occupational therapist and social worker.

Mycetoma

31. A, B, D

Mycetoma is a chronic specific, granulomatous, progressive, destructive inflammatory disease that involves subcutaneous tissues spreading to the skin and deeper structures. The causative organism may be true fungi when the condition is called eumycetoma; when caused by bacteria it is called actinomycetoma. The pathognomonic feature is the triad of painless subcutaneous mass, multiple sinuses and seropurulent discharge. It causes tissue destruction, deformity, disability and, in extreme cases, death. The condition predominantly occurs in the 'mycetoma belt' that lies between the latitudes 15° south and 30° north. The route of infection is inoculation of the organism, resident in the soil, through a breach in the skin continuity. Although in the vast majority there is no history of obvious trauma, the site of entry is always an area of minor unrecognised trauma in a bare-footed individual; hence, the foot is the most common site affected. The foot is affected in 70% and hand in 12%.

32. B, C, E

Ultrasound can differentiate between eumycetoma and actinomycetoma and between mycetoma and other conditions. In eumycetoma, the grains produce numerous sharp, bright hyper-reflective echoes. There are multiple thick-walled cavities with absence of acoustic enhancement. In actinomycetoma, the findings are similar but the grains are less distinct. The size and extent of the lesion can be accurately determined ultrasonically, a finding useful in planning surgical treatment. Deep biopsy is obtained under general or regional anaesthesia, although the chance of local spread is high. The biopsy should be adequate, contain grains and be fixed immediately in 10% formal saline. Deep biopsy is obtained under general or regional anaesthesia, although the chance of local spread is high.

In Type I, a layer of polymorphonuclear leukocytes usually surrounds the grains. In Type II tissue reaction, the neutrophils largely disappear and are replaced by macrophages and multinucleated giant cells which engulf grain material. Type III reaction is characterised by the formation of a well-organised epithelioid granuloma with Langhan's type giant cells. The centre of the granuloma sometimes contains remnants of fungal material. Fine-needle aspiration cytology (FNAC) can yield an accurate diagnosis and helps in distinguishing between eumycetoma and actinomycetoma. The common serodiagnostic tests are immunoelectrophoresis and ELISA, while culture can be used to isolate and grow the microorganisms.

33. A, D

Management of this condition should be a team effort between the physician and surgeon. In actinomycetoma, combined drug therapy with amikacin sulphate and co-trimoxazole in cycles is the treatment of choice. Amoxicillin, clavulanic acid, rifampicin, sulphonamides, gentamicin and kanamycin are used as a second line of treatment. Long-term drug treatment may have serious side effects.

In eumycetoma, ketoconazole, intraconazole and voriconazole are the drugs of choice. They may need to be used for up to 1 year. Use of these drugs should be monitored closely by the physician for side effects. While not curative, these drugs help to localise the disease by forming thickly encapsulated lesions which are then amenable to surgical excision. Medical treatment for both types of mycetoma must continue until the patient is cured and also in the postoperative period.

Surgery is indicated in small, localized lesions, resistance to medical treatment, or for better response after medical treatment in patients with massive disease. Excision may need to be much more extensive than suggested at first on clinical appearance, because the disease may extend to deeper planes that are not clinically apparent.

The surgical options are wide, local and debulking excisions and amputations. Amputation, used as a life-saving procedure, is indicated in advanced mycetoma refractory to medical treatment with severe secondary bacterial infection. The amputation rate is 10% to 25%. Postoperative medical treatment should continue for an adequate period to prevent recurrence, local or regional, which is 25% to 50%. Recurrence is usually due to inadequate treatment.

Poliomyelitis

34. A, C, E

Poliomyelitis is an enteroviral disease that enters the body by ingestion or inhalation. The disease targets the anterior horn cells, causing lower motor neuron paralysis. It does not cause sensory loss, a fact that distinguishes it from the Guillain–Barré syndrome, which also presents with fever and muscle weakness.

Tropical chronic pancreatitis

35. A, C, D, E

The disease is not caused by alcohol ingestion but by derivatives of cyanide in cassava (tapioca), which is eaten as a staple diet; hence, it is a disease present in families. Patients present with abdominal pain, thirst, polyuria, weight loss due to malnutrition and features of gross pancreatic insufficiency. ERCP is used as a therapeutic procedure. Surgery is necessary for intractable pain, particularly for stones in a dilated pancreatic duct. The choice of procedure is usually a lateral pancreaticojejunostomy. Resectional surgery is used as a last resort for intractable pain.

Tuberculosis of the small intestine

36. A, B, D

Typically when a patient with pulmonary tuberculosis swallows infected sputum, the organism colonises the lymphatics of the terminal ileum, causing transverse ulcers with undermined edges. The other variety, called the hyperplastic type, occurs when the host's resistance is stronger than the virulence of the organism. It is often caused by drinking infected unpasteurised milk. There is a marked inflammatory reaction, causing hyperplasia and thickening of the terminal ileum because of the abundance of lymphoid follicles. Transmural inflammation with a propensity for fistula formation is not a feature of tuberculosis but Crohn's disease.

37. A, B, C, D

A patient with tuberculosis of the intestine may present with weight loss, vague abdominal pain and evening rise of temperature. As an emergency the patient presents with distal small-bowel obstruction or peritonitis from perforation. There may be multiple perianal fistulae, sometimes causing a typical water-can perineum. Caseation on histology is the *sine qua non* of tubercular infection. Abdominal examination gives a doughy feel from the area of localised ascites. There may be a mass in the right iliac fossa.

38. A, B, E

Tuberculosis is often endemic in developing countries in patients from a poor socioeconomic background. There is often co-existent pulmonary tuberculosis. While tuberculosis may affect multiple sites of the intestine, 'skip lesions' are characteristic of Crohn's disease. Narrowing of the terminal ileum on a barium study is present in Crohn's disease as in tuberculosis. However, because of intense fibrosis of the intestine and around draining lymph nodes, the caecum in tuberculosis often gets pulled up into the subhepatic position.

39. E

Tuberculosis affects various sites of the intestine, and therefore all the noted surgical procedures may be carried out for a patient with intestinal tuberculosis depending upon the extent, site, number of lesions and length of healthy bowel in between affected parts of the intestine.

40. B, D

There should be a high index of suspicion for tubercular perforation. Rarely, patients present with features of peritonitis and, because of a localised perforation due to adhesions gas under the diaphragm is often absent. These patients sometimes present very late. While laparotomy is almost always indicated, resection and anastomosis may not be feasible in a septic, undernourished patient with severe adhesions. In these individuals, resection and exteriorisation is carried out as a first step. A few weeks later this is followed by restoration of bowel continuity after completion of antituberculous chemotherapy.

Typhoid

41. B, C, D, E

The bacillus is ingested in contaminated food and drinks and is a result of poor hygiene and inadequate sanitation. The clinical features and a history of a visit to an endemic area should raise suspicion about the disease.

42. A, C, D

The Widal test, mostly obsolete, tests for the presence of agglutinins to O and H antigens of the *Salmonella typhi* and *paratyphi* in the patient's serum. The risk of a perforation is high in cases of untreated typhoid fever. Therefore, a patient who has abdominal symptoms and shows signs of deterioration in the second or third week should be investigated appropriately, using an erect chest x-ray or abdominal x-ray in lateral decubitus, if the patient is very sick, to exclude free gas in the abdomen.

43. A, C, D, E

Metronidazole, cephalosporins and gentamycin are used in combination in the treatment of typhoid perforation. Chloramphenicol, though very specific for typhoid infection is used very sparingly, because it can cause aplastic anaemia. Surgical options for treatment of typhoid perforation can vary, including closure of the perforation after freshening the edges, wedge resection of the perforated segment, resection of bowel with anastomosis or exteriorisation of ileum or colon and closure of the perforation with and side-to-side ileo-transverse anastomosis. Delayed wound closure is an accepted procedure as is creating a laparostomy in the presence of rampant infection.

Answers to extended matching questions

1. J Actinomycetoma
Of the two types of mycetoma, actinomycetoma is characterised by earlier and more extensive invasion of deeper tissues as compared with eumycetoma. The swelling is variable in its physical characteristics, which are firm and rounded, soft and lobulated, rarely cystic and often mobile. Multiple secondary nodules may evolve; they may suppurate and drain through multiple sinus tracts. The sinuses may close transiently after discharge during the active phase of the disease. Fresh adjacent sinuses may open, while some of the old ones may heal completely. They coalesce and form abscesses, the discharge being serous, serosanguinous, or purulent.

During the active phase of the disease the sinuses discharge grains, the colour of which can be black, yellow, white, or red depending upon the organism. Pain occurs when there is secondary bacterial infection. Local spread occurs predominantly along tissue planes. The organism multiplies, forming colonies that spread along the fascial planes to skin and underlying structures. Lymphatic spread occurs to the regional lymph nodes. During the active phase of the disease, these lymphatic satellites may suppurate and discharge. Lymphatic spread is more common in actinomycetoma; lymphadenopathy may also be due to secondary bacterial infection. Spread by bloodstream can occur.

X-ray may show multiple large cavities with well-defined margins and periosteal reaction typical of eumycetoma. Periosteal reaction with new bone spicules may create a sun-ray appearance and Codman's triangle, not unlike in osteogenic sarcoma. However, clinical appearance is completely different in the latter where bony swelling rather than subcutaneous nodules are the predominant picture. MRI of the involved joint usually shows multiple 2–5 mm lesions of high signal intensity, which indicates the granuloma, interspersed within a low-intensity matrix denoting the fibrous tissue. The 'dot-in-circle sign', which indicates the presence of grains, is highly characteristic. Kaposi sarcoma may be associated with swollen foot, multiple soft tissue nodules and destruction of the bones of the foot, making it sometimes difficult to differentiate from mycetoma.

2. B Amoebic liver abscess
Amoebiasis is caused by *Entamoeba histolytica*. The disease is common in the Indian subcontinent, Africa and parts of Central and South America where almost half the population is infected. The majority remain asymptomatic carriers. Amoebic liver abscess, the most common extraintestinal manifestation, occurs in less than 10% of the infected population and, in endemic areas, is much more common than pyogenic abscess.

The typical patient with amoebic liver abscess is a young adult male with a history of pain and fever and insidious onset of non-specific symptoms such as anorexia, fever, night sweats, malaise, cough and weight loss, which gradually progress to more specific symptoms of pain in the right upper abdomen, shoulder-tip pain, hiccoughs and a non-productive cough. A past history of bloody diarrhoea or travel to an endemic area raises the index of suspicion.

Examination reveals a patient who is toxic and anaemic. The patient will have upper abdominal rigidity, tender hepatomegaly, tender and bulging intercostal spaces, overlying skin oedema, pleural effusion and basal pneumonitis – the last feature being a late manifestation. Occasionally, a tinge of jaundice or ascites may be present. Rarely, the patient may present as an emergency due to the effects of rupture into the peritoneal, pleural, or pericardial cavity.

3. L Ascariasis
Ascaris lumbricoides, commonly called the roundworm, is the most common intestinal nematode to infect humans and affects one-quarter of the world's population. The parasite causes pulmonary symptoms as a larva and intestinal symptoms as an adult worm.

The adult worm can grow up to 45 cm long. Its presence in the small intestine causes malnutrition, failure to thrive and abdominal pain. Small intestinal obstruction can occur, particularly in children, due to a bolus of adult worms incarcerated in the terminal ileum. This is a surgical emergency. Rarely, perforation of the small bowel may occur as a result of ischaemic pressure necrosis from the bolus of worms.

A high index of suspicion is necessary so as not to miss the diagnosis. If a person from the tropics, or one who has recently returned from an endemic area, presents with pulmonary, gastrointestinal, hepatobiliary and pancreatic symptoms, roundworm infestation should be high on the list of possible diagnoses. Increase in the eosinophil count is common, in keeping with most other parasitic infestations. Stool examination may show ova. Sputum or bronchoscopic washings may show Charcot–Leyden crystals or the larvae.

4. F Filariasis

Filariasis is chiefly caused by the parasite *Wuchereria bancrofti*, which is carried by the mosquito. A variant of the parasite called *Brugia malayi* and *Brugia timori* is responsible for causing the disease in about 10% of sufferers. The condition affects more than 90 million people worldwide, two-thirds of who live in India, China and Indonesia.

It is chiefly males who are affected, because females in general cover a greater part of their bodies, thus making them less prone to mosquito bites. In the acute presentation, there are episodic attacks of fever with lymphadenitis and lymphangitis. Occasionally, adult worms may be felt subcutaneously.

Chronic manifestations appear after repeated acute attacks over several years. The adult worms cause lymphatic obstruction, resulting in massive lower limb oedema. Obstruction to the cutaneous lymphatics causes skin thickening, not unlike the 'peau d'orange' appearance in breast cancer, thus exacerbating the limb swelling. Secondary streptococcal infection is common. Recurrent attacks of lymphangitis cause fibrosis of the lymph channels, resulting in a grossly swollen limb with thickened skin, producing the condition of elephantiasis. Bilateral lower limb filariasis is often associated with scrotal and penile elephantiasis. Early on, there may be a hydrocele underlying scrotal filariasis.

Eosinophilia is common, and a nocturnal peripheral blood smear may show the immature forms or microfilariae. The parasite may also be seen in chylous urine, ascites and hydrocele fluid.

5. C Hydatid disease

Commonly called dog tapeworm, hydatid disease is caused by *Echinococcus granulosus*. While it is common in the tropics, in the United Kingdom the occasional patient may come from a rural sheep farming community. The dog is the definitive host and, as a pet, is the most common source of infection transmitted to the intermediate hosts, including humans, sheep and cattle.

As the parasite can colonise virtually every organ in the body, the condition can be protean in its presentation. When a sheep farmer, who is otherwise healthy, complains of a gradually enlarging painful mass in the right upper quadrant with the physical findings of a liver swelling, a hydatid liver cyst should be considered. The liver is the organ most often affected. The lungs are the next site most commonly affected. The parasite can affect any organ or several organs in the same patient.

The disease may be asymptomatic and discovered incidentally at postmortem or when an ultrasound or CT scan is done for some other condition. Symptomatic disease presents with a swelling causing pressure effects. Thus, a hepatic lesion causes dull pain from stretching of the liver capsule, and a pulmonary lesion, if large enough, causes dyspnoea.

The patient may present as an emergency with severe abdominal pain following minor trauma when the CT scan may be diagnostic. Rarely, a patient may present as an emergency with features of anaphylactic shock without any obvious cause.

6. D Hyperplastic ileocaecal tuberculosis

Infection by *Mycobacterium tuberculosis* is common in the tropics. Any patient, particularly one who has recently arrived from an endemic area and who has features of generalised ill health and altered bowel habit, should arouse the suspicion of intestinal tuberculosis.

Patients present electively with weight loss, chronic cough, malaise, evening rise in temperature with sweating, vague abdominal pain with distension and alternating constipation and diarrhoea. As an emergency, they present with features of distal small-bowel obstruction from strictures of the small bowel, particularly the terminal ileum. Rarely, a patient may present with features of peritonitis from perforation of a tuberculous ulcer in the small bowel. Examination shows a chronically ill patient with a 'doughy' feel to the abdomen from areas of localised ascites. In the hyperplastic type, a mass may be felt in the right iliac fossa.

Some patients may present late as an emergency from intestinal obstruction. Abdominal pain and distension, constipation and bilious and faeculent vomiting are typical of such a patient who is in extremis.

Raised erythrocyte sedimentation rate (ESR) and C-reactive protein (CRP), anaemia and a positive Mantoux test are usual, although the last is not significant in a patient from an endemic area. Sputum for culture and sensitivity (the result may take several weeks) and staining by the Ziehl–Neelsen method for acid-fast bacilli (the result is obtained much earlier) should be done. A barium meal and follow-through (or small-bowel enema) will show strictures of the small bowel, particularly the ileum, typically with a high subhepatic caecum with the narrow ileum entering the caecum directly from below upward in a straight line rather than at an angle.

In the patient presenting as an emergency, urea and electrolytes show evidence of gross dehydration. Plain abdominal x-ray shows typical small-bowel obstruction– valvulae conniventes of dilated jejunum and featureless ileum with evidence of fluid between the loops.

7. G Leprosy

Leprosy, also called Hansen's disease, is a chronic infectious disease caused by the acid-fast bacillus, *Mycobacterium leprae* that is widely prevalent in the tropics. Globally, India, Brazil, Nepal, Mozambique, Angola and Myanmar (Burma) account for 91% of all the cases.

The disease is broadly classified into two groups, lepromatous and tuberculoid. In lepromatous leprosy, there is widespread dissemination of abundant bacilli in the tissue with macrophages and a few lymphocytes. This is a reflection of the poor immune response, resulting in depleted host resistance from the patient. In tuberculoid leprosy, on the other hand, the patient shows a strong immune response with scant bacilli in the tissues, epithelioid granulomas, numerous lymphocytes and giant cells. The tissue damage is proportional to the host's immune response.

The disease is slowly progressive and affects the skin, upper respiratory tract and peripheral nerves. In tuberculoid leprosy, the damage to tissue occurs early and is localised to one part of the body with limited deformity of that organ. Neural involvement is characterised by thickening of the nerves, which are tender. There may be asymmetric well-defined anaesthetic hypopigmented or erythematous macules with elevated edges and a dry and rough surface – lesions called leprids.

In lepromatous leprosy, the disease is symmetrical and extensive. Cutaneous involvement occurs in the form of several pale macules that form plaques and nodules called lepromas. The deformities produced are divided into primary, which are caused by leprosy or its reactions, and secondary, which result from effects such as anaesthesia of the hands and feet.

There is loss of eyebrows and destruction of the lateral cartilages and septum of the nose with collapse of the nasal bridge and lifting of the tip of the nose. There may be paralysis of the branches of the facial nerve in the bony canal or the zygomatic branch.

The hands are typically clawed because of involvement of the ulnar nerve at the elbow and the median nerve at the wrist. Anaesthesia of the hands makes these patients vulnerable to frequent burns and injuries. Similarly, clawing of the toes occurs as a result of involvement of the posterior tibial nerve. When the lateral popliteal nerve is affected, it leads to foot drop, and the nerve can be felt to be thickened behind the upper end of the fibula. Anaesthesia of the feet predisposes to trophic ulceration, chronic infection, contraction and auto-amputation. Involvement of the testes causes atrophy, which in turn results in gynaecomastia.

8. H Poliomyelitis

Poliomyelitis is an enteroviral infection that affects children in developing countries. The virus enters the body by inhalation or ingestion. Clinically, the disease manifests itself in a wide spectrum of symptoms, from a few days of mild fever and headache to the extreme variety consisting of extensive paralysis of the bulbar form that may not be compatible with life because of involvement of the respiratory and pharyngeal muscles.

The disease targets the anterior horn cells, causing lower motor neuron paralysis. Muscles of the lower limb are affected twice as frequently as those of the upper limb. Only 1% to 2% of sufferers develop paralytic symptoms, but, when they do occur, the disability causes much misery. When a patient develops fever with muscle weakness, Guillain–Barré syndrome needs to be excluded. The latter has sensory symptoms and signs, and cerebrospinal fluid (CSF) analysis should help to differentiate the two conditions. The regional anatomical deformities are as follows:

Foot and ankle: The most common deformities are claw toes, cavovarus foot, dorsal bunion, talipes equines, talipes equinovarus, talipes cavovarus, talipes equinovalgus and talipes calcaneus.

Knee: Flexion contracture, quadriceps paralysis, genu recurvatum and flail knee.

Hip: Common problems are flexion and abduction contractures, hip instability due to paralysis of the gluteal muscles and paralytic hip dislocation.

Trunk: Unbalanced paralysis causes scoliosis along with pelvic obliquity.

Shoulder, elbow, wrist and hand: Common problems are shoulder weakness, wrist drop and claw hands.

9. I Psoas abscess

Psoas abscess is a condition in which an abscess develops in the fascial sheath of the psoas major muscle. The source of infection may be from the adjacent lumbar vertebrae (tuberculosis of the spine is the most common), haematogenous, or from the overlying peritoneal cavity.

The abscess remains silent for a long time due to the deep-seated location of the muscle. At this time the patient may have systemic features of the infection, such as fever or malaise, or may have symptoms attributable to the spine such as backache or neurological complaints. The infection tracks along the muscle sheath and may involve the iliacus muscle, which joins the psoas for a common insertion, to form an iliopsoas abscess. This may be palpable as a lump in the iliac fossa. Rarely, the abscess may point on the medial side of the thigh at the point of insertion of the muscle on the femur. The affected muscle may go into spasm, causing flexion deformity of the hip joint.

Clinical signs may include tenderness of the affected vertebrae, fullness of the paravertebral space and scoliosis with concavity toward the affected side, mass in the iliac fossa, flexion deformity of the hip and lump on the upper medial thigh with cross-fluctuation of the abscess (cold abscess). An x-ray of the dorsolumbar spine or US or CT scan help in arriving at a diagnosis.

10. A Tropical chronic pancreatitis

Tropical chronic pancreatitis is a disease affecting the younger generation seen mostly in southern India. The aetiology remains obscure, with malnutrition, dietary, familial and genetic factors being possible causes.

Cassava (tapioca) is a root vegetable that is readily available and inexpensive and is therefore consumed as a staple diet. Several members of the same family have been known to suffer from this condition; this strengthens the theory that cassava toxicity is an important cause, because family members eat the same food.

The patient, usually male, is almost always younger than 40 years and usually from a poor background. The clinical presentation is abdominal pain, thirst, polyuria and features of gross pancreatic insufficiency, causing steatorrhoea and malnutrition. The patient looks ill and emaciated.

Initial routine blood and urine tests confirm that the patient has type 1 diabetes mellitus. Plain abdominal x-ray shows typical pancreatic calcification in the form of discrete stones in the duct. Ultrasound and CT scan of the pancreas confirm the diagnosis.

11. K Tubercular peritonitis

Infection by *Mycobacterium tuberculosis* is common in the tropics. Any patient, particularly one who has recently arrived from an endemic area and has features of generalised ill health and altered bowel habit, should arouse the suspicion of intestinal tuberculosis.

Patients present electively with weight loss, chronic cough, malaise, evening rise in temperature with sweating, vague abdominal pain with abdominal distension and alternating constipation and diarrhoea. As an emergency, they present with features of distal small-bowel obstruction from strictures of the small bowel, particularly the terminal ileum. Rarely, a patient may present with features of peritonitis from perforation of a tuberculous ulcer in the small bowel. Examination shows a chronically ill patient with a 'doughy' feel to the abdomen from areas of localised ascites. In the hyperplastic type, a mass may be felt in the right iliac fossa.

Because this is a disease seen mainly in developing countries, patients may present late as an emergency from intestinal obstruction. Abdominal pain and distension, constipation and bilious and faeculent vomiting are typical of such a patient who is in extremis.

Raised ESR and CRP, low haemoglobin and a positive Mantoux test are usual, although the last is not significant in a patient from an endemic area. Sputum for culture and sensitivity (the result may take several weeks) and staining by the Ziehl–Neelsen method for acid-fast bacilli (the result is obtained much earlier) should be done. A barium meal and follow-through (or small-bowel enema) will show strictures of the small bowel, particularly the ileum, typically with a high subhepatic caecum with the narrow ileum entering the caecum directly from below upward in a straight line rather than at an angle.

In the patient presenting as an emergency, urea and electrolytes show evidence of gross dehydration. Plain abdominal x-ray shows typical small-bowel obstruction – valvulae conniventes of dilated jejunum and featureless ileum with evidence of fluid between the loops.

12. E Typhoid perforation

Typhoid fever is caused by *Salmonella typhi*, which is also called the typhoid bacillus. This is a Gram-negative organism. The organism gains entry into the human gastrointestinal tract as a result of poor hygiene and inadequate sanitation. It is a disease normally managed by physicians, but the surgeon is called upon to treat the patient with typhoid fever because of perforation of a typhoid ulcer.

A typical patient is from an endemic area or someone who has recently visited such a country and suffers from a high temperature for 2 to 3 weeks. The patient may be toxic with abdominal distension from paralytic ileus. The patient may have melaena due to haemorrhage from a typhoid ulcer; this can lead to hypovolaemia.

In the second or third week of the illness, if there is severe generalised abdominal pain, this heralds a perforated typhoid ulcer. The patient, who is already very ill, deteriorates further with classical features of peritonitis. An erect chest x-ray or a lateral decubitus film (in the very ill, as they usually are) will show free gas in the peritoneal cavity. In fact, any patient being treated for typhoid fever who shows a sudden deterioration accompanied by abdominal signs should be considered to have a typhoid perforation until proved otherwise.

7 Principles of laparoscopic and robotic surgery

C R Selvasekar

Multiple choice questions

→ **Advantages of minimal access surgery (MAS)**

1. Which of the following statements are true?

A Decrease in wound size.
B Decreased postoperative pain.
C Reduced operating time.
D Improved vision.
E Reduced operating theatre costs.

→ **Limitations of MAS**

2. Which of the following statements are true?

A Technically more demanding.
B Loss of tactile feedback.
C Extraction of large specimens.
D Difficulty with haemostasis.
E Surgery following previous multiple operations.

→ **Gas used in pneumoperitoneum**

3. Which of the following statements are true?

A It should be a supporter of combustion.
B It should be highly soluble in blood.
C It should be rapidly excreted by the body.
D There should be low risk of embolism.
E It should have low diffusion co-efficient.

→ **Complications of pneumoperitoneum**

4. Which of the following statements are true?

A Hyperthermia.
B Acidosis.
C Cardiac arrhythmias.

D Gas embolism.
E Compromised cardiac return.

5. Which of the following statements are true regarding complications associated with creating pneumoperitoneum?

A Bleeding.
B Visceral injuries.
C Gas dissection in the abdominal wall.
D Injury to the blood vessels.
E Omental tears.

→ **Energy sources in MAS**

6. Which of the following energy sources are used in minimal access surgery?

A Monopolar diathermy.
B Bipolar diathermy.
C Laser.
D Ultrasound energy.
E Vapour plasma coagulation (VPC).

→ **Robotic surgery**

7. The following are the advantages of robotic surgery except:

A 3-D vision.
B Articulated instruments allowing precise dissection.
C Cost effectiveness.
D Steep learning curve.
E Surgery can be performed in a confined space.

8. What are the benefits of robotic surgery over laparoscopic surgery?

A Better ergonomics.
B Reduces the need for assistants.
C Precise dissection and motion scaling.
D Shorter operating time.
E Shorter learning curve.

9. **What are the current drawbacks of robotic surgery?**

A Increased costs.
B Prolonged learning curve.
C Increased operating time.
D Socioeconomic implications.
E Loss of tactile feedback.

Bleeding in MAS

10. **How can bleeding from the trocar site be controlled?**

A By applying upward and lateral pressure with the trocar.
B By using a percutaneous monofilament suture loop.
C Suturing.
D Application of Foley catheter balloon.
E Diathermy.

Risk of electrosurgery in MAS

11. **Which of the following statements are true in relation to the risks of electrosurgery in minimal access surgery?**

A Majority of injuries occur following the use of monopolar diathermy.
B The incidence is about one to two cases per 1000 procedures.
C All the injuries are recognised at the time of surgery.

D The injuries are minor.
E Bipolar diathermy is equally dangerous.

Electrosurgical injuries in laparoscopic surgery

12. **What are the main causes of electrosurgical injuries in laparoscopic surgery?**

A Inadvertent touching or grasping of tissue during application.
B Direct coupling.
C Insulation breaks.
D Indirect coupling.
E Passage of electricity from recently coagulated tissue.

Natural orifice transluminal surgery (NOTES)

13. **Which of the following are used as access points for natural orifice transluminal surgery (NOTES)?**

A Mouth.
B Vagina.
C Umbliicus.
D Anus.
E Retroperitoneum.

Extended matching questions

Complications of laparoscopy include the following:

1 Bowel injury
2 Major vessel injury
3 Port-site bleeding
4 Port-site hernia
5 Port-site metastasis
6 Referred pain
7 Thromboembolic complications

Scenarios of complications

Match the diagnoses with the clinical scenarios that follow:

A A 64-year-old male who had laparoscopic colectomy for cancer presents with a lump at the port site. The lump is painless and hard. There is no cough impulse and it is not reducible.
B A 36-year-old female who had laparoscopic cholecystectomy two days ago is brought to A&E with increasing abdominal pain and distension. On examination she is very unwell and shows signs of peritonitis.

C A 32-year-old female had an uneventful laparoscopy 4 hours previously. The nurses observe that the dressings are soaked with blood despite repeated changing. The woman has tachycardia but is otherwise well. The abdomen is soft and not distended.

D A 40-year-old female who underwent laparoscopic cholecystectomy the previous day complains of pain over the right shoulder. She is otherwise stable and her abdomen is soft and non-tender.

E A 55-year-old male who had laparoscopic cholecystectomy two years ago presents with a slowly increasing lump over the substernal scar. This gets more prominent on sitting and coughing. It is causing local discomfort. Clinical examination reveals a 2 cm soft lump over the area. It is reducible and has cough impulse.

F A 70-year-old obese female who had a laparoscopic cholecystectomy 1 week ago is admitted with chest pain and shortness of breath. A CT pulmonary angiogram confirms the diagnosis.

G A 34-year-old thin female undergoes a diagnostic laparoscopy for unexplained pelvic pain. The woman collapses after the introduction of the first trocar. The surgeon could not visualise any structures in the peritoneal cavity, as the view is 'red out', The abdomen is distended with free blood in the peritoneal cavity.

Answers to multiple choice questions

1. A, B, D
The other advantages are reduced wound pain and wound-related complications such as infection, bleeding, hernias and nerve entrapment. In the long-term there is possibility of decreased adhesions and incisional hernia. MAS is complimentary to enhanced recovery programme (ERP) in reducing postoperative hospital stay and improving patient experience.

2. A, B, C, E
The other limitations are reliance on remote vision and operating and dependence on hand-eye coordination. The set-up costs and operating theatre costs can be high. However, the overall hospital costs are less.

3. B, C, D
The gas used for pneumoperitoneum should not be combustible or supportive of combustion, because this can cause fire with the use of diathermy. It should have a high diffusion coefficient to minimise the risk of embolism.

4. B, C, D, E
The other complications include hypothermia and referred shoulder-tip pain.

5. A, B, C, D, E
The procedure to create pneumoperitoneum can be associated with major risks, hence utmost care needs to be employed. Risks can be reduced by avoiding a blunt puncture and taking extra care in difficult cases, such as with those who have had previous operations. Gas dissection within the abdominal wall can be avoided by confirming, without doubt, placement of trocars in the peritoneal cavity before starting insufflation and correlating pressures generated with the volume of gas insufflated. Injury to major vessels is life threatening and should be promptly recognised. Laparotomy performed without delay and expert help, if needed and damage repaired.

6. A, B, C, D
Monopolar diathermy is the common energy source used. This has potential risks, thus needs to be used with caution. Argon plasma coagulation (APC) is used to augment the coagulation effect of the diathermy, but there is a potential for lateral spread and care should be exercised in its use. Biploar energy devices are safer to use. A modern energy device commonly used is ultrasound, which can generate heat and thus must be used with caution.

7. C

In robotic surgery, the robot is used as a tool to perform the MAS. The advantages are the magnified 3-D vision with articulated instruments, which provide precise dissection. The fixed traction is also of benefit, however, the current robot technology does not allow procedures to be performed in multiple quadrants easily and in dealing with mobile structures.

8. A, B, C, E

Robotic surgery has shorter learning curve for those already practising laparoscopic surgery and allows open surgeons to take up minimal access surgery.

9. A, C, D, E

Despite these drawbacks, robotic surgery has a role in single-quadrant disease such as in the pelvis. Currently robotic surgery is mainly used for prostatectomy and hysterectomy, as well as in the surgery for rectal cancer. Robotic surgery is also used in cardiothoracic surgery in performing anastomosis and valve replacement.

10. A, B, C, D, E

This recognised complication can be reduced by inserting and removing trocars under direct vision and avoiding the path of the epigastric vessels.

11. A, B

These injuries can be potentially serious. They are often not recognised at the time of operation and patients may present 3 to 7 days after injury with pyrexia and nonspecific abdominal pain. Bipolar diathermy is safer than monopolar diathermy, as there is no lateral spread of current.

12. A, B, C, D, E

Awareness of electrosurgical injuries is essential in minimal access surgery. Injuries can be avoided by having an optimal visual image, employing safer surgical technique by avoiding excessive diathermy use and using alternative energy sources.

13. A, B, D

This is also called scarless or incisionless surgery. In this technique, the peritoneal cavity is entered via a natural orifice and surgery is carried out with specialised instruments. This technology is still in its developmental stage not used as a recognised technique.

Answers to extended matching questions

1. B Bowel injury

Bowel injury is a recognised complication after laparoscopic surgery. This can be due to bowel handling or diathermy injury. Only bowel graspers should be used to handle bowels and all graspers should be kept under vision. This complication is suspected if a patient presents with signs of peritonitis a few days after surgery.

2. G Major vessel injury

This is a major life-threatening complication and requires immediate recognition and laparotomy. This complication can be caused by both verres needle and the trocars. Trocars should be inserted cautiously.

3. C Port-site bleeding

Port-site bleeding can present with overt wound bleeding or signs of shock due to internal bleeding. The bleeding from epigastric vessels or vessels in the falciform ligament can cause significant bleeding, and this complication can be identified by removing the ports under direct vision.

4. E Port-site hernia

Port-site hernia has a 1% to 2% incidence. It is important all the ports of 1 cm and above are closed. Lateral ports made using bladeless trocars are associated with lower incidence of hernia formation.

5. A Port-site metastasis

Port-site recurrences are a potential complication following laparoscopic surgery for cancer. In colorectal cancer this is reported as 1%, which is similar to open procedures. This incidence can be reduced by using wound protectors and endobag for specimen retrieval, and by allowing the gas to escape through the ports, avoiding chimney effect, and cleaning the port sites prior to closure.

6. D Referred pain

Referred pain to the shoulder is not uncommon after laparoscopic surgery. This is referred from the diaphragm, should subside within a couple of days and can be reduced by ensuring that all the CO_2 is removed from the peritoneal cavity prior to waking the patient up. Sometimes administration of local anaesthetic in the peritoneal cavity can decrease the referred pain.

7. F Thromboembolism

Deep vein thrombosis (DVT) and pulmonary embolism are potential complications following minimal access abdominal surgery. All patients should receive appropriate DVT prophylaxis based on the current NICE (England) or SIGN (Scotland) guidelines.

Principles of paediatric surgery

Pradip K Datta

Multiple choice questions

→ ## Anatomy and operative surgery

1. Which of the following statements are true?

A For open surgery, vertical midline incisions give better access.

B The ribs are more horizontal and flexible.

C The liver and bladder are intra-abdominal.

D The infant's head constitutes 20% of the surface area.

E The infant has a large tongue, the epiglottis projects backwards and the larynx is high.

→ ## General surgical management

2. Which of the following statements are false?

A A neonate is a baby up to 4 weeks old.

B The urinary bladder is an intra-abdominal organ in infants and children.

C An infant's head accounts for 20% of the body surface area.

D Gluconeogenesis in infants is as good as in adults.

E The infant's immune system is immature.

3. Which of the following statements are true?

A Children are regarded as small adults, and therefore their surgical management is adjusted according to their size.

B Attention to thermoregulation is very important.

C Postoperative management requires extreme care, because of inadequate stress response.

D Postoperatively, children do not recover as quickly as adults.

E Minimal access surgery (MAS) can be used at all ages.

→ ## Paediatric trauma

4. Which of the following statements regarding paediatric trauma are true?

A Follow usual Advanced Trauma Life Support (ATLS) rules as in an adult.

B The usual rules of resuscitation apply.

C Blunt trauma is more common than penetrating trauma.

D Splenic injury in the majority should be treated by splenectomy.

E Consideration must be given to non-accidental injury (NAI).

→ ## Inguinoscrotal swellings

5. Which of the following statements about inguinoscrotal swellings are false?

A A hydrocele is a patent processus vaginalis, as is a hernia.

B Hernia is always indirect.

C Hernia can be direct or indirect.

D In incarcerated hernia, reduction should be attempted by taxis followed by operation 24 hours later.

E A hydrocele always needs an operation.

→ ## Undescended testis

6. Which if the following are true for undescended testis?

A Orchidopexy in a subdartos pouch is the treatment of choice.

B The operation is recommended at the age of 2 years.

C When a testis is impalpable and therefore intra-abdominal, laparotomy should be done.

D Laparoscopy is the gold standard procedure for an intra-abdominal testis.

E Orchidopexy reduces the chance of malignancy.

→ Acute scrotal pain

7. **Which of the following statements are true with regard to acute scrotal pain?**

A Acute testicular pain can be from torsion of the testis, torsion of the hydatid of Morgagni, or acute epididymitis.

B Pain of testicular torsion may originate in the groin or suprapubic area.

C Doppler ultrasound should be done in suspected testicular torsion.

D Incarcerated hernia may cause similar symptoms.

E In case of any doubt, exploration of the scrotum must be carried out.

→ Surgical treatment

8. **What is the operation for congenital hypertrophic pyloric stenosis called?**

A Hartmann's

B Whipple's

C Heller's

D Ramstedt's

E Ivor-Lewis'

Extended matching questions

→ Vomiting

1 Congenital hypertrophic pyloric stenosis

2 Incarcerated inguinal hernia

3 Intussusception

Match the diagnoses with the clinical scenarios that follow:

A A 2-year-old boy has been sent in as an emergency with vomiting for 24 hours. According to the parents, the vomitus was greenish to start with but over the past few hours has consisted of dirty brownish fluid. There has been no bowel action. On examination the child looks toxic and is dehydrated – sunken eyes, depressed fontanelles, loss of skin turgor. There is a tympanitic abdomen with a red, irreducible swelling in the left groin not noticed by the parents.

B Jonathan, a 5-week-old boy, has been vomiting intermittently for 2 weeks. This has become incessant for the past 24 hours. The vomitus is clear fluid. The infant seems hungry and takes its feed only to bring it up within a short while. The mother noticed some twitching of muscles. The baby is dehydrated. The paediatrician felt a lump in the upper abdomen when Jonathan was being fed by his mother.

C Mary-Ann, a 10-month-old girl, has been brought in with occasional vomiting for a couple of days. The parents noticed that the vomitus is sometimes green and at other times brownish. They feel that Mary-Ann is in pain intermittently, because she screams, flexing her knees and elbows, denoting spasms. They noticed that the nappy has bloodstained mucus. On examination she looks ill and dehydrated, and the right side of the abdomen feels empty.

→ Acute abdomen

1 Acute appendicitis

2 Nonspecific abdominal pain

3 Urinary tract infection

Choose and match the correct diagnosis with each of the scenarios that follow.

A George, a 10-year-old boy has been brought in with abdominal pain, vomiting, pyrexia and diarrhoea for the past 24 hours or so. He has been off his food for a couple of days. He has pyrexia of 39°C, tachycardia, looks toxic and has marked lower abdominal tenderness, rigidity and rebound tenderness, and the abdominal wall does not move with respiration.

B Kerry, a 5-year-old girl, has been brought in by her parents with generalised abdominal pain, which has been recurrent over 6 months or so. On this occasion she looks ill, out of sorts and anorexic, and she has been vomiting. She has marked urinary frequency. On examination she has a temperature of 100°C, looks toxic, listless and dehydrated and has generalised abdominal and bilateral loin tenderness.

C Millie, a 10-year-old girl, has been admitted with generalised abdominal pain, vomiting and anorexia for 2 days. She has missed school a few times because of similar attacks of abdominal pain in the past, which has subsided on its own within 24 hours. On this occasion it has persisted. Examination revealed a well-looking introspective child with generalised abdominal tenderness without any rigidity or rebound tenderness, with the abdominal wall moving freely with respiration.

Congenital malformations

1 Biliary atresia
2 Congenital diaphragmatic hernia
3 Duodenal atresia
4 Hirschsprung's disease
5 Intestinal malrotation
6 Necrotising enterocolitis
7 Tracheo-oesophageal fistula

Choose and match the correct diagnosis with each of the scenarios that follow.

A A 2-month-old Down's syndrome baby has been brought in with gradual abdominal distension and intermittent bilious vomiting with a history of delayed passage of meconium. The parents feel that the baby is unduly constipated. Examination shows a baby that has not been thriving normally, with a hugely distended abdomen and gross dehydration.

B A prenatal ultrasound scan alerted the paediatricians to a congenital abnormality affecting the abdomen and chest. The premature neonate has been born with severe respiratory compromise and is on ventilatory support in the neonatal ICU.

C A neonate is born with frothy saliva and episodes of cyanosis. Any attempt to feed makes the symptoms worse. A fine orogastric tube is arrested. A plain x-ray shows that the tube is curled up in the chest and there is gas in the abdomen. The condition was suspected on prenatal ultrasound.

D A mother who suffered from polyhydramnios has given birth to a baby who has Down syndrome. The baby has bilious vomiting. The plain abdominal x-ray shows a 'double-bubble' appearance, and the condition was suspected on prenatal ultrasound.

E A neonate has bile-stained vomiting with passage of blood-stained stools. The baby is very sick, and a contrast meal shows the bowel mostly on the right side with a subhepatic caecum.

F A 2-week-old neonate who was born with jaundice has exhibited increasing yellowish discoloration of skin and conjunctiva ever since birth. There are some superficial skin bruises.

G A few days after birth, a neonate has developed abdominal distension, blood-stained stools and bilious vomiting. The baby is toxic with septic shock.

Answers to multiple choice questions

→ Anatomy and operative surgery

1. B, C, D, E

In infants and small children, the ribs are more horizontal and flexible. This means that ventilation needs greater diaphragmatic movement. The flexibility of the ribs means that rib fractures are rare and, therefore, should an infant have a fractured rib, non-accidental injury (NAI) should be suspected. The liver and urinary bladder are intra-abdominal structures and hence more liable to get damaged in blunt upper abdominal trauma.

The infant's head constitutes 20% of the body surface area (as opposed to 9% in the adult), an important fact in thermoregulation and when calculating the total body surface area in burns. A large tongue, backward projecting epiglottis and high larynx are important anatomical landmarks about the airway. This is significant, as the tongue can obstruct the airway and impede laryngoscopy in the unconscious. The anatomy of the epiglottis and larynx requires the use of a straight-bladed laryngoscope in those under 1 year of age. Uncuffed tubes should be used to prevent irritation and subglottic stenosis, as the cricoid is the narrowest part.

For open surgery, transverse abdominal incisions give better access than longitudinal incisions because children have a wide abdomen and a broad costal margin.

→ General surgical management

2. D

In paediatric surgery, it is important to have a clear idea about the various age groups. A baby born before 37 weeks is called a preterm; a baby born between 37 and 42 weeks is full term. A baby is called a neonate up to four weeks in age; an infant up to 1 year; a pre-school child below 5 years; and a child and adolescent up to 16 years.

Because infants and small children have a shallow pelvis, the urinary bladder is intra-abdominal. The head in infants accounts for 20% of body surface, and this does not equal an adult proportion of 9% until the age of 14 years.

The ability for gluconeogenesis is much impaired in infants, which renders them hypoglycaemic very easily in the postoperative period. An immature immune system renders them more susceptible to infection, which may manifest with nonspecific features.

3. B, C, E

Children should never be regarded as small adults. Conditions that afflict children by and large are different from those in adults. In children, the thermoregulatory system is immature. Children have little subcutaneous fat (hence no natural insulation) and an undeveloped vasomotor centre. Therefore, the theatre must be well heated, their head and neck well covered (the head is almost one-fifth of the body's surface area), infusions need to be warmed, a warm air blanket used and the core temperature closely monitored.

The metabolic response to stress is inadequate because of the immature neurohormonal and immune systems. The effects of clotting deficiencies need to be prevented with intramuscular vitamin K. Ability to concentrate urine and conserve sodium is impaired; therefore, fluid and sodium needs are high. Gastro-oesophageal reflux may result in aspiration, causing pulmonary problems.

With meticulous attention to detail along with good pain relief, children recover more quickly than adults under similar circumstances. Intravenous fluids – 0.45% saline with 2.5% dextrose or isotonic saline – help to maintain optimum fluid and electrolyte balance. Minimal access surgical techniques have all the advantages, as seen in the adults; obviously, the instruments and insufflation pressures have to be tailored.

Paediatric trauma

4. B, C, E

In the western world, injury is the most common cause of death and disability in childhood; most of the deaths are avoidable. Adult ATLS guidelines cannot be followed because of the smaller body mass of children. Therefore, trauma results in a larger force applied per unit of body area. The effects are far more serious because the body has less fat, less elastic connective tissue, a poor thermoregulatory system and there is proximity of vital organs to the skin. Because of the elasticity of the child's skeleton, underlying solid organs can be damaged without overlying skeletal damage. Cardiac, pulmonary, hepatic, pancreatic and splenic injury can occur without any fractured ribs or sternum.

Blunt, rather than penetrating, trauma is more common. If the child is stable, contrast-enhanced computed tomography (CECT) is the investigation of choice. Liver, pancreatic, splenic and renal injuries are usually managed conservatively with close clinical monitoring supplemented by serial CECT or ultrasound. The team must be prepared to anticipate the need for immediate operation, as the child who is being observed can suddenly deteriorate.

A child's blood volume is 80 mL/kg. In shock (systolic blood pressure falls after loss of 25% of blood volume), 20 mL/kg Ringer's lactate solution is used as a bolus to be repeated judiciously. Interosseous access into the upper tibia may be necessary in infants.

When the severity of trauma is at variance with the degree of injury, when there has been undue delay in seeking medical advice following trauma, or when there is repeated trauma and inconsistent history between family members, NAI should be strongly suspected and paediatricians should be involved forthwith.

Inguinoscrotal swellings

5. C, E

An inguinal hernia in a child is indirect as it occurs in a patent processus vaginalis. Sometimes it may be incarcerated, resulting in vomiting and irreducibility. In the early stages of obstruction, manual reduction under analgesia (taxis) can be attempted so that the operation can be done as an elective procedure 24 hours later to allow the oedema to settle down. However, if the infant is ill, dehydrated and toxic with a distended abdomen, strangulation is imminent or present. This requires IV fluid resuscitation followed by emergency operation.

A congenital hydrocele is a patent processus vaginalis where the patency at the internal ring is too narrow to allow any bowel through; only normal peritoneal fluid comes into the scrotum, causing the hydrocele. This does not require any surgical treatment. If it is persistent after the age of 2 years, the persistent processus is ligated through a groin incision.

Undescended testis

6. A, B, D

When a testis is arrested in the normal path of descent, it is called an undescended testis. On the other hand, when the testis is found at a site away from its normal path of descent, such as in the superficial inguinal pouch, root of the scrotum, or femoral triangle, it is then regarded as an ectopic testis.

When the scrotum is empty but well developed, and the testis can be coaxed down into the scrotum, the infant has a retractile testis. This does not require any treatment except reassurance to the parents. When a testis is palpable in the line of descent and is not a retractile testis, the child requires an orchidopexy operation. This is ideally carried out before the age of 2 years, and the testis is fixed in a subdartos pouch.

When the testis is not palpable, it means that the testis is intra-abdominal. Laparoscopy is the procedure of choice. The testis can then be localised and mobilised as a staged procedure for orchidopexy. A maldescended testis should be brought down to prevent torsion, trauma, and infertility, and to enable earlier diagnosis of a tumour when any abnormality of a scrotal testis is much more easily identifiable. Orchidopexy does not reduce the chance of malignancy but increases the chances of early detection.

Acute scrotal pain

7. A, B, D, E

Torsion of the testis can occur at any age. There may be a history of intermittent pain in the past. On clinical suspicion, the scrotum should be explored as an emergency forthwith. Colour Doppler ultrasound, an investigation not usually carried out, to show reduced blood flow may be used, provided it does not compromise promptness of treatment. Torsion of the testicular appendage occurs in prepubertal boys. Sometimes, the bluish appendage can be seen on top of the testis. It can be left alone if the diagnosis is certain. Excision is preferable because it results in early cure of the problem, while at the same time excluding the serious condition of testicular torsion. Incarcerated hernia will present with vomiting and abdominal distension from intestinal obstruction.

Surgical treatment

8. D

The operation for congenital hypertrophic pyloric stenosis is called Ramstedt's operation. After full resuscitation for hypochloraemic, hypokalaemic alkalosis, the operation is carried out under general anaesthetic through a transverse right-upper-quadrant incision. The pyloric tumour is delivered out into the wound and held between the thumb and index finger, and the hypertrophied muscle incised to allow the mucosa to bulge. Great care is taken not to damage the mucosa, which is most vulnerable to inadvertent damage distally because the hypertrophy abruptly ends there, and at the duodenal end the mucosa doubles on itself to form a fornix **(Figure 8.1)** making it particularly prone to damage.

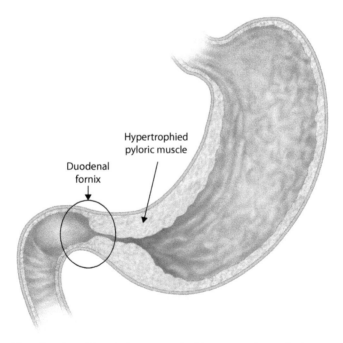

Hypertrophied
pyloric muscle

Duodenal
fornix

Figure 8.1   The duodenal fornix in congenital hypertrophic pyloric stenosis, which is most vulnerable to iatrogenic perforation during Ramstedt's pyloromyotomy.

Answers to extended matching questions

→ ## Vomiting

1. B Congenital hypertrophic pyloric stenosis

Jonathan suffers from congenital (idiopathic) hypertrophic pyloric stenosis. This occurs during the first 6 weeks of life, usually in a first-born male infant. Typically, the baby has non-bilious vomiting, is hungry and, in late cases, may have muscle spasms from alkalotic tetany. Examination shows a dehydrated baby with a hard mass ('pyloric tumour') felt in the epigastrium on test feed. Confirmation, if necessary, may be obtained on ultrasound or a gastrograffin swallow **(Figure 8.2)**.

The biochemical abnormality of hypochloraemic, hypokalaemic, metabolic alkalosis is corrected. After optimum resuscitation, a Ramstedt's pyloromyotomy (an operation that German surgeon Wilhelm Conrad Ramstedt [1867–1963] first performed in 1911) is done through a transverse right-upper-quadrant incision. For operative details, please see the previous section.

2. A Incarcerated inguinal hernia

Bilious vomiting in an infant is a sign of intestinal obstruction. An irreducible lump in the groin indicates as the cause as an incarcerated inguinal hernia. Incarceration indicates intraluminal obstruction, whereas strangulation means compromise of the blood supply to the bowel. As the child is toxic, incarceration may be proceeding to strangulation. Brownish or feculent vomitus is a sinister sign. The infant should be resuscitated with intravenous fluids, nasogastric suction and prophylactic antibiotics. Once optimised, an emergency operation should be carried out.

3. C Intussusception

Mary-Ann suffers from intussusception. This is the invagination of a proximal part of the bowel into the adjacent distal part, resulting in strangulating intestinal obstruction. Usually, the ileum invaginates into the caecum and ascending colon. The outer bowel is called the intussuscepiens, while the part that invaginates is called the intussusceptum **(Figure 8.3)**. There is bloodstained mucus from the anus ('redcurrant jelly stools') and an empty right

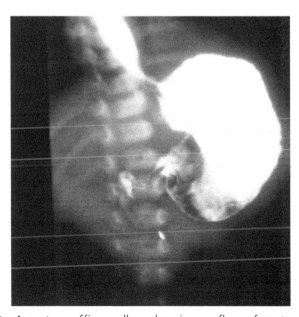

Figure 8.2 A gastrograffin swallow showing no flow of contrast past the pylorduodenal junction: congenital hypertrophic pyloric stenosis.

Pathology of intussusception

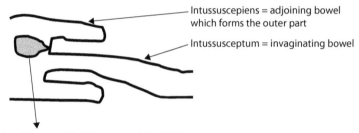

Intussuscepiens = adjoining bowel which forms the outer part

Intussusceptum = invaginating bowel

Lead point - Hypertrophied Peyer's patch in children
- Polypoid carcinoma in adults

Figure 8.3 Showing the formation and cause of an intussusception.

iliac fossa, and, sometimes, a sausage-shaped mass may be felt, which might migrate with concavity toward the umbilicus. Confirmation is by ultrasound or a gastrograffin enema, which shows a typical crab claw deformity **(Figure 8.4)**.

After full resuscitation, radiological reduction with air or contrast enema is undertaken. Successful reduction (occurs in more than 70%) is diagnosed when contrast is seen to reflux into the terminal ileum. If unsuccessful, laparotomy is undertaken and manual reduction by milking is carried out. If unsuccessful, or there is evidence of bowel infarction, limited ileocolic resection and end-to-end anastomosis is carried out.

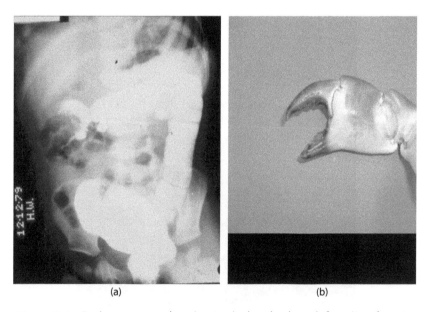

(a)   (b)

Figure 8.4 Barium enema showing typical crab-claw deformity of acute ileocaecocolic intussusception.

Acute abdomen

1. A Acute appendicitis

George has acute appendicitis. In children, the history may be atypical. Diarrhoea denotes a pelvic position of the appendix. The abdominal signs are typical of peritonitis. Perforation in children is common because of their inability to localise intra-abdominal infection as a result of poorly developed omentum. Complete examination of the chest should be done in all cases of acute abdominal pain in children to exclude right lower-lobe pneumonia.

Acute appendicitis is a clinical diagnosis. In doubtful cases, Alvarado's scoring system can be useful. The patient should undergo an emergency appendicectomy.

2. C Nonspecific abdominal pain

Millie has features suggestive of nonspecific abdominal pain – recurrent attacks, generalised abdominal symptoms, no signs of peritonism and missing school on more than one occasion, the latter denoting psychosocial problems. This is a diagnosis made in 30% to 50% of children admitted to hospital with acute abdomen. Sometimes constipation may be a cause.

3. B Urinary tract infection

Kerry has urinary tract infection. Children usually have an underlying urinary tract abnormality, such as pelviureteric junction obstruction or vesicoureteric reflux. Such conditions should be diagnosed and treated promptly to prevent long-term deleterious effects of renal scarring from ascending pyelonephritis. Clinical examination usually does not reveal any abnormality. Urine examination and renal ultrasound are the initial investigations. This is followed by micturating cystogram or isotope renogram.

Congenital malformations

1. F Biliary atresia

Congenital biliary atresia should be suspected if the jaundice in the newborn does not subside within 2 weeks. The incidence is 1 in 17,000. In the presence of conjugated hyperbilirubinaemia, coagulopathy is a problem which needs to be combated with vitamin K. An ultrasound scan, radioisotope scan and liver biopsy are the investigations of choice.

2. B Congenital diaphragmatic hernia

This is a congenital diaphragmatic hernia (**Figure 8.5**). Respiratory embarrassment is the key presentation with an empty feeling of the abdomen. The diagnosis is usually made prenatally; therefore, the team is ready to intervene soon after birth. Respiratory support is the keynote in the initial management. Repair is carried out only if adequate oxygenation is obtained on full ventilatory support. Almost one-third of cases succumb to respiratory failure due to severe pulmonary hypoplasia.

3. D Duodenal atresia

This is duodenal atresia, which may be a part of intestinal atresia. The 'double-bubble' appearance on simple x-ray is diagnostic (**Figure 8.6**). Bile-stained vomiting differentiates it from congenital hypertrophic pyloric stenosis. A complete membrane causes it. The operation is duodenoduodenostomy.

4. A Hirschsprung's disease

Congenital megacolon, first described by Harald Hirschsprung in 1911, occurs due to congenital absence of intramural ganglion cells causing large bowel obstruction. In three out of four patients, the abnormality is restricted to the rectum and colon. Enterocolitis is a dreaded complication. The diagnosis is established by a contrast enema, which shows the exact site and extent of the diseased segment; it is confirmed by biopsy.

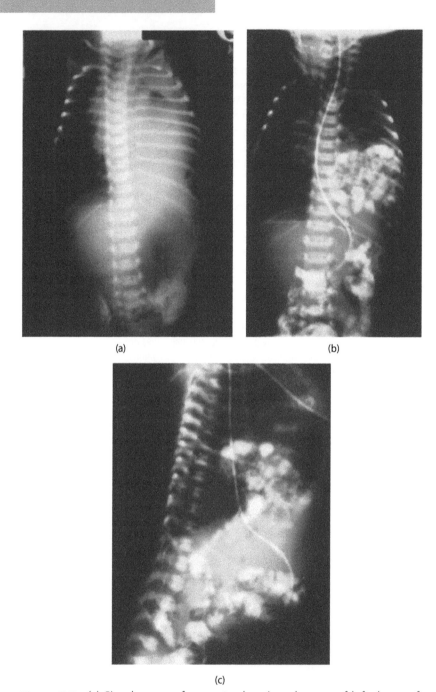

(a)

(b)

(c)

Figure 8.5 (a) Simple x-ray of neonate showing absence of left dome of diaphragm and collapsed left lung with gas shadows in the left hemi-thorax. (b) Antero-posterior view of a gastrograffin swallow showing loops of bowel in the left hemithorax: congenital diaphragmatic hernia. (c) Lateral view of a gastrograffin swallow showing loops of bowel in the left hemi-thorax: congenital diaphragmatic hernia.

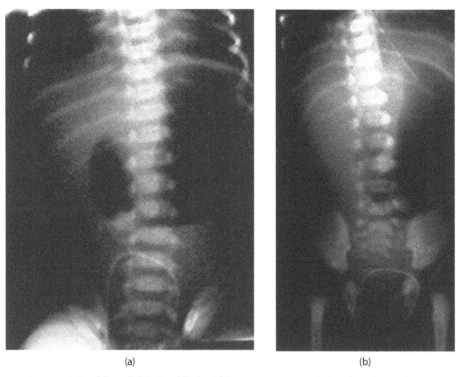

(a)   (b)

Figure 8.6   (a) and (b) Double-bubble appearance of duodenal atresia on plain abdominal x-ray.

5. E Intestinal malrotation

The neonate has bile-stained vomiting, which is a sign of intestinal obstruction. A contrast meal shows a high caecum with the duodenojejunal flexure on the right side. The small bowel mesentery has a narrow base predisposing to a midgut volvulus.

6. G Necrotising enterocolitis

Necrotising enterocolitis is an inflammatory bowel disease occurring in the premature neonate. The baby presents with features of toxic shock, abdominal distension, bloodstained stools and bilious vomiting and aspirate. A variable length of the intestine is affected.

7. C Tracheo-oesophageal fistula

Soon after birth when a neonate presents with frothy saliva and cyanosis, oesophageal atresia is the diagnosis, the most common variety being a blind proximal pouch with a distal tracheo-oesophageal fistula. Associated anomalies affecting the heart, kidneys and skeletal system may be present. After confirmation of diagnosis, referral to a paediatric surgeon is made. Operation is carried out within a day or two of birth.

9 Principles of oncology

Pradip K Datta

Multiple choice questions

→ Malignant transformation

1. **Which of the following statements are true regarding characteristics that cells should acquire before they are fully malignant?**
   A Establish an autonomous lineage.
   B Develop apoptosis.
   C Ability to invade.
   D Ability to disseminate and implant.
   E Ability to change energy metabolism.

2. **The following statements are true about cancer cells except:**
   A Obtain immortality.
   B Acquire angiogenic competence.
   C Acquire genomic stability.
   D Tumour-related inflammation promotes malignant change.
   E The major part of cell growth has occurred before the tumour is clinically apparent.

→ Causes and management of cancer

3. **Which of the following statements are true?**
   A Environmental factors have been the cause in >80% of cancers.
   B Genetic inheritance has a role in 20% of cancers.
   C Certain cancers can be prevented.
   D Screening aims at detecting disease in an asymptomatic stage.
   E Accurate diagnosis is the key to successful management.

→ Principles of cancer surgery

4. **Which of the following statements are not true?**
   A The extent of the disease, local and distant, should be mapped by staging.
   B Once diagnosed, the cancer should be radically excised at the earliest.
   C Non-surgical treatment of cancer can be expressed in reproducible units, unlike surgery.
   D Radiotherapy works by damage to the DNA of cells and targeting gene expression.
   E Chemotherapy acts by selective toxicity.

5. **Which of the following statements are true?**
   A Ultraradical surgery for local control of cancer has little effect on metastatic disease.
   B Surgery for metastatic disease is appropriate in certain circumstances.
   C Overall treatment of cancer consists of surgery, chemotherapy and radiotherapy.
   D The goal of palliative treatment is the relief of symptoms.
   E Palliative care is the same as end-of-life care.

Extended matching questions

→ ## Clinical scenarios and diagnoses

1 *Bone secondary*: A 54-year-old man complains of a swelling in the front of his thigh with throbbing pain of 6 weeks duration. The swelling is 4 cm across, warm to the touch, tender and pulsating. Three years ago, he underwent a right nephrectomy for carcinoma.

2 *Carcinoma of breast*: A 58-year-old woman complains of a hard, mobile lump in her left breast, which is 3 cm in diameter. Triple assessment confirmed a carcinoma without palpable axillary lymph nodes. A sentinel lymph node biopsy confirmed positive axillary lymph nodes.

3 *Carcinoma of descending colon*: A 65-year-old man complains of increasing constipation and colicky left-sided abdominal pain for 6 weeks. Investigations confirmed a carcinoma of the mid-descending colon, and staging showed no distant spread and the cancer confined within the colonic wall. A radical left hemicolectomy was done, which came back as Dukes' Stage B.

4 *Carcinoma of head of pancreas*: A 78-year-old woman presents with severe itching and jaundice. She has scratch marks all over her body with an enlarged nodular liver, palpable gallbladder and ascites. CT scan confirms the diagnosis of disseminated cancer of head of pancreas.

5 *Carcinoma of prostate*: A 75-year-old man complains of severe backache of 2 months duration. One year ago, he underwent radiotherapy for a carcinoma of the prostate. A bone scan shows hot spots all over the lumbar vertebrae and pelvis.

6 *Carcinoma of rectum:* A 62-year-old man complains of early morning spurious diarrhoea with rectal bleeding of 6 weeks duration. Clinical examination, investigations and staging showed an adenocarcinoma 5 cm from the anal verge, which has spread locally to the lateral pelvic wall without any distant metastases.

7 *Medullary thyroid carcinoma*: A 56-year-old woman complains of a diffuse thyroid swelling of 6 months duration. She has sporadic diarrhoea without any toxic symptoms. Core biopsy showed amyloid stroma, and a diagnosis of medullary thyroid carcinoma was made.

8 *Multiple liver metastases*: A 72-year-old woman complains of severe diarrhoea, colicky abdominal pain, flushing attacks and jaundice. On examination she has an enlarged, hard, nodular liver. Seven years ago she underwent a right hemicolectomy for a carcinoid tumour of the ileum.

9 *Pulmonary secondaries*: A 32-year-old man presents with two episodes of haemoptysis. Eight years ago, he underwent a right orchidectomy following which he was given a course of chemotherapy. Three years ago, he was given the 'all clear' and discharged. A current chest x-ray shows two shadows in his right lung.

10 *Thyroid lymphoma*: A 32-year-old woman complains of malaise for 4 months. Three months ago, she noticed a lump in front of her neck. She underwent fine-needle aspiration cytology followed by core biopsy. A diagnosis of lymphoma was made. Full staging did not show disease anywhere else in the body.

Match the clinical scenarios and diagnoses with the most appropriate management, bearing in mind that the same management may be used in more than one of the above diagnoses:

→ ## Modalities of treatment in malignancy

A Interventional radiological technique
B Minimal access surgery
C Neoadjuvant chemoradiotherapy followed by surgery

D Radiotherapy alone
E Radiotherapy +/− hormonal manipulation
F Surgery alone
G Surgery followed by chemotherapy
H Surgery followed by radiotherapy

Answers to multiple choice questions

→ ## Malignant transformation

1. A, C, D, E

The cancer cell is independent of signals that control the process of multiplication, thus distinguishing it from the normal cell. In normal wound healing, cellular proliferation is coordinated in an orderly manner such that the process occurs when it is needed, as in injury, and ceases when healing is complete. Cancer cells are free from such constraints, causing them to grow and proliferate and thus demonstrating their autonomous nature. In the human body, there are aberrant forms of normal cellular genes, called oncogenes, responsible for malignant change.

Cancer cells do not respect tissue planes and have the ability to break into the basement membrane and invade blood and lymphatic vessels, which form the perfect transport system to metastasise. The cells secrete enzymes, collagenases and proteases, which dissolve the boundaries formed by extracellular matrix, thus helping their invasion and spread.

Having gained access to the lymphatics and blood vessels, the body's natural transport system, the cancer cell develops the propensity to disseminate throughout the body. The 'seed and soil hypothesis' of Stephen Paget explains the ability of certain host organs to 'invite' clinical metastases. Although the cancer cell (seed) may settle into an organ (soil), the cell may not grow to form a clinical metastasis. When the soil is fertile, as in liver, lungs, bone, brain and lymphatics, implantation of the cancer cell occurs, producing overt metastases. This is done by the cancer cells producing inflammatory cytokines, making the soil fertile enough to allow the seed to grow into a 'plant or sapling' (metastasis).

Blood flow within a tumour is haphazard. This may result in the cancer cell living in an environment of hypoxia or at times where there is profuse vascularity when oxygen is abundant. In the latter situation there is aerobic (oxygenated) glycolysis causing the pyruvate to go to the mitochondria ultimately producing lactate. The cancer cells use this to produce energy. This phenomenon is called the Warburg effect, which was first described by Otto Warburg, a Nobel Laureate. The phenomenon of aerobic glycolysis is used in the technique of positron emission tomography (PET) scanning, which uses radiolabelled glucose to see tumours.

Apoptosis is programmed cell death seen in the normal human and is a physiological process that is a self-regulatory mechanism in growth and development. Cancer cells evolve mechanisms to prevent apoptosis. For example, the *p53* gene is a tumour suppressor gene that activates apoptosis. Loss of function in such a tumour suppressor gene will contribute to malignancy.

2. C

It is genomic instability that contributes to cancer development. As the pathogenesis of cancer involves multiple genetic events, genomic instability contributes to mutations in the DNA of tumour cells. The most important factor of genomic instability is chromosome instability.

A normal cell in the human body undergoes a finite number of divisions. This limitation is caused by shortening of the end of the chromosome (telomere) every time the cell divides. With each cell division there is telomeric attrition, which ultimately causes cell death. But cancer cells produce an enzyme telomerase that extends the length of the telomeres, thus allowing continued cell division thereby conferring on the cancer cell the quality of immortality. Along with the ability of immortality, cancer cells have the unique ability in a tumour to form new blood vessels, a phenomenon termed 'angiogenic competence'.

Another aspect that perpetuates the growth of malignancy is the ability of a tumour to provoke an inflammatory response. This produces cytokines that help to elaborate growth factors, angiogenic factors (see previous section) and anti-apoptotic factors, all of which contribute to the progression of a tumour. A certain feature of cancer biology is the unpredictable nature of the condition. The unpredictable nature of cancer is obvious by the clinical application of the Gompertzian growth factor (Gompertz being an insurance actuary). The major part of the growth of a tumour has occurred before it is clinically detected; when tumours are detected they have passed their stage of most rapid growth, thus making them less amenable to chemotherapy. In many patients at presentation cancer has already become a systemic disease.

Causes and management of cancer

3. A, B, C, D, E

The aetiology of cancer can broadly be divided into two causes – environmental factors (80%) and genetic inheritance (20%). The environmental contributions as a cause of cancer are manifold and include smoking (lung), alcohol (oesophageal, liver), ultraviolet exposure (skin), ionising radiation (lymphomas), viral infection (cervix), parasitic infection (Bilharziasis in urinary bladder, H. pylori in stomach), chemicals (aniline dye in bladder, immunosuppression in Kaposi's sarcoma, tamoxifen in endometrium) and obesity (breast and others). Genetic factors are in the vast majority from an autosomal dominant inheritance. They are familial adenomatous polyposis coli (*APC* gene), hereditary non-polyposis coli cancer (DNA mismatch repair genes) also associated with endometrial, stomach, ureter and renal pelvis, MEN syndrome 2A causing medullary thyroid cancer (*RET* gene), familial breast cancer (*BRCA1* and *2*) and other less common cancers. The purpose of knowing the aetiology is to provide strategies to prevent the disease by changing the environmental and behavioural factors and offering genetic counselling.

Screening, prevention, accurate diagnosis, staging, treatment and rehabilitation should form the overall management of cancer. Once diagnosed, it is a 'cancer journey' that the patient has to take. Several criteria for screening are set out. The disease should be common; early treatment should make a difference in enhancing the longevity; the test should be sensitive, specific, inexpensive and safe; diagnostic facilities should be readily available for those with positive tests; and benefit must outweigh physical and psychological harm.

Accurate diagnosis is crucial in the management. In this regard, the cellular architecture, differentiation, lymphovascular invasion, grading and local and distant staging are necessary. These factors are often given numerical points to obtain an overall score of the cancer to accurately stratify the disease. This would enable the team to mount the most effective treatment, which may turn out to be a combination of modalities as decided by the multidisciplinary team (MDT).

Principles of cancer surgery

4. B

Once diagnosed, the cancer should not be excised at the earliest; it would be poor surgical principle to do so. The condition should be staged, scored if appropriate, discussed in a MDT and then the best form of treatment instituted. The team looking after a complex cancer patient (such as head and neck cancer) should not only be multidisciplinary but multi-professional, the latter having a larger number of members. In certain cases, surgery may not be best form of treatment at the outset.

When the diagnosis has been confirmed on histology, the extent of the disease should be staged, both locally and regionally. Technological advances in recent years have revolutionised the staging of cancer. Depending upon the particular type of cancer and the organ involved, contrast enhanced CT scan, MRI, PET scan, ultrasound (US), laparoscopy +/– US and sentinel node biopsy (using radiolabelled colloid) all have an important role in mapping the disease as accurately as possible. Tumour markers have an important place also in follow up.

Surgery is one of tri-modal methods of treating cancer, the other two being radiotherapy and chemotherapy. The latter two can be expressed in reproducible units. For example, in the case of drugs, milligrams, and Grays (Gy) in the case of radiation; but, for example, it is not possible to describe in units of measure an operation such as a hemicolectomy.

Radiotherapy acts by producing damage to the DNA of dividing cells. While this explains the biological effects, radiation also has effects on gene expression thereby working as a targeted form of gene therapy. Chemotherapy acts by selective toxicity and often is used for palliation rather than cure. Therefore, in its use one must make sure that the effect of the treatment is not worse than the disease. Cytotoxic drugs are usually used in combination and often along with radiotherapy. When choosing a combination of drugs, the principles are to use drugs with distinct mode of action; use drugs against the disease; and use drugs with non-overlapping toxicities.

5. A, B, C, D
Radical cancer surgery entails removal of the primary tumour, as much of the surrounding tissue as possible and lymph nodes to achieve local control. Ultraradical surgery, which used to be done for breast cancer, has hardly any effect on the development of metastatic spread. Meticulous surgical technique with minimal handling of the primary tumour is the key to good surgery that would prevent local recurrence.

Surgical excision of metastases must be considered under certain circumstances. Excision of liver metastases from colorectal cancer and pulmonary secondaries from testicular cancer, which is usually seen in the younger patient, gives good palliation. Overall management of cancer in general consists of all three modalities – surgery, radiotherapy and chemotherapy – depending upon the patient, type of cancer and stage. Neoadjuvant therapy (chemotherapy and radiotherapy) is used to downstage the tumour prior to surgery.

When radical surgery cannot be carried out, palliative treatment is the answer. This would be in a patient who has distant metastases with a resectable primary, for example, a colorectal carcinoma with liver secondaries. Palliative care is not the same as end-of-life care. Patients may survive for months, if not years, with palliative care and good symptomatic control. End-of-life care is different from palliative care. It concerns the last few months or weeks of a patient's life. This may entail non-medical issues such as bereavement counselling (with family and friends), spirituality, alternative therapies and community support at home.

Answers to extended matching questions

1. Bone secondary: H surgery followed by radiotherapy
This patient who underwent a nephrectomy for renal carcinoma has a typical bone secondary in a long bone (femur in this case). Bone secondaries in renal carcinomas characteristically are osteolytic and very vascular. He needs an operation of internal fixation of the secondary to be followed by radiotherapy in the postoperative period.

2. Carcinoma of breast: G surgery followed by chemotherapy
This patient would undergo the appropriate surgery for local treatment of her breast carcinoma (mastectomy +/– reconstruction or breast conservation surgery) followed by chemotherapy for her node-positive lymph nodes.

3. Carcinoma of descending colon: G surgery followed by chemotherapy
This patient has undergone a radical left hemicolectomy. Postoperative staging is Dukes' stage B, which means that the growth has extended to extra-colonic tissues without lymph-node metastasis. Such patients benefit from a course of chemotherapy. (Dukes' staging initially was instituted for rectal carcinoma but later extended to all large bowel cancers).

4. Carcinoma of head of pancreas: B minimal access surgery
This patient requires palliation from her itching. This is ideally achieved by inserting a stent endoscopically into the common bile duct. Failing this, external biliary drainage can be carried out by interventional radiology. Sometimes, if the patient has gastric outlet obstruction, he or she may need a stent insertion into the pylorus. If, for technical reasons, none of these methods are successful, then the patient will need the palliative operative procedure of triple bypass.

5. Carcinoma of prostate: E radiotherapy +/– hormonal manipulation
This patient has multiple bone secondaries from a prostatic carcinoma. He is best treated by palliative radiotherapy. This can be supplemented by hormonal manipulation by performing bilateral subcapsular orchidectomy or carrying out a chemical castration with drugs.

6. Carcinoma of rectum: C neoadjuvant chemoradiotherapy followed by surgery
This patient has a locally advanced rectal carcinoma that has spread to the lateral pelvic wall. The patient should undergo a course of neoadjuvant chemoradiotherapy over a period of 6 weeks. This should downstage the tumour, following which an anterior resection with total mesorectal excision should be carried out.

7. Medullary thyroid carcinoma: F surgery alone
This patient should undergo a total thyroidectomy with resection of central and bilateral cervical lymph nodes. Follow up should entail serum calcitonin at regular intervals.

8. Multiple liver metastases: A interventional radiological technique
This patient has multiple liver secondaries from a carcinoid tumour excised in the past. The liver secondaries are producing the hormone serotonin, giving the patient carcinoid syndrome with distressing symptoms. This can be palliated well by the interventional radiological technique of chemoembolisation thus destroying the secondaries, which will not be able to produce serotonin.

9. Pulmonary secondaries: G surgery followed by chemotherapy
This young man has developed lung secondaries from treated testicular teratoma. He should be discussed in a MDT where the outcome would certainly be resection of the secondaries (metastasectomy). Consideration should be given to postoperative chemotherapy. The management of testicular tumours is changing all the time. He might even be considered for preoperative chemotherapy, to be followed by surgery.

10.Thyroid lymphoma: D radiotherapy alone
This patient with a proven thyroid lymphoma, which is localised to the thyroid, is treated by external beam radiotherapy.

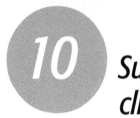

Surgical audit and clinical research

CR Selvasekar

Multiple choice questions

→ **Audit**

1. **Which of the following statements are true?**

A It addresses clearly defined questions, aims and objectives.
B It measures against a standard.
C It may involve randomization.
D Re-audit is not necessary.
E There is no allocation to intervention group.

→ **Service evaluation**

2. **Which of the following statements are true?**

A Designed and conducted to define the current standard of care.
B Measures current service without reference to a standard.
C Involves an intervention only.
D Involves analysis of already collected data, but may include simple interviews or questionnaires.
E Involves allocation to intervention and randomization.

→ **Research studies**

3. **Which of the following statements are true?**

A A cross-sectional study is one where a series of patients with a particular disease or condition are compared with matched control patients.
B Type 1 error is when benefit is perceived when really there is none (false positive).
C Randomised trials are essential for testing new drugs.
D It is a common practice to set the level of power for the study at 80% with a 5% significance level.

E A single blind study is when the clinician is unaware of the treatment allocation.

→ **Statistical analysis in research**

4. **Which of the following statements are true?**

A Range is the value with the highest frequency observed.
B Unpaired t test is used to compare two groups, which are numerical and normally distributed.
C A confidence interval that includes zero usually implies lack of statistical significance.
D A p-value of <0.5 is commonly taken to imply true difference.
E Chi-square tests are useful in comparing two groups that are categorical.

→ **Research**

5. **Which of the following questions should be answered before undertaking research?**

A Why do the study?
B Will it answer a useful question?
C Will there be any financial incentives?
D Is it practical?
E What impact will it have?

→ **Evidence-based surgery**

6. **Which of the following acronyms are not associated with publications in surgery?**

A CONSORT
B PRISMA
C IMRAD
D TREND
E TNM

Extended matching questions

→ Types of research study

1 Case-control
2 Cross-sectional
3 Longitudinal
4 Observational
5 Randomised
6 Randomised controlled double-blind

Match the correct study with each of the descriptions that follow:

A Two randomly allocated treatments are compared.
B Series of patients with a particular disease or condition are compared with matched control patients.
C A condition or treatment is evaluated in a defined population. This study can be prospective or retrospective.
D This study involves a control group that receives standard treatment.
E Measurements are made on a single occasion, not looking at the whole population but selecting a small similar group and expanding results.
F Measurements are taken over a period of time, not looking at the whole population but selecting a small similar group and expanding results.

→ Statistical tests

1 Chi-square test
2 Mann-Whitney U-test
3 Paired t-test
4 Unpaired t-test
5 Wilcoxon's signed-rank test

Choose and match the correct test with each of the scenarios that follow:

A To compare two groups, which are numerical but not normally distributed?
B To compare two groups, which are categorical?
C To assess whether a variable has changed between two time points in numerical and normally distributed data.
D To assess whether a variable has changed between two time points in numerical but not normally distributed data.
E To compare two groups, which are numerical and normally distributed?

Answers to multiple choice questions

→ Audit

1. B, E

Clinical audit is a process used by the clinicians who seek to improve patient care. The process involves comparing aspects of care (structure, process and outcome) against explicit criteria. An audit study is designed and conducted to produce information to inform the delivery of best care. This is designed to answer the question 'Does the service reach a pre-determined standard?' This does not involve randomisation or allocation to intervention group, which is seen in a research study. It usually involves analysis of existing data but may include administration of simple interviews or questionnaires. Re-audit is an important part to close the loop.

→ ## Service evaluation

2. A, B, C, D

Service evaluation is done to assess the quality of care provided without reference to a standard. Here, a retrospective analysis of the service provided is performed. This, in future, can be used to set a standard.

→ ## Research studies

3. B, C, D

Research is designed to generate new knowledge and might involve testing a new treatment or regimen. A research study addresses clearly defined questions, aims and objectives. It is of two broad types, quantitative and qualitative. Quantitative research is designed to test a hypothesis, which may involve evaluating or comparing interventions, particularly new ones. The study design may involve allocating patients to intervention groups. Qualitative research identities or explores themes following established methodology and usually involves the way in which interventions and relationships are experienced. This uses a clearly defined sampling framework underpinned by conceptual or theoretical justifications.

A single blind study is when the patient is unaware of the treatment allocation. A case-control study is one in which a series of patients with a particular disease or condition are compared with matched control patients. A cross-sectional study is one in which measurements are made on a single occasion, not looking at the whole population but selecting a small similar group and expanding results.

→ ## Statistical analysis in research

4. B, C, E

Mean (average) is the result of dividing the total by the number of observations. Median is the middle value with an equal number of observations above and below – used for numerical or ranked data. Mode is the value with the highest frequency observed – used for nominal data collection. Range is the largest to the smallest value.

The most important difference between analysis is whether the distribution of results is normal, i.e., parametric or non-parametric. Normally distributed results have a symmetrical bell-shaped curve. The mean, median and mode all lie at the same value.

When analysing numerical or normally distributed data (e.g., blood pressure), a t-test is used to compare two groups and a paired t-test to assess if a variable has changed between two time points. When analysing numerical but not normally distributed data (e.g., tumour size), a Mann-Whitney U-test is used to compare two groups and Wilcoxon's signed rank test to assess if a variable has changed between two time points.

When dealing with categorical data (e.g., admission to ITU), a chi-square test is used to compare two groups.

A p value <0.05 is commonly taken to imply a true difference. This simply means that there is only one in 20 chance that the difference between the variables would have happened by chance when there was no real difference.

→ ## Research

5. A, B, D, E

The other questions to be asked are, 'Can it be accomplished in the available time and with the available resources? What are the expected findings?'

→ Evidence-based surgery

6. E

In scientific publications, IMRAD (Introduction, Methods, Results and Discussion) is an accepted format for presenting a research or audit.

The CONSORT statement (Consolidated Standards of Reporting Trials) is a checklist for reporting randomised controlled trials. This assists with improving the quality of reporting; similarly, PRISMA (Preferred Reporting Items for Systematic Reviews and Meta-Analyses) is an evidence-based minimum set of items (27 point checklist and four flow diagrams) for reporting systematic reviews and meta-analysis.

The TREND (Transparent Reporting of Evaluation with Nonrandomised Designs) statement is a 22-item checklist specifically designed to guide in standardising the reporting of non-randomised controlled trials.

TNM (Tumour, Node and Metastasis) is a pathological classification used for staging malignant tumours and is not relevant to scientific publishing.

In scientific publications, one of the important concepts is impact factor. This is the average number of citations of recent articles in a particular journal. For example, an impact factor of year 3 will be the number of times the published articles in a journal in year 1 and 2 were cited in peer-reviewed journals in year 3 divided by the number of published articles in the journal in year 1 and 2. This is one of the quality measures of the journals.

Answers to extended matching questions

→ Types of research study

1. E Case control

This is a retrospective research study in which the investigators compare the exposure between subjects with particular condition (cases) to those without the condition (control) to investigate the effect of particular exposure to developing a certain condition. The study is reported using odds ratio, risk ratio and rate ratios.

2. A Cross-sectional

In this type of research study the investigators assess all individuals in a sample at the same time point to examine the prevalence of exposure or risk factors or disease. The studies may be analysed similar to cohort or like case-control study.

3. D Longitudinal

These are otherwise called cohort studies in which subjects are followed prospectively. The aim is to compare subjects who are unexposed with those who are exposed or to compare individuals or groups with different categories of exposure to determine whether exposure predisposes to developing certain conditions.

4. F Observational

These include the cohort, case-controlled and cross-sectional studies. These make up the large proportion of medical literature. These study designs are often used to answer important questions about the cause of disease, benefits and harms of medical interventions and rate of late adverse effects of treatment.

5. B Randomised

These are study designs used to assess the effect of an intervention. The aim is to minimise selection bias and allocation bias. These studies allow valid inferences of cause and effect. There are several methods used for randomisation, including computer-generated random numbers for allocation of patients into the study.

6. C Randomised controlled double-blind

In these studies there is a control group where, apart from the intervention, the subject characteristics are similar between both groups being compared. This means the results of the study can be attributed to the intervention.

In evidence-based surgery, the evidence is categorised into four levels.

Level 1a, which includes meta-analysis of RCTs and 1b, which includes single RCT.

Level 2a has a well-designed non-randomised study, whereas 2b includes well-designed cohort study.

Level 3 includes descriptive studies such as case-controlled studies, whereas level 4 includes case reports and expert opinion.

Based on these levels there are four grades of recommendations.

→ Statistical tests

1. B Chi-square test

This test is used to compare large group of nominal data. If the groups are small, Fisher's exact test is preferred.

2. A Mann-Whitney U-test

This test is used to compare unpaired, two sample where ordinal data is used, e.g. ordered or ranked data such as ASA, tumour grade.

3. C Paired T-test

In a study if the subjects are studied at two different occasions, the two samples of measurements are then considered to be paired. Alternatively, when we have two different groups of subjects who have been individually matched then we should treat the data as paired.

4. E Unpaired t-test

In normally distributed data, if there is no pairing, a two-sample t-test or unpaired t-test is used.

5. D Wilcoxon's signed-rank test

This test is used to compare paired two samples where ordinal data is used, e.g. ordered or ranked data such as ASA, tumour grade.

Statistical tests are used to deal with the chances that the observations between populations are different and should be dealt with with caution. Clinical results should show the difference, and this can be further augmented by statistics. Caution should be exercised if the statistical significance is shown when clinically the results are not clear, and various statistical tests are used based on the study design and data collected.

Surgical ethics and the law

Pradip K Datta

Multiple choice questions

→ ### Informed consent

1. Which of the following statements are true?

A Consent should be obtained by the person doing the operation.

B The written communication should always be in English.

C Consent is necessary before physical examination of a patient.

D Every possible hazard, however remote the possibility, should be explained in detail.

E Legally, a signed consent from a patient is proof that valid consent has been properly obtained.

→ ### Consent in difficult situations

2. Which of the following statements are true?

A There is no need to explain to children the procedures for which consent has already been given by their parent or guardian.

B Children can unconditionally refuse treatment.

C The child's views should be taken into account where possible.

D In patients who cannot give consent because of their illness, e.g., they are unconsciousness or there is psychiatric illness, their legal guardian can give consent.

E Therapy can proceed after consent from a carer in an unconscious patient irrespective of any previous wishes of the patient.

3. For consent to be valid, which of the following statements are true?

A The patient must be competent to give it.

B The patient must not be coerced into decision making.

C The patient must be given sufficient information.

D If competence is severely compromised, the patient's carer should assume responsibility.

E If a patient has a legally valid advanced directive refusing treatment, the decision must be honoured.

→ ### Matters of life and death

4. Which of the following statements are true?

A The surgeon is always obliged to provide life-sustaining treatment.

B A decision to withhold treatment should be taken along with another senior clinician and recorded in detail.

C In palliation for pain in advanced malignancy, a potential lethal dose of analgesia is appropriate.

D Confidentiality is absolute.

E All research activity must be externally validated.

Answers to multiple choice questions

→ Informed consent

1. A, C

The surgeon who will carry out the operation should take the consent. The obtaining of consent should not be delegated to a junior member of the team who has not performed the procedure. Informed consent must be obtained before starting treatment. Informed consent denotes that patients understand the nature of the procedure to which they are consenting. Patients must be given information and choices so that they can make subsequent plans and decisions in future. They must be given appropriate and accurate information to agree to undergo surgical treatment and in a language they can understand. Information should consist of the condition and reason for the operation, type of operation, prognosis with anticipated side effects, unexpected complications, any alternative but successful treatment and the outcome of not having the procedure carried out. Patients should be given the chance to ask questions and voice any misgivings.

The communication need not always be in English, as the patient may not speak or understand English. Written and verbal communication in the patient's preferred language, by use of an interpreter, should be given with adequate time for patients to mull over the advice given to be able to make up their own minds.

Prior to touching a patient for physical examination, consent must be obtained; otherwise it constitutes battery. However, this is unnecessary every time a patient is to be touched while under the care of the surgeon. Implied consent will have been given by the patient once an initial consent has been taken.

It is not necessary to inform patients of every possible hazard, however remote the possibility. Surgeons should inform patients of hazards that any reasonable person in their position would like to know. A signed consent form is no proof that a valid consent has been properly obtained. Patients can and do sometimes deny that they were given appropriate information. Surgeons should therefore record in the notes details of information given, particularly about complications.

→ Consent in difficult situations

2. C, D

The surgeon must take care to explain to children in layperson's terms the proposed treatment, and, where possible, their views should be sought. This is in keeping with patient autonomy, for both adults and children. 'Under English law, children can provide their own consent to surgical care, although they cannot unconditionally refuse it until they are 18 years old.' Notwithstanding this statement, the surgeon must respect the child's autonomy with regard to the surgical management.

In the presence of psychiatric illness or mental handicap, the legal guardian can give consent. In patients who are detained for compulsory psychiatric care, their competence to consent to surgical treatment should be assumed and hence consent sought. If they are incompetent to provide consent, then life-saving surgical treatment can proceed. If adult patients are permanently incompetent to give consent for surgery, treatment can proceed to save life or prevent disability. The exception to this rule is when the patient has already drawn up a legally valid document refusing specific intervention – 'a living will'.

3. A, B, C, D, E

In considering competence of a patient to give consent, the patient must be able to understand explanations given in lay terms and remember them. When choices of treatment are given, the patient should be able to deliberate them and make an informed choice. If a patient seems unsure about the choices, he or she should never be coerced into making a particular decision; instead, the patient should be given more time for deliberation. The patient may prefer more information and has the right to receive it to make a choice based on the understanding of the pros and cons of a particular type of treatment.

In instances where competence may be compromised, as in psychiatric patients needing essential surgical treatment, the legal carer must assume responsibility. After consultation with the carer, if it is concluded that the patient is incompetent to provide consent, then surgery to prevent death or serious disability can proceed without consent in the best interest of the patient. In a situation where a patient has made a legally advanced decision to decline treatment of a specific kind, that decision must be respected, provided it pertains to the current clinical situation.

Matters of life and death

4. B, C, E

The surgeon is not obliged to provide or continue life-sustaining treatment in the following cases: If doing so is futile; death is imminent and irreversible; or there is permanent brain damage. A decision to withhold treatment should be taken in consultation with a senior colleague. All details of decisions and conversations should be recorded.

There are circumstances when palliation for disseminated and inoperable cancer is becoming increasingly difficult. The management of pain under such circumstances may require analgesia in doses that may cause respiratory depression, thus hastening death. This is legally justifiable on the premise of 'double effect' – pain relief and death might follow.

A surgeon must not discuss a patient's clinical condition with anyone else without the patient's explicit consent; to do so would incur the wrath of the General Medical Council. Nevertheless, this is not absolute. Surgeons may communicate with other members of the multidisciplinary team should this information help in the patient's management. When patients consent to a treatment plan, they have given implied consent. Confidentiality cannot be strictly adhered to if doing so poses a serious threat to the health and safety of others or if there is a court order, or in an attempt to prevent serious crime or protect individuals who may be at risk.

While it is accepted that the boundaries of surgical endeavour must be extended by research, certain protocols must be mandatory before undertaking research. These should include external regulation, approval of research ethics committees, full- informed patient consent and evidence that any known risk to patients is far outweighed by the potential benefits.

12 Patient safety

Iain J Nixon

Multiple choice questions

→ Incidence and aetiology

1. Which of the following statements are true?

A One in 100 patients are estimated to be at risk of preventable harm in the hospital setting.

B A near miss is an event that reaches the patient but results in no injury.

C Poor communication is a common cause of adverse events.

D Human fallibility combined with complex health systems greatly increases the potential for errors.

E It is estimated that there are around 10 near misses for every patient injury.

→ Strategies for patient safety

2. Which of the following statements are false?

A The World Health Organisation plays a leadership role in patient safety.

B Both developed and developing countries share the same issues with patient safety.

C The routine use of information technology systems has been shown to reduce medical errors.

D Radical system redesign is likely to result in higher rates of patient harm.

E Individual training is critical to decreasing medical errors.

→ Patient safety at the coal face

3. Which of the following statements are true?

A Following an adverse event, open disclosure should be a priority.

B Competence or fitness to practice refers only to skills and knowledge.

C Complaints provide an opportunity to highlight a problem.

D Fatigue and medical errors are not associated.

E Safe prescribing requires knowledge of the patient, the patient's condition, the medication and the dose.

→ Patient safety and the surgeon

4. Which of the following statements are true?

A Introduction of surgical safety checklists has been associated with a reduction in major surgical complications of up to 30%.

B The surgical safety checklist calls for specific checks at two key time points.

C The transition from conscious to unconscious control is called the learning curve in surgery.

D A failure due to 'misinterpretation' relates to the misreading of a two-dimensional image.

E The surgeon involved in an adverse incident may be considered the second victim.

Extended matching questions

Potential causes of adverse events

→ Factor

1 Complexity of health care environment
2 Deficiencies in training
3 Inadequate safety review systems
4 Inadequate staffing levels
5 Lack of coordination at handovers

Identify the factor that most predisposes the patients below to adverse events:

→ Clinical scenarios

A A 64-year-old lady following a low anterior resection is discharged back from surgical recovery to the general ward. Half-hourly observations are requested, but the ward has only 4 trained nurses for 36 patients.

B An 18-year-old man is admitted with right lower quadrant abdominal pain, fever and abdominal guarding. The emergency room physician diagnoses acute appendicitis and refers to the surgical middle grade on call. Tonight, a junior trainee has been asked to 'act up' and cover one of his senior colleagues despite not having taken an acute abdomen to theatre in the past.

C A 45-year-old man is admitted with abdominal pain of unknown origin at 5 p.m. Investigations including bloodwork and an erect chest x-ray are ordered by the doctor, who is working until 6 p.m.

D An 80-year-old lady is admitted for total hip replacement. The operating surgeon plans to perform their standard procedure using the regular prosthesis. The previous three patients who received this prosthesis under the care of different surgeons in the hospital went on to develop significant operative site infections.

E A 24-year-old man is admitted to neurosurgical intensive care. The night before admission he was involved in a road traffic accident resulting in significant injury to the thorax, cervical spine and brain. An 8-hour procedure, which included thoracotomy and craniotomy, was required and the patient now requires invasive ventilation and support, including intracranial pressure monitoring.

Answers to multiple choice questions

→ Incidence and aetiology

1. C,D,E

The World Health Organisation estimates that 1 in 10 patients in the hospital is at risk of preventable harm. These rates highlight the importance of recognising the importance of patient safety in modern medicine. While an adverse event results in actual patient harm, a near miss is an incidence that fails to reach the patient. A non-harm event is an incident that reaches the patient but does not result in harm. The factors that contribute to patient safety incidents are shown in **Table 12.1**. Poor communication is amongst the most common causes underlying adverse incidents. Although humans make mistakes, the complexity of modern medical systems substantially increases the potential for harm. The problem can be seen on a personal level (understanding why an individual made a mistake) or a systems level. Most errors result from a series of failures, and systems should be set up to minimise the chance of such a series resulting in patient harm. It is important to understand that there are estimated to be around 300 near misses for every 29 minor injuries and one major injury (**Figure 12.1**). It is for this reason that near misses are reported. These provide the best method for assessing the integrity of systems designed to protect patients from preventable harm.

Table 12.1   Factors that contribute to patient safety incidents

Human factors	Inadequate patient assessment; delays or errors in diagnosis
	Failure to use or interpret appropriate tests
	Error in performance of an operation, treatment, or test
	Inadequate monitoring or follow up of treatment
	Deficiencies in training or experience
	Fatigue, overwork, time pressures
	Personal or psychological factors, e.g., depression or drug abuse
	Patient or working environment variation
	Lack of recognition of the dangers of medical errors
System failures	Poor communication between health care providers
	Inadequate staffing levels
	Disconnected reporting systems or overreliance on automated systems
	Lack of coordination at handovers
	Drug similarities
	Environment design, infrastructure
	Equipment failure, due to lack of parts or skilled operators
	Cost-cutting measures by hospitals
	Inadequate systems to report and review patient safety incidents
Medical complexity	Advanced and new technologies
	Potent drugs, their side effects and interactions
	Working environments – intensive care, operating theatres

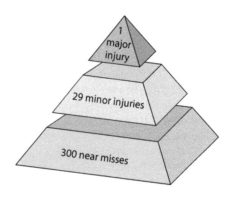

Figure 12.1   The relationship between near misses, minor injuries and major injuries (Heinrich's pyramid).

Strategies for patient safety

2. B, D, E

The WHO has taken an international leadership role in patient safety, championing, amongst other initiatives, surgical checklists (**Figure 12.2**). Although aspirations of developing and developed countries are similar, the challenges they face differ significantly. While developed countries have systems such as physician licensure, patient safety education programmes and national level agencies to monitor safety issues, developing countries have significant challenges relating to equipment availability and basic training.

There are many ways that health care systems can improve safety, but for most, radical system redesign is required to institute significantly reduced patient harm. One example shown to improve patient safety is the increasing reliance on information technology. Not only does this allow more efficient reporting of outcomes, but technologies such as computerised physician prescribing have been shown to reduce medical errors. Although training on an individual level is important, almost all heath care is delivered by teams. It is critical that training in patient safety is delivered throughout the team to improve communication and decision-making behaviours.

Patient safety at the coal face

3. A, C, E

Although the natural tendency after a clinical error is to avoid the patient and the subject, open disclosure is important. Good communication is critical as part of a patient-centred approach. Although an assessment of competence includes knowledge and skills, it also includes aspects such as attitude and health. Competence can be demonstrated using a system of credentialing and revalidation. Complaints can be stressful to handle, but they allow a health care system to identify problems that can lead to patient harm. Modern health care systems are designed to make the process of complaining easier via patient advocacy units. The environment in which health care is provided is critical. Tired surgeons make more errors and can be linked to personal health problems, which can further undermine patient care. All physicians are involved in prescribing medicines. Not only is in-depth knowledge of the patient and the drug required, legible handwriting is also important in accurate prescribing.

Patient safety and the surgeon

4. A, C, D, E

Surgical safety checklists are now a mandatory part of surgical practice in many countries. They have been shown to reduce complication rates, and a fall from 11% to 7% (36%) in major complications has been demonstrated. The checklist is used at three time points: before anaesthesia, before the incision and before the patient leaves the operating room (**Figure 12.2**). Failures in operative technique include errors of judgement, procedure, execution, or misuse of instrumentation. The term misinterpretation is used to describe the function of misreading a two-dimensional image and is unique to minimally invasive surgery. Not all errors will be evident at the time of surgery, and the team must remain vigilant for missed iatrogenic injuries, which may present at a later date. Although the patient is a clear victim of the error, the surgeon involved in the incident may also be considered a victim. Coping with the impact of an error may be challenging, and support structures should be in place to help manage this stressful situation.

Surgical safety checklist (first edition)

Before induction of anaesthesia

SIGN IN

☐ Patient has confirmed:
 • identity
 • site
 • procedure
 • consent

☐ Site marked/not applicable

☐ Anaesthesia safety check completed

☐ Pulse oximeter on patient and functioning

Does patient have a:

Known allergy?
☐ No
☐ Yes

Difficult airway/aspiration risk?
☐ No
☐ Yes, and equipment/assistance available

Risk of >500 ml blood loss
(7 ml/kg in children)?
☐ No
☐ Yes, and adequate intravenous access and fluids planned

Before skin incision

TIME OUT

☐ Confirm all team members have introduced themselves by name and role

☐ Surgeon, anaesthesia professional and nurse verbally confirm
 • patient
 • site
 • procedure

☐ Anticipated critical events

☐ Surgeon reviews: what are the critical or unexpected steps, operative duration, anticipated blood loss?

☐ Anaesthesia team reviews: are there any patient-specific concerns?

☐ Nursing team reviews: has sterility (including indicator results) been confirmed? Are there equipment issues or any concerns?

Has antibiotic prophylaxis been given within the last 60 minutes?
☐ Yes
☐ Not applicable

Is essential imaging displayed?
☐ Yes
☐ Not applicable

Before patient leaves operating room

SIGN OUT

☐ Nurse verbally confirms with the team:

☐ The name of the procedure recorded

☐ That instrument, sponge and needle counts are correct (or not applicable)

☐ How the specimen is labelled (including patient name)

☐ Whether there are any equipment problems to be addressed

☐ Surgeon, anaesthesia professional and nurse review the key concerns for recovery and management of this patient

Figure 12.2 World Health Organisation (WHO) Surgical Safety Checklist.

➡ Potential causes of adverse events

When considering the causes of adverse events in surgery, multiple factors often contribute and no one issue can be singled out. There is often overlap of personal and system failures and errors can be made at an individual, team, or institutional level.

1. E Complexity of health care environment

Modern medical systems are complex. Patients may require multi-system support, input from many specialties and close monitoring. All of these requirements increase the risk to the patient, in addition to the critical clinical condition faced by patients with such needs.

2. B Deficiencies in training

In this example, a junior is left to manage at a level he or she cannot achieve. Training is inadequate to prepare him or her for the level of clinical responsibility he or she requires. Although the institution may consider this a deficiency in training, this should not be interpreted as a personal failing of the trainee. The system in which he or she works should not allow this situation to arise, and analysis of how this scenario was allowed to develop should be undertaken. Such situations are common, and often no harm comes to the patient. However, surgeons should remember that for every one major injury, there are more than 300 near misses.

3. D Inadequate safety review systems

It is impossible for a single surgeon to know everything that goes on in his or her department, let alone across a complex hospital. For this reason, it is critical that all adverse events are recorded and reviewed to protect future patients. In this example, there should be concern about the sterility of the current batch of prostheses. Problems such as these require robust systems of reporting and review to identify that an issue exists, to identify its cause and to act to prevent future occurrences.

4. A Inadequate staffing levels

Staffing levels are controversial and apply throughout health care systems. As the needs of sick patients increase, so does the need for staff to care for them. Improvements in technology aid in meeting these complex needs, but without adequate staffing levels, patients remain at risk. At the same time, health care providers are asked to ration resources and minimize expenditure on staff wherever possible. Clearly, this results in pressures on all departments to provide more with less.

This example can be seen in a number of ways. Staffing levels are too low on a general ward to provide the requested care. There may be deficiencies in training, which led to the surgeon discharging the patient to this unsafe environment or to the nurse in charge accepting the patient. If the hospital environment does not provide adequate facilities, such as a high-dependency unit, this institutional failure should be addressed to minimize risk to patients.

5. C Lack of coordination at handovers

Clinical handovers are an increasingly important part of modern medicine. Whether at junior or senior level, they represent a critical time for the patient, even though the patient is not present. Thorough clinical handovers are important and require a structured approach. Nursing staff have great experience of handing over between shifts. In contrast, medical staff have been required to develop these skills in a shorter time. Many departments now have systems in place to promote high-quality handover of patients to minimise patient risk at this critical time point.

Investigation and diagnosis

13 *Diagnostic imaging*

Pradip K Datta

Multiple choice questions

→ ## Hazards of imaging and radiation

1. Which of the following statements are true?

A Low-osmolality contrast media (LOCM) are safer than their higher-osmolality counterparts.

B Routine steroid prophylaxis is recommended before use of contrast in the high-risk patient.

C In the diabetic, metformin should be stopped before using contrast.

D The majority of ionising radiation comes from medical exposure from investigations.

E Portable x-ray machines use much more radiation to achieve the same result.

→ ## Diagnostic imaging

2. Which of the following statements is false?

A Conventional x-rays will delineate different soft tissue reliably.

B Conventional x-rays can be manipulated.

C Dedicated transducers can help in endocavitary ultrasound (US).

D Change in the frequency of an US wave can be caused by red blood cells.

E The higher the frequency of the US wave, the greater the resolution of the image.

3. Which of the following statements are true?

A US has no disadvantages.

B Computed tomography (CT) scan has a higher resolution than plain radiographs.

C Magnetic resonance imaging (MRI) scans give excellent contrast resolution.

D MRI scan has no disadvantages.

E Radionuclide imaging allows function to be studied.

→ ## Responsibilities

4. The following statements are true except:

A The clinician referring the patient must balance risk against benefit.

B The clinician must give as much information as possible.

C Use portable machines and fluoroscopy wherever possible.

D Take all precautions when using an image intensifier.

E The lungs, heart and pancreas are especially vulnerable to irradiation.

→ ## Orthopaedic imaging

5. Which of the following statements is false?

A Synovitis can be detected by plain x-ray.

B MR arthrography is the ideal imaging for articular cartilage damage.

C MRI is the ideal method for local staging of a malignant bone tumour.

D X-ray is the first investigation in destructive bone lesions.

E US is used to examine mass lesions of soft tissues.

→ ## Imaging in trauma

6. Which of the following statements are false?

A In a multiply injured patient, CT of head and spine should be the first line of imaging.

B Focused assessment with sonography for trauma (FAST) helps in detecting intraperitoneal fluid and cardiac tamponade.

C CT should not be used when a patient is unstable.

D US is useful for diagnosing occult pneumothorax.

E CT is the main imaging method for intracranial, intra-abdominal and vertebral injuries.

→ Imaging in the acute abdomen

7. The following statements are true except:

A US is a good first-line investigation.

B CT is the best investigation for acute diverticulitis.

C Plain x-ray of KUB (kidney, ureter, bladder) is the best imaging for suspected ureteric colic.

D US and CT can diagnose the cause and site of intestinal obstruction.

E Plain x-ray is the first-line investigation for suspected perforation or obstruction.

→ Imaging in oncology

8. Which of the following statements is false?

A Early disease is best staged by endoscopic US (EUS).

B Accurate preoperative nodal involvement is possible by EUS.

C Liver and lung metastases are best detected by US and CT.

D Intraoperative US is used in liver resection.

E PET/CT is an important tool in oncological staging.

Extended matching questions

→ Imaging techniques

1 Contrast enhanced computerised tomographic scan (CECT scan)
2 Endoluminal (endoscopic) ultrasound (EUS)
3 Intraoperative ultrasound (IOS)
4 Magnetic resonance imaging scan (MRI scan)
5 Plain x-ray
6 Positron emission tomography scan/CT (PET/CT scan)
7 Radionuclide imaging
8 Ultrasound (US)

Match the imaging techniques with the clinical scenarios that follow as the most appropriate initial imaging to be used:

→ Clinical scenarios

A A 68-year-old man complains of increasing dysphagia of 3 months duration. He is unable to swallow any solids, and liquids go down with difficulty. He has lost 25 kilogrammes in weight during this period. What should be the first investigation?

B A 78-year-old man complains of gnawing backache associated with urinary frequency and poor stream for 4 months. Transrectal ultrasound (TRUS) biopsy showed a carcinoma of prostate.

C A 32-year-old man while skiing sustained an injury to this right ankle following which it became very painful and grossly deformed.

D A 45-year-old woman sustained a blunt injury to her lower chest and upper abdomen while horse riding. She was brought in with hypovolaemic shock. Having been resuscitated according to the ATLS protocol, she is now stable.

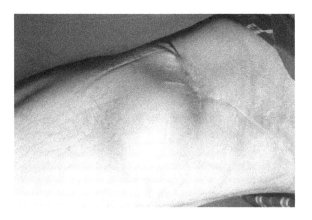

Figure 13.1 Clinical picture of soft tissue sarcoma.

E A 70-year-old man is undergoing a laparotomy for liver resection for metastases from colorectal carcinoma.

F A 55-year-old woman presented with a lymph nodal lump over her right supraclavicular area. Excision biopsy showed a non-Hodgkin's lymphoma.

G A 35-year-old woman has been admitted as an emergency with right upper quadrant pain, pyrexia and vomiting. On examination she is toxic, with a positive Murphy's sign.

H A 62-year-old man presented with a large soft-tissue mass on the medial aspect of his left femoral triangle of 4 months duration. The mass is hard, immobile and tender **(Figure 13.1)**.

Answers to multiple choice questions

→ Hazards of imaging and radiation

1. A, E
For contrast-enhanced computed tomography (CECT) scan, LOCM are much safer than the higher-osmolality agents. The Royal College of Radiologists (RCR) in the United Kingdom does not recommend routine steroid prophylaxis for high-risk patients. The use of LOCM and close observation of the patient for 30 minutes after injection is recommended with the cannula still in situ. Most reactions occur shortly after injection.

The RCR recommend that metformin can be continued and no more than 100 mL of LOCM can be given in the presence of normal renal function. A recent serum creatinine should be performed, as all contrast media are nephrotoxic. In patients with a history of iodine allergy, gadolinium diethyltriaminepentacetic acid (DTPA) can be used. Mild reactions can occur in 1:200 and severe reactions in 1:10,000 patients.

The majority of ionising radiation in the human comes from natural sources, with medical exposure accounting for only 12%. Portable x-ray machines should be avoided as much as possible. Along with fluoroscopy, such imaging equipment uses much more radiation to obtain the same result.

→ Diagnostic imaging

2. A

Different soft tissue cannot be reliably distinguished, as all soft tissue contains the same quantity of water. In certain circumstances, however, such as mammography, by manipulating the x-ray systems and x-ray energies, differentiation between the different types of soft tissue can be obtained.

Ultrasound is the second most common method of imaging. Special transducers have been developed for intracavitary imaging, such as transvaginal, transrectal and endoscopic (of oesophagus and stomach). The latter not only allows imaging of the wall of the viscus but also of the adjacent structures, such as mediastinal lymph nodes in oesophageal US and the pancreas in gastric US. The higher the frequency of the US wave, the greater is the resolution of the image.

A change in the frequency of the US wave can be caused by moving objects, such as red blood cells. This change in frequency helps to measure the speed and direction of movement – the principle of Doppler US (Christian Johann Doppler, a Viennese professor of experimental physics, articulated this principle in 1842), which can record the speed of blood flow through a vessel or a solid organ – thus diagnosing stenosis within a vessel wall.

3. B, C, E

Ultrasound has its drawbacks. It is very operator-dependent; the information is mostly useful during the actual scanning process so that images cannot be reliably reviewed by looking at static pictures; it does not go through air and bone; resolution depends upon the machine used; and the process has a long learning curve.

CT scan has a high-contrast resolution, allowing the assessment of tissue with similar attenuation characteristics. The injection of contrast allows images at various phases of the blood supply, the early arterial phase, for example, in vascular liver lesions and the delayed pictures for solid renal lesions.

Magnetic resonance imaging gives excellent contrast resolution without any radiation hazard. It lends itself to imaging particularly of tissue with relatively little natural contrast. MRI does have some downsides, however. There is limited availability because of expense; it is time consuming; and the patient needs to be motionless, making it difficult in those with pain. Patients with metallic implants cannot be examined, because the investigation entails the use of high-strength magnetic fields.

The use of a radionuclide allows the study of function. The chosen radionuclide – technetium, gallium, thallium, iodine – is coupled with other compounds and administered intravenously for it to be tracked by a gamma camera, thus forming a functional image. Positron emission tomography (PET) is a similar imaging method, which is useful in detecting recurrent cancer, particularly when combined with CT (PET/CT).

→ Responsibilities

4. C, E

Portable machines and fluoroscopy units should be avoided whenever possible. Such equipment uses much more radiation to achieve the same result. Besides staff, patients in the next bed are at risk. Moreover, the results from portable x-ray machines are of poor quality. The organs particularly vulnerable to irradiation are the gonads, eyes and thyroid. Hence, whilst using the image intensifier, the use of lead aprons, thyroid shields, lead glasses and radiation badges is mandatory.

Requests for diagnostic imaging by the clinician must be done after carefully considering the risks against the benefits. The request form must have as much information as possible, while at the same time a discussion with the radiologist as to the correct imaging technique to be used can be most helpful.

Orthopaedic imaging

5. A

Plain x-ray is not the choice of imaging to confirm synovitis. This is best detected by gadolinium DTPA-enhanced MRI, which will show up synovial thickening. MRI is the best way to detect articular damage. MR arthrography, where a scan is performed after gadolinium DTPA is injected into the joint, is 'the gold standard'. MRI is the best investigation for staging of bone or soft-tissue malignant tumours. Image-guided (US, CT, or MRI) needle biopsy in consultation with the surgeon is then carried out. Bone scan or whole-body MRI is particularly necessary when multiple lesions are suspected.

A plain x-ray is the first imaging technique when a destructive bone lesion is suspected. It also shows up soft-tissue calcification in muscle, tendon and fat. Careful interpretation is essential to distinguish malignant from benign lesions. When malignancy is suspected, further investigations are mandatory to establish a firm diagnosis.

Ultrasound is diagnostic in the majority of mass lesions of soft tissue. When the lesion is cystic, it obviates the need for further imaging. However, if the lesion has a solid element to it, then MRI is performed. In soft-tissue lesions, the routine should be US on all palpable lesions; when there is an unidentifiable mass or the mass is partly solid, then MRI is used.

Imaging in trauma

6. A

Initially, plain x-rays and not CT will give a rapid assessment of major injuries. Although the areas to be x-rayed will depend upon the mechanism of injury and the condition of the patient (intubated or not), the initial radiographs are x-rays of the chest, an antero-posterior view of the pelvis and the cervical spine (C/S).

FAST, although operator-dependent, is extremely efficient in detecting intraperitoneal fluid and cardiac tamponade. It may not be helpful in the presence of bowel gas or extensive surgical emphysema. A repeat FAST may be used when the initial test has been negative.

The unstable patient needs to be treated forthwith according to the clinical needs and no time should be lost in arranging a CT, which should only be considered in a patient who is stable after adequate resuscitation.

Pneumothorax in a supine chest x-ray can be difficult to see. An US using a high-resolution probe will detect the pleura as an echogenic stripe and its movement can be assessed; the sliding motion of the pleura is lost in a pneumothorax; haemothorax can also be diagnosed.

CT is the ideal method of imaging intracranial and intra-abdominal injuries and vertebral fractures. Using a multidetector scanner, a comprehensive examination of the entire body can be completed in 5 minutes – in far less time than it takes to organise the investigation. Hence, this imaging modality should be reserved only for the stable patient.

Imaging in the acute abdomen

7. C

Ultrasound is a good initial imaging for most acute abdominal conditions – biliary colic, acute cholecystitis, acute appendicitis, acute pancreatitis and pelvic diseases.

When patients present with left iliac fossa pain and a diagnosis of acute diverticulitis is made, CT is the investigation of choice – showing thickening of the bowel wall, paracolic collection, or abscess. CT-guided drainage of an abscess can also be done.

In suspected ureteric colic (wrongly called renal colic because one cannot get colic in a solid organ), plain x-ray of the KUB area is of limited value. Faecoliths cannot be distinguished from ureteric stones. Unenhanced helical CT is the most sensitive imaging procedure for ureteric colic.

In intestinal obstruction, US and CT are useful in showing dilated fluid-filled loops and can often identify the site and cause of obstruction. CT colonography is increasingly being used in the confirmation of acute large-bowel closed-loop obstruction from carcinoma.

Clinical suspicion of perforation of a hollow viscus is best confirmed by an erect chest x-ray or abdominal x-ray to include the diaphragmatic domes or lateral decubitus film (if the patient is too ill).

⇥ ## Imaging in oncology

8. B

Accurate preoperative nodal staging cannot be obtained by EUS. While the size of nodes (pararectal in rectal cancer or mediastinal in oesophageal cancer) gives an idea of nodal involvement, one cannot be absolutely certain, as the enlargement can be due to metastasis or reactive hyperplasia.

In the staging of early carcinoma (T1 and T2) of distal large bowel, endoluminal ultrasound (EUS) is the imaging of choice. The same is true of early oesophageal cancer. Biopsy is carried out at the same time; however, this should be done only after US so as not to distort the US images.

Ultrasound (US) and CT are the ideal imaging methods to detect haematogenous spread to the lungs and liver. CT is the most sensitive technique for pulmonary deposits. However, occult lesions may be overlooked in 10% to 30% of patients.

Intraoperative US is a routine during liver resection for metastasis. Deep-seated impalpable secondaries may be missed by the conventional preoperative US and CT, particularly if they are smaller than 1 cm. Good high-resolution imaging will detect secondaries as small as 0.5 cm – a finding that will influence the definitive management.

Positron emission tomography (PET)/CT is a technique increasingly used as a functional and anatomical imaging tool. The procedure reflects tumour metabolism and detects occult metastases. It is particularly used in lymphoma, non-small cell lung cancer and potential resectable liver metastases.

Answers to extended matching questions

Please note that in the following answers, only the most appropriate initial imaging technique is discussed and not the whole gamut of investigations for the particular diagnosis. To learn about the investigations in detail for the particular diagnosis, the reader should refer to the relevant chapter.

1. D Contrast enhanced computerised tomographic scan (CECT scan)

CT scanning is the investigation to be carried out in this patient who is stable following resuscitation for upper abdominal and lower thoracic injury. With multidetector scanners a comprehensive examination of the head, spine, chest, abdomen and pelvis can be done in 5 minutes. However, to organise this investigation it would easily take half an hour or more. Hence, this investigation should only be contemplated in the stable patient.

2. A Endoluminal (endoscopic) ultrasound (EUS)

EUS is the investigation to be done for an oesophageal carcinoma. The first investigation is oesophagogastroduodenoscopy (OGD) when carcinoma of oesophagus is suspected. When the lesion is seen, initially an EUS is done, which gives an accurate idea about the local spread while at the same time diagnoses enlarged mediastinal lymph nodes. Biopsy should only be taken after EUS, so as not to distort the US images.

3. E Intraoperative ultrasound (IOS)

IOS is carried out during planned liver resection for liver metastasis. It provides high-resolution imaging for detection of small liver secondaries (5 mm) in the depths of the liver parenchyma that will not be picked up by the usual imaging techniques.

4. H Magnetic resonance imaging scan (MRI scan)

This patient has a suspected soft tissue sarcoma. MRI is the gold standard for diagnosing soft tissue sarcoma and local staging.

5. C Plain x-ray

This is clinically a fracture-dislocation of the ankle. The investigation of choice is a plain x-ray of the ankle. However, this should only be carried out after the fracture-dislocation has been reduced under sedation and a back slab applied. Nothing is gained by doing the x-rays before reduction, because precious time may be lost during which neurovascular compromise may occur and the patient may develop skin blisters.

6. F Positron emission tomography scan/CT (PET/CT scan)

This patient has a histologically proven non-Hodgkin's lymphoma. A PET/CT shows active disease and detects occult disease.

7. B Radionuclide imaging

This patient has proven prostate carcinoma. His symptoms are from bone metastases. Therefore, a whole-body bone scintigraphy is highly sensitive and allows functional imaging of the whole body **(Figure 13.2)**.

8. G Ultrasound (US)

This patient clinically is suffering from acute cholecystitis. US of the abdomen is the first investigation of choice to confirm the diagnosis. It will show a thickened gallbladder with pericholecystic fluid and gallstones. It may also show whether there is any dilatation of the common bile duct.

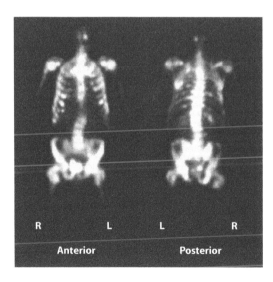

Figure 13.2   Bone scan showing hot spots from multiple secondaries from prostate cancer.

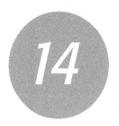

14 Gastrointestinal endoscopy

CR Selvasekar

Multiple choice questions

→ **Conscious sedation**

1. Which of the following statements are false?

A Sedation has no significant dangers and can be used without restrictions.

B All sedated patients require secure intravenous access.

C Co-administration of opiates and benzodiazepines has a synergistic effect and opiates administered wherever possible before benzodiazepines.

D Use of supplemental oxygen is essential in sedated patients.

E All sedated patients require pulse oximetry to monitor oxygen saturations.

→ **Prophylactic antibiotics**

2. In which of the following should antibiotic prophylaxis not be considered?

A Prosthetic heart valves.

B Previous history of endocarditis.

C Severe neutropenia.

D Chronic liver disease undergoing variceal sclerotherapy.

E Previous cholecystectomy.

→ **Capsule endoscopy**

3. It is not used in which of the following situations?

A Diagnosis of obscure gastrointestinal bleeding.

B Diagnosis of small bowel Crohn's disease.

C Assessment of coeliac disease.

D Screening and surveillance of polyps in familial polyposis syndrome.

E Assessment of small bowel obstruction.

→ **General issues in endoscopy**

4. Which of the following statements are true?

A It is easy to get views beyond the ligament of Treitz during an oesophagogastroduodenoscopy (OGD).

B Current endoscope is fibreoptic endoscope.

C It is not necessary to stop clopidrogel before colonoscopic polypectomy.

D Verbal consent is an accepted practice.

E Perforation and haemorrhage are uncommon but significant complications of the procedure.

→ **Post-ERCP pancreatitis**

5. Which of the following are not risk factors for post-ERCP (endoscopic retrograde cholangiopancreatography) pancreatitis?

A Young age.

B Difficult cannulation.

C Increased bilirubin.

D Pancreatic sphincterotomy.

E Balloon dilatation of biliary sphincter.

→ **Colonoscopy**

6. In which of the following conditions is colonoscopy indicated?

A Assessment of rectal bleeding with loose stools.

B Management of iron deficiency anaemia.

C Assessment of chronic diarrhoea (> 6 weeks).

D Follow up of colorectal cancer and adenomatous polyp.

E Diagnosis of fulminant colitis.

→ ## Endoscopic ultrasound (EUS)

7. Which of the following statements are true?

A In the staging of upper gastrointestinal track malignancies (oesophagus, stomach, liver and biliary system).

B Diagnosis of choledochal microlitithasis.

C Biopsy of paraoesophageal lymph nodes.

D Biopsy of pancreaticobiliary mass and in assessment of neuroendocrine tumours.

E Transgastric drainage of pancreatic pseudocyst.

→ ## Recent trends in endoscopy

8. Which of the following developments are false?

A Chromoendoscopy involves the use of pigments and stains to improve tissue localisation.

B Narrow band imaging relies on an optical filter technology that radically improves the visibility of veins and capillaries in the superficial layers.

C High-resolution magnification endoscopy achieves near cellular definition of the mucosa.

D Capsule endoscopy acquires video images during natural propulsion through the gut.

E Balloon enteroscopy permits visualisation of the small bowel but is unable to perform therapeutic procedures.

Extended matching questions

→ ## Endoscopic diagnosis

1 Barrett's oesophagus
2 Carcinoma of the oesophagus
3 Gastrointestinal stromal tumour (GIST)
4 Hiatus hernia
5 Linitis plastica
6 Mallory-Weiss tear
7 Oesophageal varices
8 Peptic stricture
9 Rectal cancer
10 Reflux gastritis

Match the diagnoses with the endoscopic findings that follow:

→ ## Endoscopic findings

A Abnormal veins are seen in the lower end of the oesophagus, which are dilated and grape like.

B A smooth, tapering stricture is seen at the lower end of the oesophagus along with inflammation and ulceration.

C A mucosal tear is seen at the cardia with some fresh blood.

D The pylorus is seen to be wide open with plenty of bile in the stomach. The antrum shows streaks of erythema.

E The stomach is difficult to distend and appears to have low capacity. The mucosa appears stretched but no mucosal lesion is seen.

F A submucosal lump is seen. The mucosa is stretched over this lump but is otherwise normal. The mucosal biopsies are normal.

G There is an ulcerated and polypoidal mass at the lower end of the oesophagus causing obstruction.

H There is evidence of gastro-oesophageal reflux disease (GORD) and a linear tongue of erythematous mucosa extending for a few centimetres into the oesophagus proximally.

I The gastro-oesophageal junction is at 34 cm with prolapsing fundal mucosa and increased oesophageal fluid. The diaphragm is located at 39 cm.

J A large polypoidal mass is noted in the lower rectum in a patient not fit for major surgery.

→ Endoscopic complications

1 Aspiration
2 Bleeding
3 Dental injury
4 Perforation
5 Sedation overdose

Choose and match the correct diagnosis with each of the scenarios that follow:

A An 80-year-old man who has just had an OGD after local anaesthetic spray has severe coughing and breathing problems after eating a sandwich in the recovery room.

B A 71-year-old patient collapses and is found to be hypotensive after an endoscopic polypectomy.

C A 70-year-old male is rushed to the emergency 8 hours after an endoscopic dilatation of an oesophageal stricture, complaining of severe chest pain and change in voice.

D An 86-year-old woman has severe pain and bleeding from the mouth following an uneventful OGD.

E An 80-year-old woman patient has severe bradycardia and low PO_2 and is difficult to arouse.

Answers to multiple choice questions

→ Sedation in endoscopy

1. A

Sedation should be used cautiously. The risk is higher in elderly and those with comorbidities. Pharyngeal anaesthesia may increase the risk of aspiration in sedated patients. The use of supplemental oxygen and pulse oximetry is essential in all sedated patients. A trained assistant should be present to monitor the patient throughout the procedure. Resuscitation equipment and reversal agents must be readily available. Increasingly, nitrous oxide is used for lower gastrointestinal examinations. CO_2 use instead of air for the procedure is known to decrease the need for sedation.

→ Antibiotic prophylaxis in endoscopy

2. E

The majority of the endoscopic procedures are performed safely, without the need for antibiotic prophylaxis. However, certain procedures are associated with significant bacteraemia. The risk of bacteraemia after colonoscopy, diagnostic OGD and ERCP for obstructed CBD are 2% to 4%, 4% and 11%, respectively. In fact, the incidence of bacteraemia can be between 34% and 54% after oesophageal dilatation. Patients with high-risk conditions, such as severe neutropenia, prosthetic heart valves, or a previous history of infective endocarditis, should have prophylaxis for all endoscopic procedures. Patients with moderate-risk conditions, such as mitral valve prolapse with leaflet disease and regurgitation, require antibiotics for procedures, which causes significant bacteraemia. The antibiotic regimen depends on local policies, but a standard protocol is 1 g amoycillin and 120 mg gentamycin IV 5 to 10 minutes prior to the procedure (Teicoplanin 400 mg IV if allergic to pencillin).

Capsule endoscopy

3. E

Capsule endoscopy (CE) is the investigation of choice in patients with persistent obscure gastrointestinal bleeding who have a negative gastroscopy and colonoscopy. In addition to assisting with the diagnosis of Crohn's disease, CE is useful in assessing the extent and in the diagnosis of recurrence following resection. CE may be used in the diagnosis of complications of coeliac disease. The main complication of CE is retention. Hence is contraindicated when obstruction is suspected.

General issues in endoscopy

4. E

A diagnostic OGD usually examines up to the second part of the duodenum. The fibreoptic endoscope was the originally used, however, the charge-coupled device (CCD) has been in use since 1960s. The CCD allows the creation of a digital electronic image, which is processed by a computer and transmitted to a TV monitor. The patient needs to stop clopidrogel prior to colonoscopic polypectomy to minimise the risk of bleeding. Although endoscopy is safe, it is still associated with rare but potentially life-threatening complications such as bleeding, perforation, missed lesions, incomplete examination and sedation-related problems. It is hence mandatory to explain clearly the procedure and complications to the patient and obtain a fully informed consent prior to the procedure. Approximately 1% of medical negligence claims in the United States are related to endoscopic procedures.

Post-ERCP pancreatitis

5. C

The incidence of post-ERCP pancreatitis is around 4.3%. The additional risk factors for this complication include suspected sphincter of oddi dysfunction, normal bilurubin, prior ERCP-related pancreatitis and pancreatic duct contrast injection. Possible factors also include female sex, absent CBD stone and low volume of ERCP performed.

Colonoscopy Indications

6. A, B, C, D

Colonoscopy is the gold standard investigation for large-bowel mucosal lesions. It allows in the diagnosis (visualisation and biopsy) of benign and malignant lesions of the colon and rectum. Polyps can be snared or removed by endoscopic mucosal resection (EMR) if appropriate. Colonoscopy is indicated in patients with loose stools where biopsies can assist in the management. Colonoscopy in indicated in the screening and surveillance of colorectal cancer and inflammatory bowel disease. Colonoscopy is contraindicated when severe fulminant colitis is suspected, as the risk of perforation is high.

Endoscopic ultrasound (EUS)

7. A, B, C, D, E

EUS allows traditional mucosal imaging and also depicts clearly intestinal layers and proximate extraintestinal structures. EUS has revolutionised the staging and management of upper gastrointestinal and hepatobiliary malignancies. EUS allows sampling of paraoesophageal and celiac lymph nodes and drainage of peripancreatic abscess or pseudocysts. The complications are similar to other endoscopic examinations.

→ Recent trends in endoscopy

8. E

Balloon enteroscopy allows the direct visualisation and therapeutic intervention of the entire small bowel and may be attempted via the oral or rectal route.

Answers to extended matching questions

→ Endoscopic diagnosis

1. H Barrett's oesophagus

This is becoming increasingly important, as it is associated with increasing the risk of malignancy. The incidence of adenocarinoma of the lower end of the oesophagus is increasing. Barrett's oesophagus showing dysplastic changes needs regular surveillance. There is still some debate about its management, but most agree that severe dysplastic changes would be a strong reason for surgery. Invasive carcinoma may be found in almost half of these cases.

2. G Carcinoma of the oesophagus

This causes profound weight loss and rapidly progressive dysphagia. Staging investigations such as endoscopic US, computerised tomography (CT) scan and laparoscopy are important before embarking on major resections. Prognosis still remains poor.

3. F Gastrointestinal stromal tumour (GIST)

This may be an incidental finding but can cause upper gastrointestinal bleed, which draws attention. Prognosis, though variable, is a lot better than adenocarcinoma. Even advanced cases respond to tyrosine kinase inhibitors such as imatinib.

4. I Hiatus hernia

A small hiatus hernia may be an incidental finding. Some are associated with features of reflux oesophagitis. This can rarely present with complications such as incarceration, necrosis and perforation.

5. E Linitis plastica

The mucosa may appear deceptively normal (though a bit stretched) and biopsies may be negative because the pathology is submucosal. The stomach will be very contracted and non-distensible. Special biopsy forceps are necessary to get the required tissue. Patients usually present late and hence this carries a very poor prognosis.

6. C Mallory-Weiss tear

Patients present with severe epigastric pain, retching and mild haematemesis. The clinical differential diagnosis includes duodenal perforation, acute pancreatitis, myocardial infarction and oesophageal perforation. Endoscopy confirms the diagnosis, which is self-limiting.

7. A Oesophageal varices

This may be seen in patients with portal hypertension presenting with haematemesis. The varices are usually injected or banded. More rarely, embolisation or vasopressin may be used. Surgery is almost never indicated nowadays, except in desperate situations.

8. B Peptic stricture

This is a complication of long-standing GORD. Barrett's oesophagus may be present. The diagnosis is confirmed on histology, where intestinal metaplasia is seen. Smooth tapering and absence of shouldering differentiate this from malignancy.

9. J Rectal cancer

Large rectal polyp in an otherwise unfit individual is assessed by taking a detailed history, followed by thorough clinical examination. This is followed by endoscopic assessment and biopsies. If the biopsies show dysplasia, there still may be a focus of cancer. Hence, MRI of pelvis and CT chest abdomen and pelvis are performed. To assess the local T staging, EUS may be beneficial.

EUS is used in the lower gastrointestinal tract in the assessment of low rectal polyps to differentiate between T1 and T2 lesions, and in the assessment of perirectal lymph nodes. EUS is also indicated in the assessment of fistula in ano and in assessment of anal sphincter complex in faecal incontinence. However, EUS is an investigation that is operator dependent.

10. D Reflux gastritis

This is a complication of long-standing GORD. Barrett's oesophagus may be present. The diagnosis is confirmed on histology, where intestinal metaplasia is seen. Smooth tapering and absence of shouldering differentiate this from malignancy.

2. Endoscopic complications

A Aspiration

B Bleeding

C Dental injury

D Perforation

E Sedation overdose

Endoscopic complications can be divided into cardiovascular and respiratory, which are usually related to sedation and mainly affect the elderly. In extreme cases, an anaesthetic opinion may be needed. The other complications are those related to the procedure and are surgically oriented.

Sedation must be used with caution in the elderly. Procedure-specific complications include bleeding, perforation and infections. Patients on anticoagulants should be assessed for their risk of thromboembolism against the risk of bleeding if a therapeutic procedure is planned. If bleeding is encountered during the procedure, combined modality using adrenaline injection, mechanical methods such as clips and snares and thermal methods such as argon plasma coagulation (APC) are used. Caution should be exercised when using APC, because there is a risk of perforation. Perforation should be suspected following upper gastrointestinal procedure if the patient complains of severe chest pain and has haemodynamic instability. On examination there may be subcutaneous emphysema or peritonitis. Early recognition and treatment is essential to reduce the risk of mortality.

15 Tissue diagnosis

Pradip K Datta

Multiple choice questions

Specimens for histology

1. The following statements are true except:

A Specimens must always be sent fixed in formalin.

B Specimens can be obtained by fine-needle aspiration cytology (FNAC).

C Specimens are classified as biopsies and resections.

D Frozen section histology has many disadvantages.

E Both macroscopic and microscopic findings are reported.

Cytology

2. Which of the following statements are true?

A It gives as much information as histology.

B In some instances, an invasive method has to be used to obtain material.

C Fluids may be useful in establishing diagnosis.

D A negative cytology has no value.

E There is risk to laboratory personnel associated with cytology and histology.

Principles of microscopic diagnosis

3. Which of the following statements are true?

A Malignancy is diagnosed histologically by invasion, architectural changes and cytological features.

B Dysplasia indicates microscopic features of cancer.

C False-positive diagnosis can occur.

D Tissue assessment helps in prognosis.

E Hyperplasia indicates an increase in cell size.

Inflammation and cytology

4. Which of the following statements is false?

A Inflammatory conditions are characterised by the predominant cell type.

B Cytology has some advantages over histology.

C In an ulcerated tissue, ideally cytology and biopsy should be taken from the centre of the lesion.

D Additional techniques may be necessary to elucidate the diagnosis.

E Special stains may sometimes be necessary.

Immunohistochemistry

5. Which of the following statements are true?

A This is a special staining method.

B It relies on the use of a specific antibody to detect a specific antigen.

C It helps to determine cell type and differentiation.

D It has a role in the determination of treatment and prognosis.

E This process has no role in other than neoplasms.

Special techniques

6. Which of the following statements is false?

A Electron microscopy is routinely used in histology.

B Polymerase chain reaction (PCR) is a useful investigation to detect microorganisms.

C PCR is a method that can be used to detect gene mutations.

D Study of chromosomes (cytogenetics) can be done using fluorescence in situ hybridisation (FISH).

E Autopsy can only be done with the coroner's permission.

Specimens for histology

1. A, B

All specimens need not be sent fixed in formalin (10% formaldehyde). Samples for routine histology are sent fixed. Fresh tissue samples are sent for frozen section, and when microbiological assessment is necessary as in suspected tuberculosis. In such a situation, a part of an excised lymph node is sent fresh and the remainder is fixed in formalin.

Fine-needle aspiration cytology only gives cytology; compared with histology, FNAC has a limited value. Cytology gives an idea about the cell type. FNAC is an invasive method and is helpful in breast and thyroid lumps and in lymphadenopathy. In certain situations, FNAC needs to be carried out under CT or ultrasound guidance.

While biopsy means any tissue sample, histology specimens are classified as biopsies and resections. Types of biopsy include punch biopsy, as in skin lesions, and core biopsy, as in Tru-Cut of breast lump or a prostatic nodule. Biopsy following a resection is usually also therapeutic as in small, ulcerated skin lesions.

The speed of a diagnosis after frozen section is outweighed by many disadvantages. The patient will not have a preoperative diagnosis and so cannot make an informed choice with regard to the definitive treatment; the tissue is not fixed and so there is a risk of infection to laboratory staff; the quality is inferior, thereby compromising diagnostic accuracy; and the procedure is time consuming.

Any specimen sent for histology is first sliced up into parts depending upon the size and fixed in formalin. After about 24 hours, a description of the macroscopic appearance is reported. Slices for microscopic examination are then reported. Report from a malignant specimen will include resection margins, tumour, lymph nodal status and neighbouring non-neoplastic tissue.

Cytology

2. B, C, D, E

Cytology does not give as much information as histology. It is a study of cells and gives an idea about the presence of malignancy. Therefore, in a breast lump, cancer can be established by FNAC. A Tru-Cut biopsy gives histological tissue, which helps to grade the tumour, may show the presence of perivascular and lymphovascular invasion, and gives an idea of the oestrogen receptor status. Fluids may be sent for cytological assessment; for example, urine may be sent when transitional cell carcinoma of bladder is suspected or sputum for bronchogenic carcinoma. However, a report of absence of cancer cells does not have any value.

In some instances, cells for cytology can be obtained only by invasive techniques, e.g., CT guidance for mediastinal lymph nodes, transbronchial fine-needle aspiration for mediastinal masses, or fine-needle aspiration of liver, pancreas and kidney. A negative cytology has no value. Absence of cancer cells from FNAC may mean that the incorrect tissue has been needled. There is always a risk for transmissible infection, such as hepatitis B or tuberculosis, particularly when fresh tissue is being sent.

Principles of microscopic diagnosis

3. A, B, C, D

Features confirming a histological diagnosis of malignancy are invasion of neighbouring tissue, blood vessels and lymphatics; architectural changes; atypical mitotic figures; and nuclear abnormalities of hyperchromatism and pleomorphism.

Dysplasia is a term used to indicate microscopic features of cancer without invasion. It is graded as mild, moderate and severe. Severe dysplasia is regarded by most as indicating carcinoma in situ, e.g., colorectal carcinoma in inflammatory bowel disease, oesophageal carcinoma in Barrett's oesophagus, or cervical intraepithelial neoplasia.

False-positive diagnoses can occur from contamination or interchanging of tissue, pitfalls in interpretation that are best avoided by good clinical details. A history of previous radiotherapy must be disclosed to the pathologist, as radiotherapy changes may mimic cancer.

Prognosis can be determined by tissue assessment. Stage is the important prognostic factor according to the UICC (Union Internationale Contre le Cancer). Grade is determined microscopically: Low-grade, well-differentiated tumours have a good prognosis as opposed to poorly differentiated, high-grade tumours. Vascular and perineural invasion with positive resection margins carry a poor prognosis.

Hyperplasia indicates an increase in cell number while an increase in cell size is referred to as hypertrophy. Examples of the former are seen in the breast (epithelial hyperplasia) and the prostate (benign prostatic hyperplasia). Examples of hypertrophy can be due to physiological causes, such as hypertrophied muscles as seen in bodybuilders, or pathological, such as occurs in the colon proximal to an annular obstructing carcinoma.

Inflammation and cytology

4. C
A sample from the centre of an ulcer may only show necrosis and nonviable tissue. Therefore, when taking a piece of tissue for biopsy (incision biopsy), it should be taken from the periphery with some apparently normal tissue. This enables interpretation of invasiveness and architectural changes. Superficial biopsies may fail to distinguish dysplasia.

The type of cell does determine the type of inflammation. Polymorphonuclear leucocytosis indicates acute inflammation. Presence of lymphocytes and plasma cells are seen in chronic inflammation. Eosinophilia indicates parasitic infestation or allergy. Granulomas, a collection of epithelioid histiocytes, are seen in mycobacterial infection (tuberculosis and leprosy), fungal infection and as a foreign body reaction.

Cytology does have some advantages over histology. Cytology allows a wider area to be sampled; it is less invasive, fast and cheap; and non-medical staff can be trained in its interpretation.

In a minority of difficult situations, further specimens may need to be obtained from deeper levels with extra blocks, as in linitis plastica. Special stains and immunohistochemistry are additional techniques available.

Special stains are used when routine stains do not provide the answer. For example, the periodic acid-Schiff (PAS) stain demonstrates glycogen and mucin; a diastase PAS (D-PAS) stain shows up mucin in adenocarcinoma. Iron accumulation, as in haemochromatosis, is demonstrated by Perls' Prussian blue stain. Fibrosis is shown up by reticulin stain, while Congo red shows up amyloidosis.

Immunohistochemistry

5. A, B, C, D
This technique is a special staining method. It detects a specific antigen using a specific antibody, which is labelled with a dye and, when bound to its target antigen, is seen as a coloured stain. It determines confirmation of neoplasia, site of origin, cell type and differentiation. This method can be applied to fixed and frozen tissue and cytological preparations.

The method has a role in the selection of treatment and in prediction of prognosis. Examples of this are seen in breast carcinoma where assessment for oestrogen, progesterone and HER-2 status is routine. Lymphomas are subjected to a panel of markers, while the management of endocrine tumours is enhanced by the assessment of Ki67 proliferative index.

It also has a role in infections. There are antibodies to many infective agents such as cytomegalovirus (CMV), Epstein–Barr virus (EBV), herpes virus, *Helicobacter pylori* and hepatitis B.

Special techniques

6. A, D

Electron microscopy is time consuming, labour intensive and expensive, and is used only selectively. Polymerase chain reaction (PCR) amplifies DNA, yielding innumerable copies from a single copy of a selected target. The amplified DNA is detected using techniques such as electrophoresis. The technique, which is highly sensitive, fast and safe, is used to detect chromosomal abnormalities and microorganisms. Several different tumours have been tested for mutation of the *APC* gene, which can reside in colorectal carcinoma.

In cytogenetics, the analysis of chromosomal changes is done using the fluorescent in site hybridisation (FISH) technique. For example, along with immunohistochemistry, FISH will detect HER2 amplification in breast cancer. Autopsy does not always require coroner's permission; it can be done for the purpose of medical education and audit with the consent of the next of kin.

PART 3

Perioperative care

Preoperative preparation

Ian Leeuwenberg

List of abbreviations

HRT	Hormone replacement therapy	VTE	Venous thromboembolism
IHD	Ischaemic heart disease	COPD	Chronic obstructive pulmonary disease
BMI	Body mass index	CXR	Chest X-ray
ECG	Electro cardiogram		

Multiple choice questions

→ ## Preoperative fasting

1. **Which of the following statements about preoperative fasting are true?**

A Clear fluids are allowed up to 2 hours before surgery.

B Cow and formula milk are allowed up to 3 hours before surgery.

C Pain, opiates and trauma increase gastric emptying time.

D Hiatus hernias increase the risk of aspiration.

E Routine medication can be given within 2 hours of surgery.

→ ## Tests of coagulation

2. **Which of the following drugs will cause derangement of a standard coagulation screen?**

A Low-molecular-weight heparin

B Unfractionated heparin

C Clopidogrel

D Warfarin

E Aspirin

→ ## Coronary artery disease

3. **Which of the following statements are true regarding coronary artery disease?**

A Dual antiplatelet therapy can be safely stopped after 6 months in patients with a drug-eluting coronary stent.

B Aspirin should be stopped 7 days prior to surgery with a high risk from bleeding.

C The risk of stopping dual antiplatelet therapy in people with bare metal coronary stents is significantly reduced after 6 weeks.

D There is a significant mortality risk associated with coronary stent thrombosis.

E Elective surgery should be postponed for 1 year following a myocardial infarction.

→ ## Predictors of difficult airways

4. **Which of the following factors increases the likelihood of difficulty obtaining and securing the airway under anaesthesia?**

A Obesity

B Dentures

C Reduced neck movement

D Mallampati grade 1 and 2

E Previous radiotherapy to the neck

→ ## Preoperative investigation

5. **With regard to preoperative investigation prior to elective surgery, which of the following statements are true?**

A Preoperative chest x-rays are routinely required in patients with chronic obstructive pulmonary disease (COPD).

B A full blood count is routinely required in all patients.

C An ejection fraction of less than 30% on echocardiography is associated with an increased risk of perioperative mortality.

D Patients over the age of 60 should usually have an electrocardiogram (ECG) performed preoperatively.

E Cardiac stress testing has a high negative predictive value and a low positive predictive value.

Obesity

6. **Which of the following is a problem associated with surgery in obese patients?**

A Deep vein thrombosis
B Pressure sores
C Postoperative respiratory failure
D Nerve injury
E Pain control

Consent

7. **Regarding consent for surgery which of the following statements are true?**

A Jehovah's Witnesses will never accept blood transfusions.
B It can be assumed that a patient with a mental illness will not have the capacity to give informed consent.
C All treatment options, including doing nothing, should be discussed.
D Children under the age of 16 can never give consent.
E All complications with an incidence of 1% or more should be discussed with the patient.

Preoperative preparation

8. **Which of the following statements regarding preoperative preparation prior to elective surgery are true?**

A Hormone replacement therapy (HRT) should be stopped 6 weeks prior to surgery.

B Elective surgery should be postponed for 6 weeks following a respiratory tract infection.
C A patient taking 5 mg of prednisolone will require perioperative steroid supplementation.
D Patients with a body mass index (BMI) of less than 15 have a significantly increased risk of hospital mortality.
E Patients with a haemoglobin of 8 should be transfused prior to surgery.

Diabetes

9. **Regarding patients with diabetes undergoing surgery, which of the following statements are true?**

A Tight glucose control is recommended to prevent infection.
B Diabetic patients should be prioritised on the theatre list.
C Diabetic patients have an increased risk of cardiac events.
D HbA1c reflects glucose control over the preceding 8 to 12 weeks.
E Poor wound healing is more common in diabetic patients.

Risk factors for thrombosis

10. **Which of the following is a risk factor for thrombosis?**

A Pregnancy
B Young age
C Smoking
D Trauma
E Malignancy

Answers to multiple choice questions

Preoperative fasting

1. A, C, D, E

The aim of fasting a patient preoperatively is to reduce the gastric contents and thereby minimise the risk of aspiration during anaesthesia. Fasting guidelines are 6 hours for solids and cow's milk, 3 hours for breast milk and 2 hours for clear fluids. A normally functioning gastro-oesophageal sphincter is also required to prevent normal residual gastric secretions (~30-40 mLs) from being regurgitated. Factors that cause dysfunction of the gastro-oesophageal sphincter include reflux disease, hiatus hernia and pregnancy. Patients can take all their usual medications, with a small sip of water if required, unless withheld for a specific reason. These guidelines are less helpful in patients who have increased gastric emptying times secondary to factors such as opiates, trauma, acute abdomen, acute pain and alcohol intoxication.

Cow's milk is treated as a solid because it curdles when mixed with gastric secretions and forms a thick flocculate.

Tests of coagulation

2. B, D

Warfarin inhibits the vitamin K dependent clotting factors II, VII, IX and X, which are part of the extrinisic pathway in the coagulation cascade. This is measured by the prothrombin time. Unfractionated heparin exerts its effects on the coagulation cascade by binding to and potentiating the action of antithrombin 3 (AT3). AT3 inhibits factors IIa (thrombin), Xa, and XIa, and its effects are measured by the activated partial thromboplastin time, or APTT.

Low-molecular-weight heparins selectively inhibit factor Xa, and their effect can be demonstrated by monitoring factor Xa levels. Antiplatelet agents do not affect the standard coagulation screen and require specialised tests.

Coronary artery disease

3. B, C, D

Aspirin irreversibly inactivates platelets and, as the lifespan of a platelet is 7 days, would need to be stopped for 1 week prior to surgery. Coronary stent thrombosis carries a high risk of mortality; patients are therefore started on dual antiplatelet therapy following stent insertion. Bare metal stents are initially thrombogenic but become covered with vessel wall endothelium, and the risk of thrombosis after 6 weeks is therefore much reduced.

In some patients with bare metal stents, scar tissue can form leading to stent restenosis. Drug-eluting stents are coated with cytotoxics, which prevent this tissue growth. The period of thrombotic risk is therefore of a much longer duration, and dual antiplatelet therapy should be continued for at least 12 months. Surgery following a recent myocardial infarction carries a significantly increased risk of cardiovascular complications, and elective surgery should therefore be delayed for 3 to 6 months.

Predictors of difficult airways

4. A, C, E

Many different bedside measurements and scoring systems for predicting difficult airways have been described, but it remains an inexact science. One such tool, the Wilson score, aims to predict difficult intubations by assessing five factors associated with difficult intubation – obesity, reduced neck movements, reduced mouth opening, receding mandible and prominent front teeth. Previous radiotherapy to the neck has a high risk of difficult intubation as the anatomy may be distorted and the tissue can become hard and inflexible.

Dentures (particularly upper ones) can be removed to make intubation easier. The Mallampatti scores of 1 and 2 are associated with a low risk of difficult intubation.

Preoperative investigation

5. C, D, E

Poor left ventricular function is a significant risk factor for complications during the perioperative period. However, normal left ventricular function at rest does not preclude significant ischaemic heart disease (IHD). Stress echocardiograms have a high negative predictive value and a low positive predictive value when used as a diagnostic tool for IHD.

Patients with a positive result should be considered for coronary angiography. ECGs are usually recommended for patients over age 60.

Healthy patients with no or minor comorbidities do not require preoperative testing prior to day case surgery. When assessing respiratory function, a static test such as a CXR is of little use and should be reserved for patients where a problem such as a respiratory infection or concomitant heart failure is suspected. Determining how far a patient with COPD can walk before getting breathless is a better indicator of respiratory function and reserve.

Obesity

6. A, B, C, D, E

Obese patients pose many challenges to the theatre team. Obesity compromises lung function, which often leads to intra and postoperative hypoxia. Obstructive sleep apnoea is also a common problem. These issues are worsened by the prolonged sedative effects of anaesthetic agents in obese patients. Opiate analgesia suppresses respiratory function, so safe and effective pain control in morbidly obese patients can be more difficult to achieve. Regional anaesthesia techniques for suitable operations are therefore very useful. Positioning obese patients safely requires care, because they are more at risk of nerve injury and pressure sores. Obesity is also a risk factor for deep vein thrombosis, and the doses of prophylactic anticoagulants will need to be increased in relation to weight.

Consent

7. C, E

All complications with and incidence of 1% or more and all significant complications should be discussed with the patient. Benefits and risks of alternative treatment strategies, including the option of doing nothing, should also be discussed. When obtaining consent a useful acronym to remember is LED TO REASON, details of which can be found in Bailey and Love, p. 236.

Jehovah's Witnesses should not be assumed to refuse any particular blood products or cell salvage treatment. It is important to discuss and document exactly what the patient will and will not accept. The capacity to provide informed consent requires the patient to be able to understand, retain, assess the information given and communicate the decision. Mental illness does not automatically preclude a person from having this capacity. 'Gillick competence' refers to a ruling in the House of Lords Gillick vs West Norfolk and Wisbech AHA, 1986. Children under the age of 16 have capacity to make decisions if they understand the nature and implications of the proposed treatment or intervention.

Preoperative preparation

8. A, B, D

HRT is a risk factor for thrombosis and should be stopped prior to surgery. Patients with active respiratory tract infections should be postponed, as they are at higher risk of intra and postoperative respiratory complications. Malnutrition has deleterious effects on all the major organ systems and is associated with a significantly increased risk of morbidity and mortality. These include infection, poor wound healing, anastomotic breakdown, increased critical care and hospital stays.

Steroid supplementation is required in patients who are taking more than 10 mg of prednisolone per day in the 3 months before an operation. Anaemic patients must have the cause of their anaemia diagnosed and treated, if possible, prior to surgery. The need for transfusion will depend on patient comorbidities and type of surgery. The transfusion triggers for patients in critical care are usually ~9 g/dL for patients with significant cardiovascular disease and ~7 g/dL for patients without such disease.

Diabetes

9. B, C, D, E

Diabetic patients should be placed first on the theatre list, as this reduces the disruption to mealtimes and administration of antidiabetic medications. Cardiovascular, cerebrovascular and peripheral vascular disease is common in diabetic patients, and these conditions should be examined carefully as part of the preoperative assessment. Cardiac ischaemia may be 'silent'. Diabetic patients are also at increased risk of poor wound healing, pressure sores, electrolyte imbalance and infection. When glucose binds to haemoglobin in red bloods cells, HbA1c (glycosylated haemoglobin) is formed, which lasts for the lifetime of a red cell (~8 to 12 weeks).

Diabetic patients undergoing major surgery or requiring critical care should have their sugars controlled below 10 mmol/L, as uncontrolled hyperglycaemia is associated with increased morbidity and mortality, including increased rates of infection. Tight blood glucose control (4.4–6.1 mmol/L) is no longer recommended, as patients are thereby exposed to an increased risk of hypoglycaemia.

Risk factors for thrombosis

10. A, C, D, E

The following are risk factors for venous thromboembolism (VTE):

- Obesity
- Trauma or surgery
- Reduced mobility
- Pregnancy/puerperium
- Oestrogen contraceptive, hormone replacement therapy
- Smoking
- Active cancer or on treatment
- Significant medical comorbidities
- Critical illness
- Family/personal history of thrombosis

Preventable hospital-acquired VTE is a significant cause of mortality. In addition, many patients will suffer morbidity from VTE due to chronic venous insufficiency, which can cause venous ulceration, chronic pain and swelling. All patients admitted to hospital should have their VTE risk assessed and balanced against bleeding risk. VTE prophylaxis can be mechanical (anti-embolism stockings, foot-impulse devices, intermittent pneumatic compression devices) or pharmacological (unfractionated heparin, fondaparinux, low-molecular-weight heparin). Other important aspects of VTE prophylaxis include early mobilisation, avoidance of dehydration and use of regional anaesthesia, where appropriate.

17 Anaesthesia and pain relief

Ian Leeuwenberg

List of abbreviations

RSI   Rapid sequence induction
GCS   Glasgow coma scale

LMA   Laryngeal mask
LA   Local anaesthetic

Multiple choice questions

→ Local anaesthetics

1. In which of the following scenarios is the maximum safe dose of local anaesthetic calculated correctly?

A 30 mLs of 0.5% bupivacaine for a 50 kg patient.

B 7 mLs of 2% lidocaine with adrenaline for a 20 kg child.

C 28 mLs of 0.5% levobupivacaine for a 70 kg patient.

D 6 mLs of 4% prilocaine for a 60 kg patient.

E 16 mLs of 1% lidocaine for a 80 kg patient.

→ General anaesthesia

2. Which of the following statements about general anaesthesia are true?

A Rapid sequence inductions are only indicated for unfasted patients undergoing non-elective surgery.

B IV access must always be obtained prior to induction of anaesthesia.

C Nitrous oxide is a useful agent due to its analgesic effect and low risk of postoperative nausea and vomiting.

D The triad of general anaesthesia is amnesia, analgesia and muscle relaxation.

E Propofol has replaced thiopentone as the most widely used induction agent because of concerns about adrenocortical depression.

→ Ketamine

3. Which of the following advantages does ketamine have when compared with other anaesthetic agents?

A Haemodynamic stability

B Potent analgesic effect

C Low incidence of postoperative delirium

D Preservation of airway reflexes

E Fastest speed of onset

→ Local anaesthetic toxicity

4. Classical features of local anaesthetic toxicity include:

A Hypertension

B Transient blindness

C Seizures

D Cardiac arrhythmias

E Loss of consciousness

→ Bier's block

5. Which of the following statements regarding Bier's block are true?

A Lidocaine is the local anaesthetic of choice.

B The minimum duration of cuff inflation is 20 minutes.

C Bupivacaine is not recommended.

D If used on the lower limb carries a higher risk of toxicity.

E Patients do not need to be fasted.

Laryngeal masks

6. Which of the following statements are true regarding laryngeal masks?

A Modern versions of laryngeal masks provide the same level of airway protection as an endotracheal tube.

B Laryngeal masks are not suitable for airway management of a patient in cardiac arrest.

C Laryngeal masks can be used in a mechanically ventilated patient.

D Laryngeal masks are less traumatic to a patient's airway than an endotracheal tube.

E Laryngeal masks are always easy to insert.

Neuropathic pain

7. Which of the following statements about neuropathic pain are correct?

A It is classically described as 'burning', 'shooting', or 'stabbing.'

B Opiates are the mainstay of treatment.

C Allodynia describes an increased sensitivity to a normally painful stimulus.

D Tricyclic antidepressants are a useful treatment modality.

E May be due to dysfunction in both peripheral and central nerves.

Epidural analgesia

8. Which of the following statements regarding epidural analgesia are correct?

A If used intra-operatively, epidural analgesia can reduce blood loss.

B Can be safely left in situ for 5 days.

C Reduces postoperative respiratory complications following abdominal surgery.

D Patients should not mobilise with an epidural, due to the risk of postural hypotension.

E Treatment of epidural-associated hypotension includes IV fluid administration and vasopressor infusions.

Pain management

9. Which of the following statements about the WHO pain step ladder are correct?

A If simple analgesics are ineffective, they should be stopped and intermediate-strength opioids prescribed.

B The breakthrough dose of strong opiates should be approximately 1/6 of the total daily dose of long-acting opiates.

C Most patients being treated for cancer pain with strong opiates will develop addiction.

D Nausea is usually a transient problem for people on strong opiates.

E Pethidine is the recommended strong opiate.

Assessment of pain

10. Patients vary greatly in their requirement for postoperative analgesia. What is the best way to assess adequacy of pain relief?

A Measure the degree of tachycardia.

B Ask the patient to measure the pain.

C Assess the level of hypertension.

D Look for tachypnoea.

E Assess level of sedation.

Extended matching questions

Match each of the following operations with an appropriate analgesic modality from the choices that follow the list of operations. Each option may only be used once.

1 Elective abdominal aortic aneurysm repair in a 68-year-old patient with ischaemic heart disease

2 Elective laparoscopic cholecystectomy in a 37-year-old ASA 1 patient

3 Emergency sigmoid colectomy for perforated diverticulitis in a 76-year-old patient

4 Mastectomy with axillary node clearance in a 57-year-old patient with stage 4 chronic kidney disease

5 Open cholecystectomy in a 42-year-old patient with mild asthma

6 Open inguinal hernia repair in a 65-year-old patient with severe COPD

A Intercostal nerve blocks
B Opiate patient controlled analgesia (PCA)
C Oral morphine
D Oral non-steroidal anti-inflammatory drugs (NSAIDs)
E Spinal anaesthesia
F Thoracic epidural

Answers to multiple choice questions

1. B, C, E

To convert to mg/mL from %, simply move the decimal point one digit to the left, i.e., 1% = 10 mg/mL.

Maximum doses of local anaesthetics are:

Lidocaine 3 mg/kg (7 mg/kg with adrenaline)
Bupivacaine/levobupivacaine 2 mg/kg
Prilocaine 6 mg/kg (9 mg/kg with adrenaline)

The correct calculations therefore are:

A 50 kg x 2 mg/kg = 100 mg → 100 mg/(5 mg/mL, i.e., 0.5%) = 20 mL
B 20 kg x 7 mg/kg = 140 mg → 140 mg/(20 mg/mL, i.e., 2%) = 7 mL
C 70 kg x 2 mg/kg = 140 mg → 140 mg/(5 mg/mL, i.e., 0.5%) = 28 mL
D 60 kg x 6 mg/kg = 360 mg → 360 mg/(40 mg/mL, i.e., 4%) = 9 mL
E 80 kg x 3 mg/kg = 240 mg → 240 mg/(10 mg/mL, i.e., 1%) = 24 mL

The doses above refer to administration into tissues with a poor blood supply. Local anaesthetics are more likely to cause toxicity if injected into vascular tissues, and the previously mentioned doses could well be fatal if inadvertently injected intravascularly.

2. D

The aims of anaesthesia are analgesia amnesia and muscle relaxation.

Rapid sequence inductions (RSI) are indicated in unfasted patients to reduce the risk of pulmonary aspiration. Even patients who are fasted will have a small amount of residual acidic gastric fluid, so patients who have severe GORD, for example, may also need an RSI. While IV access is desirable, induction of anaesthesia with an inhaled anaesthetic agent is often used in children or severely needle-phobic patients. Nitrous oxide is less commonly used for several reasons, including an increased risk of nausea and vomiting. It does however provide analgesia and is used for pain relief in labour as a first-line agent. Propofol is the most commonly used induction agent due to its reduced hangover effect compared with thiopentone and because it facilitates the insertion of laryngeal masks being a potent suppressor of laryngeal reflexes. Etomidate causes adrenal suppression.

3. A, B, D

Ketamine is an ideal anaesthetic agent for field anaesthesia and severely shocked patients, as it preserves laryngeal reflexes, maintains airway patency and also has a positive inotropic effect, thus minimising hypotension. By inhibiting NMDA receptors, it also provides potent analgesia. In a monitored environment it can be administered as a low-dose infusion as part of a pain management strategy in patients whose pain is insufficiently controlled by IV opiates.

Unfortunately there is a significant incidence of unpleasant postoperative delirium and hallucinations, which precludes routine use. It takes longer to act than other IV induction agents but has the advantage of also being able to be administered intramuscularly.

4. C, D, E

Local anaesthetics (LA) act by reversibly blocking Na+ channels in nerves, preventing depolarisation. Toxic effects occur when LA enters the circulation and blocks Na+ channels in the heart and brain. Initial symptoms are often nonspecific; a patient may complain of 'feeling strange' or of light-headedness. Other symptoms include tinnitus, tingling lips and a metallic taste. Severe effects include arrhythmias, seizures, reduced GCS and cardiac arrest. Treatment of these severe effects should proceed according to standard resuscitation algorithms, with one key difference – the administration of Intralipid®20% IV should be started as soon as possible. Intralipid is a lipid emulsion, which acts as a reservoir for lipophilic LA molecules, effectively removing them from the circulation and causing LA to dissociate from Na+ channels. Intralipid should be immediately available in all settings where potentially toxic doses of LAs are administered.

Transient blindness and hypertension are not symptoms of LA toxicity.

5. B, C, D

The minimum duration of cuff inflation is 20 minutes when performing a Bier's block. Bupivacaine must not be used, as it has a high affinity for cardiac Na+ channels with an increased risk therefore of cardiac toxicity. Bier's blocks on the lower limb are less frequently used due to an increased risk of LA toxicity.

Patients undergoing a procedure under Bier's Block should be fasted, as occasionally conversion to GA is required due to patient discomfort. Prilocaine is the local anaesthetic of choice due to its low toxicity and short duration of action.

6. C, D

Laryngeal masks (LMAs) cause less trauma and irritation of the airway than endotracheal tubes and hence present a lower incidence of postoperative sore throats and laryngospasm in patients. LMAs can be used in spontaneously breathing and mechanically ventilated patients.

Modern LMA designs provide a better seal and increased protection against gastric aspiration than the original LMA. However, LMAs do not provide the same level of airway protection as endotracheal tubes. LMAs are usually easy to insert and provide a patent airway that can be maintained by one person. Their use is therefore encouraged in cardiac arrest situations where there is not a skilled intubator present, as minimal training is required to place an LMA correctly.

7. A, D, E

Neuropathic pain is a complex and incompletely understood phenomenon that occurs due to dysfunction of both peripheral and central nerves. There may be a trigger, such as trauma or surgery, but neuropathic pain often continues even after the original tissue damage has healed. Burning, shooting and stabbing are adjectives classically used to describe neuropathic pain. Tricyclics, ketamine and anticonvulsants are a few examples of drug treatment modalities.

Neuropathic pain is often very resistant to treatment with opiate analgesia. Several terms are used to describe the abnormal sensations that accompany neuropathic pain: Allodynia describes a painful sensation to a stimulus that is not normally painful such as light touch; hyperalgesia describes an increased sensitivity to painful stimuli; and dysaesthesia describes spontaneous unpleasant abnormal sensations.

8. A, C, E
The resultant sympathetic blockade following epidural local anaesthesia causes vasodilation, reduced venous pressure and, thereby, reduced venous bleeding intraoperatively. Epidurals can provide excellent postoperative analgesia, facilitating chest physiotherapy and have been shown to reduce the incidence of postoperative chest infections following major surgery.

Epidural catheters should be removed after 72 hours, as the risk of epidural infection increases markedly if left in situ for longer. Catheters should not be removed if the patient has significant coagulation abnormalities, as there is a risk of epidural haematomas forming on removal as well as insertion. Epidurals facilitate early, even same-day, mobilisation, and are a key component of enhanced recovery care pathways. The treatment of epidural-associated hypotension requires replacing any intravascular volume deficit and potentially commencing a vasopressor infusion (e.g., phenylephrine, noradrenaline) to counteract vasodilation. Reducing the dose of local anaesthetic must be done cautiously to prevent pain.

9. B, D
In general, patients on long-acting opiates should have breakthrough doses prescribed of around 1/6 of the total daily amount of long-acting opiate; smaller doses are likely be to ineffective due to tolerance. Nausea is usually a transient problem with long-term opiate use.

Many patients will develop features of dependence following long-term opiate administration (i.e., tolerance and withdrawal symptoms on cessation); however, addiction, a psychosocial phenomenon, is not usually a problem when opiates are prescribed appropriately. Pethidine is no longer recommended for severe continuing pain due to the risk of neurotoxicity, arrhythmias and severe cor pulmonale that can occur from accumulation of toxic metabolites. The underlying principle for treating severe pain is combining several classes of drugs to achieve a synergistic effect. Therefore, simple analgesics should be continued for patients on strong opiates.

10. B
In general, the patient is the best person to assess his or her own pain and analgesia. This can be done by using verbal rating scales such as 0 to 10 or mild/moderate/severe, or by getting the patient to mark where he or she thinks is best on a 10 cm line (visual analogue scale) where one end denoted as 'no pain' and the other end as 'worst pain'. Trends in pain scores are more useful than isolated measurements, as they allow clinicians to assess whether an intervention to reduce pain is working.

Clinicians can also be guided by other signs of adequate analgesia, e.g., if a patient can cough and breathe deeply without distress following abdominal surgery. Tachycardia, hypertension, agitation and tachypnoea are nonspecific features of inadequate analgesia.

Answers to extended matching questions

1. F Thoracic epidural
Thoracic epidurals can provide excellent analgesia for major surgery and prevent the adverse effects of parenteral opiates. The main contraindications are patient refusal, local or systemic sepsis, coagulopathy, or administration of anticoagulant drugs.

All patients with epidurals should be managed in a monitored environment. They allow patients to comply with physiotherapy, and thereby reduce postoperative pneumonias and enable mobilisation.

The epidural mixture is usually a low concentration of bupivacaine (0.0625%–0.125%) with a small amount of added opiate (e.g., 2 mcg/mL fentanyl). It may be administered as a continuous infusion, patient-controlled epidural analgesia (PCEA), or a combination of both. Typical infusion rates are 6–15 mL/hour.

Epidurals should generally be removed after 3 days to minimise the risk of infection. Timing of catheter removal will also depend on concurrent anticoagulant administration and coagulopathy.

Complications and problems include the following:

- **Inadequate analgesia** – May require epidural top-up, catheter adjustment, epidural resiting. Discuss problems early with the on-call anaesthesia team.
- **Hypotension** – Replace any intravascular volume deficit and consider vasoconstrictor infusion.
- **Urinary retention** – May require short-term catheterisation.
- **Headache** – A common symptom. Rule out post-dural puncture headache (PDPH), which has an incidence of less than 1:100. PDPH can be treated effectively with an epidural blood patch.
- **Epidural haematoma/abscess** – A rare but serious complication. If suspected, requires an emergency MRI scan and neurosurgical assessment. IV antibiotics must also be started immediately if infection is suspected.
- **Nerve/spinal cord injury** – Very rare. Fully document any deficit and make appropriate referrals.

2. D Oral non-steroidal anti-inflammatory drugs (NSAIDs)

Oral NSAIDs have potent analgesic, anti-inflammatory and antipyretic properties. They act by inhibiting the cyclooxygenase enzyme, which converts arachidonic acid to prostaglandins. Oral NSAIDs should be considered as part of any analgesic regimen, however, their use is limited by several of the following adverse effects:

- Gastric ulceration, perforation and bleeding.
- Impaired platelet function.
- Renal injury, especially in the context of dehydration, chronic kidney disease, or concomitant use of ACE inhibitors.
- A small minority of asthmatics experience exacerbations following administration.

3. B Opiate patient controlled analgesia (PCA)

Opiates have a relatively narrow therapeutic window between plasma levels that provide effective analgesia and levels that cause significant side effects. Compounding the issue is the large variation in opiate requirements between individual patients. Patient-controlled analgesia delivery systems aim to circumvent this problem by allowing the patient to self-administer the drug.

A bolus of morphine 1–2 mg or fentanyl 10–30 mcg followed by a five to 10 minute lockout are standard regimens. A low-dose background infusion may be added with caution, as this increases the risk of overdose.

All patients should have 2 L of supplemental O_2 administered and should have at least hourly observations, with particular attention paid to sedation scores and respiratory rate.

4. C Oral morphine

All opiates act by inhibiting mu, delta and kappa receptors, which are found in the brain and spinal cord. A typical starting oral morphine dose would be between 5 and 20 mg, the main determinant being the patient's age, with elderly patients being more sensitive to the effects. Peak effect following oral administration of the immediate release preparations is around 30 to 60 minutes.

NB! When converting between IV and oral formulations of morphine remember that 10mg PO and 3mg IV are equipotent doses. This is because the oral bioavailability of morphine is 30%.

Twelve- and 24-hour sustained release versions of morphine are also available. In general, the PRN dose should be 1/6 of the total daily sustained release dose.

The most serious potential side effects of opiates are sedation and respiratory depression – naloxone is an opiod antagonist. For life-threatening opiate overdose, 0.4–2 mg IV repeated at intervals of 2 to 3 minutes up to a total dose of 10 mg can be administered. The duration of action is around 40 minutes, so a continuous infusion may need to be started. Naloxone will also reverse all analgesia, so for mild overdose consider more cautious administration in 40 mcg increments.

Other adverse effects are nausea, constipation, pruritus and urinary retention.

5. A Intercostal nerve blocks

Intercostal nerve blocks are a simple yet effective mode of analgesia in a variety of situations. Indications include the following:

- Fractured ribs
- Thoracotomy
- Open cholecystectomy
- Renal surgery
- Breast surgery

Technique:

In general, the nerves from T2 to T11 may be blocked. It is important to block the nerves before they give off the lateral cutaneous branch; aim to be at or proximal to the angle of the rib.

Positioning can be either leaning forward with arms crossed, or in the lateral position with the arm pulled across the chest. This keeps the scapula out of the way and enables access to T2 to T6.

As with all blocks asepsis is important.

Palpate each rib with two fingers and insert the needle perpendicularly between them until you hit bone. Then walk off the bottom of the rib, and just under it, until you feel a slight loss of resistance. Aspirate prior to injection, as the intercostal artery runs in close proximity to the nerve, and then deposit 3–5 mLs of local anaesthestic.

The block should work within 5 to 10 minutes and lasts for 8 to 12 hours.

The main complications are pneumothorax, bleeding and intravascular injection.

6. E Spinal anaesthesia

Spinal anaesthesia is a useful for abdominal and lower limb surgery. The main contraindications are the same as for epidural analgesia – patient refusal, local or systemic sepsis, coagulopathy, or administration of anticoagulant drugs.

The main advantages of spinal anaesthesia are avoidance of general anaesthesia, reduced intraoperative blood loss and reduced incidence of DVTs.

Following a single dose of local anaesthetic, a spinal can be expected to provide anaesthesia for 2 to 3 hours. For prolonged analgesia, a small dose of opiate may be added such as 0.1–0.3 mg of morphine or diamorphine. This provides excellent analgesia for 12 to 16 hours. Continuous analgesia with spinal catheters is used uncommonly.

Potential problems include the following:

- Delayed respiratory depression if spinal opiates are used. The patient will require hourly observations for 24 hours postoperatively.
- Hypotension
- Nerve damage
- Post dural puncture headache
- Urinary retention

18 Care in the operating room

Ian Leeuwenberg

Multiple choice questions

→ **Surgical infection**

1. **Which of the following interventions prevent surgical infection?**

A Administration of prophylactic antibiotics less than 1 hour before surgery.

B Preparing the skin from the incision site outwards.

C Meticulous surgical scrub technique.

D Maintaining the patient's temperature above 36°C.

E Avoiding hyperglycaemia.

→ **Theatre environment**

2. **Which of the following statement regarding the operating theatre environment are correct?**

A The relative humidity is kept at 50% to 60% to minimise the risk of surgical site infections.

B Theatres should have at least 10 air changes per hour.

C Optimal ambient temperature is 16–18°C.

D The operating theatre is kept at positive pressure relative to the surroundings.

E Filtered air should be introduced at ceiling height and exhausted near the floor.

→ **Tourniquets**

3. **Which of the following statements regarding use of a tourniquet are true?**

A A tourniquet can be safely inflated for 2½ hours.

B Distal neurovascular status must be checked before and after its use.

C The tourniquet must be placed as proximally as possible.

D Tourniquets are contraindicated in patients with Sickle cell disease.

E When used on the upper arm the cuff pressure should be 50 mmHg above systolic blood pressure.

→ **Patient positioning**

4. **Which of the following statements are true regarding the transfer and positioning of patients?**

A Universal precautions should be maintained by all staff during transfer.

B Obese patients are at higher risk of nerve injury.

C Ointment, tape, or protective pads may be used to prevent eye injury.

D Limbs not involved in surgery during lengthy operation should be moved during prolonged procedures.

E The nerve most at risk of injury when leg supports are used is the tibial nerve.

→ **Diathermy**

5. **Which of the following statements with regard to diathermy are true?**

A Should not be applied over scar tissue, bony prominences and implanted metalwork.

B The diathermy plate site should be free of hair.

C Monopolar diathermy should be used in preference to bipolar in patients with implanted defibrillators.

D Place the plate as close as possible to the operative site.

E Ensure that all metal surfaces with which the patient is in contact are earthed.

→ Surgical scrubbing

6. With regard to surgical scrubbing, which of the following statements are true?

A If the surgeon has a suspected infected lesion, it is sprayed with iodine and covered with a sterile dressing before gloving.

B 7.5% povidone-iodine scrub solution has the longest duration of effect.

C The first scrub of the day should take about 5 minutes, from start to drying.

D A sterile scrubbing brush and nail cleaner are used for 1 to 2 minutes at the first scrub, provided the surgeon stays within the theatre suite in between cases.

E Allergic reactions occur with povidone-iodine, but not chlorhexidine.

→ WHO safety checklist

7. Which of the following statements regarding the WHO safety checklist are true?

A The prelist briefing is an optional part of the safety checklist.

B The patient should confirm his or her identity, site of surgery, procedure and consent at 'sign in'.

C 'Time out' should occur just before the procedure starts.

D 'Sign out' checks are the responsibility of the scrub nurse.

E Clear postoperative instructions must be completed immediately after surgery.

Answers to multiple choice questions

1. A, B, C, D, E

These simple interventions all reduce the risk of surgical infections. Antibiotic prophylaxis, where appropriate, as well as meticulous asepsis are key components. Perioperative hypothermia not only increases the risk of infection but also impairs wound healing, glucose control and coagulation pathways. Hypothermic patients are also more likely to experience cardiac events. Blood sugar control is discussed in Chapter 18.

2. D, E

The theatre is kept at a positive pressure to prevent ingress of infective material. Airflow in theatre is from ceiling to floor to prevent stirring up dirt and dust from floors, which can contaminate the operative field.

Theatre humidity is kept at 50% to 60% to minimise the risk of static electrical charge build up. Twenty air changes per hour is the minimum requirement. Optimal ambient temperature is 20–24°C, which represents a compromise between reducing the risk of patients becoming hypothermic and allowing comfortable operating conditions.

3. B, C, D

Distal vascular status should be assessed prior to use of a tourniquet, as it is contraindicated in patients with peripheral vascular disease. Postoperatively, the return of circulation should also be noted. Tourniquets should be placed as proximally as possible to allow access to the operative site. Sickling of red blood cells in patients with sickle cell disease occurs in response to hypoxia, and tourniquets are therefore contraindicated in these patients.

The maximum safe tourniquet inflation time is 1.5 hours. Longer times risk irreversible ischaemic damage to muscle, nerves and vasculature. Tourniquets should be inflated to 100 mmHg above systolic BP for the arm and 150 mmHg for the leg.

4. A, B, C, D

Universal precautions to prevent contamination with blood or other body fluids must be maintained in all patient care situations. Obese patients are difficult to position safely and are therefore at increased risk of nerve injuries and pressure sores. The risk of corneal abrasions under general anaesthesia is around 1 in 2800. Tape, ointment and protective pads can prevent this occurring. During prolonged surgery, limbs not involved in surgery should be moved regularly to prevent pressure sores and nerve injuries.

The incidence of significant nerve damage under general anaesthesia is less than 1 in 2000. The nerves most commonly affected are the ulnar nerve in the arm and common peroneal nerve in the leg. Common peroneal nerve injury can lead to numbness over the dorsum of the foot and foot drop.

5. A, B, D

With monopolar diathermy, the entire surface area of the plate should be in contact with skin over tissues with a good blood supply to prevent burns. It should therefore not be placed on bony prominences, scar tissue and hairy skin. The plate should also not be placed over implanted metal work to avoid heating effects. The current path should be short and not travel through susceptible tissue or medical devices. Therefore, the pad should be placed close to the operative site.

Ideally bipolar diathermy should be used in patients with pacemakers or implantable cardiodefibrillators, as the current is confined to the instrument tip. The patient must not be in contact with any other metal surfaces. The risk of electrocution increases if they are earthed, because current can flow between the diathermy and the earthed appliance.

6. C, D

Surgeons should not scrub if they have an open wound or infected lesion. 2% Chlorhexidine has the longest duration of effect and, like povidone-iodine, is a cause of allergic reactions.

7. B, C, E

It is essential that the patient confirms the identity and details of the planned procedure prior to the start of anaesthesia. At this point, the patient's name-bands should also be checked. A further 'time out' check just prior to starting surgery should be done once the patient is anaesthetised.

One of the main aims of the surgical safety checklist is to encourage communication between members of the theatre team. It encourages team members to speak out when potential problems are detected and improves list efficiency. The 'pre list brief' is therefore arguably one of the most important parts of the five-step WHO process, and is not optional. Ensuring that the sign-out checks are completed is the responsibility of the entire theatre team. Clear, written postoperative instructions must be completed in a timely manner for when the patient leaves theatre.

Perioperative management of the high-risk surgical patient

Ian Leeuwenberg

Multiple choice questions

→ Cardiac risk factors

1. Which of the following are risk factors in the revised cardiac risk index of Lee?
A Morbid obesity
B Severe COPD
C Ischaemic heart disease
D Diabetes mellitus
E Renal insufficiency (creatinine >177 mmol/L)

→ Assessment of fitness

2. Regarding assessment of physical fitness, which of the following statements are true?
A Patients who cannot exercise at four metabolic equivalents of task (METS) are at a significantly higher risk of mortality.
B Four METS is equivalent to climbing two flights of stairs.
C An anaerobic threshold of 15 is used as a cut-off for placing patients in a high-risk category.
D Cardiopulmonary exercise testing (CPET) involves measuring inspired and expired respiratory gases while undergoing incrementally more demanding exercise.
E CPET is quick and easy to perform.

→ Goal-directed therapy

3. Regarding goal-directed therapy, which of the following statements are true?
A Goal-directed therapy requires estimation of the cardiac output.
B Goal-directed therapy has been shown to reduce postoperative morbidity.
C Sustained use of goal-directed therapy in patients with established critical illness is beneficial.
D Goal-directed therapy requires a pulmonary artery catheter.
E It is a term used to describe the perioperative administration of intravenous (IV) fluids and inotropic agents to achieve a predefined 'optimal' goal for oxygen delivery to the tissues.

→ Myocardial ischaemia

4. Which of the following increases the risk of myocardial ischaemia?
A Tachycardia
B Hypertension
C Pain
D Anaemia
E Beta blockers

→ **High-risk patients**

5. **Which of the following statements about the management of high-risk patients are true?**

A All patients undergoing major surgery should be started on beta blockers on the day of surgery.

B Long-term beta blockers can be safely withheld on the day of surgery.

C The oesophageal Doppler accurately measures cardiac output.

D Better fluid management can reduce postoperative ileus after abdominal surgery.

E Early return to enteric feeding is associated with reduced hospital stay.

→ **Respiratory disease**

6. **Regarding preoperative management of patients with severe respiratory disease, which of the following statements are true?**

A A course of antibiotics should always be given in patients with chronic sputum production.

B Stopping smoking prior to surgery is of little benefit.

C Regional anaesthesia should be considered where possible.

D A course of steroids prior to surgery may be necessary in patients with chronic obstructive airway diseases.

E Preoperative physiotherapy has no role.

Answers to multiple choice questions

1. C, D, E
Lee's risk factors are ischaemic heart disease, heart failure, cerebrovascular disease, diabetes and renal impairment. In general, if a patient is undergoing low-risk surgery or has an exercise tolerance of greater than four METS or has none of the previously mentioned risk factors, then surgery can proceed without further cardiac interventions. Patients outwith these criteria should be considered for initiation of beta blocker therapy prior to surgery and, if it would change management, invasive cardiac stress testing. These decisions should be discussed with an anaesthestist or cardiologist with an interest in preoperative care.

While morbid obesity is not a risk factor in Lee's scoring system it is associated with respiratory, cardiac and metabolic disease. Patients with COPD are at risk of postoperative respiratory failure and often have cardiovascular comorbidities. Obese patients and patients with COPD often benefit from regional anaesthesia techniques.

2. A, B, D
As discussed above, patients who cannot achieve four METS (two flights of stairs) without symptoms are significantly higher risk. A maximum exercise capacity of four METS corresponds roughly to a VO2 max of 15 mL/kg/minute. To put this in perspective an average untrained young male can exercise to around 12 METS or a VO2 max of 45 mL/kg/minute, which is equivalent to playing squash or running 8 miles per hour. World record VO2 max measurements of over 90 mL/kg/minute are generally obtained by cross-country skiers and long-distance cyclists.

An anaerobic threshold of 11 mL/kg/minute is generally used as an indicator of a high-risk patient. CPET testing is time consuming and requires a skilled clinician to interpret the test.

3. A, B, E
Tissue oxygen delivery = cardiac output (stroke volume x heart rate) x oxygen content of the blood ($\approx$ Hb g/dL x 1.34 x SpO2%).

Goal-directed therapy relies on being able to measure cardiac output and see the response to fluid challenges and inotrope administration. Ensuring an adequate amount of well-saturated haemoglobin is also of paramount importance to allow maximum tissue oxygen delivery. Goal-directed therapy has been shown to improve outcomes in high-risk surgery, as fluid therapy can be optimally managed and inotropes started early when indicated.

Goal-directed therapy does not require a pulmonary artery catheter; oesophageal Doppler and pulse contour analysis of the arterial pressure waveform (uncalibrated or calibrated) are less invasive options. Goal-directed therapy might be harmful to patients with established critical illness.

4. A, B, C, D

Tachycardia, hypertension and therefore pain all increase myocardial oxygen demand and may precipitate ischaemia in patients with cardiovascular disease. Anaemia reduces myocardial oxygen delivery.

Beta blockers reduce the heart rate and force of contraction, thus reducing myocardial oxygen demand, which is beneficial in patients with cardiac disease. They also reduce cardiac output, however, which may explain the increased mortality and stroke rate seen in the POISE trial.

5. D, E

Excessive fluid administration has been shown to not only cause an increased incidence of ileus but also an increase in mortality. It can be challenging to judge whether a patient has received an optimal amount of fluid; CVP, urine output and MAP are of limited use. Minimally invasive cardiac monitoring has been shown to be an effective tool to guide fluid administration. Early NG or oral feeding has also been shown to improve outcomes.

Single measurements with the oesophageal Doppler are inaccurate, but trends and measured responses to interventions are useful. Beta blockers, where indicated, should be titrated to effect over the course of a few weeks prior to elective major surgery. Patients for emergency surgery with unstable angina, myocardial ischaemia, or pathological tachyarrythmias may require STAT IV beta blockade. Withholding long-term beta blockers increases mortality significantly.

6. C, D

Patients with severe respiratory disease benefit from regional anaesthesia, as the requirement for opiates is minimised and they can avoid the harmful effects of general anaesthesia on respiratory function. Patients with severe respiratory disease should have had their treatment reviewed by a respiratory physician prior to surgery. COPD patients may require a course of steroids to reduce airway inflammation.

Antibiotics should be given only if there is evidence of infection, i.e., purulent sputum or consolidation on a CXR. Routine antibiotic therapy merely encourages resistant organisms. All patients must be encouraged to stop smoking. After 24 hours of cessation, the amount of carboxyhaemoglobin and the deleterious cardiovascular effects of nicotine are markedly reduced. Initially after stopping, patients may experience an increase in cough and airway reactivity, but this tends to reduce after a few weeks. Preoperative physiotherapy should be considered for patients with significant respiratory disease undergoing surgery.

20 Nutrition and fluid therapy

Nandini Rao

Multiple choice questions

Physiology

1. Which of the following statements are true?

A Following a 12-hour fast, plasma insulin rises.

B The liver stores all of the glycogen in the body.

C Proteins and fats are broken down when starvation is prolonged.

D Except in trauma and sepsis, breakdown of protein can be prevented by administration of glucose.

E Energy expenditure is higher in starvation.

Nutritional assessment

2. Which of the following statements are true?

A Serum albumin is not a measure of nutritional status.

B Unintentional weight loss of > 20% in the preceding 6 months is indicative of a poor outcome.

C Body mass index (BMI) is a better indicator than weight in critically ill patients.

D Anthropometry is an indirect measure of energy and protein stores.

E A Malnutrition universal screening tool (MUST) score of 1 suggests a high risk of malnutrition.

Fluids and electrolytes

3. Which of the following statements are true?

A Bilious secretions have electrolyte contents similar to normal serum.

B Gastric outlet obstruction can cause hypochloraemic metabolic alkalosis.

C An infusion of 5% dextrose provide an electrolyte content similar to plasma.

D Albumin infusions are helpful when the haematocrit is < 30%.

E A normal adult requires 50 mmol/day of potassium.

Nutritional requirements

4. Which of the following statements are false?

A Most stable patients in hospital require 20–30 kcal/kg per day.

B The physiological maximum for glucose oxidation is 4 mg/kg per day.

C Essential fatty acids are made by the body.

D Providing energy as a mixture of glucose and fat is preferred.

E Protein requirements decline during periods of metabolic stress.

Fluid and nutritional consequences of intestinal resection

5. Which of the following statements are true?

A Normally bowel motility is significantly lower in the ileum than in the jejunum.

B Resection of 50% of the proximal jejunum causes fluid, electrolyte and nutritional imbalances.

C Short bowel syndrome occurs when > 200 cm of short bowel is resected with a colectomy.

D Patients with a jejunostomy must be encouraged to drink plain water to overcome losses.

E Renal stones may occur in short bowel syndrome.

Artificial nutritional support

6. Which of the following statements are true?

A Any patient who has inadequate intake for 5 to 7 days must be considered for nutritional support.

B Polymeric feeds contain intact protein.
C If the requirement for enteral feeding exceeds 1 week, then percutaneous endoscopic gastrostomy (PEG) is preferred to the nasogastric (NG) route.
D Jejunostomy feeding is associated with reduced aspiration.
E Diarrhoea occurs in more than 30% of patients receiving enteral nutrition.

B TPN is best delivered via a dedicated central venous catheter.
C Patients on TPN have lower hospital length of stay when compared to enteral nutrition.
D A weight gain of more than 3 kg per day suggests fluid retention.
E Abnormalities in liver function tests are common with TPN usage.

Total parenteral nutrition

7. Which of the following statements are true?

A Total parenteral nutrition (TPN) should be offered to malnourished who have an inappropriate or disrupted gastrointestinal tract.

Extended matching questions

Nutritional screening and care planning using the Malnutrition Universal Screening Tool (MUST)

1 Consider parenteral nutrition.
2 High risk of refeeding syndrome and requires slow calorie replacement.
3 Increase oral/enteral nutrition.
4 MUST score is low and the patient can be observed.
5 MUST score is medium and repeat screen on a monthly basis.

Match the options of nutritional requirements with the following scenarios:

A A 47-year-old male is admitted with acute renal failure. He is HIV positive and is on antiretroviral medications. He was recently recruited into a clinical trial and started on trial medication. He has been unwell since and has noticed blood in his urine and low urine output. His BMI is 20. He has been unable to eat properly for 1 week because of a poor appetite.
B A 79-year-old female suffers from depression and long-standing arthritis. She used to weigh 66 kg 6 months ago and is now 62 kg. Her BMI is 22.
C A young man has undergone extensive bowel resection for Crohn's disease 2 days ago. He is in intensive care and his BMI is 25. Blood test shows Na 142 mmol/L, K 3.7 mmol/L, urea 8.9 mmol/L and creatinine 98 µmol/L.
D An 18-year-old girl presents to A&E having collapsed at home. She is very slim and has a BMI of 15. She is weak, thin and has poor dentition, nails and hair. Systemic examination is normal. Blood tests show Na 142 mmol/L, K 2.2 mmol/L, urea 6 mmol/L, creatinine 50 µmol/L and glucose 6.7 mmol/L.
E A 70-year-old female with a past history of large bowel cancer has recently moved to a care home and staff is concerned that she may be malnourished. Her BMI is 25. Her appetite is normal and there is no history of weight loss.

Answers to multiple choice questions

1. C, D

When fasting exceeds 24 hours, gluconeogenesis takes place in the liver. Amino acids such as glutamine and alanine are broken down in skeletal muscles followed by breakdown of fat to generate ketone bodies, which the brain begins to adapt and use as an energy fuel. Fats provide 10 kcal/g, while proteins and carbohydrates provide 4 kcal/g. In simple starvation, muscle breakdown can be reduced by providing calories in the form of glucose. The typical responses to starvation are low plasma insulin, hepatic glycogenolysis, protein catabolism, hepatic gluconeogenesis, protein catabolism and adaptive ketogenesis. In contrast, stress and trauma cause increases in adrenaline, growth hormone, cortisol and more, and associated insulin resistance and glucose intolerance.

The liver stores nearly 200 g of glycogen. When this runs out and starvation continues, muscle glycogen is broken down to lactate, which in turn is converted to glucose in the liver (Cori's cycle). Muscles contain about 500 g of glycogen. Starvation brings about reduced resting energy expenditure from 25–30 kcal/kg per day to 15–20 kcal/kg per day.

2. A, D, E

While low serum albumin levels can reflect poor dietary intake, its levels are affected by liver disease, fluid balance and renal loss. Further, its half-life is long (1 month). Proteins with shorter half-lives, such as transthyretin and retinol-binding proteins, are likely to be better markers of poor intake or absorption. Measurement of mid-arm circumference gives an indication of tissue bulk, and skin-fold thickness gives an indication of fat stores. Serially and appropriately measured, they are good markers of nutritional status.

MUST is a five-step screening tool to identify adults who are malnourished or at risk of malnutrition (**Table 20.1**).

Steps 1 and 2: Gather nutritional measurements (height, weight, BMI and recent unintentional weight loss).

Step 3: Consider the effect of acute disease.

Step 4: Determine the overall risk score or category of malnutrition.

Step 5: Form an appropriate care plan using management guidelines.

Table 20.1 'MUST' score and suggested management guidelines for adults

MUST score (BMI + weight loss + acute disease effect)	Overall risk of malnutrition	Action
2 or more	High	**Treat** – Unless detrimental or no benefit from nutritional support (e.g., terminal illness).
1	Medium	**Observe** – Or treat if approaching high risk or if rapid clinical deterioration is anticipated.
0	Low	**Routine care** – Unless major clinical deterioration expected.

Source: Adapted from http://www.bapen.org.uk.

Unintentional weight loss of 10% in the preceding 6 months is indicative of a poor outcome and is a tool used in MUST. A BMI <18.5 suggests nutritional impairment, whereas a BMI of <15 is associated with hospital mortality. However, it is affected by changes in fluid balance, post op, dialysis and critical illness, making it unreliable in these circumstances.

3. A, B, E
Bile and ileal secretions are similar to serum electrolyte concentration and contain approximately 140 mmol/L of sodium, 5 mmol/L of potassium and 100 mmol/L of chloride. Pancreatic fluid is rich in bicarbonate secretions. Anion gap is the difference between anion and cation in plasma: (Na + K) – (HCO3 – Cl). It is normally <16 mmol/L. In gastric outlet obstruction, vomiting causes a loss in chloride and the kidneys conserve HCO3 to maintain the anion gap. Gastric secretions are rich in potassium. A normal adult requires 50 mmol of potassium per day and an estimated 30–40 ml/kg of maintenance fluids.

An infusion of 5% dextrose is a source of water replacement with modest calorie supplement (1L of 5% dextrose contains 400 kcal), hence the need to supplement with potassium. If the haematocrit is <21% then blood transfusion is required. There is no role for albumin infusion.

4. C, E
Essential fatty acids such as linoleic and linolenic acid cannot be synthesized in vivo and have to be provided. Protein and hence nitrogen requirements increase during metabolic stress to 0.20–0.25 g/kg per day (normal is 0.10–0.15 g/kg per day). However, provision of nitrogen in excess of 14 g per day is unlikely to be beneficial.

Patients with normal or moderately increased needs require 20–30 kcal/kg per day. Total calorie intake in excess of 2000 kcal per day is rarely required. Up to 1500 kcal per day (4mg/kg/minute) of glucose can be oxidised. Non-oxidised glucose is converted to fat. Avoidance of hyperglycaemia is essential and a mixture of glucose and fat 'dual energy' is provided in all types of feeds. This minimizes fluid retention and metabolic complication related to nutrition.

5. A, C, E
The ileocaecal valve slows transit through the ileum, and gut motility is three times longer here than the jejunum. Loss of even 100 cm of ileum causes increased gastric motility, peptic ulceration, increased intestinal transit and steatorrhoea, as the colon receives bile salts (further reducing its ability to reabsorb water). Patients with short bowel syndrome and jejunostomy are divided into the following: Net absorbers, which have >100 cm of residual jejunum and conserve water and sodium better; Net secretors, which have <100 cm of residual jejunum and conserve water and sodium poorly. Renal complications of short bowel syndrome include hyperoxalurea and renal stones as a result of increased intestinal absorption of oxalate.

In health, if the jejunal cellular junctions are leaky fluid absorption is inefficient. Resection of the proximal jejunum results in no alteration in fluid and electrolyte levels, as the ileum and colon perform this function more efficiently. Jejunostomy losses can exceed 4L/day. If hypotonic fluids (tea, water) are consumed, there is net efflux of sodium from plasma into the bowel lumen, worsening outputs from the bowel. Patients are encouraged to take glucose and saline replacement solutions, which contain at least 90 mmol/L of sodium.

Unintentional weight loss of 10% in the preceding 6 months is indicative of a poor outcome and is a tool used in MUST. A BMI <18.5 suggests nutritional impairment, whereas a BMI of <15 is associated with hospital mortality. However, it is affected by changes in fluid balance, post op, dialysis and critical illness, making it unreliable in these circumstances.

6. A, B, D, E
Patients with sustained inadequate intake for 5 to 7 days or lesser period in persons with pre-existing malnutrition must be considered for artificial nutritional support. Nutritional support by enteral means through oral supplementation (sip feeding) or NG/PEG or feeding via the

duodenum or jejunum is considered. All feeds vary with respect to their energy content, osmolality, fat, nitrogen content and nutrient composition. Polymeric feeds contain intact protein and hence require digestion. Monomeric or elemental feeds contain nitrogen in the form of peptides or free amino acids.

When enteral feeding is required for prolonged periods (4 to 6 weeks) then a PEG is considered because it minimises complications related to NG feeding. Rarely necrotising fasciitis, intra-abdominal abscess formation and persistent gastric fistula are the potential problems associated with PEG. Jejunostomy enables post-pyloric feeding and may be associated with reduced aspiration and enhanced tolerance to enteral nutrition.

7. A, B, E

Patients with an inaccessible or nonfunctional gastrointestinal tract require TPN. For short-term feeding (e.g., < 30 days) a non-tunnelled subclavian line and for long-term feeding a tunnelled line is used. Intrahepatic cholestasis, hepatic steatosis and hepatomegaly are commonly reported with TPN usage. Reducing the fat content of TPN may help. If a patient continues to deteriorate, temporary discontinuation works. Other metabolic complications with TPN are overfeeding, hyperglycaemia and peripheral insulin resistance.

Patients on TPN are at risk of complications related to the central line, sepsis, overfeeding and nutrient deficiencies. Parenteral nutrition is associated with longer length of hospital stay. A weight gain of > 1 kg per day suggests fluid retention.

Answers to extended matching questions

➡ ## Nutritional screening and care planning using the MUST tool

1. C Consider parenteral nutrition

TPN is the provision of nutrition by means of the intravenous route without the use of the gastrointestinal tract. The most common indication is nutritional support for patients who have undergone massive resection of the small intestine, who have intestinal fistula or prolonged intestinal failure.

Complications of TPN are related to the following:

Nutrient deficiencies – Hypoglycaemia, hypocalcaemia, hypophosphataemia, or refeeding syndrome, mineral and trace element deficiencies.

Overfeeding – Excess glucose in feeds cause hyperglycaemia, hyperosmolar dehydration, hepatic steatosis, fluid retention and electrolyte abnormalities. Excess fat can cause hypercholesterolemia and raised triglycerides. Excess amino acids are associated with acidosis and uraemia.

Sepsis – Catheter-related sepsis and an increased predisposition to systemic sepsis are well-recognised complications.

Central venous catheter – At the time of central line insertion, there is an increased risk of pneumothorax, air embolism, thoracic duct damage, pleural effusion and cardiac tamponade. Long-term usage could predispose to occlusion and venous thromboembolism.

2. D High risk of refeeding syndrome and requires slow calorie replacement

Refeeding syndrome occurs when the body switches from a catabolic state to an anabolic state, resulting in transcellular shifts of electrolytes and nutrients. The following conditions predispose to the development of refeeding syndrome.

Patient has **one or more** of the following:

- BMI less than 16 kg/m².
- Unintentional weight loss greater than 15% within the last 3 to 6 months.

- Little or no nutritional intake for more than 10 days.
- Low levels of potassium, phosphate or magnesium prior to feeding.

Or

Patient has **two or more** of the following:

- BMI less than 18.5 kg/m².
- Unintentional weight loss greater than 10% within the last 3 to 6 months.
- Little or no nutritional intake for more than 5 days.
- A history of alcohol abuse or drugs including insulin, chemotherapy, antacids, or diuretics.

http://www.nice.org.uk/CG032NICEguideline

Patients at high risk of refeeding syndrome must be identified and prescribed 10 kcal/kg per day, increasing calories slowly to meet full nutritional requirements in four to seven days. Using half the calories suggested may be required in extreme cases. Oral thiamine is always replaced before and during the first 10 days of feeding to prevent the onset of Wernicke's encephalopathy, related to Vitamin B1 deficiency.

3. A Increase oral/enteral nutrition

Generally a patient with a MUST score of < 2 can be observed, whereas those with a score > 2 should be treated, preferably by the enteral route.

Acute disease effect such as following elective procedures, sepsis, pancreatitis, acute renal failure and major surgery are all additional stress factors that increase the risk of malnutrition. Poor oral intake due to depression, polypharmacy, nausea and inadequate or poor quality of foods are additional risk factors.

4. B MUST score is low and the patient can be observed

The patient has lost around 6% of her body weight but her BMI is normal and she does not have any acute illness. Hence her MUST score is 1 and she has medium risk of malnutrition.

5. E MUST score is medium and repeat screen on a monthly basis

MUST is a rapid, simple and general procedure that can be used by medical, nursing, or other health professional staff who come in contact with a patient. Screening may need to be repeated as a subject's clinical and nutritional problems change, especially as they move though care settings.

21 Postoperative care

Tessa Housden

Multiple choice questions

→ **System-specific postoperative complications**

1. Which of the following answers regarding post-op respiratory complications are false?

A Delivery of oxygen is the first line of management to a drowsy patient who is snoring, with oxygen saturations of 85% in the first line of management.

B Hypoxia in recovery is always caused by atelectasis.

C Adequate analgesia following abdominal or thoracic surgery is vital to ensure adequate ventilation and clearance of secretions.

D Patients with pre-existing lung disease are more vulnerable to respiratory complications post-operatively.

E Early mobilisation helps to reduce postoperative respiratory complication.

2. Which of the following answers regarding deep vein thrombosis (DVT) are true?

A All types of surgical procedure increase the risk of DVT equally.

B DVTs are more likely in patients with malignancy.

C With preventative treatment, DVTs are rare in the postoperative period.

D DVTs are simple to diagnose.

E Epidural and spinal anaesthesia are protective against lower limb DVTs.

3. Which of the following answers regarding hypotension are false?

A Hypotension is only important if urine output drops below 30mL/hour.

B Hypotension associated with epidural use is always due to sympathetic blockade.

C Mean arterial pressure is equal to cardiac output multiplied by systemic vascular resistance.

D Mean arterial pressure above 60 mmHg is adequate.

E Bleeding always causes a fall in blood pressure.

4. Which of the following answers regarding postoperative bleeding are true?

A Postoperative bleeding can be difficult to diagnose.

B Postoperative bleeding is not significant unless Hb drops below 8g/dL.

C Patients should be resuscitated with warmed fluids where possible.

D Postoperative bleeding is only significant if losses are over 1 L.

E Patients should have a valid group and save prior to major surgery.

5. Which of the following answers regarding postoperative renal complications are false?

A Renal failure increases mortality in the postoperative period.

B Acute renal failure is associated with a creatinine of over 150 L.

C Patients are more likely to go into retention if they have had a spinal anaesthetic.

D Comorbidities such as diabetes and cardiovascular disease increase the risk of acute renal failure.

E All patients should have urea and electrolytes checked postoperatively.

→ General postoperative problems and management

6. Which of the following answers regarding postoperative nausea and vomiting (N&V) are true?

A Patients need anti-emetics routinely in the perioperative period to prevent N&V.

B N&V is more frequent in thin patients.

C Vomiting may cause the patient to aspirate.

D Adequate pain relief with multimodal analgesia helps to prevent N&V.

E The risk of N&V does not vary with the procedure performed.

Extended matching questions

→ Diagnoses

1 Anaphylaxis
2 Abdominal compartment syndrome (ACS)
3 Acute respiratory distress syndrome (ARDS)
4 Deep vein thrombosis (DVT)
5 Hypovolaemic shock
6 Local anaesthetic toxicity
7 Pulmonary embolus
8 Renal failure
9 Sepsis
10 Fat embolism

Match the diagnoses with the clinical scenarios that follow:

→ Clinical scenarios

A A fit 35-year-old man fell from a second floor balcony and sustained a severe blunt upper abdominal trauma. He had a splenectomy for ruptured spleen and partial hepatectomy for torn liver. On the third postoperative day he became oliguric, had cardiorespiratory compromise, type 2 respiratory failure and gross abdominal distension.

B A frail 75-year-old woman, ASA category 3, underwent an Ivor Lewis with pain control managed with an epidural. On the first postoperative evening, the nurses have been worried as the patient has been agitated and confused. They call you urgently following an epidural top up, as the patient is convulsing.

C A 60-year-old man underwent an emergency laparotomy for ischaemic bowel. On the second postoperative day, while still in ITU, his urinary output has reduced to 10 mL an hour. The catheter is not blocked.

D A 55-year-old female nurse is admitted with right upper quadrant pain. She undergoes a difficult laparoscopic cholecystectomy. At the end of the operation, a urinary catheter is inserted prior to extubation. Soon afterwards the patient's blood pressure drops to 50/30 mmHg, her heart rate is 170/minute and she becomes difficult to ventilate.

E A 65-year-old woman had a hip replacement 10 days ago. She is ready to be discharged. She went to the toilet just prior to leaving the ward for home. She collapsed in the toilet.

F A 66-year-old man underwent laparotomy, pancreatic necrosectomy, feeding jejunostomy and drainage of the lesser sac in severe acute pancreatitis with infected pancreatic necrosis. In ITU he is intubated and ventilated but remains hypoxic despite increasing inspired oxygen concentrations. Chest x-ray shows diffuse bilateral infiltrates.

G A 60-year-old man of ASA 1 anaesthetic risk underwent a total gastrectomy for cancer stomach. While in the ITU, 12 hours postoperatively, his blood pressure has fallen to 80 mm Hg systolic, he is peripherally cold and his capillary refill time is 5 seconds. You note he has been oliguric for the last 3 hours.

H A 62-year-old man underwent an anterior resection for rectal carcinoma. On the first postoperative day he has a pyrexia of 39°C and a swollen, tender right calf with shiny skin.

I A 35-year-old woman underwent an emergency appendicectomy for acute perforated appendicitis. Having had an uneventful appendicectomy and being discharged home after 2 days, she returned to hospital 1 week later feverish with a temperature of 41°C, lower abdominal pain and a tachycardia. She looks ill and toxic.

J A fit 28-year-old motorcyclist involved in a road traffic accident was admitted with a femoral fracture and a fracture-dislocation of his elbow treated by internal fixation. On the second postoperative day he is hypoxic, confused, and agitated and has developed a petechial rash.

Answers to multiple choice questions

1. A, B
Respiratory complications are common postoperatively. Risks are higher in those with pre-existing respiratory disease and obesity, and those having abdominal or thoracic procedures. The anaesthetist will identify high-risk patients and an epidural may be sited to achieve excellent analgesia without the sedative effects of opioids. Adequate analgesia is vital to prevent atelectasis and pneumonia by enabling the patient to expand his or her lungs and clear secretions. Early mobilisation and chest physiotherapy has been shown to reduce respiratory complications postoperatively.

Hypoxia in recovery has a number of causes, and an anaesthetist must review the patient urgently. If there are signs of partial obstruction (snoring), the airway must first be opened using a jaw thrust or head-tilt chin-lift manouvre before oxygen therapy should be administered. Nasopharyngeal and oropharyngeal airways are useful to maintain the airway. Oxygen is useful only if the airway is patent.

2. B, E
DVTs are common, underdiagnosed and cause many preventable deaths each year. The risk of DVT is increased for all patients in the postoperative period. The exact risk is multifactorial and depends on patient factors (e.g., obesity, increasing age, pregnancy, malignancy, dehydration), type of surgery (trauma > abdominal > cardiothoracic) and anaesthetic factors (regional technique). The use of epidural and spinal anaesthesia reduces the risk of DVT. The sympathetic blockade causes vasodilatation, which improves blood flow and reduces pooling in the legs.

It is important to identify risk factors in each patient and prescribe appropriate DVT prophylaxis. Prophylaxis may be physical, using calf compression stockings, or pharmacological. No one method is foolproof and DVTs occur despite preventive measures. DVTs may present with unilateral leg swelling, tenderness and redness. However, most show only subtle signs or are completely asymptomatic. A duplex ultrasound or venography is necessary to make the diagnosis.

3. A, B, D, E
Hypotension in the postoperative period is commonplace and the causes are extensive. It causes a reduction in tissue perfusion, which may cause organ dysfunction if left untreated. Urine output (UO) can be used to assess kidney perfusion. Kidney perfusion is adequate if an hourly urine volume exceeds 0.5 mL/kg; therefore a urine output of 30 mL/hour is only acceptable if the patient weighs less than 60 kg.

Hypertensive patients are used to higher perfusion pressures, therefore, even 'normal' mean arterial pressures (MAP) may be inadequate. Young patients are particularly good at compensating for hypovolaemia, and haemorrhage and hypotension can be a late sign. Blood pressure may only drop after significant losses (up to 30% of blood volume) have occurred.

It is useful to consider the following:

MAP = cardiac output (CO) x systemic vascular resistance (SVR)

CO = stroke volume (SV) x heart rate (HR)

Therefore:

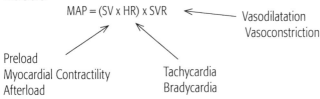

$$MAP = (SV \times HR) \times SVR$$

Vasodilatation

Vasoconstriction

Preload

Myocardial Contractility

Afterload

Tachycardia

Bradycardia

4. A, C, E

Postoperative bleeding can be frank or occult. Patients who are high risk for bleeding or who are undergoing major surgery should have Group and Save samples taken. If the patient needs fluid resuscitation, appropriate warmed fluids (crystalloid, colloid, or blood products) should be used where possible to try to prevent coagulopathy.

The question of when to transfuse is controversial. Historically, patients with ischaemic heart disease have been transfused to a haemoglobin (Hb) of 10 g/dL, and those without were transfused to a Hb of 8 g/dL. Recently, the trigger for transfusion in healthy asymptomatic individuals has been lowered to 7 g/dL. Blood products carry the risk of both morbidity and mortality, and so pros and cons should be considered for each patient.

When thinking about the 'significance' of losses, one must calculate the proportion of circulating blood that has been lost. Total blood volume = Weight (kg) x 70.

5. B, E

Evidence shows that acute renal failure adversely affects clinical outcome, increasing morbidity and mortality. High-risk patients must be identified and steps taken to try to prevent acute renal injury. Patients at particular risk are those with diabetes, pre-existing renal disease, heart failure, liver failure and those on nephrotoxic medication. These patients must have urea and electrolytes monitored postoperatively. This monitoring is not indicated for healthy patients attending for minor procedures, who are able to tolerate oral fluids soon after surgery.

An increase in serum creatinine of 1.5 times baseline or a 25% drop in eGFR indicate real injury and Stage I renal failure. It is vital that reversible causes be corrected and fluid balance be optimised.

Spinal and epidural anaesthesia puts patients at higher risk of urinary retention. These patients are often managed with a short-term urinary catheter.

6. C, D

With advancement in anaesthetic drugs and techniques, the rate of postoperative nausea and vomiting (PONV) has decreased. Patient factors (female sex, obesity, nonsmoker, motion sickness), anaesthetic factors (use of opioids) and surgical factors (squint correction, ear operations, GI manipulation) all contribute to risk. If patients are considered low risk, routine prophylaxis with antiemetics is not necessary.

Although the risk of PONV is increased with opioid analgesia, pain itself is a cause of nausea and vomiting. A multimodal approach to analgesia is important, as simple analgesics like paracetamol and non-steroidal anti-inflammatory drugs have opiate-sparing effects. A multimodal approach must also be adopted to treat PONV. Choose a combination of anti-emetics that work at different receptors in those at high risk or suffering from PONV.

Answers to extended matching questions

→ ## Scenario A: Abdominal compartment syndrome (No. 2)

Normal intra-abdominal pressure is approximately 5-7 mmHg. Abdominal compartment syndrome (ACS) occurs at intra-abdominal pressures >20 mmHg associated with new organ dysfunction. Adequate perfusion pressure to abdominal organs is required to maintain normal function. Abdominal organ perfusion pressure can be calculated as the mean arterial pressure (MAP) minus the intra-abdominal pressure.

Presentation is vague, but abdominal pain and distension are features combined with the following:

Cardiovascular:	Respiratory:
↓ Venous return, cardiac output	↑ Atelectasis, PaCO2, V/Q mismatching
↑ Systemic and pulmonary vascular resistance	↓ PaO2

Gastrointestinal:	Renal:
↓ Organ perfusion	↓ Renal perfusion
↑ Bacterial translocation	↓ Urine output

Diagnosis is difficult and a high degree of clinical suspicion is important. Patients considered at high risk should have intra-abdominal pressures monitored. Patients are at high risk if they fulfill two or more of the following:

• Diminished abdominal wall compliance (e.g., abdominal surgery with tight wound closure)
• Increased intra-luminal contents (e.g, ileus)
• Increased abdominal contents (e.g., ascites)
• Capillary leak/fluid resusciation (e.g., pancreatitis, trauma, burns)

Management is either supportive or surgical. Supportive treatment involves measures to increase cardiac output and reduce intra-abdominal pressure to ensure organ perfusion pressure >60mm Hg. A combination of inotropes and fluid resuscitation (aiming for normovolaemia) is used to boost MAP.

Surgical decompression by means of a laparotomy may be necessary if supportive treatment fails. For those at risk of ACS undergoing a laparotomy, consideration to leaving the abdomen open in the first instance should be undertaken. For patients who have developed ACS, decompression occurs as an emergency procedure.

→ ## Scenario B: Local anaesthetic toxicity (No. 6)

Local anaesthetic (LA) toxicity may manifest itself with predominant central nervous (CNS) system or cardiovascular (CVS) effects. Signs and symptoms are a result of sodium channel blockade and include tinnitus, dizziness, circumoral numbness, drowsiness, convulsions, apnoea, ECG changes, bradycardia, hypotension, asystole and cardiac arrest.

LA toxicity may occur due to an accidental overdose or an inadvertent intra-vascular injection. Particular caution should be taken in patients of low body weight and dose adjustment must be undertaken. The following dose limits should not be exceeded:

Bupivacaine	2 mg/kg
Lidocaine	3 mg/kg without adrenaline
	7 mg/kg with adrenaline

If suspected LA toxicity occurs, take the following steps:

- Stop giving LA.
- Call for urgent help (including anaesthetics).
- ABC pattern of resuscitation.
- Treat convulsions/arrhythmias.
- Reassess and monitor for circulatory arrest.
- Arrange for safe transfer to ICU.

Should circulatory arrest occur, cardiopulmonary resuscitation should commence according to standard protocols. Lipid emulsion therapy should be used in patients with LA toxicity who are in cardiac arrest. Guidelines for use are available on the AAGBI website, and management should be overseen by a consultant anaesthetist. Arrhythmias due to LA toxicity are often refractory to treatment and prolonged resuscitation attempts of more than one hour may be necessary. Cardiopulmonary bypass can be useful.

Scenario C: Renal failure (No. 8)

Acute kidney injury (AKI) in the perioperative period is a common complication of major surgery. AKI is associated with significant morbidity and mortality, and patients often require prolonged hospital stays. Patients may also progress to chronic renal failure and end-stage renal failure, requiring dialysis.

It is important to be proactive and identify patients at risk of AKI in the perioperative period. Risk factors can be split into patient factors and iatrogenic factors (**Table 21.1**). Urea and electrolytes should be carefully monitored in those at risk, and any deterioration in glomerular filtration rate should prompt careful patient assessment.

Table 21.1 The risk factors for acute kidney injury (AKI)

Patient risk factors	Iatrogenic risk factors
Acute	
Hypovolaemia	Cardiac surgery
Haemorrhage	Vascular surgery
Sepsis	Emergency surgery
Rhabdomyolysis	
Intra-abdominal hypertension	Nephrotoxic agents, e.g.:
	• ACE inhibitors
Chronic	• NSAIDs
	• IV contrast
Advancing age	• Aminoglycosides
Diabetes mellitus	
Chronic renal impairment	
Chronic liver failure	
Chronic heart failure	
Cardiac and Peripheral vascular disease	

The aetiology of renal failure is traditionally split into prerenal, renal and postrenal causes. In the perioperative period, prerenal and renal (most commonly acute tubular necrosis) are the most common causes of AKI. The key treatment strategies are the following:

- Appropriate intravascular volume expansion with fluids to maintain renal blood flow.
- Maintenance of renal perfusion pressure with an adequate cardiac output and blood pressure.
- Avoidance of nephrotoxic agents.
- Careful glycaemic control.
- Referral to critical care/renal physicians for appropriate management of AKI and other postoperative complications.

Scenario D: Anaphylaxis (No. 1)

Health care workers and others exposed frequently to latex are at risk of developing a Type I hypersensitivity reaction on subsequent exposure.

Anaphylaxis is likely when all three of the following criteria are met:

1. Sudden, rapidly progressing symptoms
2. Life-threatening airway or breathing or circulatory problems
3. Skin or mucosal changes

Skin and mucosal changes can be absent or subtle and do not indicate anaphylaxis if present in isolation. Gastrointestinal symptoms like vomiting and diarrhoea may also occur.

When managing a patient with anaphylaxis, an early call for help and an ABCDE approach is useful. If the trigger is apparent, it should be removed. In adults, 0.5 mg (0.5 mL of 1 in 1000 adrenaline) intramuscularly should be given and repeated every 5 minutes if the patient does not respond. Oxygen and fluid therapy should be given as soon as they are available. Bronchodilators can be useful in those presenting with asthma-like symptoms in isolation. After initial resuscitation, steroids and antihistamines can be given.

Mast cell tryptase is specific for mast cell degranulation and is helpful to confirm the diagnosis of anaphylaxis. Timing is important. Ideally, three samples should be taken but they should not delay initial resuscitation. The first sample should be at the earliest opportunity after resuscitation has commenced. The second should be 1 to 2 hours after the start of symptoms and the last should be after 24 hours. The patient should be referred to an allergy clinic in due course to try to isolate the causative allergen.

Scenario E: Pulmonary embolus (No. 7)

Venous thromboembolism (VTE) in postoperative period is common. Risk factors can be split into patient factors, surgical factors and anaesthetic factors (See **Table 21.2**). If patients are high risk, it is vital that appropriate prophylaxis is prescribed – calf compression with stockings or pneumatic devices, or anticoagulation.

Pulmonary emboli (PE) are classified into the categories nonmassive, submassive and massive. Nonmassive (70%) are often clinically silent. Submassive (25%) are haemodynamically stable but have evidence of right heart strain on echocardiography. Massive (5%) (including saddle PEs) cause haemodynamic instability, hypotension and cardiac arrest.

Table 21.2   The risk factors for pulmonary embolism

Patient factors	Surgical factors	Anaesthetic factors
Increased risk:	**Increased risk:**	**Increased risk:**
Increasing age Smoking, obesity Pregnancy Oral contraceptive use Hormone replacement therapy Immobility, trauma Malignancy Varicose veins Previous VTE Thrombophilias Genetic predisposition	All surgery especially pelvic, malignancy, trauma	Inadequate correction of hypovolaemia **Decreased risk:** Spinal anaesthesia Epidural anaesthesia

Decreased risk:

Appropriate prophylaxis

Investigations and management depend on the category of PE (See **Table 21.3**) Other than imaging, investigations include D-Dimer, arterial blood gas and electrocardiography (ECG). D-Dimer has little value in hospitalised patients, as a raised result is likely to be multifactorial and patients are unlikely to have a normal assay. ECG may show atrial fibrillation, tachycardia, R heart strain, R ventricular overload, R axis deviation, or S1Q3T3 pattern (< 20%).

➡ Scenario F: Acute respiratory distress syndrome (No. 2)

Acute lung injury (ALI) is characterised by acute severe hypoxia that is not a result of fluid overload or heart failure. ALI represents a disease spectrum, with acute respiratory distress syndrome (ARDS) being a severe form.

ARDS is a clinical and radiological diagnosis and can be difficult to differentiate from other acute lung conditions. Patients are critically ill and have acute respiratory failure, with diffuse bilateral infiltrates on chest x-ray (noncardiogenic pulmonary oedema). There is a genetic predisposition to ARDS, which is triggered by the following direct and indirect causes:

Direct:	Indirect:
Pneumonia	Sepsis
Aspiration	Blood transfusion
Pulmonary embolism	Trauma
Drowning	Pancreatitis
Pulmonary contusion	Burns

Diagnostic criteria include the following:

- Acute onset
- Bilateral infiltrates on CXR consistent with pulmonary oedema
- Clinical absence of left atrial hypertension/fluid overload
- Hypoxaemia with PaO2/FiO2 < 40 for ALI or < 27 for ARDS

Table 21.3 Categories of pulmonary embolism

Category of PE	Diagnosis	Management
Massive	Bedside urgent echocardiography	CPR if cardiac arrest Resuscitation Thrombolysis
Submassive	CTPA Echocardiography	Anticoagulant therapy (e.g., heparin) Thrombolysis should be considered
Non-massive	CTPA	Anticoagulant therapy

The mainstay of treatment is supportive care within a critical care environment. Conservative fluid management is necessary as excessive fluid therapy causes gas exchange to deteriorate. This is due to increased capillary permeability causing pulmonary oedema. Corticosteroids have been in and out of favour, but current evidence suggests no survival benefit.

The majority of patients with ARDS will be mechanically ventilated. An intensivist should manage ventilator settings and aims are to optimise oxygenation whilst preventing ventilator-induced lung trauma. Prone positioning, nitric oxide and oscillatory ventilation are all treatment strategies used in sicker patients. If patients fail to respond, extracorporeal membrane oxygenation (ECMO) has been used for patients with life-threatening hypoxaemia.

→ ## Scenario G: Hypovolaemic shock (No. 5)

Surgical patients are often hypovolaemic. They may have inadequate intake or excessive losses, or be bleeding postoperatively. Hypovolaemic shock can be categorised in the four following stages (See **Table 21.4**).

An ABCDE approach is useful. If there are concerns, help should be called and the patient should be fully monitored. If critical care or theatre is needed, these departments should be alerted urgently. Wide-bore intravenous access should be placed and blood should be taken for full blood count, urea and electrolytes, coagulation screen and group and save.

The cause of hypovolaemia or haemorrhage should be sought whilst fluid resuscitation is underway. Aggressive resuscitation should be undertaken if the patient is shocked, and boluses of 10 mL/kg warmed crystalloid should be started and the patient monitored for his response. If there is significant bleeding, a cross match should be arranged.

Treatment goals include a urine output of >0.5 mL/kg, a mean arterial blood pressure of >65 mmHg and a central venous pressure of 8–12 mmHg.

→ ## Scenario H: Deep vein thrombosis (No. 4)

Patients are at high risk for venous thromboembolism in the postoperative period. Surgical patients should have their risk of thromboembolism assessed on admission, and appropriate prophylaxis must be prescribed. Many patients are asymptomatic or have only very subtle symptoms and signs. Others have a warm, red, swollen, painful calf. The most serious complication of a DVT is a pulmonary embolus, which can be life threatening. About one-third of DVTs are complicated by post-thrombotic leg syndrome, characterised by leg pain, swelling and skin ulcers.

Table 21.4   The stages of shock

Stage of shock	Clinical findings
Stage 1: 0%–15% losses	Well compensated especially in young patients Normal HR, BP, RR Normal capillary refill time Normal urine output
Stage 2: 15%–30% losses	↑ HR and RR Normal systolic BP, ↑ diastolic BP Cool clammy skin, ↑ capillary refill time ↓ urine output
Stage 3: 30%–40% losses	HR ↑ and RR ↑ BP < 100 mmHg systolic Cold sweaty skin, capillary refill time ↑ Anxious, altered mental status
Stage 4: > 40% losses	HR ↑ pulse feels weak BP ↓ ↓ conscious level Extreme pallor Absent capillary refill No urine output

The diagnosis is made using imaging. The gold standard is contrast venography, however, this is rarely performed, as it is invasive and expensive. Other options include ultrasound scans (proximal compression ultrasound, whole-leg ultrasound, or Doppler ultrasound), or CT/MRI venography.

Currently, the mainstay of treatment is anticoagulation.

→ Scenario I: Sepsis (No. 9)

Sepsis is common in the perioperative period, and early recognition and goal directed treatment is vital to improve patient outcomes. Sepsis is systemic inflammatory response syndrome (SIRS) in response to a known or likely infection. SIRS is present if two or more of the following criteria are met:

- Temperature < 36°C or > 38°C
- Heart rate > 90 beats per minute
- Respiratory rate > 20 breaths per minute
- White cells < 4 x 10^9/L or > 12 x 10^9/L

Sepsis is further categorised into severe sepsis and septic shock. Severe sepsis is sepsis with sepsis-induced organ dysfunction. Septic shock is severe sepsis with tissue hypoperfusion that is unresponsive to fluid resuscitation.

Organ dysfunction can progress to multi-organ dysfunction:

- Lungs: Acute lung injury and adult respiratory distress syndrome
- Heart: Hypotension and reduction in contractility
- Kidneys: Acute kidney injury, oliguria and renal failure
- Brain: Agitiation, delirium
- Liver: Disorders of coagulation

Early treatment and referral to critical care is vital. The surviving sepsis campaign bundle (Box 21.1) is used in the U.K. to aid treatment:

Box 21.1   The following should be completed within 3 hours:

1. Measure lactate level.
2. Obtain blood cultures prior to administration of antibiotics.
3. Administer broad-spectrum antibiotics.
4. Administer 30mL/kg crystalloid for hypotension or lactate > 4mmol/L

The following should be completed within 6 hours:

5. Apply vasopressors to maintain mean arterial pressure > 65mmHg.
6. In the event of persistent hypotension despite volume resuscitation (septic shock) or initial lactate > 4mmol/L:
   a. Measure central venous pressure (target >8 mmHg).
   b. Measure central venous oxygen saturations (target >70%).
7. Remeasure lactate if initial lactate was elevated.

Source: Reprinted from Dellinger, RP, Levy, MM, Rhodes, A. et al. 2013. *Crit Care Med.*, 41:580–637.

→ Scenario J: Fat embolism (No. 10)

The majority (95%) of fat embolism occurs after major trauma. It is most common after closed long bone and pelvic fractures. The incidence increases with the number of bones involved. Fat embolism can also occur with soft tissue trauma, liposuction and bone marrow harvest.

Fat embolism syndrome typically occurs 24 to 72 hours after major trauma. Patients present with the following typical triad:

1. Respiratory changes:
   Dyspnoea, tachypnoea, hypoxia and ARDS requiring intubation and ventilation.
2. Neurological abnormalities:
   Confusion, agitation, focal neurological signs, seizures.
3. Petechial rash:
   Occurs on upper anterior aspect of body, especially neck, axilla and conjunctiva.

Anaemia, thrombocytopenia, tachycardia and pyrexia may also be seen. Diagnosis is clinical and can be difficult, because the only pathognomonic sign is petechial rash, which is present in less than 50% of cases. Early fixation of long bones is an important prophylactic measure and methods to reduce intraosseus pressure during orthopaedic fixation have been shown to reduce fat emboli syndrome. Steroids are controversial and have been used with some success, but the mainstay of treatment is supportive care. Mortality is up to 15%.

Day case surgery

Sarah M Lloyd

Multiple choice questions

Day surgery selection criteria

1. Which of the following make a patient unsuitable for day surgery?

A Age over 75 years.

B American Society of Anaesthesiologists (ASA) grade 3.

C Body mass index (BMI) of 35.

D Procedure is expected to last 90 minutes.

E Journey time home of 2 hours.

Anaesthesia

2. Which of the following are suitable to be used as part of a multimodal analgesic technique for day surgery patients?

A Infiltration of the wound with short-acting local anaesthetic.

B Oral Ibuprofen given preoperatively.

C Intramuscular morphine given during the procedure.

D Oral paracetamol given preoperatively.

E Intravenous fentanyl given during the procedure.

Day surgery

3. Which of the following statements are true?

A For some specialties, 90% of procedures are suitable to be done as day cases.

B A day case is admitted and discharged within 23 hours.

C The day surgery pathway includes input from the patient's general practitioner (GP).

D Day cases should be scheduled after complex inpatient procedures on the same list.

E The choice of anaesthetic agents is less important than the skill of the anaesthetist.

Complications

4. Which of the following are true?

A Persistent nausea or vomiting are common reasons for unplanned admission after day surgery.

B Risk of reactionary haemorrhage is a reason to keep a patient in hospital overnight.

C Surgical technique, including the extent of tissue handling and tension, contributes to the risk of unplanned admission.

D Risk of secondary haemorrhage is a reason to keep patients in hospital overnight.

E Patients should be reviewed by a member of the surgical team to decide whether they are fit for discharge.

Preoperative assessment

5. The following statements are true except:

A Assessment must be carried out by the anaesthetist who is going to do the list.

B Assessment should be carried out early in the patient pathway.

C Basic health screen includes BMI, BP, past medical history and medication.

D Appropriate investigations are performed to ensure patient fitness.

E Patient and carer must be given verbal and written information.

Perioperative management

6. Which of the following statements are true?

A Day case surgery is best performed with inpatient cases on mixed lists.

B Major day case surgery should be placed early on the list.

C Multimodal approach is the key to
successful day surgery analgesia.
D Pain levels should be routinely assessed
in the recovery area.

E Long-acting local anaesthetic infiltration
helps in giving optimal analgesia.

Extended matching questions

Following is a list of operations to be done as a day case. All patients are ASA 1 or 2. Match
the operations with the analgesic scenarios that follow, bearing in mind that you may use the
same technique in more than one procedure.

→ Operations

1 Breast lump excision
2 Carpal tunnel decompression
3 Circumcision
4 Fistula-in-ano – excision and laying open
5 Laparoscopic cholecystectomy
6 Laparoscopic inguinal herinorrhaphy

A One hour before surgery, oral administration of paracetamol and ibuprofen. General anaesthesia with spontaneous breathing, including a small dose of short-acting opiate, e.g., fentanyl.
Local infiltration of long-acting local anaesthetic by surgeon to wound(s).
B One hour before surgery, oral administration of paracetamol and Ibuprofen. General
anaesthesic technique with ventilation, including intravenous morphine. Local infiltration of
long-acting local anaesthetic by surgeon to wound(s).
C A nerve block carried out by the anaesthetist or surgeon, using a mixture of short- and long-
acting local anaesthetic agents.
D General anaesthesia, using a small dose of short-acting opiate, e.g., fentanyl. A nerve block
using long-acting local anaesthetic carried out at the beginning of the procedure.

Answers to multiple choice questions

1. E

While the comfort of the journey is also important, a maximum travelling time of 1 hour is
recommended.

Modern-day surgery practice concentrates on assessing each patient as an individual.
There is no upper age limit for day surgery. ASA 3 patients with stable, well-controlled comorbidities and those with a BMI up to 40 can be successfully treated as day cases. With
minimally invasive techniques and appropriate anaesthesia, procedures lasting up to two
hours can be managed as a day case.

2. B, D, E

Multimodal analgesia where several drugs and routes are used to maximise analgesia
while minimising side effects is key to successful day case anaesthesia. Preoperative oral
medication with paracetamol and nonsteroidal anti-inflammatory drugs such as ibuprofen
are recommended. Opiates given intravenously as part of a balanced anaesthetic technique
should be short-acting drugs such as fentanyl or alfentanil.

Wound infiltration with long-acting local anaesthetic can make a significant contribution
to a patient's postoperative analgesia. The use of large doses of long-acting opiates such as
morphine carry a significant risk of postoperative complications, including sedation, nausea and

vomiting, which can result in unplanned admission. If morphine is used, small intravenous bolus doses should administered to ensure that the minimum dose is used to achieve analgesia.

3. A, C, E

In some specialties, up to 90% of procedures could be undertaken as day cases. Day surgery is a patient pathway, not a surgical procedure, and extends from first patient contact with the GP to after discharge. To ensure the highest quality outcome and reduce unplanned admissions, both the surgeon and anaesthetist have to be highly skilled in adapting techniques to individual patients and procedures.

Day surgery is defined as the admission and discharge of a patient for a procedure within the 12-hour working day; where a patient requires an overnight admission the term '23-hour stay' should be used. Mixed lists of inpatients and day cases are not ideal. However, if they are planned, the day cases should be operated on first allowing time for recovery and reducing the risk of unplanned admission.

4. A, C

Nausea and vomiting are common following surgery and the management of postoperative pain needs to be managed actively to reduce the incidence of unplanned admission. However, such factors remain a significant cause of patients being unable to go home. Meticulous surgical technique with attention to haemostasis and minimising tissue handling is essential for successful day surgery.

The risk of postoperative haemorrhage is often given as a reason for not undertaking procedures as a day case. However, most reactionary haemorrhage occurs 4 to 6 hours after surgery while a day case is still in the unit, and secondary haemorrhage occurs after 24 hours when even an overnight stay patient will have been discharged home. While postoperative review by the surgical team is encouraged, the assessment of when a patient is fit for discharge is best done by trained day surgery nurses using strict discharge criteria.

5. A

The assessment does not need to be made by the specific anaesthetist who is going to do the list. Dedicated specialist nursing teams with anaesthetic support are allocated to do the assessment, which should be carried out early in the patient pathway. Basic health screen includes BMI, blood pressure, past medical history and current drug history. Appropriate investigations, such full blood count and biochemistry, are carried out along with an ECG if clinically indicated. Finally the patient and the carer should be given verbal information, which should be doubled up with written confirmation. The latter is particularly important, as most patients retain only a part of the information imparted to them at the consultation. Written guidelines are an essential part of day case surgery.

6. B, C, D, E

Major operations on a day case basis should be placed early on the list to enable the patient maximum recovery time. Multimodal analgesia should be planned and started from the preoperative period (see the following section); this may be supplemented by long-acting local anaesthetic to the incision site.

Pain levels should be assessed routinely in the recovery room and appropriately treated. Ideally, day case surgery should not be mixed with inpatient surgery. To obtain the optimum outcome, most NHS day case lists are performed separately in a dedicated day case unit. When inpatient surgery has to be mixed with day case surgery, the day case should be scheduled first. If not, the day case may be cancelled if the complex case takes longer than expected or could result in an unplanned overnight stay.

1. A Breast lump excision
Multimodal analgesia aims to achieve maximum postoperative pain relief whilst reducing the impact of side effects. Infiltration of long-acting local anaesthetic significantly reduces the need for intra and postoperative opiates.

2. C Carpal tunnel decompression
Carpal tunnel decompression is most commonly performed in an awake patient using a brachial plexus or more peripheral nerve blocks. These techniques not only provide excellent conditions for surgery but also prolonged postoperative analgesia.

3. D Circumcision
Hydrocoele repair can be carried out awake using a local anaesthetic nerve block technique (C). When it is to be under a general anaesthetic, if the same local anaesthetic block is used at the beginning the amount of anaesthetic and opiate required is minimal and patients wake pain free.

4. A Fistula-in-ano – excision and laying open
Multimodal analgesia aims to achieve maximum postoperative pain relief whilst reducing the impact of side effects. Infiltration of long-acting local anaesthetic significantly reduces the need for intra and postoperative opiates.

5. B Laparoscopic cholecystectomy
Laparoscopic cholecystectomy is a challenging procedure to manage as a day case and usually requires morphine; this is best given intravenously during the operation rather than postoperatively when nausea, vomiting, or sedation may result in an unplanned admission.

Trauma

23 Introduction to trauma

Andrew D Duckworth

Multiple choice questions

→ Trauma

1. Regarding trauma, which of the following statements are true?

A It is the fifth most common cause of death overall.

B It is the second most common cause of death and disability below 40 years of age.

C One-year mortality following a proximal femoral fracture in patients over 65 years is 30%.

D Trauma is predominantly secondary to high-energy injuries.

E < 25% of children who die of abuse have had previous contact with health or social services.

→ Assessment of trauma

2. Regarding trauma assessment, which of the following statements are false?

A The patient, mechanism of injury and injury are the keystones of management.

B It is as essential to identify obvious injuries as it is to identify the occult (hidden) injuries.

C High-velocity bullet injuries are associated with cavity formation.

D Blunt injuries can be direct (impact) or indirect (force transmission).

E Knife injury over a limb is easy to evaluate.

→ Blunt injuries

3. In relation to blunt injuries, which of the following statements are false?

A The mechanisms are direct or indirect.

B In indirect injury, associated injuries may be present and should be sought.

C In chest injuries damage to abdominal organs is rare.

D Overt injury should lead the clinician to look for a covert injury as well.

E Proper exposure is essential so as not to miss other injuries.

→ Covert injuries

4. In relation to coverts injuries, which of the following statements are true?

A A deductive approach is not necessary.

B A look-everywhere approach is not helpful.

C A focused approach that limits the scope of your assessment is not useful.

D Head to pelvis CT is part of a look-everywhere approach.

E Screen patients where clinical signs are obvious.

5. In relation to coverts injuries, which of the following statements are false?

A Electrocution = burn (obvious) and posterior dislocation of the shoulder (covert).

B Dashboard = patella fracture (obvious) and posterior dislocation of the hip (covert).

C Inhalational injury = facial burns (obvious) and laryngeal oedema (covert).

D Left-side impact RTA = left pneumothorax with chest wall contusions (obvious) and liver laceration (covert).

E Flexion-distraction = head injury (obvious) and cervical spine fracture (covert).

→ Non-accidental injuries (NAI)

6. In relation to NAI in children, which of the following statements are false?

A History is inconsistent with the injury sustained.

B There is a changing history.

C There are likely to be injuries of differing ages or duration.

D There may be aggressive behaviour from the carers.

E A femoral shaft fracture in a 6-month-old is not suspicious of NAI.

→ Polytrauma

7. Which of the following statements are false with regard to a polytrauma patient?

A A drop in body temperature occurs.

B There is a generalised immune response.

C The patient has compensatory mechanisms to blood loss.

D The early management is protocol-driven.

E Diversion from protocol should be avoided.

Answers to multiple choice questions

→ Trauma

1. C

Trauma is the most common cause of death and disability in patients below 40 years of age and is the third most common cause of death overall. Low-energy fragility fractures represent a large workload to health services, with elderly patients following simple falls being the most frequent trauma admissions in the United Kingdom. The 1-year mortality following a proximal femoral fracture in patients over 65 years of age is 30%, with approximately 70,000 proximal femoral fractures a year in the United Kingdom. Health care professionals must always be vigilant for non-accidental injury (NAI) in children, with 66% of children who die of abuse having had previous contact with health or social services.

→ Assessment of trauma

2. E

The patient, mechanism of injury and resulting injury are the keystones of trauma assessment and management (patient + mechanism = injury). It is essential to identify occult injuries, with certain injuries associated with specific covert injuries. In day-to-day practice, the two most common mechanisms of injury are blunt or penetrating injuries. Blunt injuries are routinely caused by falls, sports, or road traffic accidents and can be direct or indirect. Penetrating injuries are commonly secondary to weapons such as knives or low-velocity firearms. Low-velocity bullet injuries behave like knife injuries, whereas high-velocity bullet injuries are associated with permanent or temporary cavity formation. Knife injuries over a limb are not always easy to evaluate, as penetration of the joint may not always be obvious, with thorough assessment required if this is felt to be possible.

→ Blunt injuries

3. C

Blunt injuries are direct or indirect. In direct blunt trauma, the injury is concentrated at the site of impact and the effects on the soft tissue are at the injured site. In indirect injury, damage away from the site of injury should be sought. For example, fracture of the shaft of the ulna could be caused by direct trauma, e.g., nightstick blow to arm, or by indirect trauma, e.g., from a fall on an outstretched hand (overt injury). In this situation, there may also be a covert injury of a dislocated upper end of head of radius (Monteggia fracture-dislocation).

Anatomically, the abdominal contents extend into the chest. Therefore, in blunt trauma to the lower chest, liver and splenic injuries are common.

→ Covert injuries

4. D

Ideally screening of at-risk patients should be carried out before clinical signs are obvious (**Table 23.1**). This can be done by the deductive approach, e.g., assessing for classical covert injuries. A look-everywhere approach is essential in an unconscious patient to exclude further injury once initial life-saving assessment and management is complete. The primary survey in ATLS includes radiographs of the C-spine, chest and pelvis. The term 'secondary survey' in the ATLS protocol is part of a look-everywhere approach and the threshold for further imaging, e.g., CT head to pelvis, is now low in many centres. A focused-exclusion approach is mandatory for life-threatening injuries (e.g., CT scan in suspected extradural haematoma, echocardiography in cardiac tamponade) and non-life-threatening injuries (e.g., scaphoid fracture, posterior dislocation of the shoulder).

5. D

A left-sided impact would be associated with a splenic rupture and not a liver laceration.

→ Non-accidental injury

6. E

All health care professionals must be vigilant for NAI in children and elderly patients. Important factors to consider include the following:

- A delay in presentation.
- History inconsistent with the age of the child or injury.
- Changing history.

Table 23.1 Examples of covert injury patterns

Mechanism of injury	Obvious injuries	Covert injuries
Left-sided impact from RTA	Lateral compression fracture of pelvis Left sided pneumothorax	Splenic rupture Extradural haematoma
Right-sided impact from RTA	Lateral compression fracture of pelvis Right sided pneumothorax	Liver laceration Extradural haematoma
Electrocution	Skin burn Collapse	Posterior dislocation of the shoulder Rhabdomyolysis
Dashboard injury	Knee wound Patella fracture	Posterior dislocation of the hip
Flexion-distraction (lap belt)	Lumbar spine chance fracture Knee dislocation Head injury	Duodenal rupture Popliteal artery injury Cervical spine fracture

Source: Adapted from Table 23.1 in: Williams, N., Bulstrode, C., O'Connell, PR. (Eds.), *Bailey & Love's Short Practice of Surgery*, 26th ed., 2013.

- Aggressive behaviour of carers and abnormal interaction with child.
- Multiple fractures or injuries of different ages.
- A verbal explanation of brittle-bone disease (osteogenesis imperfecta) should not be accepted as a cause of multiple fractures, and the clinician should admit the patient for further thorough evaluation.
- Full examination reveals other signs of abuse, e.g., finger-shaped bruises.
- Posterior rib injuries.
- Long-bone fractures in a nonambulatory child.

→ Polytrauma

7. E

As a part of the metabolic response to trauma, there is a drop in body temperature, and heat loss thus should be prevented, e.g., a bear hugger. Heat loss may be due to exposure, inactivity, hypovolaemia, or loss of vasomotor control. The patient has compensatory mechanisms to blood loss with an aim to maintain perfusion of the vital organs, e.g., heart and kidneys. In most trauma cases, early management is routinely protocol-driven, which allows for easier and quicker decision making. The surgical plan will be recorded in the patient's notes, but a good method is to record all the details on a whiteboard in the theatre, outlining the proposed overall management. Whilst protocols can successfully aid the assessment and management of the patient, someone should be in the position (trauma team leader) to break protocol if it is in the best interest of the patient. Labelling of patients, e.g., 'neck of femur fracture,' should be avoided, as the focus should remain on the whole patient and pre-existing conditions and potential underlying causes need to be managed.

Early assessment and management of trauma

Andrew D Duckworth

Multiple choice questions

→ **Mechanisms of trauma**

1. Regarding mechanisms of trauma, which of the following statements are false?
   A The most common cause of blunt trauma is a motor vehicle accident (MVA).
   B A 10% increase in impact speed equates to a ~40% increase in pedestrian fatality.
   C Seat belts reduce the risk of death or serious injury for front-seat occupants by ~20%.
   D For head-on collisions, airbags reduce the risk of fatality by ~30%.
   E Motorcyclists have a higher rate of mortality than car occupants involved in a MVA.

→ **Primary survey and resuscitation**

2. Regarding airway assessment, which of the following statements are false?
   A If the patient is talking, he or she does not have an imminently compromised airway.
   B Suction of the airway may be required.
   C Nasopharyngeal and Guedal airways are useful adjuncts.
   D A GCS of 7 is not an indication for a definitive airway.
   E Cervical spine control is required throughout airway assessment and management.

3. Regarding assessing disability, which of the following can be responsible for a reduced consciousness level?
   A Head injury
   B Hypovolaemia
   C Hypoglycaemia
   D Alcohol
   E All of the above

4. Which of the following are not routine adjuncts to the primary survey?
   A Pulse oximetry.
   B Urinary catheter.
   C Bloods including FBC, U&Es, clotting screen and glucose.
   D Radiographs of the C-spine, chest and pelvis.
   E CT with or without angiography.

→ **Secondary survey**

5. Regarding the secondary survey, which of the following is not part of the AMPLE assessment?
   A Allergies
   B Medication
   C Pain assessment
   D Last meal
   E Events of the incident

→ **Paediatric trauma**

6. Regarding paediatric trauma, which of the following combination of observations are optimal for a preschool child (< 5 years of age)?
   A Pulse 160 bpm, systolic blood pressure 90, respiratory rate 40, urine output 1.5 tmL/kg/hour.
   B Pulse 160 bpm, systolic blood pressure 90, respiratory rate 40, urine output 1 mL/kg/hour.
   C Pulse 140 bpm, systolic blood pressure 80, respiratory rate 30, urine output 1 mL/kg/hour.
   D Pulse 140 bpm, systolic blood pressure 90, respiratory rate 40, urine output 1.5 mL/kg/hour.
   E Pulse 140 bpm, systolic blood pressure 90, respiratory rate 30, urine output 1.5 mL/kg/hour.

Extended matching questions

→ ## Primary survey and resuscitation

1 Cardiac tamponade
2 Haemothorax
3 Hypoglycaemia
4 Major vessel injury
5 Myocardial infarction
6 Pneumonia
7 Pneumothorax
8 Severe head injury
9 Tension pneumothorax

For each of the following cases, select the single most appropriate diagnosis from the options listed. Each option may be used once, more than once, or not at all.

A A patient presents following a fall from a third-story window and on primary survey is not maintaining adequate oxygen saturation on high-flow oxygen, is hypotensive, has a raised JVP with left tracheal deviation and the right hemi-thorax is hyper-resonant with no air entry.

B A patient with a background of known alcohol excess presents with minor abrasions to the arms but no evidence of head injury. Chest is clear and heart sounds are normal. There is a reduced GCS 9/15 (E3, V2, M4) but no evidence of haemodynamic instability. Pupils are equal and reactive.

C A patient presents with evidence of significant deep penetrating trauma at the level of the fifth/sixth inetercostal space in left hemi-thorax. The patient has a raised JVP and muffled heart sounds, and is haemodynamically unstable with a tachycardia and hypotension.

Answers to multiple choice questions

→ ## Mechanisms of trauma

1. C
Mechanisms of trauma include blunt, penetrating, blast, crush and thermal. The most common cause of blunt trauma is a motor vehicle accident (MVA), with speed of impact an important factor in determining the outcome; a 10% increase in impact speed equates to a ~40% increase in pedestrian fatality. Seat belts reduce the risk of serious injury or death for front-seat drivers or passengers by approximately 45%. Seat belt marks are associated with an increased rate of thoracic and abdominal trauma. For head-on MVA collisions, airbags do reduce the risk of fatality by almost one-third, although the airbag can be associated with injuries and children under 12 years of age should be in the rear seat with a belt on. Rear-facing infants under 1 year of age should never be in the front seat with a collision-activated airbag. Motorcyclists have a significantly higher rate of mortality and lower-extremity injuries than car occupants involved in a MVA.

→ ## Primary survey and resuscitation

2. D
The primary survey in ATLS includes:

A Airway with cervical spine control.
B Breathing and ventilation.

C Circulation with haemorrhage control.
D Disability and neurological status.
E Exposure (completely expose patient and assess for injuries).

A patient who is talking by definition has a patent airway. This does not mean it could become compromised and reassessment is paramount. Suctioning and removal of foreign bodies is an essential next step, ensuring not to push objects further down the airway. Useful airway adjuncts, if they can be tolerated by the patient, include a nasopharyngeal or Guedal airway. A patient with GCS of ≤ 8 is an indication for attaining a definitive airway, e.g., endotracheal tube. Cervical spine immobilisation is essential. It is often done manually initially and then collar, sand bags and tape are used until the C-spine can be cleared.

3. E

A prompt and thorough neurological assessment of all trauma patients is essential. This includes assessment and regular reassessment of the patient's Glasgow Come Scale (GCS), along with pupil size and reactivity. Important causes of a reduced GCS in the trauma patient include head injury, hypoperfusion secondary to hypovolaemia, hypoglycaemia and alcohol or drug abuse.

4. E

Monitoring during the primary survey should include pulse oximetry, blood pressure measurement and pulse rate. A urinary catheter is used to assess urine output, which is a useful indicator of perfusion and degree of shock. During the primary assessment, two large-bore cannulae are placed to gain intravenous access and bloods (FBC, UEs, clotting screen, glucose) and a cross match can be taken at this time. A toxicology screen should be requested at this stage if indicated. An arterial blood gas is a useful and quick adjunct that provides information on perfusion, oxygenation, haemoglobin level and electrolyte disturbance. Trauma series imaging includes primarily radiographs of the cervical spine, chest and pelvis. CT with or without angiography would routinely be part of the secondary survey once initial assessment and resuscitation has been carried out.

Secondary survey

5. C

Once the primary survey is complete, and a thorough assessment, resuscitation and reassessment of the patient has been carried out, the secondary survey can begin. In some cases, this can be days after the patient presents due to time in theatre, reduced consciousness level and time in the intensive care unit. The aim of the secondary survey is to define all the injuries sustained by the patient through a head-to-toe inspection and examination. The AMPLE mnemonic is used to review the patient's history and includes Allergies, Medication and tetanus status, Past medical history, Last meal and Events of the incident.

Paediatric trauma

6. E

Paediatric trauma assessment follows the same ABCDE pathway as adult trauma. However, one of the major differences is that the normal ranges for vital signs in the paediatric patient are different than adults and change with age (**Table 24.1**).

Table 24.1 Optimal paediatric vital signs and urine output

Age	Pulse (bpm)	Systolic blood pressure (mmHg)	Respiratory rate (breaths per minute)	Urine output (ml/kg/hour)
Infant (< 1 year)	160	80	40	2
Preschool (< 5 years)	140	90	30	1.5
Adolescent (> 10 years)	120	100	20	1

Source: Adapted from Tables 24.2 and 24.3 in: Williams, N., Bulstrode, C., O'Connell, PR. (Eds.), Bailey & Love's Short Practice of Surgery, 26th ed., 2013.

Answers to extended matching questions

→ **Primary survey and resuscitation**

A. 9 Tension pneumothorax

A tension pneumothorax is caused when air enters the chest through a 'one-way valve', with air being sucked into the cavity on inspiration, but the valve is closed on expiration so no air can get out. It is a life-threatening injury. Clinical signs include cardiovascular instability with tachycardia, hypotension, increased respiratory rate and hypoxia. A raised JVP is often seen. In this case, there is a right tension pneumothorax with reduced air entry on that side, along with hyper-resonance and reduced expansion. The trachea deviates away from the side affected. CXR will confirm the diagnosis. Management is with urgent needle decompression using a large-bore cannula in the affected hemi-thorax at the level of the second intercostal space mid-clavicular line. A chest drain should then be placed.

B. 3 Hypoglycaemia

This patient should be assessed as per ATLS protocols with C-spine control. This patient has a reduced GCS with no signs of haemodynamic instability or head injury. The most likely cause for a reduced GCS in this patient with alcohol excess is hypoglycaemia. Other important reversible causes to consider in patients with a reduced GCS are hypoperfusion and alcohol or drug abuse.

C. 1 Cardiac tamponade

This patient most likely has a cardiac tamponade following a penetrating injury to the left hemi-thorax. Haemodynamic instability with evidence of muffled heart sounds are the key clinical findings in this scenarios. The classic triad (Beck's) of signs is hypotension, raised JVP and muffled heart sounds. Along with tachycardia, increased respiratory rate and a rapidly reducing GCS, other findings include pulsus paradoxus and Kussmaul's sign. Urgent pericardiocentesis is indicated.

25 *Emergency neurosurgery*

Harry Bulstrode

→ Pathophysiology of raised intracranial pressure (ICP)

1. Which of the following is NOT a direct result of raised ICP?

A Reduced perfusion pressure.

B Headache, vomiting and reduced conscious level.

C Tonsillar herniation.

D Loss of cerebral autoregulation.

E Displacement of CSF and venous blood from the cranium.

→ Head injury

2. The primary survey for patients with severe traumatic brain injury does NOT include:

A Management of respiratory and circulatory compromise.

B Cervical spine clearance.

C Assessment of GCS.

D Assessment of pupil reactivity.

E Blood glucose measurement.

3. According to NICE criteria, CT is indicated after mild head injury for patients with which of the following:

A An episode of vomiting.

B Ongoing headache.

C Loss of consciousness at the time of injury.

D Age over 65.

E GCS 13 or 14 at presentation.

→ Transfer to a neurosurgical centre

4. Which of the following statements are true?

A Severe traumatic brain injury (TBI) not requiring surgery is best managed in a local unit rather than by transfer to a neurosurgical centre.

B Anaesthetic escort is mandatory for transfer of all head-injured patients.

C Sedation of head-injured patients prevents assessment of the pupils.

D Early transfer is recommended to avoid primary brain injury.

E Secondary brain injury can be minimised by optimising ventilation, electrolyte balance, and sedation and by ensuring that the hard collar is loose so as not to occlude venous return.

→ Intracranial bleeding

1 Acute subdural haemorrhage
2 Chronic subdural haemorrhage
3 Diffuse axonal injury
4 Extradural haemorrhage
5 Traumatic subarachnoid haemorrhage

Match the diagnoses with the clinical presentations that follow:

→ Clinical presentations

A   A 62-year-old gentleman taking warfarin for atrial fibrillation presents with a two-week history of headaches and clumsiness of the dominant hand. He cannot recall any impact to the head.

B   A 36-year-old male driver is involved in a high-speed RTA, and is comatose at scene. Head CT is unremarkable save for several tiny foci of high density in the corpus callosum and brainstem.

C   A 24-year-old victim of a kite-surfing accident has a GCS E2 V2 M4, and a fixed dilated right pupil at admission. A lentiform focus of acute blood underlying a temporal bone fracture is evident on CT.

D   A 30-year-old victim of a road-traffic accident is GCS E1 V1 M4 with midsize reactive pupils at admission; the left fixes and dilates in the CT scanner. A diffuse concave extra-axial bleed is evident over the surface of the left hemisphere.

E   A 24-year-old male falls from a roof while intoxicated. He is admitted GCS E3V4M5, and CT demonstrates a thin layer of high density distributed diffusely over the brain surface.

→ 'Spontaneous' haemorrhage

1   Arteriovenous malformation rupture
2   Berry aneurysm rupture
3   Dural AV fistula rupture
4   Hypertensive intracerebral haemorrhage
5   Pituitary apoplexy

Match the diagnoses with the clinical presentations that follow:

→ Clinical presentations

A   A 41-year-old woman is found collapsed in her bathroom. She is lucid in the emergency department but complains of severe headache. A right complete third nerve palsy is evident.

B   A 67-year-old gentleman presents with sudden right arm and leg weakness and dysphasia, and is markedly hypertensive at admission. CT scan, as a precursor to thrombolysis for acute stroke, demonstrates a bleed in the basal ganglia.

C   A 45-year-old man presents with thunderclap headache. He gives a history of longstanding right-side headaches and a rushing sound in the right ear in time with his pulse.

D   A previously well 35-year-old woman presents with sudden onset severe headache and loss of vision. Her acuity is 6/24 bilaterally on assessment in the emergency department.

E   A 43-year-old man presents with sudden right arm and leg weakness. He is normotensive. CT demonstrates a substantial haematoma in the left frontoparietal region.

→ Complications of traumatic brain injury

The following are recognised complications of traumatic brain injury. Match a likely diagnosis to the descriptions that follow:

1   Cerebral salt wasting
2   Syndrome of inappropriate ADH secretion
3   Diabetes Insipidus
4   Panhypopituitarism
5   Post-concussive syndrome

Match the complications with the clinical presentations that follow:

→ Clinical presentations

A A patient is intubated on ITU 48 hours after sustaining a severe TBI. Urine output has been 800 mL over 3 hours and the serum sodium level is 151 mEq/L.

B Five days after sustaining a moderate TBI, a patient's routine bloods reveal a serum sodium of 124 mEq/L. Clinically, the patient is euvolaemic.

C Several weeks after sustaining a severe traumatic brain injury managed medically, a 25 year old patient has been extubated but is failing to progress, with somnolence and failure to interact. Routine bloods are unremarkable.

D One week after sustaining a severe TBI, the patient remains intubated. Fluid balance has been persistently negative over 72 hours, and the serum sodium has dropped from 130 mEq/L to 122 mEq/L on the day's routine blood tests. The patient is clinically dehydrated.

E A young man who sustained a moderate TBI 3 months previously complains in clinic of persistent headaches and difficulty in concentrating on his studies. Routine bloods are unremarkable.

Answers to multiple choice questions

1. D

Cerebral autoregulation is compromised in significant TBI, and this adds to the difficulty of achieving satisfactory perfusion in the context of raised ICP. However, injured brain can exhibit deranged autoregulation without raised ICP, for example, after decompressive craniectomy.

Cerebral perfusion pressure (CPP) is directly related to ICP according to the relationship CPP = Mean Arterial Pressure (MAP) – ICP.

Headache, vomiting and reduced consciousness level are cardinal indicators of raised ICP.

Displacement of venous blood and CSF resulting from small rises in ICP acts to limit the rise in pressure during the Monro-Kellie doctrine's compensatory phase. Herniation of the cingulate gyrus under the falx, of the uncus of the temporal lobe under the tentorium and of the cerebellar tonsils through the foramen magnum, can occur as this compensation fails.

2. B

Cervical spine injury cannot be excluded as part of the primary survey in a patient with reduced consciousness level (severe TBI implies a GCS of 8 or less at resuscitation). Cervical spine x-rays traditionally form part of the primary survey, but generally a CT trauma series incorporating head, neck and chest/abdomen/pelvis is likely to be most appropriate, depending on mechanism. Since there is a risk of ligamentous injury even where the CT is normal, cervical spine precautions are often maintained as far as possible pending clinical clearance of the neck.

The ATLS primary survey comprises airway management with cervical spine control, attention to breathing and circulation and a brief neurological assessment including GCS, pupil reactivity and blood glucose measurement (to exclude a possible contribution to conscious impairment).

3. D
NICE criteria call for urgent CT scan of patients with mild head injury who are over the age of 65, or have a clotting disorder.

Other indications for scanning include the following:
- GCS <13 at any point, or GCS of 13 or 14 two hours after injury.
- More than one episode of vomiting.
- Anterograde amnesia >30 minutes.
- Focal Neurological Deficit.
- Suspected skull fracture.
- High energy mechanism.

4. E
Minimising secondary brain injury depends on achieving satisfactory cerebral perfusion. Ventilatory parameters, adequate sedation and avoidance of hyponatraemia are each important in limiting rises in ICP that lead to compromised perfusion. Sedation of head-injured patients prevents assessment of the GCS and focal neurological function, but it remains possible to assess the pupils. The collar can be loosened with care during transit to prevent venous obstruction.

U.K. trauma and audit research network guidelines point to a better prognosis for patients with severe TBI who are treated in a neurosurgical centre. Primary brain injury refers to the damage caused to the brain at impact – the goal of early transfer is access to specialist management to minimise secondary brain injury. Anaesthetic assessment of head-injured patients prior to transfer is generally recommended, but for conscious patients without significant intracranial bleeding or mass effect, a nurse escort may be sufficient.

Answers to extended matching questions

→ Intracranial bleeding

1. D Acute subdural haemorrhage
Acute subdural haematoma (ASDH) is typical of high-energy trauma in the young, and the patient may also have significant primary brain injury. The subdural blood encounters little resistance in dissecting dura from arachnoid, so spreads diffusely over the brain surface without regard to suture lines (**Figure 25.1**). Craniotomy and evacuation are the mainstay of management.

2. A Chronic subdural haemorrhage
Chronic subdural haematoma (**Figure 25.2**) without a history of trauma is common in those with deranged clotting. The presentation is typically insidious and, after correcting the clotting, evacuation through burr holes under local anaesthetic will often be a satisfactory approach.

3. B Diffuse axonal injury
Diffuse axonal injury is a post-mortem diagnosis implying shearing of axons due to rapid acceleration of the brain. However, foci of petechial haemorrhage in deep brain structures in a patient comatose from the moment of high- energy impact are strongly suggestive.

4. C Extradural haemorrhage
The classic presentation of extradural haematoma involves transient loss of consciousness, followed by recovery to normal (the lucid interval), then rapid deterioration to coma. More commonly, extradural haematoma can complicate a moderate or severe primary head injury as discussed in the context of ASDH previously, especially where a temporal bone

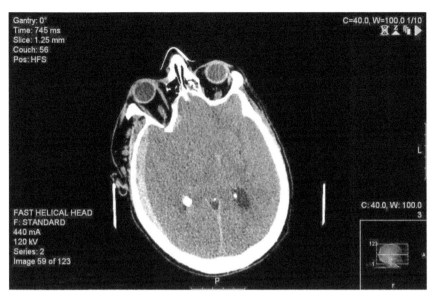

Figure 25.1   Acute subdural haematoma. A crescentic high-density collection overlies the right hemisphere. The high density visible in the occipital horn of the right lateral ventricle is likely to represent calcified choroid plexus (a normal finding) rather than haemorrhage.

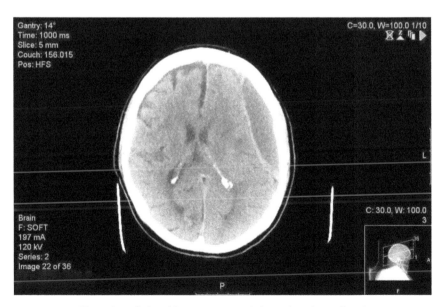

Figure 25.2   Chronic subdural haematoma. A low-density collection represents altered blood. A higher-density rim corresponding to membranes is seen frequently around long-standing collections.

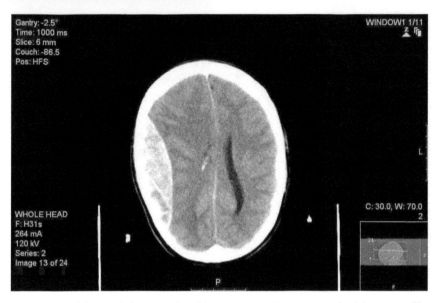

Figure 25.3 A large right extradural haematoma is associated with mass effect and midline shift.

fracture is associated with rupture of the underlying middle meningeal artery **(Figure 25.3)**. Management entails immediate craniotomy and clot evacuation.

5. E Traumatic subarachnoid haemorrhage
Traumatic subarachnoid haemorrhage **(Figure 25.4)** is the result of venous bleeding into the subarachnoid space, rather than the arterial haemorrhage of aneurysmal SAH, and is not associated with significant vasospasm.

→ 'Spontaneous' haemorrhage

1. E Arteriovenous malformation rupture
Although AVM as a cause of ICH is relatively rare compared to ICH, it has important investigation and treatment implications and the possibility of underlying AVM is a major concern in the event of attempted clot evacuation. A young patient with an ICH outside the locations typical for hypertensive bleed (e.g., basal ganglia, cerebellum) will certainly require investigation for possible AVM.

2. A Berry aneurysm rupture
Third nerve palsy associated with thunderclap headache classically represents rupture of an aneurysm compressing the posterior communicating artery. CT scan performed early is highly sensitive for SAH, but where there is a strong history and no evidence of blood, delayed lumbar puncture is indicated, with samples sent for cell count and assay for levels of the haemoglobin breakdown products oxyhaemoglobin and bilirubin, whose presence suggest prior haemorrhage. Confirmed subarachnoid haemorrhage is generally investigated with catheter angiography, and an underlying ruptured aneurysm can be managed surgically ('clipping') or by radiological embolisation ('coiling').

3. C Dural AV fistula rupture
Pulsatile tinnitus is pathonomic of dural arteriovenous fistula. Rupture of these lesions can manifest with subdural, subarachnoid, or intracerebral haemorrhage.

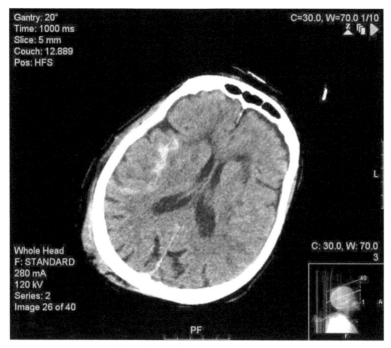

Gantry: 20°
Time: 1000 ms
Slice: 5 mm
Couch: 12.889
Pos: HFS

C=30.0, W=70.0 1/10

L

Whole Head
F: STANDARD
280 mA
120 kV
Series: 2
Image 26 of 40

C: 30.0, W: 70.0
3

PF

Figure 25.4   Traumatic subarachnoid haemorrhage is evident of the right insular cortex. The brain is generally atrophic.

4. B Hypertensive intracerebral haemorrhage

Haemorrhagic stroke is common, particularly in undiagnosed and uncontrolled hypertensives. The basal ganglia are a typical site for these bleeds. Surgery may be considered to relieve mass effect, but management is generally medical. In younger patients and those with an atypical appearance, further imaging to rule out an underlying neoplasia or vascular malformation may be indicated.

5. D Pituitary apoplexy

Pituitary apoplexy refers to the syndrome associated with acute haemorrhage or infarction of the pituitary gland (see Chapter 43). Headache, visual loss, ophthalmoplegia and variable consciousness impairment are typical. Endocrine resuscitation is the first management priority.

Complications of traumatic brain injury

In each case, diagnosis and management should be discussed promptly with a neurointensivist or endocrinologist.

1. D Cerebral salt wasting

Hyponatraemia after a brain insult should prompt consideration of cerebral salt wasting and syndrome of inappropriate ADH (SIADH). Each involves inappropriate excretion of a concentrated urine due to failure of normal pituitary control. Cerebral salt wasting leads to volume depletion, requiring prompt replacement.

2. B Syndrome of inappropriate ADH secretion

By contrast, patients suffering SIADH are clinically euvolaemic or even somewhat overfilled, because of free water retention as a result of inappropriately high ADH levels. In this case, sodium replacement and occasionally blockade of ADH activity, using demeclocycline for instance, is usually appropriate. Fluid restriction is also used but may be dangerous in the context of compromised perfusion due to raised ICP (head injury) or vasospasm (subarachnoid haemorrhage).

3. A Diabetes Insipidus
Excretion of large volumes of dilute urine resulting in hypernatraemia is another frequent complication of head injury, and reflects failure of the pituitary to secrete ADH. Administration of boluses of desmopressin/DDAVP may be used to manage this.

4. C Panhypopituitarism
Generalised pituitary dysfunction is a common sequel of TBI. It should be actively excluded in recovering patients, especially where progress is slow, by means of a pituitary function screen (9 am cortisol, free T3 and T4, oestradiol or testosterone, prolactin, IGF-1).

5. E Post-concussive syndrome
Post-concussive syndrome is a poorly defined constellation of symptoms that can interfere significantly with recovery. A head-injury rehabilitation specialist team is best placed to advise on managing these problems.

26 Neck and spine

Christopher JK Bulstrode

Multiple choice questions

→ ## Anatomy of spine injury

1. **Which of the following statements regarding spine injury are true?**

A All three columns of the spinal column must be injured for the spine to be unstable.

B The cervico-thoracic junction is especially susceptible to injury because it is a transition zone from the mobile to the rigid segment of the spinal cord.

C The size of the spinal canal in the cervical region makes the spine at this level especially susceptible to injury.

D The spinal cord in the adult ends at L5/S1.

E The stability of the cervical spine is mainly provided by the bony anatomy.

→ ## Case study: injury after fall

2. **A patient is admitted unconscious with a head injury following a 4-metre fall from the roof of a building. His blood pressure is 80/60 mmHg, his pulse 45 beats/minute and he has well-perfused extremities.**

(a) **What is the likelihood of him having a significant spinal injury?**

A < 20%

B 20%–50%

C 50%–75%

D 75%–100%

(b) **What is the safest and most reliable way to clear the cervical spine?**

A Cervical spine series of plain x-rays.

B Flexion and extension views.

C Keep him on a spine board until he recovers consciousness.

D Magnetic resonance imaging (MRI).

E There are more important things to worry about so this can be considered later.

(c) **What fluids need to be given and how?**

A A standard maintenance regimen should be started of 3 litres/24 hours, two salt, one sweet.

B Fluids can be given by naso-gastric tube at 40mL/hour.

C No fluids are needed at this stage.

D Put in a central venous pressure line and a urinary catheter. Fluids should be titrated against preload pressure and urine output.

E Two litres of saline should be given stat, and then further fluid until the systolic pressure comes above 110 mmHg.

The patient wakes up and cannot move his legs. Palpation of the spine reveals a step between T10 and T11, which is painful.

(d) **Which of the following tests are good indicators of prognosis in spinal injury?**

A A loss of power proprioception on one side with loss of temperature and pain sensation on the other side.

B Bulbocavernosus reflex.

C Distal reflexes.

D Examination for a step in the spine.

E Perianal sensation.

Examination of the lower limbs of the patient reveals sensation present in the lower limbs but no motor power.

(e) **What Frankel Grade is this patient?**

A A

B B

C C

D D

E E

→ Visualisation in neck and spine injury

3. Which of the following statements regarding visualisation are false?

A Cervical spine injuries in children are easier to visualise than in adults.

B CT scan is best at demonstrating soft-tissue haematoma in the cord.

C MRI is best for reconstructions, as they help understand the nature of the bone injury.

D Provided that the cervicothoracic junction is visualised, plain x-rays are adequate to identify cervical instability.

E Special attention needs to be paid to the cervico/thoracic and the thoraco/lumbar junctions.

→ Cervical spine injury

4. A patient is found to have an unstable cervical spine injury, with bifacet dislocation. He has a partial neurological deficit (Frankel C).

(a) What investigation is needed?

A CT.

B EMGs.

C MRI.

D No further investigation is needed. The deformity is already known, as is the extent of neurological damage.

E Tomograms.

(b) What is the optimum treatment?

A Halo traction.

B Mobilise within the limits of pain.

C Open reduction and internal fixation with bone graft plates and screws.

D Physiotherapy with manipulation until the facets relocate spontaneously.

E Stiff collar.

(c) The neurology now starts to deteriorate. What is your management plan now?

A If traction is being used, increase the traction until symptoms resolve.

B Open reduction and internal fixation with bone-graft plates and screws.

C Start high-dose steroids.

D Stiff collar and log rolling.

E This is an unavoidable complication in some cases, and nothing can be done.

Extended matching questions

→ Fractures, dislocations and subluxations

1 Anterior cranio-cervical dislocation
2 Atlanto-axial instability
3 Burst fracture
4 Chance fracture
5 Facet dislocation
6 Hangman's fracture
7 Jefferson's fracture
8 Spinal cord injury without radiographic abnormality (SCIWORA)
9 Teardrop fracture
10 Wedge fracture

Choose and match the correct fracture/dislocation/subluxation for each of the scenarios that follow:

A A child spontaneously develops a wry neck with a cock robin appearance.

B A child sustains a high-speed flexion injury. There is a neurological deficit but no abnormality visible on x-ray.

C A patient has a fracture, which is effectively a spondylolisthesis of C2 on C3.

D A patient has a hyperextension injury. X-ray shows a small chip of bone off the front of a vertebral body next to the disc space.

E A patient has a hyperflexion injury combined with axial loading. X-ray shows C3 subluxed forward on C4.

F A patient has a hyperflexion injury. The x-ray shows that the vertical height of C4 vertebra is 50% less at the front than the back.

G A patient is found to have a Power ratio of more than one.

H A patient presents having fallen on his head from a height. The atlas is fractured and expanded.

I A patient presents having fallen on his head from a height. The C4 vertebra is fractured and expanded.

J A patient sustains a flexion distraction injury at the thoracolumbar junction following a high-speed road-traffic accident where he was wearing a seat belt.

Answers to multiple choice questions

→ Anatomy of spine injury

1. B

The spinal canal in the cervical region is very spacious, so relatively large displacements of the vertebrae of the cervical spine can occur without compromise to the spinal cord itself. The cervical spine is very mobile in several planes and so there is very little bony stability. Instead, the stability is provided by the ligaments connecting the motion segments. In contrast, the thoracic spine is relatively rigid. The transition between mobile and stiff segments in any mechanical structure is the area most vulnerable to extreme loads, and so the cervicothoracic junction (the area most difficult to visualise) is also the very area most likely to be fractured or dislocated.

The anatomy of the spinal column provides stability through the following three columns: anterior (the front of the vertebral body and intervertebral discs), middle (the back of the vertebral body and the anterior longitudinal ligaments) and posterior (the spines with their interspinous ligaments and the facet joints with their pedicles). Disruption of one column does not produce instability, but disruption of all three does. Where there is disruption of two columns, the spine is usually stable but not always.

At birth the spinal cord extends the length of the spinal canal, but by adulthood the conus medullaris (the end of the spinal cord) stops at T12/L1. From then on, the spinal roots (cauda equina) pass down to exit below their vertebral bodies.

→ Case study: injury after fall

2. (a) B

The likelihood of a significant cervical injury accompanying a head or facial injury is around 30%.

2. (b) B

As the patient is unconscious, it can be difficult to 'clear' the cervical spine. Plain x-rays will not be adequate, and flexion and extension views carry an unquantified risk of causing further damage. The patient should certainly not be left on a spine board any longer than absolutely necessary, because of the risk of bed sores. An MRI would be the safest and most reliable way of ruling out an unstable spine injury.

2. (c) D

The vital signs are highly suggestive of neurogenic shock with low blood pressure, bradycardia and well-perfused periphery. Fluids should be administered with great care here because of the risk of flooding the patient. Using a CVP line to measure pre-load, and a urinary catheter to measure renal function, fluids can be titrated in to ensure adequate perfusion while minimising the risk of overloading the patient's circulation.

2. (d) A, E

The bulbocavernosus reflex returns in 24–48 hours after spinal transection. It is no indicator of prognosis. It merely indicates that the period of spinal shock has ended and that tests of prognosis can now be performed reliably. Return of perianal sensation indicates a good prognosis. A loss of power proprioception on one side with loss of temperature and pain sensation on the other side is the Brown-Sequard syndrome and also carries a good prognosis. Distal reflexes are no indicator of prognosis. A step in the spine merely indicates that there is a displaced fracture and gives no clue to the extent of neurological damage.

2. (e) B

The American Spinal Injury Association measures muscle power using the MRC grading system (0–5) and sensation in each dermatome. These are then combined into the Frankel grade. Grade A is absent sensory and motor. Grade B is sensory present, motor absent (this patient). Grade C is sensory present with motor function, which is not good enough to be useful (MRC grade less than 3). Grade D is sensory present with useful but not normal motor function. Grade E is normal function.

→ Visualisation in neck and spine injury

3. A, B, C, D

Plain x-rays will only diagnose 85% of significant spinal injuries, and even that is only true provided there is good visualisation of the cervicothoracic junction. If the cervicothoracic junction cannot be visualised with conventional films then a 'swimmer's view' may need to be taken. CT is best for diagnosing bony injury in the spine and can also prove valuable in understanding the nature and extent of the bone injury using reconstructions. MRI is always much better for soft-tissue injuries, so will show up oedema and haematoma of the cord. However, MRI is trumped by CT for planning bone reconstruction. Spine fractures in children are difficult to visualise as bones are not fully ossified, so are not clearly visible. Ligaments are also more lax, so tolerances for displacement are greater. Special attention needs to be paid to both the junctions in the spine between flexible and rigid sections, as these are stress raisers.

→ Cervical spine injury

4. (a) C; (b) C; (c) B

A facet dislocation is effectively an unstable fracture and cannot be left untreated. It can be treated in traction using halo traction (until closed reduction is achieved) or, better still, by open reduction and internal fixation. Either way it is best to get an MRI to make sure that there is not a prolapsed intervertebral disc that might compress the cord when reduction is achieved. The best treatment is open reduction, as the patient can then be mobilised safely, minimising the risks of other complications, such as bed sores, developing. The indications for surgery are relative if the neurology is stable, but if the neurology is deteriorating then the indication for surgery is absolute – surgery offers the only option. If the neurology deteriorates then surgery must be considered urgently. Increasing traction would only be likely to make the neurology worse. Syrinx is a late complication of spinal injury, and even that requires surgical decompression.

1. G Anterior cranio-cervical dislocation

The Power ratio measures the degree of subluxation of the occiput on the axis. A ratio of more than 1 indicates anterior translation, and a ratio of less than 0.75 indicates a posterior one. The ratio is the distance from the front of the foramen magnum (occiput edge) to the front edge of the back of the atlas over the distance between the back edge of the front of the axis (front of spinal canal) to the front of the back edge of the foramen magnum. Craniocervical dislocation is usually fatal.

2. A Atlanto-axial instability

A child with a cock robin neck may just have sternomastoid spasm but can also have a spontaneous onset of atlantoaxial instability. Halter traction should lead to reduction.

3. I Burst fracture

At any other level C2, this fracture is simply known as a 'burst' fracture. The fragments can be displaced into the spinal canal, causing cord damage. These fragments will need to be removed at open reduction and stabilisation.

4. J Chance fracture

The thoracolumbar junction is especially susceptible to injury, and the introduction of seat belts has produced a characteristic flexion or distraction injury at this level, which is called the Chance fracture.

5. E Facet dislocation

If hyperflexion is combined with axial compression then one (uni-) or both (bi-) facets may dislocate and lock over the front of the facet below, locking into position. There is often damage to the intervertebral disc and also neurological damage. Before reduction is undertaken, an MRI should be performed to make sure there is not a prolapsed intervertebral disc.

6. C Hangman's fracture

The Hangman's fracture is effectively a spondylolisthesis of C2 on C3 caused by traumatic hyperextension.

7. H Jefferson's fracture

The classic fracture from landing on the top of the head is the C1 burst fracture, otherwise known as a Jefferson's fracture, which can be stable or unstable.

8. B SCIWORA

SCIWORA is a spinal cord injury without objective radiological abnormality. This occurs in young children with a hyperelastic spine where the deformity at the time of trauma produces haematoma of the cord (visible on MRI) without any apparent musculoskeletal damage.

9. D Teardrop fracture

Hyperextension pulls off a small fragment of bone on the front of the vertebral body. This is known as a teardrop fracture. Its mild appearance belies a severe and unstable fracture.

10. F Wedge fracture

Osteoporotic flexion wedge fractures are common in the elderly following minor trauma. They are usually stable, but the pain and deformity can be helped with vertebroplasty performed under image-intensifier control.

27 *Maxillofacial trauma*

Andrew Hobkirk

Multiple choice questions

→ ## Mandibular fractures

1. Which of the following are common features of fractures of the mandible?

A Difficult intubation during general anaesthesia.

B Altered sensation of the skin overlying the angle of the mandible.

C A step deformity in the occlusal plane.

D Sublingual haematoma.

E Deviation away from the side of the fracture on mouth opening.

→ ## Retrobulbar haemorrhage

2. Which of the following are signs of retrobulbar haemorrhage?

A Enophthalmos

B Pain

C Decreasing visual acuity

D Normal afferent pupillary reflex

E Retinal pallor

→ ## Fractures of the facial skeleton

3. Which of the following statements are true?

A Le Fort I fractures pass through the nasal bones.

B Anterior open bite is a feature of zygomatic arch fractures.

C Le Fort II fractures are often displaced superiorly.

D Traumatic telecanthus in nasoethmoidal fracture is best managed by closed reduction.

E Cerebrospinal fluid rhinorrhoea may be confirmed by beta-2-transferrin assay.

→ ## Major maxillofacial trauma

4. Which of the following are true in major maxillofacial trauma?

A Airway obstruction may be delayed.

B Chin lift should not be attempted in bilateral mandibular condylar fractures.

C Mid facial haemorrhage may be life threatening.

D Cervical spine fracture is common.

E Patients transferred in the supine position are at increased risk of airway compromise.

→ ## Avulsed teeth

5. In managing a patient with an avulsed tooth, which of the following are true?

A Alveolar fracture is a contraindication to replantation.

B Deciduous teeth should be replanted within 60 minutes.

C Milk is a good storage medium.

D Teeth with crown fractures should not be replanted.

E Traumatic avulsion occurs in up to 3% of all traumatised teeth.

Extended matching questions

➡ Diagnoses

1 Aspiration of foreign body
2 Blow out fracture
3 Epiphora
4 Frontal sinus fracture
5 Haemarthrosis
6 Tattooing
7 Orbital apex syndrome
8 Zygomatic fracture

Match the diagnoses with the clinical scenarios that follow:

➡ Clinical scenarios

A A 27-year-old man is hit on his left chin with an elbow during a football game. Later he is unable to bring his teeth together on the right side. There is no fracture.

B A 19-year-old woman fell from her bicycle onto a tarmac road surface. She had abrasions to her left cheek and forehead. The wounds were irrigated with normal saline and she was discharged. She returned 2 months later with several dark patches on her facial skin.

C A 14-year-old boy falls from a swing and sustains a blow to his face. He is knocked out for 1 minute but makes a rapid and full neurological recovery. His upper central incisors are avulsed.

D A 38-year-old man is punched in the face during a fight. He has marked left periorbital ecchymosis and oedema and left subconjunctival haemorrhage with no posterior limit. There is palpable movement at the left frontozygomatic suture.

E A 24-year-old man is stabbed in the face and sustains a deep wound extending from his right medial lower eyelid to his mid cheek.

F A 57-year-old woman is kicked by her horse. She has a large central forehead haematoma and CSF rhinorrhea.

G A 12-year-old boy is hit in his left eye with a ball. There is minimal soft tissue injury and no palpable deformity. Eye movement is painful and restricted on upward gaze.

H A 48-year-old man falls 2 meters from scaffolding onto a flat paved surface. He presents with significant right facial ecchymosis and oedema, loss of vision in his right eye, ptosis and ophthalmoplegia. CT scanning shows a comminuted fracture of the lateral orbital wall and sphenoid bone.

Answers to multiple choice questions

1. C, D

The teeth are precisely aligned and we perceive even minute changes in dental occlusion. Displaced fractures of the mandible alter this alignment and vertical discrepancies can be seen, and felt, as a step deformity. Bleeding from the site of fracture, and especially the rich lingual plexus, spreads easily in to the sublingual space, resulting in ecchymosis and haematoma.

The limited mouth opening seen with a fractured mandible is often due to pain rather than mechanical obstruction. Mouth opening is one predictor of difficult intubation during general anaesthesia however in these patients it can often simply be managed with analgesia. The inferior dental (ID) nerve supplies sensation to the lip, chin and mandibular gingivae and teeth. It courses through the mandible from the mandibular foramen to the mental foramen in the ID canal. Injury results in loss of, or altered, sensation. By contrast, the skin overlying the angle of the mandible is supplied by the great auricular nerve, which is rarely involved. Mandibular displacement is typically toward the side of fracture as a result of the loss of resistance to muscle tension.

2. B, C, E
Retrobulbar haemorrhage can lead to acute orbital compartment syndrome. This is a surgical emergency and delay in treatment can rapidly lead to blindness in the affected eye. Visual acuity reduces, and ophthalmoplegia develops as intra-orbital pressure increases. Optic nerve nutrient vessels are compressed and later retinal artery ischaemia is seen with retinal pallor. Proptosis of the globe tensions the optic nerve and patients report severe pain. In this situation urgent decompression with lateral canthotomy and then, if necessary, cantholysis is indicated. Medical management alone (with steroid, mannitol and acetazolamide) is not sufficiently rapid or efficacious.

The afferent pupillary reflex is reduced and then lost. In an intact orbit, the contents can only move anteriorly and proptosis (exophthalmos) is seen. The globe feels tense on palpation.

3. E
Beta-2-transferrin is a protein found exclusively in cerebrospinal fluid and perilymph. Levels can be assayed in suspected CSF leak yielding a diagnostic sensitivity and specificity approaching 100%, making it the gold standard investigation. The classic 'rail track sign' is caused by the flow of CSF preventing blood clotting centrally bordered by 'tracks' of clotted blood.

Le Fort I fractures, the lowest level, pass through the nasal piriform aperture, the walls of the maxillary sinus and low through the pterygoid plates. Le Fort II fractures pass through the nasal bridge, infero-medial orbital floor, inferior orbital rim, through the maxillary sinus walls and to the superior part of the pterygoid plates. Le Fort III fractures, the highest level, separate the facial skeleton from the skull base. The fracture also passes through the nasal bridge but continues through the medial, inferior and lateral orbital walls, zygomatico-frontal suture, zygomatic arch and pterygoid plates superiorly.

Zygomatic arch fractures, by themselves, do not alter the dental occlusal relationship. Lateral excursion of the mandible can be restricted by impingement of the coronoid process and temporalis muscle. Le Fort fractures often displace posteriorly and inferiorly as they are forced along the downward sloping skull base. The posterior teeth will then come into contact first, giving the classic sign of an anterior open bite with intact mandible.

Naso-ethmoidal fractures often comminute and are difficult to treat. The nasal bridge is depressed and nasal tip upturned. Telecanthus is seen when the anterior and posterior limbs of the medial canthal ligament are disrupted. Open reduction and fixation of the fractures, and reattachment of the ligament, are indicated.

4. A, C, E
Maxillofacial fractures induce a marked inflammatory response and significant oedema may develop within 60–90 minutes; a cause of delayed airway obstruction. Patients should be observed closely and might need early intubation or a surgical definitive airway. Hypovolaemic shock from maxillofacial haemorrhage alone is uncommon, and other sources of bleeding should always be assessed. Mid-facial haemorrhage can be difficult to control, particularly with mobile fractures. In the supine position a patient may not be able to protect his or her own airway. Placed semi-prone, blood and saliva can drain out of the mouth and the tongue will fall forward. Whilst cervical spine fracture is uncommon, the cervical spine should *always* be protected until fracture is excluded.

There are four pairs of intrinsic tongue muscles. Genioglossus is attached to the superior genial tubercle on the lingual surface of the anterior part of the mandible, and contraction protrudes the tongue. Displaced bilateral mandibular fractures allow the tongue to fall back, which can obstruct the airway. Chin-lift and jaw-thrust are important basic airway management techniques and are not contraindicated.

5. C, E

The key to success in the management of avulsed teeth is *early replantation*. Tooth roots are formed of dentine, with a surface layer of cementum. Periodontal ligament fibres are inserted into this layer and attach the root to the alveolar bone of the tooth socket. They are very susceptible to drying, so if a tooth cannot be immediately replanted it should be placed in a physiological storage medium such as milk or physiological saline. After 60 minutes, few teeth will survive. Once replanted, the tooth is splinted in place for 7 to 14 days and the patient will need ongoing dental care. The upper central incisor teeth are the most readily traumatised, and the most commonly avulsed, with peak incidence in the 7–9-year-old age group. Tooth avulsion occurs in 0.5% to 3% of dento-alveolar trauma to permanent teeth.

Fractures of the alveolus should be reduced and are not a contraindication to tooth replantation, although tooth splinting may be required for longer. Deciduous teeth are not replanted to minimise risk to the ongoing development and eruption of the permanent dentition. Most crown fractures can be restored and should not delay replantation.

Answers to extended matching questions

1. C Aspiration of foreign body

Avulsed teeth can be aspirated, particularly in children or when there is loss of consciousness. The aspiration may cause an immediate threat to life with airway compromise or initially go unrecognised. Chest radiography is indicated if teeth are unaccounted for. The main bronchial angles show good symmetry up to the age of 15. It is only later that the right main bronchus becomes more vertical and hence the predominant side of aspiration. If left in situ, obstructive pneumonitis and abscess formation may develop so aspirated teeth should always be retrieved; this is often possible with a bronchoscope.

2. G Blow out fracture

The orbital floor is formed by the orbital plates of three bones – maxilla, palatine and zygoma. It is the most commonly fractured wall. Most orbital floor fractures in adults can be managed electively, whereas in children they are a surgical emergency. Soft tissue herniating through the classic narrow trap door greenstick fracture becomes incarcerated, and ischaemia can rapidly progress to necrosis. Permanent ocular motility restriction can ensue, especially if extra ocular muscles are involved. Subconjunctival haemorrhage is often not seen, hence the 'white eye', while the restricted upward gaze causes diplopia. The oculovagal reflex can be stimulated by traction on the extra ocular muscles or pressure on the globe. Afferent signals are transmitted via the ophthalmic division of the trigeminal nerve to the motor nucleus of the vagus nerve. Vagal cardiac stimulation leads to bradycardia and hypotension, which can, ultimately, lead to cardiac arrest. General malaise, nausea and vomiting are seen, and can be mistaken for signs of head injury, delaying diagnosis and treatment. A high index of clinical suspicion should prompt CT scanning of, or to include, the orbits and orthoptic assessment.

3. E Epiphora

The drainage apparatus of the eye consists of the lacrimal puncta (which can be seen on the lid margin about 6 mm lateral to the medial angle of the eye), canaliculi, lacrimal sac and nasolacrimal duct, which opens into the inferior meatus of the nose. This intricate system can be disrupted by direct injury, such as the incised wound here, or indirectly by fracture displacement. Compromised drainage leads to epiphora, and it is important to recognise this as delayed repair is complex. Surgical management depends on the site of injury and includes stenting and dacryocystorhinostomy.

4. F Frontal sinus fracture

The frontal sinus is related to the skull vault and skull base. The posterior wall separates the sinus from the anterior cranial fossa, and the floor is continuous with the naso-ethmoidal complex. The anterior wall is stronger than the posterior wall but resists direct impact poorly. If fractured in isolation the only indication for surgery is cosmesis. The key to managing posterior wall fractures is prevention of complications, which can be life threatening and delayed. These include sinusitis, mucocele, mucopyocele, osteomyelitis, meningitis and cerebral abscess. Dural tear causes CSF leak. Displaced posterior wall fractures are treated by cranialisation of the sinus and dural repair. Floor fractures can be left untreated, and repair of the frontonasal duct is no longer considered necessary.

5. A Haemarthrosis

Acute force transmitted through the mandible can cause temporomandibular joint soft tissue injury with internal derangement and haemarthrosis. The increased fluid volume widens the joint space and might cause ipsilateral lateral open bite. The inflammatory response can cause joint effusion, cartilage degeneration and, later, adhesion formation and hypomobility. Treatment with nonsteroidal anti-inflammatory drugs, soft diet and physiotherapy to increase range of movement is effective and reduces the risk of TMJ ankylosis, a serious late complication.

6. B Tattooing

Contaminated facial wounds need careful assessment and thorough exploration, cleaning and debridement. General anaesthesia might be required to achieve this. Delay in treatment increases the risk of wound infection, and progressive oedema makes accurate apposition of tissue more difficult. Road grit and other contaminants cause soft tissue tattooing, which is very difficult to remove as a secondary procedure.

7. H Orbital apex syndrome

The superior orbital fissure is bounded by the greater and lesser wings of the sphenoid bone and transmits the lacrimal, frontal, trochlear, nasociliary, oculomotor and abducent nerves and ophthalmic veins. Compression of all of these structures causes superior orbital fissure syndrome (SOFS) with ophthalmoplegia, cycloplegia, mydriasis, ptosis, exophthalmos (due to impaired venous drainage) and forehead and upper eyelid sensory deficit. Incomplete SOFS is more common. In orbital apex syndrome there is additionally involvement of the optic nerve, and this has a poor prognosis. If CT scanning shows a bone fragment compressing the optic nerve, surgical exploration might be indicated.

8. D Zygomatic fracture

Symptoms and signs of fracture of the zygomatic complex include pain, ecchymosis, oedema, flattening of the malar process, displacement of the frontozygomatic suture, step deformity, diplopia on upward gaze, paraesthesia or anaesthesia of the infraorbital nerve, subconjunctival haemorrhage without a posterior border and limitation of mandibular range of movement.

28 Torso trauma

Pradip K Datta

Multiple choice questions

Injury mechanism associated with torso trauma

1. Which of the following statements are true?

A Management of injury to a junctional zone is a surgical challenge.

B Injury to the mediastinum is extremely high risk.

C CT scan should be carried out in all patients.

D For abdominal trauma the best diagnostic modality is diagnostic peritoneal lavage (DPL).

E The retroperitoneum is subdivided into three zones.

Critical physiology

2. The following statements are true except:

A Resuscitation should follow ATLS protocol.

B Bleeding and its effects are always obvious.

C Bleeding occurs from five major sites.

D Physiological parameters must be sought.

E A rising serum lactate is an indicator of ongoing bleeding.

Thoracic injury

3. Which of the following statements are correct?

A Thoracic injury accounts for 25% of all severe injuries.

B An intercostal drain (ICD) is both diagnostic and therapeutic.

C CT scan is the most reliable investigation.

D 80% of chest injuries can be managed without an operation.

E In an open pneumothorax, close the pneumothorax and then insert ICD.

Immediate life-threatening injuries

4. Which of the following statement/s is/are incorrect?

A On suspicion of a tension pneumothorax an immediate chest x-ray must be taken.

B The differential diagnosis of a tension pneumothorax is pericardial tamponade.

C The CVP is always elevated in pericardial tamponade.

D The most common cause of bleeding in massive haemothorax is torn intercostal vessels.

E Hypoxia in flail chest is due to paradoxical respiration.

Potential life-threatening injuries

5. Which of the following statements are true?

A Thoracic aortic disruption is a common cause of sudden death in a RTA.

B Severe and rapid subcutaneous emphysema suggests tracheobronchial injury.

C Blunt myocardial injury is diagnosed by ECG changes.

D Blunt diaphragmatic rupture can be easily missed.

E Oesophageal injury is usually due to penetrating trauma.

→ Emergency thoracotomy

6. The following statements are true except:

A Emergency department thoracotomy (EDT) should be performed for most cases that require control of haemorrhage from the heart or lung.

B Definitive correction of a trauma problem should be carried out in the operating theatre.

C Left anterolateral thoracotomy is the approach for thoracic aorta, left lung and lower oesophagus.

D Right anterolateral thoracotomy is carried out to approach thoracic trachea, superior vena cava and upper oesophagus.

E 'Clamshell thoracotomy' is the preferred approach for the surgeon who enters the chest only occasionally.

→ Abdominal injury and investigations

7. Which of the following statements are true?

A Patients with abdominal trauma can be categorised into three groups, depending upon their physiological status after resuscitation.

B In torso trauma, the best investigation is contrast enhanced CT (CECT) scan.

C FAST (focused abdominal sonar for trauma) is used to assess presence of free blood.

D DPL (diagnostic peritoneal lavage) is used to assess presence of blood in the peritoneal cavity.

E DL (diagnostic laparoscopy) or thoracoscopy is useful in penetrating trauma.

Extended matching questions

→ Diagnoses

1 Abdominal compartment syndrome (ACS)
2 Cardiac tamponade
3 Diaphragmatic injury
4 Flail chest
5 Liver injury
6 Massive haemothorax
7 Open pneumothorax
8 Pancreatic injury
9 Renal injury
10 Splenic injury
11 Tension pneumothorax

Match the diagnoses with the clinical scenarios that follow:

→ Clinical scenarios

A A 40-year-old van driver has been brought to the accident and emergency (A&E) department with severe shortness of breath. He was involved in a road-traffic accident (RTA) when there was a head-on collision while not wearing a seat belt. There is bruising over his sternum. His neck veins are distended, with a systolic pressure of 80 mmHg and pulse rate of 130/minute. The trachea is in the midline, but breath sounds are difficult to discern because there is a lot of noise in the A&E department. The pulse oximeter shows an oxygen saturation of 92%.

B A 25-year-old motorcyclist has been brought to the A&E department in a panicky state, as he is unable to breathe properly and is intensely hypoxic (oxygen saturation of 90%). The trachea is shifted to the right, the left hemithorax does not move and there is hyper-resonance over the left chest wall. The noise in the A&E department makes listening to breath sounds difficult.

C Following an injury at a building site where a piece of heavy masonry fell on his chest, a 35-year-old man has been sent to the A&E department with severe pain in his chest and marked bruising of the chest wall on the left. On examination his blood pressure is 80/50 mmHg, the left chest is dull on percussion and there is no air entry.

D A 22-year-old rugby player has been brought to the A&E department with severe left-sided chest pain following blunt injury sustained in a match about 2 hours ago. He is very tachypnoeic and extremely tender over the central part of his left hemithorax. The skin over the ribs looks badly bruised, and the chest wall is unstable when he coughs or tries to take a deep breath.

E A 15-year-old boy has been brought into the A&E department having been stabbed on the left side of his axilla. He is gasping for breath and his pulse oximeter shows a saturation of 90%. There is an open wound in the region of the fifth left interspace, through which a sucking sound can be heard.

F A fit 35-year-old man who was working on a building site sustained severe blunt upper abdominal trauma. He had a splenectomy for ruptured spleen and partial hepatectomy for torn liver. On the third postoperative day, while still in the ITU, he became oliguric, had cardiorespiratory compromise, type 2 respiratory failure and gross abdominal distension.

G A 30-year-old man sustained an injury at a building site when a heavy piece of masonry fell on his lower abdomen. He is tachypnoeic and in hypovolaemic shock, with a pulse of 130/minute and a blood pressure of 80/60 mmHg. He has been resuscitated by the ATLS protocol and is stable after 4 hours, has a pulse of 100/minute, blood pressure of 130/90 mmHg and CVP of 4 cm H_2O. He continues to be short of breath, with an oxygen saturation of 92%. He has an indwelling catheter, two IV cannulae with crystalloids and blood and a nasogastric tube. A chest x-ray shows the tip of the nasogastric tube next to the heart in the left chest.

H A 9-year-old boy sustained a kick in the left side of his abdomen and loin while playing rugby. After a brief period of rest, he finished his game. In the changing room when he passed urine, it was haematuria. He was brought to the A&E department. He was stable with a pulse of 90/minute and blood pressure of 110/80 mmHg. On examination he had bruising over the left lumbar region and left loin with some obliteration of the loin curve.

I A 50-year-old man was brought to the A&E department having been viciously assaulted by being kicked in his upper abdomen and lower right chest. He is in very severe pain and short of breath with tachycardia. His pulse is 110/minute, blood pressure is 90/70 mmHg and clinically he has fracture of his right fifth to ninth ribs. Abdominal examination shows Cullen's sign with marked tenderness and bruising in the right upper quadrant. Following resuscitation by the ATLS protocol, his blood pressure is 120/90 mmHg and his pulse rate is 100/minute. His CVP is 5 cm H_2O.

J Following a severe RTA, a 35-year-old female passenger in the back seat of a car had to be extricated. She has been brought in with generalised abdominal pain across the site of the seat belt. She is breathless and complaining of pain in the left upper quadrant and left shoulder, which had impacted against the front seat. Her pulse is 110/minute and blood pressure is 100/60 mmHg. She is very tender over the left upper quadrant and clinically there is no shoulder injury. She has fracture of her left 9th, 10th and 11th ribs.

K A 10-year-old girl has been brought to the A&E department complaining of upper abdominal pain of 10 days' duration. She has not been feeling well, with nausea and occasional vomiting and a feeling of listlessness and she has been off school. On examination she has a distended upper abdomen where there is a suggestion of a smooth firm mass in the epigastrium where the skin is bruised. When asked about the skin bruising, she said that it occurred 10 days ago when she fell off her bicycle and the handlebar struck her epigastrium.

Answers to multiple choice questions

→ Injury mechanism associated with torso trauma

1. A, B, E

As trauma is always unpredictable and does not respect anatomical regions, injury to a junctional zone presents huge challenges requiring teamwork from different specialists. The key junctional zones are between neck and thorax, between thorax and abdomen and between abdomen and pelvis (including groin). Injuries affecting the lower neck usually extend down to the mediastinum. The latter with its major vessels and heart is a very high-risk area.

Injuries in the area of the lower chest should arouse suspicion of diaphragmatic damage with potential injury to both the thoracic and abdominal cavities. Pelvic injury can be the cause of major haemorrhage because of the rich vascular plexus of arteries and veins. Retroperitoneal injury is often difficult to diagnose, because it is associated with other intra-abdominal injuries. For management purposes, it is divided into the following three zones: zone 1 – central involving major vessels requiring exploration; zone 2 – lateral involving kidneys usually managed conservatively; and zone 3 – pelvis–haematomas, which are best left undisturbed. The junctional zones therefore can be summarised as neck, mediastinum, diaphragm, groin and retroperitoneum.

Much as spiral CT scan is the best diagnostic modality, it cannot be used in the unstable patient. Similarly for abdominal injuries, DPL is not the best method to make a diagnosis, as a negative result has no significance and it has a morbidity; moreover, DPL is considered when the patient is stable when the ideal investigation should be a CT scan.

→ Critical physiology

2. B

The physiological effects of bleeding are not always obvious. Clinically, one looks for tachycardia, tachypnoea and hypotension – the usual clinical effects. These will not be obvious, particularly in the young fit individual. In any patient with trauma, the initial management should be according to the Advanced Trauma Life Support (ATLS) principles of resuscitation, which consists of **ABCDE**: **A**irway, **B**reathing, **C**irculation, **D**isability, **E**nvironment and **E**xposure. One should look for bleeding from five major sites – external (which would be obvious), thoracic, abdominal, pelvic and extremity fractures. Biochemically there is increase in serum lactate, which is due to type A lactic acidosis arising from hypoperfusion and hypoxaemia from haemorrhage.

→ Thoracic injury

3. A, B, C, D

Thoracic trauma contributes to 25% of all severe injuries. In a further 25%, it contributes significantly to the cause of death because of chest-related complications that can be attributed directly to the thoracic trauma. A chest x-ray is the first investigation of choice. However, in certain situations, insertion of an ICD may not only be therapeutic but also diagnostic, for example, in a patient with haemothorax. This is because an inflated lung will float and hence sound normal on auscultation from the front.

Contrast-enhanced CT scan with 3-D reconstruction will define fractures, show haematomas and pneumothoraces and lung contusion. In case of penetrating trauma the track can be seen. Once thoroughly resuscitated and accurately investigated, 80% of thoracic injuries can be managed conservatively. In the case of an open pneumothorax, an ICD should be inserted first before fully closing the sucking chest wound. However, the defect can be closed with a sterile occlusive plastic dressing taped on three sides to allow the dressing to act as a flutter-valve.

Immediate life-threatening injuries

4. A, C, E

Tension pneumothorax is a clinical diagnosis. On clinical suspicion, one should never wait for a chest x-ray. The patient requires an immediate needle thoracostomy. The differential diagnosis is pericardial tamponade. While a rise in central venous pressure is usual in pericardial tamponade, it is not always present because there may be coincidental hypotension from severe haemorrhage at other sites such as the abdomen and pelvis. When there is flail chest, hypoxia occurs. This is not due to paradoxical respiration but is the result of underlying lung contusion and splinting of the chest wall due to severe pain.

The differential diagnosis of tension pneumothorax is pericardial tamponade, particularly in a shocked patient with distended neck veins. In pericardial tamponade the heart sounds will be muffled along with tachycardia and raised jugular venous pressure. However, it must be appreciated that in a busy A&E department normal heart sounds may be difficult to discern. In massive haemothorax the most common source of bleeding is torn intercostal artery or arteries; occasionally, damaged internal mammary artery may be the source.

Potential life-threatening injuries

5. A, B, C, D, E

Instantaneous death in a road-traffic accident (RTA) is often from traumatic aortic rupture, resulting from shear forces due to sudden high-energy impact disrupting the walls of the aorta. In the rare instance when the adventitia is intact, a stable patient may arrive in the hospital. The condition is suspected when there is discrepancy in the systolic blood pressure between the upper and lower limbs, wide pulse pressure and thoracic wall contusion. A CT scan will confirm the diagnosis, and the patient needs to be treated in a cardiovascular unit.

A patient who develops severe rapid and extensive surgical emphysema should be suspected to be having tracheobronchial injury. Chest drains are inserted, which would be both therapeutic and diagnostic. Bronchoscopy is diagnostic and is followed by intubation; subsequent management has to be in a thoracic unit. If after blunt chest injury, the patient's ECG is abnormal cardiac contusion should be excluded by echocardiography and warrants urgent referral to a cardiothoracic surgeon.

Diaphragmatic rupture following blunt injury can be missed easily, as it is silent unless there is evidence of injury to neighbouring organs. If the patient has a nasogastric tube, the tip of which can be seen in the chest, diaphragmatic rupture should be strongly suspected. The best confirmatory investigation is video-assisted thoracoscopy (VATS) or laparoscopy. Oesophageal injuries are usually due to penetrating injuries and present with subcutaneous or mediastinal emphysema. The upper gastrointestinal or thoracic surgeon should be involved.

Emergency thoracotomy

6. A

Emergency department thoracotomy (EDT) should hardly ever be performed. Most thoracotomies for trauma should be performed in the operating theatre. EDT should be reserved for those with penetrating injury in whom signs of life are still present. EDT in patients with penetrating trauma in whom the blood pressure (BP) is rapidly falling in spite of resuscitation have a survival rate of 60% if the BP is > 60 mmHg; if it is < 40 mmHg the survival rate is 3%.

Emergency thoracotomy for a definitive correction of a trauma problem should be carried out in the operating theatre. The approach chosen will depend upon the organ injured. Approach to the thoracic aorta, left side of heart, left lung and lower oesophagus is best obtained by a left anterolateral thoracotomy. A right anterolateral thoracotomy should be the approach to the superior vena cava, azygos vein, right lung and thoracic trachea. A 'clamshell incision' is a combined right- and left-sided thoracotomy, which gives good exposure for the surgeon who enters the chest very occasionally.

→ Abdominal injury and investigations

7. A, B, C, D, E

In abdominal injuries, after resuscitation, triaging them into the following groups helps in their management:

- Haemodynamically normal patients whose treatment can await completion of investigations.
- Haemodynamically 'stable' patients in whom investigations are urgent and are needed to decide whether management will be nonsurgical or surgical.
- Haemodynamically 'unstable' patients who need to be taken to theatre immediately to arrest bleeding.

The 'gold standard' in torso trauma is CECT, provided the patient is stable, and belongs to the second category as detailed previously. Intravenous contrast is used. In suspected duodenal injury, oral contrast is used, and in suspected rectal injury, rectal contrast is used. FAST is a useful and readily available investigation ideal for diagnosing blood or fluid in the abdomen and pericardium. The great advantage is that it is portable and can be done while resuscitation is being carried out; the disadvantage is that it is highly operator dependent.

DPL is a means of excluding intra-abdominal bleeding in the unstable patient with polytrauma. However, it has been superseded by FAST and CT scan. DL is a useful investigation. The stable patient with a penetrating injury is suitable for this invasive investigation, particularly to avoid exploratory laparotomy and to diagnose diaphragmatic injury. The procedure can be used therapeutically if suitable.

Answers to extended matching questions

1. F Abdominal compartment syndrome (ACS)

Patients who have undergone major surgery following trauma are prone to the complication of abdominal compartment syndrome (ACS). This is a major cause of mortality and morbidity in the patient with multiple injuries. Quite often it is not recognised. All the clinical features result from raised intra-abdominal pressure, which compresses the individual organs, thereby causing deterioration of their individual functions. Renal failure, decreased cardiac output from reduction in preload and increase in afterload, respiratory embarrassment from raising of the diaphragm and reduction in visceral perfusion account for this complication.

Measurement of intra-abdominal pressure by measuring the intravesical pressure through the indwelling catheter will help in making a diagnosis. An intra-abdominal pressure of more than 25 mm Hg is sinister, and the patient requires immediate abdominal decompression. Some surgeons following major surgery after severe abdominal trauma leave the abdomen open, covered with a plastic mesh (Bogota bag). Definitive surgery is carried out later. The condition has a high mortality of about 60%.

2. A Cardiac tamponade

This van driver is a shocked patient with distended neck veins following direct blunt and penetrating chest injury. Any patient with a penetrating injury near the heart who is shocked is deemed to have pericardial tamponade unless otherwise proved. The classic triad consists of low systolic pressure, raised jugular venous pressure (JVP) and muffled heart sounds (Beck's triad). The last sign may not be reliable, as it may be difficult to interpret because of noise in the busy surroundings of an A&E department. If the patient has lost a large amount of blood elsewhere, the JVP and central venous pressure (CVP) may not be elevated.

A chest x-ray, FAST, echocardiography and a rising CVP might help if the diagnosis is in doubt. Pericardiocentesis under ECG control is the emergency treatment. Withdrawal of 10–15 mL of blood will result in marked improvement and is a life-saving emergency measure before a formal thoracotomy is carried out by a cardiac surgeon. However, if the patient has lost a large amount of blood elsewhere, the JVP and CVP may not be elevated.

3. G Diaphragmatic injury

This patient has suffered a blunt injury to his abdomen and pelvis, resulting in a compression force. This nature of injury should alert one to the possibility of a diaphragmatic injury. On the chest x-ray, the tip of the nasogastric tube next to the heart confirms the injury. As the patient is stable, VATS is the investigation of choice. A DL is also useful if only to exclude intra-abdominal injury. Surgical repair is carried out in all cases. The abdominal route is preferred so that injury to abdominal organs is excluded and repaired if necessary.

4. D Flail chest

This rugby player, having sustained a blunt injury to the left side of his chest, has an unstable segment of chest wall on the left side. This is typical of a flail chest. A flail chest is defined as a segment of the chest wall that is discontinuous with the rest of the thoracic cage. It occurs when there are more than three ribs fractured at more than two sites. On inspiration the loose segment of chest wall moves inwards and on expiration it moves outwards – paradoxical respiration. This is a clinical diagnosis made on observation when the patient breathes or coughs. Hypoxia is primarily caused by the inevitable underlying lung contusion and lack of chest wall movement due to pain; paradoxical respiration contributes only a minor part to the hypoxia.

Pneumothorax or haemothorax is a complication. The treatment is mechanical ventilation to help internally splint the flail segment. Intercostal nerve block to relieve pain is a good alternative to opiates. Some surgeons perform internal operative fixation in selected cases to stabilise the chest.

5. I Liver injury

This badly assaulted patient's injuries are mostly on the right lower chest and abdomen. He has Cullen's sign which is a telltale finding of liver injury, because blood from the torn liver tracks to the umbilicus through the ligamentum teres. Liver is damaged typically as a result of blunt trauma. This patient is resuscitated according to the ATLS protocol. He is now reasonably stable. A CECT scan is carried out to determine the exact degree of liver injury and exclude other solid organ damage.

If the patient remains stable, he is treated conservatively, as most liver injuries are. If the patient becomes unstable, laparotomy is undertaken. Liver injury can be graded by various systems. The principles of surgery in liver injury can be summarised by the four Ps – push, Pringle's method, plug, pack. In very severe injuries, after packing the damaged liver, the patient should be transferred to a tertiary hepatobiliary unit.

6. C Massive haemothorax

This patient's type of injury typically will produce a massive haemothorax, the bleeding occurring from intercostal vessels or internal mammary artery. The patient suffers from haemorrhagic shock with collapsed neck veins, absence of breath sounds, hypoxia and dullness on percussion on the left side.

Massive haemothorax is defined as an initial drainage of more than 1.5 L of blood or more than 200 mL of blood per hour over 3 to 4 hours. Urgent vigorous resuscitation for the haemorrhagic shock followed by insertion of an intercostal drain is carried out. This is followed by an urgent thoracotomy by a cardiothoracic surgeon.

7. E Open pneumothorax

This young boy has an open pneumothorax, or a sucking chest wound. The wound should be closed immediately with a plastic Opsite dressing taped only on three sides to create a valve so that the air can escape out and not cause a tension pneumothorax. A formal intercostal drain (using as large a drain as possible) is inserted. The drain may be attached to a low-pressure suction. An early referral to a cardiothoracic surgeon is mandatory, as a thoracotomy might be needed.

8. K Pancreatic injury

This 10-year-old girl has the classical manifestation of a traumatic pseudocyst of the pancreas. The most common cause of acute pancreatitis in a child is from blunt trauma to the abdomen from a cycle handlebar injury. This girl sustained such an injury 10 days ago. At the time she suffered from traumatic acute pancreatitis, which obviously was not clinically bad enough to seek hospital help. Over the ensuing 10 days, she has developed a mass in the epigastrium typical of a pseudocyst.

This should be confirmed by ultrasound scan, which would show a cyst behind the stomach. Depending upon the size and the patient's symptoms, it should be managed accordingly. A cyst larger than 6 cm will need to be drained. A cystogastrostomy is performed by the endoscopic route.

9. H Renal injury

This young boy has right renal injury as a result of blunt abdominal and loin trauma. He is stable. After instituting ATLS resuscitation policy, an emergency intravenous urogram (IVU) is carried out (Figure 28.1). This is mainly done to ensure that the other kidney is normal. A renal ultrasound is done to gauge the size of the perirenal haematoma and repeated if necessary in a few days' time to make sure that it is reducing in size. Some may do a CECT scan. But as the same information can be obtained from a US scan, unnecessary radiation is avoided particularly because the patient is 9 years old.

The vast majority of renal injuries are treated conservatively (Figure 28.2). Every time the patient passes urine, some of it is saved in a transparent jar and the time of passing urine is noted (Figure 28.3). This gives an idea if the haematuria is getting better. In selected cases, if the haematuria does not improve while the patient is still stable, there is a place for selective renal angiogram with a view to renal artery embolisation. Haematuria following minor trauma should alert the surgeon to the possibility of injury to a pathological kidney, such as a congenital hydronephrosis or horseshoe kidney.

10. J Splenic injury

This female back-seat passenger in a car has had blunt trauma over the left lower chest and abdomen. She has fractured left lower ribs and referred pain to her shoulder tip due to diaphragmatic irritation from blood under the left dome from a ruptured spleen. A CECT scan will confirm the diagnosis. The patient is observed if she continues to be stable. Otherwise, a laparotomy is done at which a splenectomy or splenorrhaphy or splenic preservation by placing it in a mesh bag is attempted. Postoperatively she will require prophylaxis against opportunist post-splenctomy infection (OPSI).

11. B Tension pneumothorax

This motorcyclist has a left tension pneumothorax. He has intense hypoxia, is tachypnoeic, has a deviated trachea, a hyper-resonant percussion note and probably no breath sounds, which may be difficult to hear in a busy A&E department. This is an absolute emergency, which needs to be dealt with immediately by inserting a large-bore needle into the second intercostal space in the midclavicular line. This allows one to buy time for some 20 minutes or so, during which the definitive procedure of insertion of an intercostal drain in the fifth intercostal space in the anterior axillary line is carried out.

The usual causes are penetrating or blunt chest trauma with lung injury, causing air leak or iatrogenic lung puncture while inserting a CVP line through the subclavian route. This occurs when air leaks through a one-way valve from the lung. Air is forced into the chest cavity without any route of escape, causing complete lung collapse. There is a decrease in the venous return, causing engorgement of neck veins. The differential diagnosis is cardiac tamponade.

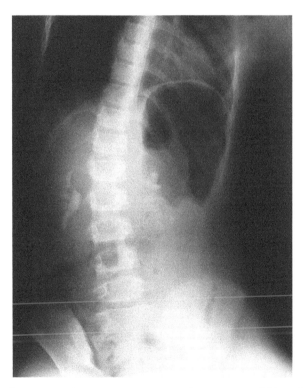

Figure 28.1 Emergency intravenous urogram in a 9-year-old boy kicked in the left side of his abdomen and back while playing rugby showing marked sco-liosis with concavity to the right, elevated left dome of diaphragm, loss of left psoas shadow, extravasation of contrast on the left side and normal excretion from right kidney. These findings are typical of a left renal injury with a perirenal haematoma.

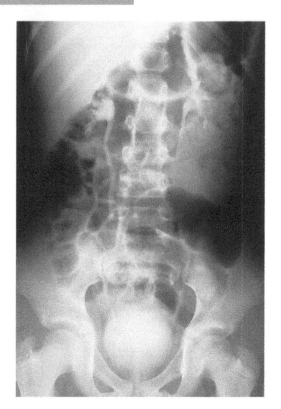

Figure 28.2 Intravenous urogram of the same patient 6 months later, showing both kidneys functioning normally after conservative management.

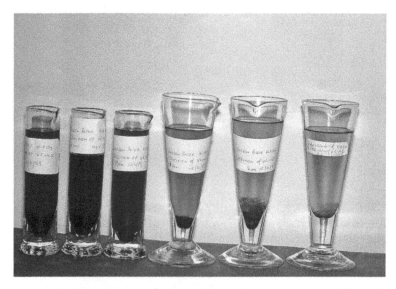

Figure 28.3 Serial specimens of urine collected from a patient with renal injury during conservative management showing the urine is becoming clear.

29 Extremity trauma

Andrew D Duckworth

Multiple choice questions

→ **Diagnosis**

1. Which of the following important injuries is notorious for not being seen on initial radiographs that appear normal?

A Anterior dislocation of the shoulder
B Supracondylar fracture of the elbow
C Hip fracture
D Scaphoid fracture
E Distal radius fracture

2. Regarding diagnostic imaging, which of the following imaging modalities would be most appropriate for assessing an x-ray confirmed L1 fracture of the spine in a polytrauma patient?

A CT
B Ultrasound
C MRI
D Bone scan
E Fluoroscopy

→ **Fracture classification**

3. What is the Gustilo and Anderson open-fracture classification for a 4 cm wound over the medial aspect of the mid-calf associated with a mid-shaft fracture of the tibia and an arterial injury, requiring repair?

A I
B II
C IIIA
D IIIB
E IIIC

4. What is the Salter-Harris fracture classification for a fracture of the distal radius that passes along the epiphyseal plate and then deviates off into the metaphysis (Figure 29.1)?

A I
B II
C III
D IV
E V

→ **Fracture healing**

5. A 50-year-old woman sustains a displaced and angulated fracture through the diaphysis of the right humerus. Following four months of treatment with initially a U-slab and then a humeral brace, the patient has persistent pain and mobility at the fracture site and check radiographs demonstrate no cortex bridging and no callus. What is the most likely diagnosis?

A Delayed union
B Atrophic non-union
C Hypertrophic non-union
D Infected non-union
E Union

→ **Fracture management**

6. Which of the following statements regarding the treatment of fractures is false?

A Not all fractures require reduction or stabilisation.
B Pain relief is a benefit of fracture treatment.
C Anaesthesia is a possible risk of fracture treatment.
D Relative stability leads to primary bone healing.
E Absolute stability leads to primary bone healing.

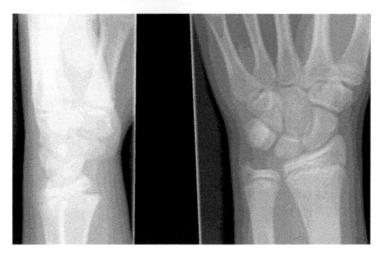

Figure 29.1 A fracture of the distal radius in a skeletally immature child.

Extended matching questions

→ Imaging

1 Bone scan
2 CT
3 Fluoroscopy
4 MRI
5 Ultrasound
6 X-ray

For each of the following cases, select the single most appropriate next investigation from the options listed. Each option may be used once, more than once, or not at all.

A A man presents after a game of squash with pain in the back of the calf and heel that was of sudden onset and difficulty weight bearing. On calf-squeeze test, the ankle does not dorsiflexion.

B A displaced intra-articular distal radial fracture is being reduced under general anaesthetic and held with a volar plate.

C A patient who had a breast cancer excised 5 years previously presents with weight loss and a pathological fracture of the femur. You want to know if there is evidence of other metastases in the body.

D A pedestrian sustains a fall from 30 feet, sustaining an open-book fracture of the pelvis. The patient is stabilised and the plan now is for reconstruction.

E A footballer has twisted his ankle in a tackle. The ankle is very tender over the medial and lateral malleolus.

F A rugby player sustains a twisting injury to his left knee during a game and subsequently complains of the knee giving way under him (instability) with episodes of locking. The knee had a significant effusion at the time or injury. X-ray is normal.

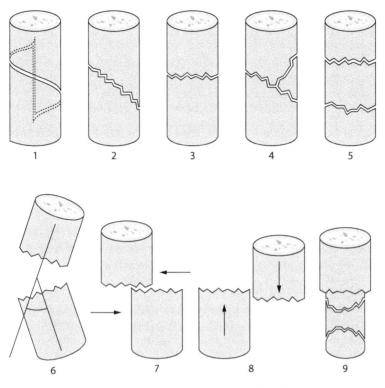

Figure 29.2 Fracture patterns and classification.

Fracture classification

1 Angulated
2 Oblique
3 Rotated
4 Segmental
5 Shortened
6 Spiral
7 Translated
8 Transverse
9 Wedge

For each of the diagrams shown in Figure 29.2, select the single most appropriate description from the options listed below. Each option may be used once, more than once, or not at all.

Fracture management

1 Cannulated screws
2 Dynamic hip screw
3 External fixation
4 Hip hemi-arthroplasty
5 Intramedullary nailing
6 K-wire fixation
7 Non-operative – collar and cuff

8 Non-operative – plaster of Paris
9 ORIF
10 Total hip arthroplasty
11 Traction
12 Wound debridement and washout
13 Wound debridement with washout and closure, fracture fixation
14 Wound debridement, washout, leave wound open and fracture fixation

For each of the following cases, select the single most appropriate management from the options listed. Each option may be used once, more than once, or not at all.

A A 32-year-old woman twists her right ankle, sustaining an isolated Weber B undisplaced lateral malleolus fracture with no displacement of the ankle mortice.

B A 17-year-old boy falls and suffers a transverse displaced midshaft fracture of the left radius and ulna. It is a closed and neurovascular intact injury.

C A 22-year-old man sustains an open fracture of his left distal radius following a heavy fall while playing football. There is 0.2 cm small puncture wound over the ulna aspect of his left wrist, with no evidence of contamination and is neurovascularly intact.

D A 71-year-old man with carcinoma of the lung and metastases presents with a pathological fracture through the upper third of the femur.

E An 81-year-old woman presents following a simple mechanical fall, and on presentation her right leg is shortened and externally rotated. She has a past medical history of ischaemic heart disease and COPD. X-rays reveal a right intertrochanteric neck of femur fracture.

F A 4-year-old girl falls from a trampoline and sustains a displaced fracture of the left distal humerus (supracondylar). It is a closed and neurovascular intact injury.

G A 68-year-old woman presents following a low-energy fall whilst out at bingo, and on presentation her right leg is shortened and externally rotated. She has a past medical history of hypertension and hypothyroidism, otherwise she is fully independent. X-rays reveal a displaced right intracapsular neck of femur fracture (**Figure 29.3**).

Answers to multiple choice questions

→ Diagnosis

1. D

Up to 30% to 40% of fractures of the scaphoid are not identified on initial four-view radiographs (**Figure 29.4**), with the clinical scaphoid fracture continuing to be a diagnostic conundrum. Posterior dislocations of the shoulder are classically (although not exclusively) associated with a seizure or electrocution, with displacement of the head in a posterior-inferior direction. Posterior dislocations (5%) are much rarer than an anterior dislocation (95%) and are easily missed on initial radiographs, with the anteroposterior (AP) view appearing normal apart from a possible lightbulb sign. A lateral or axillary view will clarify the diagnosis. Lateral condyle fractures of the elbow in children can be missed on initial radiographs, with an internal oblique view helpful. Hip fractures are identified routinely on initial radiographs of the pelvis and hip, although in cases where the diagnosis is unclear, further imaging in the form of CT or MRI can be indicated. Slipped upper femoral epiphysis in children is analogous to a posterior dislocation of the shoulder and may often appear normal on an AP pelvis view, with a frog-leg lateral view best for identifying the true extent of the slip. Distal radius fractures are routinely identified on standard AP and lateral views of the wrist.

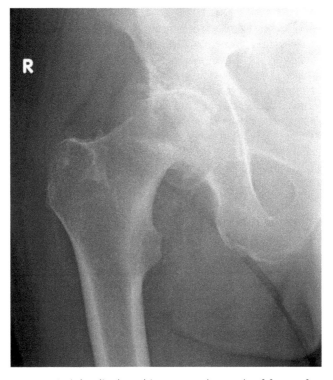

Figure 29.3 A right displaced intracapsular neck of femur fracture.

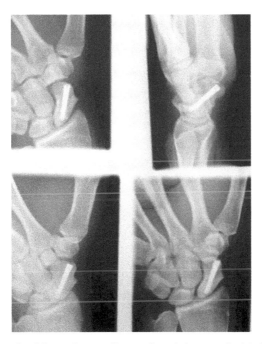

Figure 29.4 Standard four view radiographs of the scaphoid demonstrating a fracture through the waist that has been fixed with percutaneous screw fixation.

2. A

CT is the optimal imaging modality to determine the extent of any spinal fracture, e.g., number of columns involved, particularly in the polytrauma patient. The secondary survey in the ATLS protocol is part of a look-everywhere approach, and a CT head to pelvis is now used routinely in many centres. CT is also useful in planning surgery for complex peri-articular fractures, although availability and radiation dose should be considered. Ultrasound is useful for diagnosing soft tissue injuries, e.g., rotator cuff tears around the shoulder, but is operator dependent. MRI is primarily useful for assessing soft tissue injuries and some fractures. For certain spinal fractures, it may be used to assess the extent of ligamentous and/or cord injury but would not routinely be the next line of investigation. MRI is expensive and specialist equipment is needed in the ventilated patient. Bone scan is useful for assessing pathological fractures and possible metastases. Fluoroscopy is used intra-operatively.

→ Fracture classification

3. E

Any open fracture associated with an arterial injury requiring repair is a type IIIC. The Gustillo and Anderson classification **(Table 29.1)** is designed for open fractures and applies to the state of the soft tissue. The classification does not take account of the body part involved. The primary concern is the energy imparted to the soft tissue and hence its disruption, as well as the soft-tissue cover of the fracture and whether there is contamination. These factors are important to determine treatment and predict outcome.

Some injuries are classified as a grade III irrespective of wound size or soft tissue injury, e.g., traumatic amputation, segmental fracture, or heavy contamination (e.g., farming, gunshot).

4. B

Fractures involving the growth plate are classified according to shape and prognosis using the Salter-Harris classification **(Table 29.2, Figure 29.5)**.

Table 29.1 Examples of covert injury patterns

Grade	Description
I	Wound less than 1 cm, low-energy, clean, no periosteal stripping, minimal soft tissue damage
II	Wound greater than 1 cm, moderate soft tissue damage, no periosteal stripping/flaps/avulsions
IIIA	Often high-energy, extensive soft tissue damage (e.g., skin, muscle), periosteal stripping, contamination *Adequate coverage post fracture stabilisation – no flap required*
IIIB	Often high-energy, extensive soft tissue damage (e.g., skin, muscle), periosteal stripping, contamination *Inadequate coverage post fracture stabilisation – flap required*
IIIC	Open fracture associated with an arterial injury requiring repair

Source: Adapted from Table 29.3 in: Williams, N., Bulstrode, C., O'Connell, PR. (Eds.), *Bailey & Love's Short Practice of Surgery,* 26th ed., 2013.

Table 29.2 Salter-Harris fracture classification for growth plate injuries

Grade	Description
I	Rare translational fracture (sideways slip) that passes all the way along the epiphyseal plate. The metaphysis is the weakest side, and the blood supply enters from the epiphysis, so this fracture does not damage the growth potential of the plate.
II	Fracture along epiphyseal plate but exits and breaks off a fragment of the metaphysis. This fracture is by far the most common and has a good prognosis as it is along the safe (metaphyseal) side of the epiphyseal plate.
III	Similar to II, but the angulation of the fracture line is into the epiphysis and then on into the joint line. If it creates a step in the joint, there is a significant risk of the onset of premature traumatic osteoarthritis, so this fracture needs careful management.
IV	Fracture crosses from the metaphysis to the epiphysis. If there is any displacement then, when healing occurs, a bar of bone bridges across the epiphyseal plate from the metaphysis to the epiphysis. This will cause growth arrest.
V	Rare crush fracture of the epiphyseal plate that may not be obvious on x-ray. Growth arrest and deformity is common, as the growth plate has been destroyed.

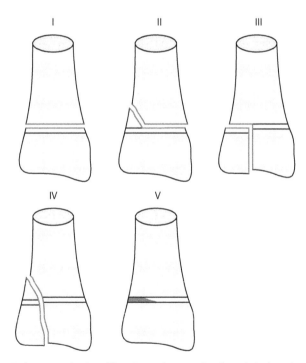

Figure 29.5 Salter-Harris classification of growth plate injuries. (Adapted from Figure 29.7 in: Williams, N., Bulstrode, C., O'Connell, PR. (Eds.), *Bailey & Love's Short Practice of Surgery,* 26th ed., 2013.)

⇒ Fracture healing

5. B

Radiological union is routinely characterised by the bridging of 3 of 4 cortices at the fracture site. Malunion is characterised by bone healing in a non-anatomical position. Generally, this is considered as an articular step of > 2mm, with angulation or rotation < 5 degrees. Delayed union is used to describe a fracture that has not healed within the expected time. Diagnosing a delayed union is fracture dependent, e.g., femoral fractures in adult can take 12–16 weeks to unite. Fractures in children unite quicker than fractures in adults, and upper-limb fractures unite quicker than lower-limb fractures. Non-union is defined as failure to develop signs of clinical and radiological healing. Following are the three types of non-union:

1 Atrophic – No callus formation, thinning of the fractures ends, associated with poor blood supply, fracture mobile.
2 Hypertrophic – Abundant callus formation, expansion of bone ends, no bridging of the fracture site, associated with poor stability or fixation.
3 Infected – Union prevented by infection, potentially catastrophic complication, multi-stage treatment may be required.
4 Risk factors for delayed or non-union include patient (age, diabetes, smoking, NSAIDs), fracture (open, severe soft tissue damage, infection, neurovascular injury) and management (inadequate fracture reduction or fixation) characteristics.

Fracture management

6. D
There are two stages in treating a fracture. The first of these is reduction, or putting the fragments back together so that the shape and alignment of the bone are correct. This is not always necessary and is dependent on both patient and fracture characteristics. If the fracture is undisplaced or the displacement does not matter, reduction is not needed. The second stage is 'stabilisation'. Not all fractures need stabilization – they might be stable once reduced, while others cannot easily be reduced or stabilised, nevertheless, they will heal. Benefits of fracture treatment include pain relief, restoration of anatomy and preservation of function, early mobilisation of the joint and the patient, prevention of infection and, potentially, reduced risk of secondary OA. Risks of fracture management include anaesthesia, possible introduction of infection, periosteal stripping, soft tissue or neurovascular damage and the need for a second operation to remove metalwork. Relative stability refers to a degree of movement at the fracture site that is expected and leads to indirect or secondary bone union with callus formation (enchondral ossification). Absolute stability occurs when the fracture has be anatomically reduced and stabilised so that there is no motion at the fracture site. The result is primary bone healing without callus formation, e.g., bone remodelling with cutting cones crossing the fracture site and lamellar bone being laid down.

Answers to extended matching questions

Imaging

A. 5 Ultrasound
The history and examination findings are classical of a ruptured Achilles tendon. Soft tissue is usually best visualised with ultrasound, especially if dynamic imaging is needed.

B. 3 Fluoroscopy
When fractures are being reduced and fixed under anaesthetic, fluoroscopy (image intensifier) is the best way of achieving this while keeping the radiation dose to a minimum.

C. 1 Bone scan
If metastases are suspected, a radioisotope bone scan allows the whole skeleton to be screened for increased lytic activity.

D. 2 CT
For complex fractures, further imaging in the form of CT, possibly with three-dimensional reconstruction of the fracture, will be helpful in planning surgery.

E. 6 X-ray
A footballer who has gone over on his ankle may have fractured the malleolus. Plain x-rays are the best way of imaging this type of injury.

F. 4 MRI
The history is classical of a soft tissue of the knee, with a ruptured anterior cruciate ligament or a torn meniscus, or both. MRI is the best imaging modality for this type of suspected soft tissue injury.

Fracture classification
A. 6 Spiral
This is a spiral fracture caused by a rotatory force.

B. 2 Oblique
This is an oblique fracture probably caused by a bending force.

C. 8 Transverse
This is a transverse fracture, caused by three-point loading (a force is applied across the fracture point, while the two ends are fixed). This injury commonly occurs in the tibia of footballers.

D. 9 Wedge
A wedge or butterfly fragment fracture occurs when the bone receives a sharp and heavy blow. The bone bends and the wedge fragment blows out on the other side.

E. 4 Segmental
This is a segmental or comminuted fracture and is associated with a high-energy mechanism of injury and is unstable. The central fragments can sometimes lose their blood supply, so non-union can be a problem.

F. 1 Angulated
This fracture is angulated, and so is likely to need reduction before fixation; otherwise a malunion will result.

G. 7 Translated
This fracture is displaced in the form of translation with one fragment moving in relation to the other. This pattern of injury is likely to need reduction before fixation otherwise a malunion may result.

H. 5 Shortened
This fracture is so displaced ('off-ended') that the two fragments have slid past each other. If this is not reduced, the fracture may still heal, but the limb will heal much shorter than before.

I. 3 Rotated
This fracture has rotated. Normally this is accompanied by a spiral fracture, in which case the fragments are usually displaced and shortened.

Fracture management
1 Cannulated screws
2 Dynamic hip screw

3 External fixation
4 Hip hemi-arthroplasty
5 Intramedullary nailing
6 K-wire fixation
7 Non-operative – collar and cuff
8 Non-operative – plaster of Paris
9 ORIF
10 Total hip arthroplasty
11 Traction
12 Wound debridement and washout
13 Wound debridement with washout and closure, fracture fixation
14 Wound debridement, washout, leave wound open and fracture fixation

A. 8 Non-operative – plaster of Paris

Ankle fractures are commonly classified according to the AO-Weber classification, which is based on AP and lateral x-rays of the ankle. This classification helps to guide treatment (**Table 29.3**).

B. 9 ORIF

Anatomic reduction with absolute stability is the optimal treatment for this patient using open reduction and internal fixation. Plates and screws are ideal for forearm fractures where a perfect reduction is needed, if full pronation and supination are to be achieved.

C. 13 Wound debridement with washout and closure, fracture fixation

Assessment and management of open fractures should start with ATLS guidelines. The first step is to lavage and photograph the wound, followed by using an iodine-soaked gauze to cover the fracture. Reduction of fracture may be necessary if there is surrounding skin or neurovascular compromise. The fracture should be immobilised for comfort and to prevent further soft tissue damage. Intravenous antibiotics should be commenced and the patient's tetanus status ascertained. The timing to theatre remains controversial, particularly for lower-grade fractures. Debridement involves wound extension and removal of all contaminated or devitalised soft tissue, followed by delivery and cleaning of the bone ends via the wound. Fracture stabilisation is then carried out. In this case primary fixation, possibly with a volar pate, would be carried out. However, temporary, e.g., external fixation may be carried out if there is concern about the soft tissue, contamination, or patient stability. For small (Grade 1) open wounds associated with a fracture, a thorough exploration, debridement and closing the wound primarily at the time of surgery would be done by many. All other open wounds would return to theatre at 48 hours for review +/- closure.

Table 29.3 The AO-Weber classification for ankle fractures

Grade	Description	Management
A	Avulsion lateral malleolus fracture Below level of syndesmosis	Stable injury – non-operative
B	Lateral malleolus fracture At level of syndesmosis	Undisplaced or stable – non-operative Displaced or unstable – ORIF
C	Lateral malleolus fracture or fibula fracture Above level of syndesmosis	ORIF

D. 5 Intramedullary nailing

The intramedullary nail is valuable in treating long-bone fractures, including pathological fractures. Combined with locking screws, it can provide adequate 'relative' stability to allow immediate weight bearing, while minimising vascular compromise.

E. 2 Dynamic hip screw

Hip fractures are best classified according to damage of the capsular blood supply to the femoral head. For extracapsular intertrochanteric or pertrochanteric fractures, there is no problem with the blood supply but strong fixation is required to allow early mobilisation. The dynamic hip screw is effectively a combination of an intramedullary nail fitted up the femoral neck, which connects to a heavy plate screwed to the side of the femur. The nail in the neck can slide into a slot in the nail so, that the fracture ends can be compressed together. This improves stability and stimulates bone healing.

F. 6 K-wire fixation

Supracondylar fractures of the elbow make up more than 50% of all paediatric elbow fractures, with the extension type most frequently seen (95%–98%). Neurovascular compromise can occur. The Gartland classification is employed, with type 1 fractures nondisplaced and effectively managed non-operatively in an above-elbow cast. Type 2 (displaced with an intact posterior cortex) and type 3 (completely displaced) fractures require closed reduction (open, if reduction not attained closed) and K-wire fixation, often using divergent lateral wires.

G. 10 Total hip arthroplasty

The intracapsular fracture of the neck of femur destroys the blood supply to the femoral head, so it requires replacement. In independent patients, total hip arthroplasty has been proved to provide a superior outcome over hemi-arthroplasty and ORIF for these injuries.

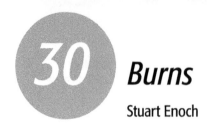

30 Burns

Stuart Enoch

Multiple choice questions

→ General

1. **Which of the following statements regarding burns in children in the United Kingdom are true?**
A The majority are electrical or chemical.
B Scalds are the most common type.
C Hot water thermostat setting at 60°C helps to improve safety in homes.
D Intravenous (IV) resuscitation in children is not required for burns up to 10% total body surface area (TBSA).
E Non-accidental injury is common in children's burns.

2. **Regarding burn injury in adults in the United Kingdom, which of the following statements are true?**
A Electrical and chemical burns are common.
B Scalds at home are more common than flame burns.
C Alcohol problems are rare in relation to burn injury.
D Effective care requires multidisciplinary input.
E Intravenous fluids are required for burns of 15% TBSA or more.

3. **Which of the following statements are true regarding epidermal burns?**
A Epidurmal burns are classified as superficial burns.
B Epidurmal burns are red in colour.
C Epidurmal burns are painless.
D Epidurmal burns are associated with a normal capillary refill time.
E Epidurmal burns heal by primary intention.

4. **The criteria for transfer of a patient with burns to a specialised burns unit include the following:**
A Partial- and full-thickness burns ≥10% of the total body surface area in patients ≤10 years or ≥50 years of age.

B Full-thickness burns involving the genitalia.
C Full-thickness burns ≥5% body surface area in any age group.
D Chemical injury.
E Inhalation burn.

→ Respiratory problems in burns

5. **Which of the following statements regarding respiratory problems in burns are true?**
A Burn injury to the lungs can be fatal.
B Injury can be due to inhalation of hot or poisonous gases.
C Burn injury is more common in the supraglottic than in the lower airway.
D Haemoglobin combines with carbon monoxide less easily than with oxygen.
E Hydrogen cyanide interferes with mitochondrial respiration.

→ Smoke inhalation

6. **Which of the following statements regarding smoke inhalation are true?**
A Inhaled smoke particles can cause a cause a chemical alveolitis and subsequent increased gaseous exchange.
B Inhaled smoke particles may be suspected with a specific situation in an enclosed space.
C Early elective intubation is contraindicated.
D Symptoms can take 24 hours or up to 5 days to develop.
E The result of carbon monoxide poisoning is a metabolic alkalosis best treated by low-inspired oxygen.

7. **Which of the following statements are true regarding carbon monoxide poisoning?**

A Carboxyhaemoglobin dissociates less readily than oxyhaemoglobin.

B The fall in PaO_2 is directly proportional to a rise in carboxyhaemoglobin levels.

C The PaO_2 levels are always reduced.

D Carbon monoxide binds with the intracellular cytochrome system and produces abnormal cellular function.

E Carboxyhaemoglobin levels of $\geq 20\%$ is manifested by ataxia and convulsions.

→ Extent of burns

8. **Which of the following statements are true in relation to burns and total body surface area (TBSA)?**

A Epidermal destruction can occur when a surface temperature of 70°C is applied for 1 second.

B A child's head comprises a smaller percentage of TBSA than that of an adult.

C According to the Lund and Browder chart, an adult with burns involving both sides of one upper limb, as well as the hand, equates to about 15% TBSA burn.

D The 'rule of nines' is widely used in the burns unit to estimate burn size in a 10-year-old child.

E In small burns the patient's whole hand is 1% of TBSA and is a useful guide to assess a burn.

9. **Which of the following statements regarding burn depth are true?**

A The depth of a burn together with percentage of TBSA and smoke inhalation are key parameters in the assessment and management of a burn.

B Alkalis, including cement, usually result in superficial burns.

C Fat burns are deeper than electrical contact burns.

D Capillary filling is not present in superficial burns.

E Deep dermal burns take a maximum of two weeks to heal without surgery.

→ Consequences of burns

10. **Which of the following statements regarding the consequences of burns are true?**

A As a result of a burn, complement causes degranulation of mast cells and, subsequently, neutrophils.

B Mast cells do not release primary cytokines.

C As a result of a burn, an increase in vascular permeability occurs.

D Following a burn, water only moves from the intravascular to extravascular space.

E In burns affecting >15% TBSA in an adult, fluid loss results in shock and the volume lost as fluids is directly proportional to the area of burn.

11. **Which of the following statements regarding burn complications are true?**

A Cell-mediated immunity is increased in major burns.

B Infections with bacteria and fungi are rare in large burns.

C Malabsorption from gut damage is a known complication in a burned patient.

D Circumferential full-thickness burns of a limb can result in ischaemia.

E A change in voice is an important clinical sign in a burned patient.

12. **The systemic effects of $\geq 50\%$ total body surface area burns in adults include the following:**

A Immunosuppression

B Increase in circulating catecholamines

C Hypoglycemia

D Hypervolaemia

E Adult response distress syndrome

→ Treatment of burns

13. **Which of the following statements regarding the treatment of burns are true?**

A Cooling of a scald for 10 minutes is sufficient to reduce the effect of acute injury.

B Other non-burn injuries may coexist with a burn.

C Major determinants of burn outcome are percentage of TBSA, depth and presence of any inhalation injury.

D Criteria for acute admission to a burn unit does not exist or is unnecessary.

E Hand burns do not need to be referred to a burn unit and can be managed in A&E setting or GP practice.

14. **Which of the following statements are true in the management of a six-month old child with burns?**

A Each leg is about 18% of TBSA in this child.

B A dark, lobster red with slight mottling is indicative of deep partial or full-thickness burn.

C The child should be fully wrapped in damp dressings until he or she reaches the burn unit.

D A urine output of 0.5 mL/kg/hour is an indicator of adequate hydration.

E A blood lactate level of >4 mmol/L suggests inadequate intravascular fluid volume.

15. **Which of the following statements are true in the early management of adult burns?**

A Clothing should not be removed immediately since it tears away burnt skin.

B Ice or cold water should be used for 20 minutes to cool the burn.

C Full-thickness burn of >5% total body surface area is an indication for transfer to the specialized burn unit.

D Application of silver sulphadiazine is recommended before the patient is transferred to the burn unit.

E Nasogastric tubes should be avoided in the early stages since they predisposes to gastric ulcers.

16. **Which of the following statements are true in the emergency management of a 33-year-old man with extensive burns to his abdomen, arms and legs?**

A Fluid resuscitation should be commenced only after accurate assessment of the total body surface area of burn.

B A urinary catheter is indicated if the burn is full-thickness covering ≥15% total body surface area.

C Leathery white appearance is suggestive of full-thickness burns.

D Intravenous access should not be secured through burned skin.

E Escharotomy should not be performed until the patient is assessed in the burn unit.

→ **Burn depth**

17. **Which of the following statements are true?**

A The depth of a burn can be assessed initially from the temperature and nature of the causative agent and time of application.

B Electric contact burns are almost certainly full-thickness.

C Superficial partial-thickness burns involve destruction of the whole dermis.

D Sensation is totally absent in a full-thickness burn.

E Tangential shaving may be a useful diagnostic and management tool in partial-thickness burns.

→ **Fluid management**

18. **Which of the following statements are true?**

A Oral fluids containing no salt are essential when given as fluid replacement in burns.

B Fluids required can be calculated from a standard formula.

C Hyponatraemia can be avoided in oral fluid management by rehydrating with a solution such as Dioralite.

D Urine output gives a major clue as to adequacy of fluid replacement.

E Three types of fluid are commonly used for IV fluid replacement in burns: Ringer's lactate, hypertonic saline and colloids.

19. **Which of the following statements are true?**

A The simplest and most commonly used crystalloid is Ringer's lactate.

B Hypertonic saline produces an excess of intracellular water shifting to the extracellular space.

C Human albumin solution is a colloid that reduces protein leak out of cells, thereby helping to reduce oedema.

D The Parkland formula is the most widely used formula in the United Kingdom and calculates the fluid replacement in the first 24 hours.

E Using the Parkland formula, the fluid requirement in the first 24 hours for a man of 70 kg with an 18% TBSA burn is about 2,800 mL.

20. Which of the following statements are true?

A In resuscitation, a urine output of 0.5 mL/kg body weight per hour does not mean that the rate of infusion should be altered.

B In resuscitation, a urine output of 1 mL/kg body weight per hour indicates the fluid rate infusion is too low.

C In resuscitation, hypoperfusion is recognised by cool extremities.

D Urine output in excess of 2 mL/kg body weight per hour is associated with a low haematocrit.

E In large burns, monitoring tissue perfusion by a central line may be required even though there is increased infection risk.

Escharotomy

21. Which of the following statements are true?

A Escharotomy is not indicated for circumferential burns to the chest.

B Significant blood loss is not a feature to be considered when escharotomy is contemplated.

C Damage to major nerves can result by placing incorrect escharotomy incisions.

D Escharotomy of the hand and fingers is best done outside of a main operating theatre.

E In the lower limb, for escharotomy, the incision should be anterior to the ankle medially.

Dressings

22. Which of the following statements are true?

A Superficial burns can be treated with simple dressings such as Vaseline gauze.

B Deep dermal burns should not be irrigated with saline since this will lead to burn contractures.

C Hydrocolloid dressings such as Duoderm can be left on for 14 days.

D Silver sulphadiazine (1%) can be used effectively as a broad spectrum-antibiotic but not for methicillin-resistant *Staphylococcus aureus* (MRSA).

E An optimal healing environment can make a difference to the outcome in borderline-depth burns.

23. Which of the following statements are true?

A Biological dressings and synthetic ones such as Biobrane do not need to be changed and are useful in deep- and mixed-depth burns.

B Amniotic membrane is an accepted treatment modality for superficial burns.

C Mepitel is a nonpermeable form of dressing.

D Honey or boiled potato peel are unusual dressings for superficial burns but can be effective.

E *Pseudomonas aeruginosa* is not treatable by 1% silver sulphadiazine cream.

Burn management

24. Which of the following statements are true?

A Paracetamol is useful in small, superficial burns.

B For large burns >10% TBSA, intramuscular (IM) injections of opiates are best.

C Removing the burn tissue and achieving healing reduce pain and are also effective in stopping the catabolic drive.

D In adults with >15% TBSA burns, extra feeding is indicated.

E The greatest nitrogen losses in burns occurs between days 14 and 21.

→ Infection control

25. Which of the following statements are true?

A Infection control requires attention to hand washing and cross-contamination prevention.

B A rise or fall in white cell count is a sign of infection.

C Swabs taken from the burn wound normally do not grow any flora.

D Antibiotics given should be ideally based on cultures and following discussion with a microbiologist.

E Catheter tips are a possible source of an infection.

→ Allied therapies

26. Which of the following statements regarding allied therapy in burn patients are true?

A Success or failure of physical and psychological care of the burn patient is dependent on intensive nursing and physiotherapy management.

B Physiotherapy can be best done after 2 to 3 weeks.

C Post-traumatic stress disorder can occur as a result of burns.

D Psychological help may be required for relatives of the burned patient.

E Elevation is of little use in hand burns.

→ Treatment of blisters and burn depth

27. Which of the following statements are true?

A Blisters should not be debrided.

B Initial cleaning of a burn wound with chlorhexidine solution is contraindicated.

C If a burn has not healed within 3 weeks, then skin grafting may be required.

D Burn of indeterminate depth should be dressed appropriately and reassessed after 2 weeks.

E Deep dermal burns may require burns tangential shaving and split-skin grafting.

→ Surgical management

28. Which of the following statements regarding surgical management of burns are true?

A The anaesthetist is of great assistance and essential in the management of a major burn.

B Blood loss is not a feature of surgery in major burns.

C Blood loss may be reduced by application of a skin graft.

D A core temperature below 36°C may affect blood clotting.

E Synthetic dermis, including Integra or homografts, may provide temporary stable cover following excision of larger burns.

→ Role of physiotherapy, escharotomy and eyelid care

29. Which of the following statements are true?

A Physiotherapy and splintage are important in maintaining range of movement and reducing joint contracture.

B It is not necessary to splint the hand after skin grafting.

C Supervised movement by physiotherapists under direct vision of any affected joints should begin after about two weeks.

D Escharotomy of the circumferential burn of the upper trunk should help respiratory function.

E Early care must be taken when eyelids are burned.

→ Surgical management

30. Which of the following statements are true?

A Early surgery is indicated in the hands and axilla.

B Contractures are best treated with split-skin grafts.

C A Z-plasty is a useful technique for reconstruction of areas with burn scarring causing restricted movement.

D Tissue expansion is useful in treating alopecia caused by a burn.

E Local flap may be indicated if the recipient site has got poor blood supply.

→ Scar management

31. Which of the following statements regarding scar management of burns are true?

A Hypertrophy of a burn scar can be treated by the use of pressure garments worn for a month.

B Intralesional steroid injection or silicon patches may be useful in small areas of burn scar hypertrophy.

C Pharmacological treatment of itchy burn scars is not important.

D Use of Integra to resurface a healed full-thickness burn scar can improve scar quality.

E Flamazine cream should not be used as a topical agent in pregnant women or nursing mothers.

→ Electrical burns

32. Which of the following statements are true?

A Low-tension electrical burn injury is most likely to be found in accidents in the home.

B Underlying heart muscle damage is likely in low-tension injuries.

C Large amounts of damage to subcutaneous tissue and muscle are associated with high-tension electrical burns.

D Myoglobinuria is a serious complication of low-tension burns.

E Severe alkalosis is common in large electrical burns.

33. Which of the following statements are true concerning electrical burns:

A Superficial burns are more common than deep burns in low-voltage electrical injuries.

B All patients with electrical burns require cardiac monitoring for at least 24 hours.

C Renal failure in electrical burns is due to rhabdomyolysis.

D A urinary output of 0.5 mL/kg/hour should be aimed for in adults with myoglobinuria secondary to electrical burns.

E Mannitol is contraindicated in electrical burns.

→ Chemical and radiation burns

34. Which of the following statements are true?

A Copious water lavage is the best first-aid measure for phosphorus burns.

B Elemental sodium burns should not be treated by water lavage.

C Damage from alkalis is usually less than with acids.

D The onset of pain may be delayed in alkali burns.

E Local radiation burns causing ulceration need excision and split-skin graft repair.

35. The following statements are true regarding chemical burns:

A Acid burns require longer irrigation than alkali burns.

B Dry powder should be brushed away before irrigation with water.

C Neutralising agents should be the first line of treatment in cement burns.

D Hydrofluoric acid burns are associated with hypercalcaemia.

E Systemic sodium chloride may be required in the treatment of burns due to hydrofluoric acid.

36. Which of the following statements are true regarding 'trench foot':

A 'Trench foot' is caused by acute exposure to temperatures between 14°C and −8°C.

B 'Trench foot' is due to microvascular endothelial damage and vascular occlusion.

C 'Trench foot' appears black even in the absence of deeper tissue destruction.

D 'Trench foot' is characterized by pruritic, red/purple lesions.

E 'Trench foot' can lead to gangrene.

Answers to multiple choice questions

→ ## General

1. B, C
The majority of burns in children are scalds with kettles, pans, hot drinks and bath water. Legislation, health promotion and appliance design, together with education of patients regarding smoke alarms and hot water thermostats kept at 60°C, have reduced the incidence of burns. IV fluids in children are required when the TBSA is 10% or more.

2. A, D, E
Most electrical and chemical burns occur in adults, while scalds are less common than flame burns. The presence of alcohol, drug abuse, epilepsy and mental disorder is common in those who have suffered burn injury. A multi-disciplined approach must be available for effective care. IV fluids in adults are required when 15% or more of TBSA is affected.

3. A, B, D
Epidermal burns include only the epidermis and are classified as superficial burns. Common causes of epidermal burns are sun exposure and minor flash injuries from explosions. Due to the production of inflammatory mediators, hyperaemia occurs; so these burns are red in colour and may be quite painful. The underlying vascular plexus is not affected and hence the capillary refill time is normal. The stratified layers of the epidermis are burnt away and healing occurs by regeneration of the epidermis (also known as epithelialisation) from the underlying intact basal layer.

4. A, B, C, D, E
According to the American Burn Association guidelines (also followed by the British Burn Association), the following patients require transfer to the specialised burn unit: (i) Partial-thickness and full-thickness burns >10% of the total body surface area (TBSA) in patients <10 years or >50 years of age; (ii) Partial-thickness and full-thickness burns >20% TBSA in other age groups; (iii) Partial-thickness and full-thickness burns involving the face, ears, hands, feet, genitalia, or perineum or those that involve skin overlying major joints; (iv) Full-thickness burns >5% TBSA in any age group; (v) Significant electrical burns, including lightning injury; (vi) Significant chemical burns; (vii) Inhalation injury; (viii) Burn injury in patients with pre-existing illnesses that could complicate management, prolong recovery, or affect mortality; (ix) Any burn-injury patient with concomitant trauma poses an increased risk of morbidity or mortality, and may be treated initially in a trauma centre until stable before transfer to a burn centre; (x) Children with burn injuries who are seen in hospitals without qualified personnel or equipment to manage their care should be transferred to a burn centre with these capabilities; and (xi) Burn injury in patients who will require special social and emotional or long-term rehabilitative support, including cases involving suspected child abuse and neglect.

→ ## Respiratory problems in burns

5. A, B, E
Burns can damage the airway and lungs with life-threatening consequences. This can occur when the face or neck are burned, when the fire causing the burn is in an enclosed space, or when hot gases or poisonous vapours are inhaled. Burn injury is more common in the lower airway than in the supraglottic airway. Carbon monoxide has an affinity 240 times greater than oxygen for combining with haemoglobin and thus blocks the transport of oxygen. Blood gas measurement can be done to confirm the diagnosis. A concentration of carbon monoxide above 10% is dangerous; 60% is likely to be lethal. Hydrogen cyanide is a metabolic toxin produced in house fires, which interferes with mitochondrial respiration.

Smoke inhalation

6. B, D

Inhaled smoke particles can cause a chemical irritation or alveolitis. This results in interference with gaseous exchange. Early elective intubation is important and is definitely not contraindicated. Symptoms might not be immediately evident and can take up to 5 days to develop. Carbon monoxide poisoning causes a metabolic acidosis and is treated by inhalation of pure oxygen.

7. A, B, D

Carbon monoxide (CO) combines very readily with haemoglobin, forming carboxy-haemoglobin (COHb). Carboxyhaemoglobin dissociates less readily than oxyhaemoglobin, and so once formed reduces the oxygen-carrying capacity of the blood, leading to tissue anoxia. The dissolved oxygen in the plasma remains unaffected and hence the PaO_2 remains normal. In addition to binding preferentially with haemoglobin, CO also binds with great affinity to other haem-containing compounds, most importantly the intracellular cytochrome system. This combination may produce abnormal cellular functioning, and in severe exposure produces a 'sick cell syndrome'. Carboxyhaemoglobin level has to reach about 50% for the patient to manifested symptoms such as hallucination, ataxia, syncope, convulsions and coma; a level of $\geq 60\%$ could lead to death.

Extent of burns

8. A, E

The first indication of burn depth comes from the history of temperature and time of application at that temperature. Burn area can be measured by a series of formulae plotted on a chart. It should be remembered that the size of a child's head is proportionally larger than in an adult. The 'rule of nines' offers only a rough guide to estimate TBSA burn and is not very accurate in children <12 years of age. The Lund and Browder chart is widely used in U.K. burn units and measures a whole arm and hand (both sides) as about 8% of TBSA. In small burns it may be useful to use the patient's whole hand–palm as 1% of TBSA **(Figure 30.1)**.

9. A

The key factors in the assessment and management of a burn are smoke inhalation, depth and percentage of TBSA affected. If oral fluids are to be used, salt must be added to counter salt loss in the stressed situation. The likely depth of any burn can be derived from the causative agent. Thus fat usually causes deep dermal burns, while full-thickness burns are more certain in electric contact injuries. The burns caused by alkalis such as cement usually produce deep dermal or full-thickness burns. Any burn that heals spontaneously within 3 weeks is superficial; deep dermal burns will take longer. Sensation and capillary filling are features of a superficial burn **(Figure 30.2)**.

Consequences of burns

10. A, C, E

As a result of a burn, complement is produced, which degranulates mast cells and leucocytes. Mast cells act on leucocytes and produce primary cytokines. There is a movement of water and salt from the intra to the extravascular compartment due to an increase in vascular permeability. The resulting shock is related to this fluid loss and in an adult becomes significant when TBSA affected is >15% **(Figure 30.3)**.

11. C, D, E

In the burned patient there is a reduction in cellular immunity, and one should have a high index of suspicion for infections with bacteria and even fungi. Damage in the gut-lining

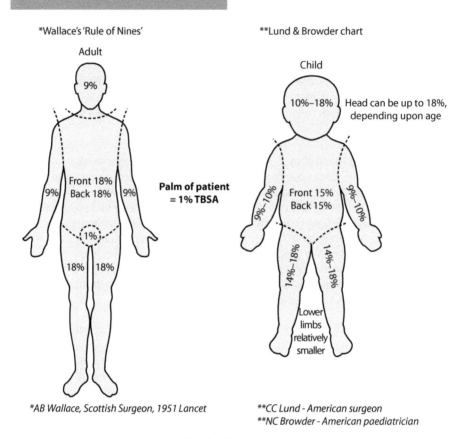

Figure 30.1   Methods of assessment of burn area.

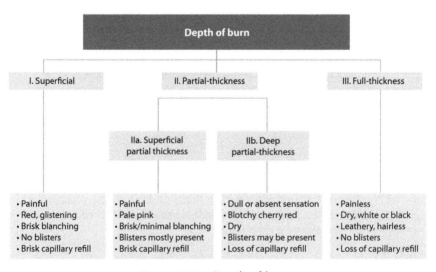

Figure 30.2   Depth of burn.

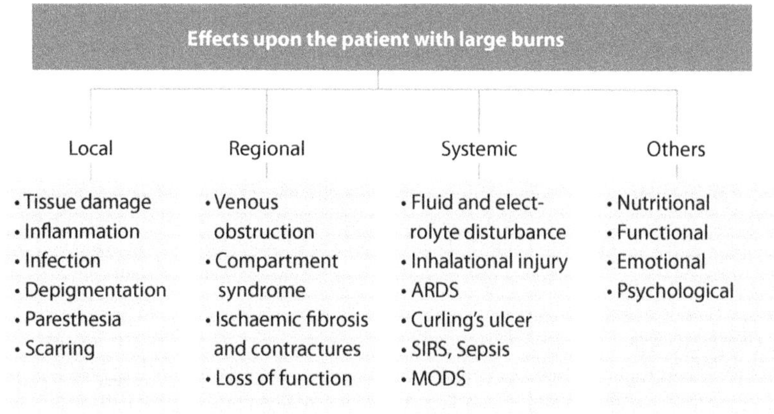

Effects upon the patient with large burns			
Local	Regional	Systemic	Others
• Tissue damage	• Venous	• Fluid and elect-	• Nutritional
• Inflammation	obstruction	rolyte disturbance	• Functional
• Infection	• Compartment	• Inhalational injury	• Emotional
• Depigmentation	syndrome	• ARDS	• Psychological
• Paresthesia	• Ischaemic fibrosis	• Curling's ulcer	
• Scarring	and contractures	• SIRS, Sepsis	
	• Loss of function	• MODS	

Figure 30.3 Effects upon the patient with large burns.

tissue might cause malabsorption. Ischaemic changes are a definite risk for full-thickness circumferential burns of the limbs as a result of swelling and a tourniquet effect. For the same reason, circumferential full-thickness burns of the chest may cause respiratory impairment. Warning signs of burns to the respiratory system include stridor or change in voice.

12. A, B, E
Virtually every organ system in the body is affected after a significant burn. This is due to alterations in the release of inflammatory mediators and neural stimulation. Immunosuppression is due to depression of many facets of the immune mechanism, both cellular and humoral. Burn injury results in a hypermetabolic state, caused by secretion of the stress hormones, including cortisol, catecholamines and glucagons. In addition, there is suppression of or resistance to anabolic hormones (growth hormone, insulin and anabolic steroids). Blood glucose is often elevated in major burns. Hypovolaemia is a characteristic feature of major burns, which is principally due to loss of protein and fluid into the interstitial space. The lungs frequently suffer from the changes of the post-burn systemic inflammatory response (adult acute respiratory distress syndrome) even in absence of inhalation injury.

Treatment of burns

13. B, C
A fresh burn should be cooled for about 20 minutes. Lowering the temperature of the agent causing the burn and the local tissue will help to reduce burn injury – this may sometimes be done by using cold water but not for every burn. Non-burn injuries may coexist with burns and should not be overlooked. Criteria for admission to each burn unit exist and advice about this and any burn is readily available. Hand burns are significant injuries due to the potential for long-term morbidity and contractures, and thus have to be managed by a specialised burn unit.

14. B, E
In a child up to 1 year of age the head and neck are 18% of the total body surface area, whereas each leg is approximately 14%. A dark, lobster red with slight mottling is indicative of deep partial or full-thickness burn. Hypothermia is a much greater risk in children than in adults. Children under 1 year of age do not have a shivering reflex. Cool water or damp dressing should only be applied to the burn surface, and the rest of the child should be kept warmly wrapped. Continuous assessment (every 30 minutes) until the child reaches the burn

unit is essential. A urine output of 0.5 mL/kg/hour is adequate in adults; however, in children of this age group, a urine output of at least 1–2 mL/kg/hour is required. Blood lactate level is a useful indicator in the management of burns and rising lactate level associated with a fall in the pH may suggest poor perfusion of the tissue secondary to inadequate intravascular volume.

15. C

All clothing should be removed as soon as possible; any skin that is adherent and peels off with the clothing is 'dead,' and it is essential to remove all dead tissue. Those whose clothing is alight should 'drop and roll'. The use of a wet blanket may facilitate extinguishing the burning clothing. The burn should be cooled with lukewarm running water for at least 20 minutes. Ice or very cold water should be avoided, as blood flow to the affected area will be reduced. This may lead to hypothermia, which is a particular risk in infants and the elderly. Among others, a full-thickness burn of >5% total body surface area is an indication for transfer to the specialised burn unit. Silver-based products render subsequent assessment difficult and therefore should not be applied without discussion with the burn team. Nasogastric (NG) tubes help to decompress the stomach and are recommended in burn patients, particularly those at risk of aspiration. NG tubes ensure mucosal integrity, thus minimising the risk of endogenous infection and bacterial translocation.

16. B, C

It might be difficult to accurately estimate the total body surface area (TBSA) of burn in an emergency situation. If a quick, initial assessment reveals a partial- or full-thickness burn of ≥15%, fluid resuscitation should be commenced immediately. The resuscitation of burns of >15% TBSA in an adult or 10% TBSA in a child should be monitored by a urinary catheter. Leathery-white or charred-black appearance is suggestive of full-thickness burns. The coagulated tissue is called 'eschar'. It does not blanch with pressure and is typically insensate. Intravenous access should be secured by any means, even through burned skin. Intravenous cut-down in the cubital fossae or on the long saphenous vein may be required if percutaneous intravenous access cannot be obtained. In children <6 years old, if intravenous access is not obtained, access should be sought through an intraosseous approach (commonly in the tibia). Emergency escharotomy may be needed to save life and thus may be indicated before the patient is transferred to the burn unit.

→ Burn depth

17. A, B, D, E

Most burns can be assessed from the history, nature and temperature of the causative agent and time of application. Electrical contact usually results in full-thickness burns. In superficial and deep partial-thickness burns, some dermal tissue is intact. Sensation is absent in full-thickness burns, as all nerve endings are destroyed. Tangential shaving using a skin-grafting knife is a useful management and diagnostic operation in partial-thickness burns – the presence of punctate bleeding after one or two shaves confirms this type of injury.

→ Fluid management

18. B, C, D, E

It is important to give salt and water in oral fluids provided for resuscitation instead of water alone, to account for salt loss. Dioralite is useful in the treatment of hyponatraemia. The output of urine gives a good indication of fluid requirements. Various formulae are available to calculate fluid requirements, which may be given as Ringer's lactate (Hartmann's solution), hypertonic saline or colloid.

19. A, C, D

Ringer's lactate is the most commonly used, and cheap, burn crystalloid fluid, while albumin is a colloid increases the intravascular oncotic pressure. Hypertonic saline also reduces oedema by producing hyperosmolarity and hypernatraemia – this reduces the shift of intracellular water to the extracellular space. The Parkland formula calculates the fluid to be replaced in the first 24 hours, with half of this volume to be given in the first 8 hours: TBSA percentage × weight (kg) × 4 = volume (mL). For a 70 kg patient with a 16% TBSA burn, the fluids required in the first 24 hours would be about 5040 mL (70 x 18 x 4).

20. C, D, E

Adequacy of fluid replacement can be assessed from measuring urine output, haematocrit and clinical status. For adults, a urine output of 0.5–1.0 mL/kg body weight per hour is normal. If it is lower than this and the haematocrit is higher than normal, more fluid should be given – there may be signs of restlessness, tachycardia and cool extremities. It is important that patients are not overresuscitated, and a urine output in excess of 2 mL/kg per hour means the rate of infusion should be reduced. Care should be taken in patients with acute or chronic cardiac problems, and the use of a central line should be considered even though there might be an increased risk of introducing infection.

Escharotomy

21. C

Escharotomy is indicated for circumferential burns of limbs or trunk – deep dermal or greater. A tourniquet effect occurs due to the increasing pressure and swelling that result. This procedure should be done early to aid respiration and prevent limb ischaemia, and can be associated with a significant blood loss. Adequate blood should be available for transfusion. Care should be taken in performing an escharotomy to prevent damage to major structures, including nerves. In the lower limb, it is also important to make the incision posterior to the ankle to prevent damage to the saphenous vein.

Dressings

22. A, B, E

Superficial burns can be dressed or left exposed. Most heal irrespective of the dressing unless they are contaminated or become infected. All burns need to be irrigated with saline and debrided, if appropriate. Irrigation of a burn does not lead to burn contractures. Vaseline gauze is a commonly used dressing. Duoderm, a colloid dressing, is useful in mixed-depth burns but should be changed every 3 to 5 days. Silver sulphadiazine (1%) is effective in cases of MRSA. It is important to remember that the optimal healing environment will provide the best chance of healing quickly and well, especially when the depth is mixed or uncertain.

23. B, D

Biobrane and amnion can be used for dressings for superficial but not deep dermal or full-thickness burns. Honey or banana has also been used around the world. Mepitel is a permeable fenestrated silicone sheet that can also be used. Silver sulphadiazine 1% is effective against *Pseudomonas* infection.

Burn management

24. A, C, D

Analgesia is a vital part of burn management. Oral paracetamol is useful in small burns, especially if they are superficial. Intravenous opiates are indicated for larger burns – not IM as absorption is uncontrolled and dangerous. Administration of this and other agents, such

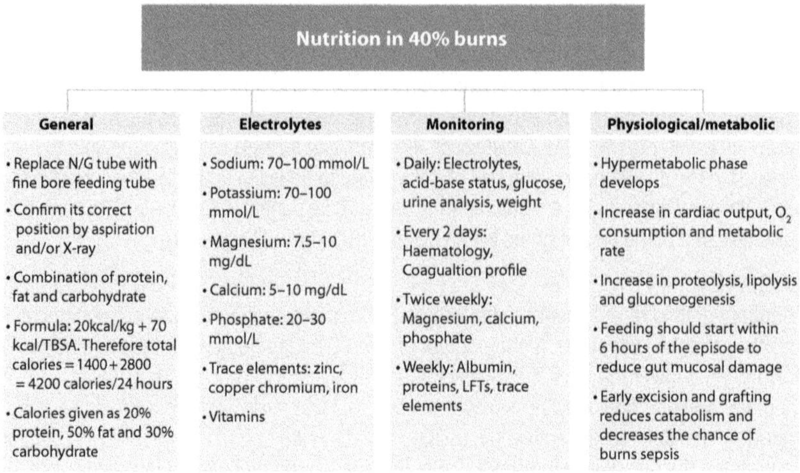

Nutrition in 40% burns			
General	**Electrolytes**	**Monitoring**	**Physiological/metabolic**
• Replace N/G tube with fine bore feeding tube • Confirm its correct position by aspiration and/or X-ray • Combination of protein, fat and carbohydrate • Formula: 20kcal/kg + 70 kcal/TBSA. Therefore total calories = 1400 + 2800 = 4200 calories/24 hours • Calories given as 20% protein, 50% fat and 30% carbohydrate	• Sodium: 70–100 mmol/L • Potassium: 70–100 mmol/L • Magnesium: 7.5–10 mg/dL • Calcium: 5–10 mg/dL • Phosphate: 20–30 mmol/L • Trace elements: zinc, copper chromium, iron • Vitamins	• Daily: Electrolytes, acid-base status, glucose, urine analysis, weight • Every 2 days: Haematology, Coagualtion profile • Twice weekly: Magnesium, calcium, phosphate • Weekly: Albumin, proteins, LFTs, trace elements	• Hypermetabolic phase develops • Increase in cardiac output, O_2 consumption and metabolic rate • Increase in proteolysis, lipolysis and gluconeogenesis • Feeding should start within 6 hours of the episode to reduce gut mucosal damage • Early excision and grafting reduces catabolism and decreases the chance of burns sepsis

Figure 30.4 Nutrition in 40% burns.

as general anaesthesia, ketamine, or midazolam, might require an anaesthetist. There are catabolic changes as long as the burn wound remains unhealed, and rapid excision of the burn and stable wound coverage are the crucial factors in reversing this. Extra feeding must be given, and this should be by nasogastric tube in burns covering >15% TBSA; 20% of kilocalories should be provided by proteins. The greatest nitrogen losses occur between days 5 and 10 (**Figure 30.4**).

Infection control
25. A, B, D, E
Control of infection begins with policies on hand washing and other cross-contamination prevention measures. A rise in white blood cell count, thrombocytosis and an increase in catabolism are warning signs in the development of infection. Swabs taken from the burn wound and sputum can help in establishing flora. The advice of a bacteriologist is of great importance in the decision on antibiotics. Catheter tips can be a source of infection.

Allied therapies
26. A, C, D
Intensive nursing, physiotherapy and psychological management of a burned patient are of importance. Psychological support might help the relatives and prevent post-traumatic stress. Physiotherapy should be started early, and in the case of hand burns this should be on day 1 and reinforced daily. All burns of the hands cause swelling, and elevation and splintage will improve the outcome.

Treatment of blisters and burn depth
27. C, E
Blisters can be debrided in a clean and controlled setting in a burn unit before application of an appropriate dressing. Initial cleaning of a burn wound can be undertaken with chlorhexidine, betadine, or saline. If a burn has not healed within 3 weeks, then further debridement and skin grafting may be indicated. All burns of indeterminate depth should be reassessed every 48–72 hours. Deep dermal or full-thickness burns may need tangential shaving and split-skin grafting.

Surgical management

28. A, C, D, E

An anaesthetist must be available for dressing or debridement of a major burn. As blood loss can be a feature of large burn debridement, facilities for blood transfusion and blood must be available. The application of limb tourniquet or topical or subcutaneous adrenaline solution – diluted 1:500,000 – will help to control or reduce bleeding. Blood-clotting irregularities can occur when the core temperature of the patient falls below 36°C; thus, the operating room must be kept warm. The use of Integra or homograft can be a useful temporary way of dressing a large burn that has been excised.

Role of physiotherapy, escharotomy and eyelid care

29. A, D, E

Physiotherapy and splintage both help considerably in preventing joint contractures. A hand splint is used in hands treated by split-skin grafts. Supervised physiotherapy for any affected joints should occur on day 1 so that early recovery can be aided. In full-thickness burns or deep dermal circumferential burns of the upper trunk, escharotomy will help to improve respiration. It is important to provide early care, including surgery if necessary, if eyelids are burned.

Surgical management

30. A, C, D, E

Early excision and grafting are indicated in burns of the axilla and hands. Contractures are usually best treated by full-thickness skin grafts. If full-thickness skin grafting is not appropriate or possible, then a Z-plasty is a useful technique to treat scar contractures. Tissue expansion may be useful in treating alopecia of the scalp caused by burns. Full-thickness grafts are useful in situations where the blood supply is good in the recipient site; and local or free flaps are useful if the blood supply to the recipient site is poor or absent (since a flap brings its own blood supply).

Scar management

31. B, D, E

Pressure garments may be effective in reducing burn scar hypertrophy but require to be fitted and worn for at least 6 months and would be ineffective if only used for 1 month. Intralesional injection of steroid or application of a silicon patch or sheet might be useful for smaller hypertrophic areas. It is important to treat any itchy areas with appropriate pharmacological agents, as a patient scratching the area may cause distress and increase the chance of introducing infection and delayed healing. The use of Integra may improve the quality of burn scars. Flamazine cream, although useful, should not be used in pregnant women or nursing mothers.

Electrical burns

32. A, C

Low-tension electrical burns are associated with electrical burns in the home due to the fact that appliances are 'low tension'. Heart damage is not a feature of low-tension burns but can be in high-tension burns, which are associated with large amounts of subcutaneous and muscle damage, resulting in myoglobinuria and renal damage. Acidosis is more common in large electrical burns and may require treatment with boluses of bicarbonate.

33. C

The energy imparted from low-voltage electrical injuries usually gives a small entry and exit wound but may cause deep dermal or full-thickness burns. Cardiac damage and myocardial arrhythmias can arise if the alternating current crosses the heart. Cardiac monitoring is indicated if cardiac injury is diagnosed; however, cardiac monitoring is not indicated if the echocardiography is normal and there was no history of loss of consciousness. Acute renal failure can arise from the myoglobin released due to rhabdomyolysis. A urinary catheter should be inserted in all patients with severe electrical burns, once the life-threatening injuries have been addressed and the patient adequately resuscitated. The presence of haemochromogens leads to a dark-coloured urine. Fluid administration should be increased to ensure a urinary output of at least 1–1.5 mL/kg/hour in an adult. If the pigment does not clear with increased fluid administration, 25 g of mannitol should be administered immediately and 12.5 g of mannitol should be added to subsequent litres of fluid to maintain diuresis.

→ Chemical and radiation burns

34. B, D
Chemical burns can be classified broadly into acids, alkalis and other specific agents including petroleum products, nitrates, phosphorous and elemental metals. With phosphorus and elemental sodium burns, washing with copious water is contraindicated. Alkali burns are generally deeper than acid burns and act for a longer time. Acid burns are generally more painful than alkali burns; however, in alkali burns, the onset of pain is delayed, which often postpones first aid and leads to more tissue damage. Radiation burns cause tissue damage associated with blood vessel necrosis – split-skin grafts will not take on avascular tissue, so vascularised flaps or free flap reconstructions are required.

35. B
The local and systemic effects of chemical burns are influenced by the duration of contact, concentration of the chemical and amount of the agent. Both acid and alkali burns should be flushed away immediately with large amounts of water for at least 20 to 30 minutes. Alkali burns require longer irritation than acid burns. If dry powder is still present on the skin, it should be brushed away before irrigation with water. In cement burns, neutralizing agents have no advantage over water lavage, because reaction with the neutralizing agent might itself produce heat and cause further tissue damage. Hydrofluoric acid burns are associated with hypocalcaemia and, following copious lavage with water, treatment with topical calcium gluconate gel (10%) is indicated. Hydrofluoric acid penetrates tissue deeply and even small burns can cause fatal systemic toxicity. Systemic calcium may be required in some patients, as hydrofluoric acid sequesters calcium with the burn.

36. B, C, E
Trench foot or cold immersion foot (or hand) is caused due to a nonfreezing injury of the hands or feet. This is typically seen in soldiers, sailors, or fishermen, who are chronically exposed to wet conditions and temperatures just above freezing, i.e., 1.6°C to 10°C (35°F to 50°F). It occurs due to microvascular endothelial damage, stasis and vascular occlusion. Although the entire foot may appear black, deep tissue destruction may not be present. An alternating arterial vasospasm and vasodilatation occurs, with the affected tissue first cold and anaesthetic, progressing to hyperaemia in 24 to 48 hours. This leads to an intense painful burning and dysaesthesia, as well as tissue damage characterized by oedema, blistering, redness, ecchymosis and ulcerations. Pruritic, red-purple skin lesions (papules, macules, plaques, or nodules) are a feature of chilblain (also known as pernio) and not of trench foot. Complications of trench foot include local infection, cellulitis, lymphagitis and gangrene. Careful protection from further exposure and proper attention to foot hygiene can prevent the occurrence of most such injuries.

31 Plastic and reconstructive surgery

Stuart Enoch

Multiple choice questions

→ **Wound healing**

1. Which of the following statements regarding wound healing are true?

A Wound healing can proceed in the absence of polymorphonuclear leucocytes.

B Monocytes are essential for wound healing.

C Collagen is formed by two polypeptide chains.

D Type IV collagen is seen predominantly in the basement membrane.

E The normal ratio of Type I to Type III collagen in the skin is approximately 4:1.

2. Which of the following statements regarding types of wound healing are true?

A Healing by primary intention happens when a wound is closed within 12–24 hours of its creation.

B Healing by secondary intention occurs by both wound contraction and epithelialisation.

C Delayed primary healing is recommended for human bite wounds.

D Myofibroblasts play a crucial role in primary wound healing.

E Split-skin graft donor sites heal by secondary intention.

→ **Keloid scars**

3. Which of the following statements regarding keloid scars are true?

A Keloid scars are predisposed by wound haematoma and infection.

B Keloid scars extend beyond the margins of the original scar.

C Keloid scars are more common in children and young adults.

D Keloid scars usually develop within weeks of initial injury.

E Keloid scars are characterised by increased collagen synthesis.

4. Which of the following treatment options are useful in the management of keloid scars?

A Topical silicone gel

B Intralesional steroid injections

C Radiotherapy

D Intralesional surgical excision

E Systemic steroids

→ **Skin characteristics**

5. Which of the following statements are true?

A The surface of the skin is an important biological layer for homeostasis.

B The epidermis regenerates from deeper follicular elements.

C Epidermal keratinocytes cannot be cultured and thus are of no value in wound management.

D The depth of skin varies in different parts of the body.

E In the absence of skin, a wound heals by secondary intention with fibrosis and contracture.

→ **Skin grafts**

6. Which of the following statements regarding blood supply to skin grafts are true?

A Skin blood supply comes from muscle and fascial perforating vessels.

B Direct cutaneous vessels can also contribute to the blood supply of the skin.

C A graft has a separate blood supply, which enables it to survive on an avascular wound.

D A full-thickness graft has the whole dermis attached with fat trimmed off.

E A composite graft is a full-thickness graft to which other structures such as hair may be added by suturing on.

7. **Which of the following statements regarding grafts are true?**

A Imbibition is not a process associated with survival of split-skin grafts in the first 48 hours.

B Gentle handling and the best postoperative care help to ensure the successful take of a full-thickness graft.

C Grafts will take on exposed tendons and cortical bone.

D Contraction occurs in all grafts used in tissue repair but is dependent on amount of dermis taken with the graft.

E The more dermis in the graft, the more is the contraction.

8. **Which of the following statements regarding grafts are true?**

A Split-skin grafts are sometimes known as Thiersch grafts.

B Full-thickness grafts are useful in small areas such as fingers, eyelids, or on the face.

C John Wolfe, an Aberdeen orthopaedic surgeon, described a composite graft in 1902.

D Split-skin grafts produce a superior cosmetic result compared with full-thickness grafts.

E Scars placed in 'the lines of election' or lines of minimal tension produce the best cosmetic results.

9. **Which of the following statements regarding full thickness skin grafts are true?**

A Full-thickness grafts require a well-vascularised recipient bed.

B Inosculation is the process of adherence of the graft to the recipient bed.

C Full-thickness skin grafts shrink less compared to split-thickness grafts.

D The texture and pigmentation of full-thickness grafts are usually quite similar to normal skin.

E The donor site of a full-thickness graft is usually left to heal by secondary intention.

10. **Which of the following statements regarding split-skin grafts are true?**

A Split-skin grafts can be cut at varying thicknesses using handheld or electrical dermatomes.

B The best donor site for getting a split-skin graft in children or females is the thigh.

C Other useful donor sites for split-skin grafts are the buttocks and scalp.

D The size and number of bleeding points in the donor tissue for split-skin grafts do not identify the thickness of the graft.

E The take of a split-skin graft is affected by a number of factors, including the presence of group A beta-haemolytic *Streptococcus*.

11. **Which of the following statements regarding mesh grafts are true?**

A Mesh grafting enables expansion of a split-skin graft to be done.

B Mesh grafting prevents release of exudates from under a split-skin graft.

C The possible donor site for a full-thickness graft is from behind the ear.

D Conditions for take of a full-thickness graft are not as critical as for a split-skin graft.

E Large full-thickness grafts when used in the face and over good facial muscle do not produce a satisfactory cosmetic result.

→ **Flaps**

12. **Which of the following statements regarding soft tissue coverage are true?**

A Full-thickness skin grafts are preferred to flaps to cover exposed bone.

B Flaps depend on their own vascular pedicle for survival.

C Random-pattern flaps rely on random cutaneous vessels for their blood supply.

D Island flaps are more mobile and versatile than random flaps.

E Free flaps require a vascular pedicle of at least 5-mm in diameter.

13. **Which of the following statements regarding flaps are true?**

A Flaps introduce blood supply into an area for reconstruction.

B Classification of flaps can be made on the basis of their blood supply.

C In a random-pattern flap, a length:breadth ratio of 3:1 is considered safe.

D Delay is a technique that can further lengthen a random flap.

E Axial flaps, based on known blood vessels, enable longer flaps to be moved over longer distances.

14. **Which of the following statements regarding flaps are true?**

A Islanding of a random flap can safely and usefully be done.

B Inclusion of fascial tissue in a skin flap does not make for greater safety.

C The design of a transposition flap demands knowledge of a pivot point.

D The transposition flap length equals the length of the defect to be covered – assuming the breadth:length ratio is no greater than permitted.

E Following the use of a transposition flap, skin grafting of the donor defect is a likely necessity though direct closure may be just possible.

15. **Which of the following statements regarding flaps are true?**

A Z-plasties are triangular transposition flaps.

B Z-plasties are able to lengthen very broad contracture scars.

C A bilobed flap is useful to close a small convex defect in the nose tip.

D Rhomboid flaps are useful in the repair of defects of the fingertips.

E Rotation flaps are used for buttock or scalp defect repairs.

16. **Which of the following statements regarding flaps are true?**

A Burrow's triangles are not of significance in the use of bipedicle flaps.

B Multiple Y to V releases are one of most effective means of managing moderate isolated burn scars over flexion creases.

C V to Y flaps are ineffective in the management of fingertip injuries.

D The key to successful random flap use is to pull available local spare lax skin into the defect, so that the closed scar lies in a good line of election.

E A disadvantage of using local flaps may be a poor cosmetic result.

17. **Which of the following statements regarding local flaps are true?**

A Limberg's flap is a type of rotation flap.

B Dufourmentel flap is a variant of V-Y advancement flap.

C Rotation flaps are useful in scalp reconstruction.

D Bilobed flaps are commonly used in lip reconstruction.

E Langenbeck's palatoplasty is an example of a uni-pedicled advancement flap.

18. **Which of the following statements regarding myocutaneous and fasciocutaneous flaps are true?**

A Myocutaneous and fasciocutaneous flaps are unreliable in plastic surgery repairs.

B The above flaps require complex equipment to be available.

C Knowledge of blood supply in the area of use is essential when these flaps are used.

D These flaps can be used without skin if required.

E Survival of the skin when used in these flaps as skin-island flaps depends on small perforating vessels.

19. **Which of the following statements regarding free flaps are true?**

A Free flaps are the best way of reconstructing major composite loss of tissue.

B Surgical expertise and equipment in microsurgery are essential for the use of free flaps.

C Debridement of the area of reconstruction is necessary for the use of free flaps.

D Donor site morbidity is a possible disadvantage in free-flap surgery.

E Latissimus dorsi muscle is frequently used as a free flap to reconstruct the breast.

20. Which of the following statements regarding complications with flaps are true?

A A pale and cold flap is a sign that the venous supply is compromised.

B Too much tension of flap inset can cause flap failure in every type of flap, including free flaps.

C Poor knowledge of anatomy and the blood supply to flap tissue will cause a flap to fail.

D Medicinal leeches can be useful as a last resort in flaps that have an arterial input problem.

E Well-controlled analgesia to reduce catecholamine output is good advice in the management of major tissue transfers.

21. Which of the following statements regarding flaps are true?

A Burrow's triangles are associated with the use of Z-plasties.

B A defect of the lower eyelid may be repaired using a 'bucket handle' flap.

C An inner canthal defect can be repaired using a transposition flap from the glabellar area.

D A bilobed flap is an example of an axial-pattern flap.

E A disadvantage of the use of local flaps used in tumour surgery might be compromise to excision.

22. The following statements about the 'Z-plasty' technique are true:

A It is widely used to increase tissue bulk in a scarred area by using local flaps.

B It is useful in reorienting the direction of a scar.

C It is a very safe technique since the flap viability is always maintained.

D A 30° Z-plasty will provide an approximate 75% gain in length of the scar.

E The commonly used angle for a Z-plasty in surgical practice is 120°.

→ Reconstructive options

23. Which of the following statements are true?

A A large scalp defect – say as much as 75% in area and involving skull excision – can be best repaired using a rhomboid flap.

B A defect in the heel may be repaired using an islanded pedicled instep flap.

C The definitive repair covering for an Achilles tendon scar problem is a split-skin graft.

D Repair of an ankle defect involving the skin can be accomplished by using a fasciocutaneous flap.

E Position of perforating vessels can be identified using a Doppler apparatus.

24. Which of the following statements are true in major tissue reconstruction?

A Nerves and tendons cannot be transferred as free, nonvascularised grafts.

B The fibula can be used in jaw reconstruction as a free flap.

C The radial forearm flap is a random-pattern flap.

D The antero-lateral thigh flap is a type of perforator flap.

E The jejunum is a useful means of free-flap repair for oesophageal defects.

25. Which of the following statements are true in free flap surgery?

A Success in repair of major tissue defects requires a team approach and meticulous planning.

B In the absence of trained staff or equipment, free-flap surgery can still be a good option.

C Free flap success is dependent on the availability of a suitable flap, good artery and venous connecting vessels in the recipient site, and no infection or local tissue induration.

D Microsurgery is best done using the increased magnification provided by loupes.

E The ischaemic time for safe transfer of free flaps is 10 hours.

D The ulnar side of the hand is more commonly affected.

E It may be associated with retroperitoneal fibrosis.

→ Miscellaneous conditions in plastic surgery

26. Which of the following statements regarding Dupuytren's disease are true?

A It is caused due to contraction of the palmar fascia.

B It is more common in Caucasians than in people of African origin.

C It most commonly affects the little finger.

27. Which of the following surgical options in the management of lymphoedema are true?

A Excision of subcutaneous tissue and dermal flap

B Circumferential excision of lymphoedematous tissue and skin grafting

C Lympholymphatic anastomosis

D Mesenteric transfer

E Lymphoarterial shunt

Answers to multiple choice questions

→ Wound healing

1. A, B, D, E

Although polymorphonuclear leucocytes (PMNL) are important in the early stages of the wound-healing process, healing can nevertheless proceed in the absence of PMNL (and also lymphocytes). However, monocytes are essential for wound healing. Blood monocytes on arriving to the wound site undergo a phenotypic change to become tissue macrophages. Collagen is a rod-shaped molecule composed of three polypeptide chains that form a rigid triple helical structure. About 28 different types of collagen have been described in the human body but the five main types are I–V. Type I collagen is found mainly in bone, skin and tendon, whilst Type III collagen is found mainly in arteries, uterus and bowel wall. The skin nonetheless contains Type III collagen as well, and the normal ratio of Type I to Type III collagen in adult skin is approximately 4:1.

2. A, B, C

Healing by primary (first) intention occurs when a wound is closed within 12–24 hours of its creation as in a clean surgical incision or a clean laceration. The wound edges may be approximated directly by sutures, tissue glue, tapes, or staples. Grossly contaminated wounds, wounds with extensive soft tissue loss, or wounds after some surgical procedures (e.g., laparostomy) are left to heal by secondary intention (secondary healing). In this type of healing, the wound closes by wound contraction and epithelialisation. Delayed primary healing is recommended for contaminated or poorly delineated wounds such as bites or abdominal wounds after peritoneal soiling. They are closed after a few days after being left open to prevent infection. The skin and subcutaneous tissue are left unapposed (sutures may be put in place but not tied) and closure is performed after the normal host defences are allowed to debride the wound. Myofibroblasts, having structural properties between those of a fibroblast and a smooth muscle cell, are thought to play a key role in wounds healing by secondary intention. Healing of split-thickness donor graft sites does not occur by secondary intention but by epithelialisation. In this type of injury, since the basal layer of cells remains uninjured, the epithelial cells within the dermal appendages, hair follicles and sebaceous glands replicate to cover the exposed dermis.

➡ Keloid scars

3. B, C, E
Keloids are dermo-proliferative disorders unique to humans. The aetiology of keloids is unclear, although various theories including familial tendency such as an autosomal dominant or recessive inheritance, hormonal influence, altered immunological response, enhanced role of TGB–β, abnormality of ketatinocyte control over fibroblasts and down-regulation of apoptosis related genes have been purported. Factors such as haematoma, infection and wound dehiscence predispose to hypertrophic scar formation (not keloids). Keloids extend beyond the original scar margins whilst hypertrophic scars are confined to the borders of the original wound. Keloids are more common in wounds that cross tension lines and in areas such as the earlobe, pre-sternal and deltoid regions. They commonly affect children and young adults, and such scars undergo rapid growth during puberty and increase in size during pregnancy. Hypertrophic scars generally develop within weeks of injury, whereas keloids can develop up to one year later. Collagen synthesis is three times higher in keloids than in hypertrophic scars and 20 times higher in keloids than in normal skin.

4. A, B, C, D
The management of keloid scars remains challenging. Various treatment options such as topical silicone gel application, intralesional excision (excision through the substance of the keloid), steroid injections and radiotherapy have been attempted and used widely but none has gained lasting or universal acceptance. However, combination of the previously mentioned treatment options is generally considered to give better results. Systemic steroids do not have any role in the treatment of keloid scars.

➡ Skin characteristics

5. A, B, D, E
Skin is important for sensation and temperature control – it is an important homeostatic tissue. Its depth varies in different parts of the body and regenerates from follicular elements of the dermis. Keratinocytes can be cultured and used in wound care. If wounds have no dermis in their base, healing occurs by secondary intention from the sides.

➡ Skin grafts

6. A, B, D
Skin blood supply comes from direct cutaneous vessels and perforators from underlying fascia and, where present, from underlying muscle. A skin graft consists of varying amounts of epidermis and dermis. It requires the bed or receiving area to be vascularised, so that ingress of capillaries into the graft can occur and revascularise it. A similar situation exists for successful take of a full-thickness graft or composite graft. The former consists of epidermis and the whole of the dermis from which fat has been removed; the latter is a full-thickness graft that contains hair follicles, cartilage, or other adnexal tissue deliberately taken as part of the complete graft and not secondarily sutured on, e.g., hair transplants or reconstruction of deficient nasal rim.

7. B, D
Imbibition is the means whereby a split-skin graft is nourished during the first 48 hours of life in its recipient site. Gentle handling is important to create the best conditions for take of a full-thickness graft. Grafts do not take on bare tendon or cortical bone, because these do not produce granulations or vascular support. Graft contraction depends on the amount of dermis in the graft and is thus greatest in split-skin grafts and least in full-thickness grafts.

8. A, B, E

Thiersch was a professor of surgery in Leipzig, Germany, who described free skin grafting in 1874. Full-thickness grafts were described by John Wolfe, a Glasgow ophthalmic surgeon, in 1875, to reconstruct an eyelid. Full-thickness grafts are useful in the repair of face and eyelids and produce a better cosmetic result than split-skin grafts. Incisions and resulting scars are best placed in lines of minimal tension to get the best cosmetic result but do not always correspond to Langer's lines.

9. A, C, D

Full-thickness skin grafts are fully detached from one part of the body (donor site) and placed on another part (recipient site). It relies solely on revascularisation from a healthy, well-vascularised wound bed. Full-thickness skin grafts initially adhere to the recipient bed by fibrin, which must be vascular enough to support the metabolism of the graft; this process is known as *imbibition*. Within 48 hours, capillaries grow from the underlying bed into the graft, and the graft becomes vascularised. This process is known as *inosculation*. Since full-thickness skin grafts contain the entire dermis, it shrinks less compared to split-thickness skin grafts. For the same reason (presence of the entire dermis), the texture and pigmentation of full-thickness skin grafts are usually quite similar to normal skin. The donor site of a full-thickness graft is usually closed primarily, whilst the donor site of a split-thickness graft is left to heal by epithelialisation.

10. A, C, E

Split-skin grafts can be cut by using a handheld, hand-powered dermatome (batteries), or one powered by electricity. The best donor site for taking a split-skin graft in a child or female is the buttock, where any problems in healing and the risk of poor scars can be hidden. Other useful donor sites are the thighs and shaved scalp. It is possible to determine the depth of split skin taken from the bleeding nature of the donor site – larger-spaced punctate bleeding points indicate a thicker graft. Graft take depends on a number of factors, including presence of infection, notably group A beta-haemolytic streptococci, shearing forces and a good blood supply in the recipient area.

11. A, C

Mesh grafting of split-skin grafts is a useful technique to expand a smaller graft. The holes in the graft also enable escape of exudates. The retroauricular tissue provides a useful donor site for full-thickness grafts – other sites include the supraclavicular neck or hairless groin skin. The take of split-skin grafts is easier than for full-thickness grafts because there is less tissue depth needing to be vascularised. If the conditions are good, the cosmetic results are superior for a full-thickness graft and the presence of active muscle underneath a full-thickness graft of the face will improve, not worsen, the result.

→ Flaps

12. B, C, D

Grafts will not 'take' on nonvascularised beds. Avascular wounds, such as bone without periosteal cover, tendon without paratenon, denuded cartilage, fracture sites and irradiated wounds, are incapable of nourishing a graft. In such instances, a flap is indicated to achieve wound coverage. A flap, by definition, remains attached to the body via a vascular pedicle and thus does not depend on the recipient site for blood or nutrients. Random-pattern flaps rely on random cutaneous vessels for their blood supply. Greater lengths of flap can be used by including the underling deep fascia, by including a perforating blood vessel in the base of the flap, and by ensuring axial blood vessels within the flap itself. Islanding a flap on its vascular pedicle allows even greater pedicle length and thus greater mobility and versatility. When there are no options for local wound cover, tissue in the form of free flap has to be imported from elsewhere in the body. Any tissue that can be isolated on a suitable vascular pedicle can be used, and a free flap might include nerve and bone. Arteries as small as 1 mm diameter can be successfully anastamosed in free-flap surgery.

13. A, B, D, E
Flaps can be classified according to the types of blood supply and, in contrast to grafts, introduce their own blood supply to the recipient area. Flaps can thus be used to reconstruct areas with no, or poor, vascularity. For a random flap, the maximum safe breadth:length ratio is 1:1.5; extending more can be done if the extra portion is 'delayed' or temporarily raised and replaced for a few weeks before the whole flap and delayed portion are used in the reconstruction. When the main vascular supply is confidently known, a longer flap can also be used at a greater distance. This is an example of an axial- pattern flap such as the groin flap.

14. C, E
A random flap cannot be islanded because the blood supply is not known precisely; this is not the case for an axial-pattern flap, which can be islanded. Inclusion of underlying muscle or fascia with a skin flap increases the flap blood supply if perforators are included. In the design of a transposition flap, it is important to take note of the pivot point as this determines the length of the flap to be used. This point is situated at the base of the flap on the side furthest away from the defect to be covered. The length of this type of flap will be longer than the length of the defect. Usually the donor defect will have to be grafted in part, though in some cases a direct closure might be possible if this is in a very lax area of skin.

15. A, C, E
Z-plasties are triangular transposition flaps that are useful in lengthening narrow, not broad, contracture bands. For tip-of-the-nose defects of about 1-cm diameter, a bilobed flap is a good alternative to a retroauricular full-thickness graft. The rhomboid flap is not a flap for use in fingertips but can be in the temple or back. Rotation flaps are mostly used in moderate-sized scalp defects or in the buttocks.

16. A, B, D
Burrow's triangles do not play any part in the design or use of bipedicle flaps. Multiple Y to V flaps are useful in treating burn scars over flexure creases, and V to Y flaps are useful in repair of fingertip defects. A good cosmetic result in random flaps can be obtained when attention in design is made to the lines of election in the located area. The cosmetic result of a flap is better than a graft because it is thicker, has a better blood supply and retains better colour and texture.

17. C
Limberg's flap or Rhomboid flap is an example of a transposition flap. The defect is converted into a rhomboid with angles of 60° and 120°, and a flap of similar dimensions is designed and transposed into the defect. Dufourmentel flap is a variant of Limberg's flap but with narrower angles. Rotation flaps are commonly used in scalp reconstruction and can be combined with scoring of the galea to enhance utility of the flap. (Forehead flap is usually used as an interpolation flap). Bilobed flaps, described by Zimany, are useful in nasal reconstruction. Langenbeck's palatoplasty is an example of a bipedicled advancement flap.

18. C, D, E
Myocutaneous and fasciocutaneous flaps have very reliable blood supply, and complex equipment and highly trained surgeons are not required. However, it is important to have a

good knowledge of anatomy and blood supply for these flaps. Skin survival depends on the perforators, especially if islanded, but the fascia and muscle can be used as flaps without the overlying skin.

19. A, B, C, D

Free-flap reconstruction is the best method for composite tissue loss but requires expertise and microsurgical instruments. The operative time for microsurgical procedures is usually longer than for other types of reconstruction. Careful debridement of the area for reconstruction is essential for success. Donor site morbidity is a recognised disadvantage in free-flap surgery, although this can be minimised with careful pre-operative planning. In breast reconstruction, the latissimus dorsi muscle is usually used as a pedicled flap (blood supply not detached) rather than as a free flap. The commonly used free flap in breast reconstruction is the deep inferior epigastric artery perforator flap (DIEP). The other free flaps used in breast reconstruction include thoraco-dorsal artery perforator flap (T-DAP) and the superior and inferior gluteal artery perforator flaps (SGAP and IGAP). The transverse rectus abdominus muscle (TRAM) free-flap surgery that was in vogue about a decade ago has been now superseded by DIEP since it spares the muscle and thus minimises weakness of the anterior abdominal wall.

20. B, C, E

A pale, cold flap has arterial input problem while a blue distended flap has a venous problem. Tension can affect all types of flaps adversely, as can failure to know the anatomy and blood supply to the flap being used. Medicinal leeches are useful in situations where venous output has been compromised but are of no value if there is an arterial problem. Each leech can only be used once on an individual patient. It is important that appropriate analgesia is given in major tissue transfers so that catecholamine production is reduced.

21. B, C, E

Z-plasties do not need to make use of Burrow's triangles. The bucket-handle flap is used in reconstruction of the lower eyelid. A glabellar transposition flap can be used to repair a defect of the inner canthus. The bilobed flap is not an axial-pattern flap, as it is not based on known vessels – if anything, it is a modified rotation or transposition flap. Compromising tumour excision to fit the design of a local flap should not be done but it is a risk. Excision of any tumour should always be the first priority, with the repair of the resulting defect by a flap designed to fit the defect created and not vice versa.

22. B

Z-Plasty is a technique used widely by plastic surgeons to lengthen or reorient a scar by transposing two Z-shaped flaps or two triangular flaps. The technique, if not executed properly, may result in complications such as haematoma under the flaps, wound infection, 'trapdoor' effect and flap necrosis. They have several applications in plastic surgical reconstruction and the theoretical gain in length depends on the angles of the 'Z'. In theory the following will occur:

- A 30° Z-plasty will provide a 25% gain in length.
- A 45° Z-plasty will provide a 50% gain in length.
- A 60° Z-plasty will provide a 75% gain in length.
- A 75° Z-plasty will provide a 100% gain in length.
- A 90° Z-plasty will provide a 120% gain in length.

However, these figures are theoretical and the actual gain in length is determined by the amount of laxity of the skin laterally. The commonly used angle for a Z-plasty in surgical practice is 60°.

→ Reconstructive options

23. B, D, E
A large scalp defect with bone tissue removed cannot be repaired by a rhomboid flap but would require reconstruction with a free flap. Heel ulcers are difficult due to their site, but can be treated by employing a pedicled instep flap. Achilles tendon wounds are not permanently and properly repaired by using split-skin grafts because of durability, vascularity and mobility problems – a flap repair is better. Wounds of the ankle and lower third of the leg can be repaired using fasciocutaneous or free flaps. Doppler apparatus is an easy and good way to identify perforating vessels on the skin surface.

24. B, D, E
Nerve and tendons can be used as free grafts – the sural nerve and, when available, the palmaris longus tendons are useful sources of donor tissue. The fibula is a useful source of free flap for bone to reconstruct the jaw. The radial forearm flap is a good example of an axial-pattern flap as it is designed around well-known vessels. The antero-lateral thigh flap is a commonly used perforator flap (musculo-cutaneous or septo-cutaneous perforator), with the vessels arising from the descending branch of the lateral circumflex femoral artery. For oesophageal defects, free-jejunum grafts offer a good way for reconstruction.

25. A, C, D
For major tissue reconstructions, meticulous planning and teamwork is essential for success. If this is to be done using a microvascular procedure, the use of loupes is not satisfactory and the best results are obtained using proper staff and apparatus. Good vessels in donor flap and recipient area, the lack of tissue induration, lack of tension and lack of infection in the area of reconstruction are also important for successful repair. The ischaemic time is dependent on the presence or absence of muscle tissue in the free flap – it is less in the case of the former. A 1- to 2-hour period is safe for muscle-containing free flaps – longer times of up to 6 hours are permissible only in skin or fascia flaps.

→ Miscellaneous conditions in plastic surgery

26. A, B, D
Dupuytren's disease is a condition of unknown aetiology characterised by contraction of the palmar or digital fascia. It affects 1% to 3% of the population of North Europe and the United States. It is rare in the Far East and Africa. It is three times more common in males. Its incidence increases with age. It has a strong hereditary disposition. The ring finger is the most commonly affected finger; the little finger is the next most commonly affected digit. The ulnar side of the hand is more commonly affected than the radial side. The following conditions are associated with Dupuytren's disease: knuckle pads (Garrod's pads), penile fibrous plaques (Peyronie's disease) and plantar fibromatosis (Lederhosen's disease). Retroperitoneal fibrosis, however, is not associated with Dupuytren's disease.

27. A, B, C
Surgical techniques for correcting lymphoedema may be excisional or physiological. Excisional techniques include circumferential excision of the lymphoedematous tissue followed by skin grafting (Charles technique), longitudinal removal of the affected segment of skin and subcutaneous tissue and primary closure (Homans technique), excision of subcutaneous tissue and tunneling of a dermal flap thorough the fascia into a muscular compartment of the leg (Thompson technique) and liposuction. Physiological techniques include lympholymphatic anastomosis (autologous lymphatic grafts to bridge obstructed lymphatic segments), lymphovenous shunt (anastomosis of lymphatic channels to veins), lymphangioplasty, enteromesenteric flap and omental transfer (pedicled portion of omentum transposed to the affected limb).

32

Disaster surgery

Christopher JK Bulstrode

Multiple choice questions

→ Characteristics of disasters

1. **Which of the following are true about man-induced disasters compared with natural disasters?**
   A They are finite in size.
   B Intrastructure such as communications are likely to be preserved.
   C They cross national boundaries.
   D Shelter is the first priority.
   E Rioting and break down of civil structure is more likely.

2. **Which of the following statements are true regarding actions and their priorities after a natural disaster?**
   A Work closely with the media.
   B Rescue work should start before the extent and size of the disaster is fully established.
   C The environment is usually hazardous but medical triage of injured is the first priority.
   D Rescue teams should not clutter themselves with food supplies and shelter. They should be able to 'live off the land'.
   E First responders should be those who are most eager to go in first and do not need any special training or experience.

→ Triage

3. **Which of the following are true concerning triage?**
   A Triage is the job of the less experienced members of the first responder team, while the experienced get on with treatment.
   B Triage cannot be started until site safety is secured.

   C Fast Triage is best performed by going quickly from patient to patient, just taking a quick look at them.
   D Triage needs to be only performed once.
   E Triage is performed as soon as possible after the sickest patients have been stabilised.

→ Evacuation of casualties

4. **Which statements are false regarding the moving of casualties?**
   A Casualties should be moved out of danger before triage.
   B Transfer of triaged casualties should be made to the nearest medical facility.
   C Transfer should be made by the fastest form to transport.
   D Drips and chest drains should be removed before transfer.
   E Trained staff must accompany major casualties during transfer.

→ Emergency care in the field hospital

5. **Which of the following statements regarding emergency care in the field hospital are true?**
   A Definitive surgery should be performed in the field when necessary.
   B Measures to control haemorrhage should be undertaken in the field.
   C Amputation of devitalised limbs and for gas gangrene should be undertaken in the field.
   D Open fractures should be cleaned in the field.
   E Repair of damaged major vessels should be attempted, if this is necessary to save a limb.

→ ## Debridement of contaminated wounds

6. **Which of the following statements regarding debridement are true?**

A The term used to mean letting out pus.

B Tissue of questionable viability can be left and reviewed later.

C It frequently involves leaving the wound open.

D It might require repeated exploration.

E It does not involve definitive treatment.

→ ## Tetanus

7. **Which of the following statements regarding tetanus are true?**

A It is caused by an organism in the *Clostridium* group.

B Its route of transmission is by ingestion.

C It thrives in aerobic conditions.

D Its spores are found everywhere.

E Heavily contaminated wounds require anti-tetanus globulin as well as tetanus toxoid.

→ ## Necrotising fasciitis

8. **Which of the following statements regarding necrotising fasciitis are true?**

A It is primarily caused a *Staphylococcus*.

B It can also be caused by infection with several different organisms.

C Necrosis is caused by the release of toxins.

D It may appear in a location remote from the main site.

E Surgery should not be undertaken even if the patient's metabolic state is deranged.

→ ## Gas gangrene

9. **Which of the following statements regarding gas gangrene are true?**

A It may be caused by several different types of *Clostridium*.

B More than one toxin is produced.

C It thrives only in poorly perfused tissues.

D It is more likely to progress if wounds are left open to the air.

E The gas produced is oxygen from haemolysed red cells.

→ ## Blast injuries

10. **Which of the following statements regarding blast injuries are true?**

A Casualties hidden behind walls or other obstructions are protected from blast injury.

B Blasts mainly affect air-filled cavities in the body.

C Penetrating wounds from fragments are deep and their borders difficult to define.

D Contamination of a wound is not an issue, as the heat sterilises any fragments.

E Patients are usually deaf so communication is a problem.

Extended matching questions

→ ## Diagnoses

1 Compartment syndrome
2 Crush syndrome
3 Frost bite
4 Gas gangrene
5 Hypothermia
6 Necrotising fasciitis
7 Tetanus

Match the diagnoses with the clinical scenarios that follow:

A A 28-year-old man is trapped under a collapsed building for 18 hours. His right arm and leg were crushed under a beam. When he is finally freed, he is confused, his pulse is faint but regular and his right arm and leg are cold, pale and pulseless. He does not appear to be able to feel or move either of them.

B   Some 10 days ago, a 60-year-old rescue worker trod on a nail while climbing over wreckage. It passed through the sole of his shoe and into his foot. He did not seek treatment and the wound healed up well. Now he presents with fever, sweating and drooling, and he is unable to open his mouth properly. Each time there is a loud noise, his muscles go into spasm and he seems to be having some difficulty breathing.

C   During the clearance of a building, which had collapsed 48 hours before, a 10- year-old boy is found trapped in the remains of a room and unable to move. He had no problems with dehydration as he was soaked from head to foot with water from a ruptured pipe. A quick survey revealed no obvious injury, but even so, he was drowsy (unable to give his name or obey verbal commands) with a slow pulse and an unrecordable blood pressure.

D   A 16-year-old girl sustains a forearm fracture caused by a falling tree branch during a hurricane. The fracture is only slightly displaced, so a simple reduction is performed and the arm is put in plaster. Twelve hours later she returns to the emergency assessment centre, with terrible pain in the arm, which cannot be controlled with analgesia. The distal pulse is normal, so is sensation in the fingers, but as soon as the fingers are extended passively, she cries out with pain.

E   After an earthquake in midwinter, high in a valley in Chitral, survivors start appearing at the road head, having walked for 2 days through the snow. Some have no shoes. They have no feeling in their feet, which feel hard and wooden to touch. They are not in any pain.

F   A terrorist bomb blast has injured a large number of people in a market three days before your team arrives on site. Your patient had several cuts on her leg and torso. One on the thigh was deep and 5 cm long. It was sutured by the local first-aid team some five hours after the blast. It is now red or purple in colour and is oozing fluid. It smells (surprisingly the smell is sweet but a little sickly). When you palpate the swelling around the wound, there is a feeling of crackling in the tissue.

G   An elderly diabetic patient had a tetanus injection as part of her treatment for a wound sustained during evacuation after a flood. Some days later she presented with a red swollen thigh. She was generally unwell, and pyrexial. The thigh in which she had been given the injection was red and swollen with an area of fluctuance. When this area was opened surgically, there was some pus to be released but the muscle appeared purple and did not contract when stimulated. The wound was extended but the muscle throughout the compartment had an identical appearance.

Answers to multiple choice questions

1. A, B

- All the increasing complexity of society and mane appeared purple and will to harm others is increasing; the sheer scale of natural disasters still outweighs by an order of magnitude the effects of accidents or deliberate damage by man.
- Natural disasters hit all aspects of society indiscriminately and so infrastructure tends to be more badly damaged in a natural disaster than a man-induced one.
- Natural disasters tend not to recognise national boundaries. Man-induced ones frequently do.
- Because of the size and indiscriminate nature of natural disasters, it is likely that more people will be left without shelter in inclement conditions than after a man-induced disaster.
- Rioting is more likely after a natural disaster because of its size. Also, damage to police and military structure as well as the prolonged delay in getting assistance due to breakdown of all civil structures all predispose to rioting.

2. A, B

- The media have the finances and communications to hire helicopters and provide vital information earlier than anyone else. They may be a nuisance at times, but they are much better used than fought.
- Rescue work should not start before work has begun on defining the extent of the problem but certainly should not wait until the extent is fully established.
- Safety of rescued and rescuers is the first priority and so comes before triage.
- Rescue teams must not be an added burden on already compromised people who may be struggling themselves to find food water and shelter. Rescue teams must only go in fully self-supporting in terms of shelter, clean water and food.
- The most senior and experienced should go in as first responders, so that they can accurately assess what is needed, and have the authority to order things accordingly.

3. B

- Triage is the job of the most experienced member of the first-responder team. Correct triage makes a big difference to the efficacy of the team and is most effectively performed by an experienced team member, however much they may wish to get involved in treating individual patients.
- Safety of rescue staff and of disaster victims takes priority, so unsafe buildings should be cleared before triage is started.
- Triage cannot be reliably performed by just glancing at the patient safe buildings should be. A brief history and swift ABC(DE) examination will give much more reliable results.
- Triage needs repeating, as the condition of patients can both deteriorate and improve over a short period of time.
- Triage is performed while quickly stabilising the sickest patients. Treatment should not delay triage but if there are obvious simple tasks to be performed, such as turning a patient into the recovery position to open his or her airway, then this should be done.

4. B, C, D

- Patients and rescue staff must move out of hazardous places as soon as possible, otherwise secondary injuries may occur. Triage is best performed with all the patients grouped together under shelter and where there is access to light, electricity and water, e.g., a school assembly area.
- Casualties should be transferred to facilities that have the skill and resources to deal with the injuries and are not already overloaded with patients.
- As a general rule the fastest transport should be used this might be true, but transport should be chosen which will not further exacerbate injuries to the patient, and where appropriate monitoring can be continued. It is almost impossble to monitor a patient during helicopter flight, so, if the patient's condition cannot be stabilised slower transport might allow stops to be made to stabilise the situation when necessary.
- Drips and chest drains may be vital to the physiological stability of a patient during transfer. However, they are easily accidentally displaced so should be securely (doubly) fixed in place.
- Staff capable of monitoring the patient's condition and taking emergency action if necessary must accompany each severely injured patient. This temporarily removes skilled staff from the disaster site, but sick patients cannot be transferred without experienced staff.

5. B, C, D, E

- Definitive surgery is best performed in an appropriately equipped centre by trained staff who do not have other emergency priorities.
- Haemorrhage control is one example of 'damage control' surgery which should be undertaken in the field.
- Amputation of a devitalised limb or one that is gangrenous cannot wait for transfer to a definitive centre as they threaten the life of the patient (from re-perfusion rhabdomyolysis or infection).

- The sooner that open fractures are cleaned, the better the chance of preventing local and systemic infection.
- An anastomosis needed to salvage a limb may be appropriate if there is time and expertise available.

6. A, C, D, E

- Its meaning was the unbridling (release) of laudable pus, one of the few useful things that surgeons living in the pre-antibiotic era could do, once a wound was infected.
- It is best to remove all dead tissue and any which is of doubtful viability, as this is unlikely to recover and once dead will act as a source of infection.
- Wounds which have been cleaned (debrided) should be left open and packed.
- They should then be reinspected and debrided again and again, until they are absolutely clean. Then and only then can delayed primary closure be contemplated.
- Definitive treatment should be left until the patient reaches a centre geared to deal with this problem.

7. A, D, E

- The organism is *Clostridium tetani,* a Gram-positive coccus belonging to the same group as gas gangrene *(Clostridium perfringens).*
- Infection is transmitted by the spores of the organism actually contaminating dead or dying tissue.
- It can only thrive in anaerobic conditions, hence the need to debride wounds thoroughly.
- The spores can be found everywhere but especially in soil contaminated with manure.
- If a wound is heavily contaminated, then support needs to be given to the activated immune system of the body.

8. B, C, D

- The primary organisms are usually a *betalytic Streptococcus*
- It commonly involves more than one infective organism.
- Exotoxins lead to microvascular thrombosis with tissue necrosis.
- Although there is rapid local spread, skip lesions may appear remote from the original site.
- Surgery must be undertaken without delay, as optimisation of the patient's condition will not be possible.

9. A, B, C

- There are several different types of *Clostridium* which may cause gas gangrene. Normally it is *C. Perfringens,* but it can be *C. bifermentans, septicum, or sporogens.*
- Several toxins are involved Alpha toxin is a lecithinase and destroys red and white cells as well as muscle cells. Phi toxin is a myocardial suppressant. Kappa toxin destroys connective tissue.
- It is an obligate anaerobe so it thrives in poorly perfused tissues. Spores can take one hour to 6 weeks to germinate but usually do so in 24 hours.
- *Clostridium* cannot germinate or thrive in the presence of oxygen, so leaving a wound open protects the tissue from developing gangrene. Even so, regular inspection is needed to remove dead tissue.
- The gas produced is hydrogen sulphide from the breakdown of proteins. It is toxic in its own right.

10. B, C, D, E

- Paradoxically, blast waves curl around solid objects, so even those apparently sheltered from the blast can be affected.
- It is the interface between a closed air-filled cavity and other tissue in the body where the most damage is seen.
- Some of the most serious damage from blast is caused by fragments propelled by the blast. They may leave wide tracks of soft-tissue damage, as they are high-energy projectiles.

- The fragments themselves may be hot and so are sterile, but they will push in with them pieces of clothing and will suck other material in behind them, all of which may be heavily contaminated.
- One of the most common air-filled cavities to cause damage is the middle ear, which might rupture the eardrum and so cause temporary deafness.

Answers for extended matching questions

1. D Compartment syndrome

Compartment syndrome is a build-up of pressure in a soft tissue compartment, which unless released quickly, will lead to its death. It can only develop where muscles are enclosed in an in-elastic fascia. The most common sites are the forearm and the lower leg, but the intrinsic muscles of the hand or foot can also be affected. It develops most commonly after a closed injury, as open injuries are able to decompress themselves. Severe or prolonged crushing of the soft tissue may be adequate to start the condition, but it develops more frequently after a fracture. Swelling of the muscles or haemorrhage into the fascial compartment leads to a rise of pressure inside that compartment. The thin-walled veins draining the compartment collapse because of the raised external pressure on their walls, and so blood fails to drain from the compartment. However, the thicker-walled arteries continue to allow blood to be pumped in. As a result, pressure continues to rise in the compartment until it is the same as in the arteries pumping blood in (mean arterial pressure). Blood flow into the compartment then stops, although blood will continue to flow through the compartment to the limb beyond the compartment (so peripheral pulses may be preserved). Compartment syndrome is diagnosed clinically by a) pain out of all proportion to the injury and b) extreme pain on passive extension of the digits distal to the compartment. Treatment is by fasciotomy of the affected compartment(s) and is a surgical emergency.

2. A Crush syndrome

Crush syndrome is a systemic injury, which occurs to the kidneys when tissue that has been deprived of blood supply for a long period is re-perfused and releases tissue breakdown products (myoglobin and vasoactive substances) into the circulation. Myoglobin blocks the kidneys, while vasoactive substances cause fluid sequestration. Both cause renal failure. Patients who are trapped should have intravenous fluids started at high volume (1–1.5 L/hour) even before they are released, and their urine output monitored to sustain a diuresis. It is equally important to try to avoid the release of the damaging molecules. Limbs that are clearly dead should be amputated rather than being allowed to reperfuse. Fasciotomy for compartment syndrome should not be undertaken when the compartment is obviously dead, because it will do more harm than good.

3. E Frostbite

Frostbite is the death of tissue which has been frozen. Normally this occurs in the extremities – toes, fingers, nose and ears. Initially the affected structure appears white and is wooden-hard to pressure. The patient and affected part should be warmed gently (to prevent heat damage) and pain relief given. Over the following days, some of the apparently dead tissue will recover while the worst affected parts will progress to dry gangrene. Provided infection does not set in, the demarcation between dead and viable tissue should be allowed to define itself without surgical interference. Only once clear and immovable demarcation has occurred should the dead tissue be excised.

4. F Gas gangrene

Gas gangrene is infection of a wound with one of the *Clostridium* bacteria, usually *C. perfringens*. The spores are everywhere, including in the human bowel, but can only germinate and thrive in anaerobic conditions. Gangrene is therefore found in contaminated wounds, which have not been laid open and cleaned as quickly as possible (debridement), and especially in wounds which are closed when there is dead or contaminated tissue inside. The bacteria produces toxins which kill tissue and so provides an environment for its own spread. It is susceptible to Penicillin, but the antibiotic cannot penetrate dead tissue. Hyperbaric oxygen may also help, but it too cannot penetrate dead tissue. Early high amputation might be the only way to save the patient.

5. C Hypothermia

Hypothermia is a decrease in body temperature below normal levels. Mild hypothermia down to 35 degrees is accompanied by shivering, but below that the patient stops shivering and becomes increasingly confused. Their periphery will be shut down and they may be bradycardic. Below 28 degrees cardiac arrhythmias may occur, and below 20 degrees cardiac arrest is likely. Hypothermia can be highly protective and so hypoxia or anoxia can be tolerated for longer periods than in a normal patient. Core temperature is difficult to measure and requires a special low-reading rectal thermometer. Rewarming should not be done too fast. A variety of methods are available, depending on facilities. These vary from blankets and buddy warming, through warm drinks (if they can swallow safely), humidified warmed oxygen, warm IV fluids and even peritoneal dialysis with warm dialysate.

6. G Necrotising fasciitis

Necrotising fasciitis is a rapidly spreading infection of fascial planes caused by a mixture of organisms, usually including β-haemolytic *Streptococci. Staphylococcus, Proteus, Pseudomonas* and *Clostridium*, amongst others, can also be involved. It can produce skip lesions, spreads very rapidly and has a very high mortality of well over 50%. The cornerstone of management is aggressive surgical excision, but high doses of appropriate antibiotics will be necessary as well as respiratory and circulatory support if severe. So, the patient may need endotracheal intubation and nursing in an intensive care unit during the acute phase.

7. B Tetanus

Tetanus or lockjaw is caused by *Clostridium tetani*, a Gram-positive coccus whose spores are found especially in manure-contaminated soil (farmyards) but can be found everywhere else too, including the human bowel. It thrives in a wound where there is anaerobic tissue and releases a toxin, tetanospasmin, which blocks the motor inhibition pathways to sensory stimuli. The first muscles affected are in the face and larynx, causing lockjaw and risus sardonicus (facial spasms producing what could be mistaken for a smile). It is perfectly possible to protect children from this condition by inoculation with tetanus toxoid. This needs repeating every 10 years. But in cases of heavily contaminated wounds, it is probably best to give immunoglobulin as well as appropriate prophylactic antibiotics. Of course, proper wound debridement with delayed primary closure is always required. Full-blown cases will need nursing away from any stimuli (to reduce spasms) and might require paralysis and ventilatory support.

Elective Orthopaedics

33 History taking and clinical examination in musculoskeletal disease

Andrew D Duckworth

Multiple choice questions

→ Musculoskeletal history

1. **Regarding history taking, which of the following are not routinely part of the process?**
   A Introduce yourself.
   B Confirm the patient's name and date of birth.
   C Obtain details of the patient's past medical history.
   D Ask about any previous surgical procedures.
   E Assess for tenderness.

→ Musculoskeletal examination

2. **Regarding the Apley system of examination, which of the following statements are true?**
   A It is a four-stage system.
   B The 'look' stage only starts once the patient has been fully exposed.
   C It requires exposure only of the affected limb and one joint above and below.
   D Assessing the skin for scars, wounds and redness is part of the 'feel' stage.
   E It requires that the distal neurovascular status be checked in all cases.

3. **Regarding the Apley system of examination, which of the following statements are false in relation to the 'move' stage?**
   A 'Move' is the third stage of the Apley system of examination.
   B The physician should move the limb first (passive movement).
   C Stability includes checking muscle power, joint stability and special tests.

D Abduction is movement of the limb away from the midline.
E Muscle power is measured on a six-level scale (0–5).

→ Spine examination

4. **Regarding examination of the spine, which of the following statements are true?**
   A Forward bend accentuates the rib hump of idiopathic thoracic scoliosis.
   B The thoracic spine normally has a lordosis.
   C A hairy tuft at the base of the spine is diagnostic of Down syndrome.
   D The Lasègue straight-leg raise test is a special test for fixed flexion deformity of the hip.
   E Palpation of the spinous processes does not detect a spondylolisthesis.

→ Hand and wrist examination

5. **Regarding examination of the hand and wrist, which of the following statements are false?**
   A Tight bands on the volar surface are indicate of Dupuytren's disease.
   B Wasting of the thenar eminence is diagnostic of an ulnar nerve palsy.
   C Froment's sign assesses the power of adductor pollicis.
   D Median nerve neuropathy can be assessed with Phalen's test.
   E Allen's test determines the efficacy of the blood supply to the hand.

→ Shoulder and elbow examination

6. Regarding examination of the shoulder and elbow, which of the following statements are true?

A The physiological carrying angle of the elbow is less than five degrees.

B Tenderness over the common flexor origin is diagnostic of tennis elbow.

C A positive Jobe's test can be indicative of rotator cuff impingement.

D Internal rotation of the shoulder is normal if the patient can reach L2.

E A painful arc is diagnostic for a rotator cuff tear.

→ Hip examination

7. Regarding examination of the hip, which of the following statements are false?

A A broad based gait can be caused by cerebellar ataxia.

B Leg-length discrepancy can be divided into true and apparent.

C Thomas's test assess for a fixed flexion deformity of the hip.

D Trendelenburg test positive is indicative of weak adductors.

E Impingement can be assessed with hip flexion, adduction and internal rotation.

→ Knee examination

8. Regarding examination of the knee, which of the following statements are true?

A The patellar tap test is a test for patellar femoral osteoarthritis.

B The lag test assesses the integrity of the flexor mechanism.

C The integrity of the collateral ligaments is assessed with the knee in full extension.

D A posterior cruciate deficient knee will have a positive Lachmann test.

E A positive apprehension test could indicate a previously dislocated patella.

→ Foot and ankle examination

9. Regarding examination of the foot and ankle, which of the following statements are false?

A Pes cavus is associated with Charcot-Marie Tooth disease.

B Loss of sensation in a glove-and-stocking distribution is associated with diabetes.

C Inversion and eversion occur at the ankle joint.

D The windlass test distinguishes physiological from spastic flat foot.

E Patients with a ruptured tendo Achilles might still be able to stand on their tiptoes.

Answers to multiple choice questions

→ Musculoskeletal history

1. E

Introduction consists of giving your own name and position, followed by checking the patient's name and date of birth. You should then explain what you are proposing to do before obtaining the patient's verbal consent to proceed. Essential aspects of the musculoskeletal history include the following:

- Presenting complaint and history
- Associated symptoms, e.g., pain, swelling, instability, other joint or bone involvement
- Past medical and drug history, e.g., warfarin, steroids
  - Previous surgical procedures or anaesthetics
  - Relevant family history
  - Allergies

- Social history
  - Smoking and alcohol
  - Occupation
  - Level of mobility including the use of aids
  - Activities of daily living

Assessing for tenderness is routinely part of the musculoskeletal examination.

Musculoskeletal examination

2. E

The Apley system is a triad (three parts) comprising 'look', 'feel,' and 'move'. This is followed by special tests and a neurovascular assessment. Looking starts as the patient enters the room for the following:

- Assess the gait and for evidence of discomfort, as well as any walking aids
- Look for any stigmata of disease, e.g., Horner's syndrome in the eyes or rheumatoid arthritis in the hands

Exposure requires removing any clothes from one joint above to the one below in relation to the affected area as well as the opposite side, so that a comparison can be made between normal and abnormal. The Apley system starts with looking at the skin, which is often best done with the patient standing, walking around the patient to make sure that no view (especially the back) is missed. Look at the following:

- Skin: scars, wounds, erythema, sinuses, rashes, ulcers, bruising, hair loss, pigmentation
- Soft tissue: swelling, lumps, muscle wasting or fasciculation
- Bones: alignment or deformity

Feel is the second stage of the Apley system and follows the same principle: skin, soft tissue and bone. It is good practice to ask the patient if there is an especially tender area, to avoid causing unnecessary discomfort. Observe the patient's face, not your hands, when palpating as it is on the patient's face that the first signs of discomfort will be found. Assessment of the distal neurovascular status is required in all cases.

3. B

Move is the third stage of the Apley system of the examination. Initially, active movement (by the patient) of the affected limb is carried out to give an overall impression of the range of movement and discomfort. The physician should then progress with passive movements and assess stability. The standard range of movement involves the following:

- Flexion (forward/anterior movement of trunk or limb)
- Extension (backwards/posterior movement)
- Abduction (away from the midline)
- Adduction (towards the midline)
- Internal rotation (rotation towards midline)
- External rotation (rotation away from midline)
- Pronation-supination (palms down/posteriorly, palms up/superiorly)
- Inversion-eversion (sole of foot moves medially, sole of foot moves laterally)

Stability has static and dynamic components that are assessed through muscle power, ligament stability and special tests. Muscle power is routinely graded on the Medical Research Council (MRC) scale, with consideration given to the action of each muscle, the peripheral nerve supply and nerve root supply (**Table 33.1**).

Table 33.1 The MRC grading of muscle power

Grade	Description
0	No contraction
1	Contraction seen
2	Active movement with gravity eliminated
3	Active movement against gravity
4	Reduced power on active movement against resistance
5	Normal power

Source: Adapted from Table 33.4 in: Williams, N., Bulstrode, C., O'Connell, PR. (Eds.), *Bailey & Love's Short Practice of Surgery*, 26th ed., 2013.

Spine examination

4. A

Examination of the spine – cervical, thoracic and lumbar – follows the same system as for any other joint. The spine should be straight in the coronal (front/back) plane with the head centred over the sacrum, but in the sagittal (side) plane the following should be seen:

- Cervical spine: concave/lordosis (range 20–40 degrees)
- Thoracic spine: convex/kyphosis (range 20–45 degrees)
- Lumbar spine: concave/lordosis (range 40–60 degrees)

Asking the patient to bend forward accentuates the rib hump (on the thoracic convex side) caused by the rotation of idiopathic thoracic scoliosis. If the curve disappears as the patient bends forward, this is indicative of a flexible curve secondary to other deformities, e.g., leg length discrepancy.

A hair tuft at the base of the spine is diagnostic of spina bifida. The Lasègue straight-leg test excludes pain arising from the hip joint and tight hamstrings, focusing on pain produced by stretching the sciatic nerve (sciatica, L5-S1 nerve roots). Palpation of the lumbar spinous processes might detect the characteristic gap and 'step-off' caused by the forward slip of one vertebral body on the one below (spondylolisthesis).

Hand and wrist examination

5. B

Dupuytren's contracture is immediately visible when inspecting the hand. The skin is contracted by tight bands, with the little and ring fingers (commonly) pulled down into a fixed flexion deformity.

Patterns of motor and sensory disturbance, along with the special tests, for median and ulnar neuropathy are detailed in **Table 33.2** (see also **Figure 33.1**). Wasting of the thenar eminence is diagnostic of median neuropathy. Abnormal sensation in the hand can be assessed using the stroke test, utilising the contralateral hand for comparison. However, for accurate delineation of the extent and severity of sensory loss, two-point discrimination is tested. When testing for carpal tunnel syndrome, Tinel's or Phalen's test can be used. Tinel's involves tapping over the suspected nerve with the tip of a finger, e.g., over the flexor retinaculum for the median nerve. A positive test is associated with pains or tingling sensation over the nerve and its distribution.

Table 33.2 The sensory, motor and special tests for detecting median and ulnar neuropathy

Nerve	Muscle wasting	Sensory loss	Special tests
Median (C8)	Thenar	Radial three and half digits	Phalen's test: wrist held in maximal flexion with elbows extended until symptoms reproduced Tinel's test (at carpal tunnel)
Ulnar (T1)	Hypothenar Intrinsics	Ulnar one and half digits	Froment's sign: See **Figure 33.1** Tinel's test (at elbow or wrist)

Source: From Figure 33.16 in: Williams, N., Bulstrode, C., O'Connell, PR. (Eds.), *Bailey & Love's Short Practice of Surgery,* 26th ed., 2013.

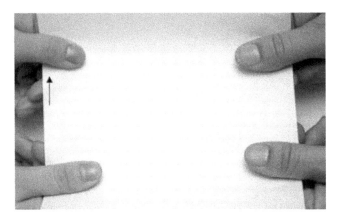

Figure 33.1 Froment's sign; the arrow illustrates the flexed posture of the thumb interphalangeal joint, indicating weakness of the ulnar nerve innervated adductor pollicis muscle.

Allen's test assesses the contribution of the ulnar and radial arteries to the palmar arch and hand. It involves occluding both arteries at the wrist, while the patient repeatedly makes a fist until the fingers go pale. Each artery is released in turn to determine the contribution.

Shoulder and elbow examination

6. C
The physiological carrying angle is the axis that the forearm makes with the upper arm when the patient stands with the elbows fully extended, palms facing anteriorly. The carrying angle reduces with elbow flexion and an abnormal angle may be associated with previous trauma, e.g., supracondylar fracture malunion. The normal carrying angle is ~7–16 degrees (~10 degrees in males, ~13 degrees in females). Tennis elbow is a painful inflammation of

the common extensor origin on the lateral side of the elbow, i.e., lateral epicondylitis. Golfer's elbow is less frequent and involves the common flexor origin, i.e., medial epicondylitis.

The movements of the shoulder with the patient standing include the following:

- Flexion (0–180°) and extension (0–45°)
- Abduction: 0–180°
  - 0–70° glenohumeral,
  - 70–150° glenohumerual and scapulothoracic
  - 150–180° glenohumerual and scapulothoracic
- Adduction
- External rotation (0–40°)
  - Arms by side, elbows at 90° flexion
- Internal rotation (T4–T9 normal range)
  - Touch back as high up as possible with dorsum of hand

The rotator cuff (supraspinatus, infraspinatus, teres minor, subscapularis) can become inflamed or damaged as it passes under the acromion. A positive Jobe's test or painful arc is indicative for impingement syndrome:

- Jobe's test for supraspinatus impingement and tear: abduct to 90°, angle forward 30°, internal rotation, thumb pointing to floor
  - 'Empty can' position
  - Push down on arm: weak = tear or impingement, pain = impingement
- Painful arc for impingement: abduct arm from side
  - Positive if pain between ~50–120°

Hip examination

7. D

Common gaits are described in **Table 33.3**. Osteoarthritis of the hip is the most common condition affecting the hip, which moves into a position of comfort (flexed and adducted). Classically, patients lose hip flexion and internal rotation, although all movements can be affected. With the leg held in a flexed adducted position, an apparently 'short' leg (because of the deformity) is found even when there is no difference in the 'real' leg lengths as measured by checking the bone lengths.

Leg lengths are best measured with the patient supine, pelvis square and legs flat and in an equal abduction angle. The true lengths are measured from the anterior superior iliac spine to the medial malleolus, with the apparent lengths measured from the xiphisternum to the medial malleolus. Galleazzi test confirms whether the discrepancy is coming from the femur or tibia.

A positive Trendelenburg test is indicative of weak abductors. You kneel in front of the patient with hands on their pelvis and ask them to stand on each leg in turn while resting their hands on your shoulders. If the abductors are weak, then as they take weight on the affected limb the pelvis will not tilt down (pelvis drops on the contralateral side) and the patient may lose balance pressing down on your shoulder to prevent them falling.

Thomas' test is used to determine the degree of fixed flexion deformity of the hip and is performed with the patient supine. One hand is placed under the lumbar lordosis, and the unaffected contralateral hip is flexed up. The lumbar lordosis should flatten out and any fixed flexion of the hip in question becomes apparent. Femoro-acetabular impingement can be assessed by the following:

1 Hip flexion to ≥ 90°, adduction, internal rotation (anterior impingement)
2 Hip flexion to ≥ 90°, full adduction, external rotation

Table 33.3 Common gait disorders

Gait	Description	Causes
Trendelenburg	Rolling, swaying or waddling gait Gluteal abductor dysfunction (weak)	CDH, coxa vara, polio, previous hip surgery, L5 radiculopathy
Antalgic	Dot-dash gait Shortened period on affected limb Pain-reducing gait	Osteoarthritis
Broad-based	Due to lack of balance Disordered rhythm	Cerebellar ataxia, alcohol intoxication, medications, stroke, peripheral neuropathy
Drop-foot	High stepping gait High knee flexion with toe contact Weak dorsiflexors	Common peroneal neuropathy Loss of proprioception
Deformity	In-toeing Tripping gait – foot catches on weight bearing limb	Persistent femoral anteversion

Source: Adapted from Table 33.11 in: Williams, N., Bulstrode, C., O'Connell, PR. (Eds.), *Bailey & Love's Short Practice of Surgery*, 26th ed., 2013.

Knee examination

8. E

Dislocation of the patella can be difficult to diagnose, as it normally relocates spontaneously. However, from then on any manual attempt to dislocate the patella laterally will cause apprehension in the patient, along with potentially pain and quadriceps contraction. Patello-femoral osteoarthritis is associated with crepitus. Following are the two common methods when assessing for a knee joint effusion:

1. Stroke or massage test: The knee is in extension, and the medial side of the knee is emptied into to the suprapatellar pouch by massaging upwards on the medial aspect of the knee. This fluid is then massaged down, filling the medial gutter.
2. Patellar tap: The knee is in extension, and fluid is squeezed from the suprapatellar pouch into the knee and with the other hand the patella is depressed and a 'tap' is felt.

The lag test is a sensitive test for weakness or rupture in the extensor mechanism of the knee. The leg is raised passively first to ensure that the knee can fully extend. The patient is then asked to perform a straight leg raise actively. A difference between passive range of movement and active indicates a positive lag test. When assessing the collateral ligaments, it is necessary to flex the knee to ~10°, to release the posterior capsule. Lachmann's test assesses the integrity of the anterior cruciate ligament, whereas the posterior draw test assesses the posterior cruciate ligament.

Foot and ankle examination

9. C

Pes cavus is defined by a high medial arch and is associated with spinal and neurological disorders, e.g., Charcot-Marie Tooth, spina bifida. Loss of sensation in the foot resulting from nerve root entrapment will be in the distribution of a dermatome, e.g., L5, but diabetes produces a glove-and-stocking distribution of sensory loss. Dorsiflexion and plantar flexion occur almost exclusively at the tibiotalar (ankle) joint, while inversion and eversion occur at the subtalar joint. When you ask a patient to stand on tiptoes, the arch of the foot should increase. This is the windlass test. If the arch does not appear or increase, then the patient has a fixed or rigid flat foot, e.g., tarsal coalition. Thompsons's or Simmonds' test is used to test the integrity of the Achilles tendon. The patient lies prone and the calf is squeezed, and the ankle should dorsiflex with an intact tendon. It is a paradox that patients with a complete rupture of the tendo Achilles might still be able to stand on their tiptoes using the long toe flexors as plantarflexors of the ankle.

Sports medicine and sports injuries

Andrew D Duckworth

Multiple choice questions

→ Tendon disease

1. **Regarding tendon injuries and repair, which of the following statements are true?**

A The strength of a damaged tendon returns to normal within 3 months following injury.

B Tendons heal by degeneration of the distal end followed by regrowth from the proximal end.

C Paratendinitis has a poor prognosis.

D Tendinosis can be painless.

E Tendons consist of type-2 collagen fibres.

→ Ligaments

2. **A patient who has a suspected anterior cruciate ligament (ACL) injury with pain around the knee and some laxity to the ACL but with a firm end-point on testing, has which grade of injury?**

A Grade 0

B Grade 1

C Grade 2

D Grade 3

E Not enough information

→ Bursae

3. **Regarding bursae, which of the following statements are true?**

A They are normal structures designed to reduce friction.

B They do not contain synovium.

C They are unable to become inflamed and infected.

D They do not have a nerve supply.

E None of the above.

→ Stress fractures

4. **Regarding stress fractures, which of the following statements are true?**

A They most frequently present acutely following a high-intensity, high-load sport.

B Pain is very well localised.

C They are easy to diagnose with radiographs.

D MRI is a useful adjunct in the diagnosis.

E They heal at the same rate as acute fractures.

→ Soft tissue injuries

5. **Regarding soft tissue injuries, which of the following statements are true?**

A Soft tissue haematomas do not resolve spontaneously.

B A cyst following a soft tissue haematoma never requires surgical excision.

C Quadriceps tears routinely affect the vastus lateralis muscle.

D Meniscal tears of the knee lead to a rapid onset effusion.

E Damaged muscle can be replaced with cartilage.

→ Ankle injuries

6. **Regarding the anatomic reduction of displaced unstable ankle fractures (Figure 34.1), which of the following statements are true?**

A It guarantees a full range of motion in the long term.

B It guarantees full strength in the ankle in the long term.

C It aims to avoid the premature onset of osteoarthritis.

D It aims to avoid the premature onset of osteoporosis.

E It aims to improve proprioception.

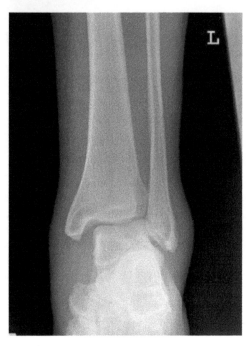

Figure 34.1 An AP radiograph of the left ankle and distal tibia. There is widening of the medial joint space, and radiographs at the knee reveal a fracture of the proximal fibula. This is a Weber C fracture (Maisonneuve type injury) and is unstable, requiring surgery to reduce and stabilise the ankle mortise.

Extended matching questions

→ Injuries associated with individual sports

1 Ballet
2 Football
3 Golf
4 Javelin Throwers
5 Kayaking
6 Marathon runners
7 Rugby
8 Swimming
9 Tennis

For each of the following cases, select the single most likely sport associated with the injury sustained from the options listed. Each option may be used once, more than once, or not at all.

A A 38-year-old woman presents with pain over the lateral aspect of her right elbow. The pain is reproduced when her wrist is extended against resistance.

B A 24-year-old man falls heavily on his right wrist when diving and complains of pain over the anatomical snuffbox. Scaphoid radiographs are initially normal. Subsequent MRI reveals an undisplaced fracture of the waist of the scaphoid.

C   An 18-year-old woman presents with a gradual worsening pain over the proximal forearm, with pain on resisted supination with 4+/5 weakness on extension of the metacarpals.

D   A 21-year-old man presents acutely with pain and tenderness over volar aspect of the distal interphalangeal joint (DIPJ) of the ring finger. On examination the ring finger has no active flexion of the DIPJ. Radiographs of the finger are normal.

→ Knee injuries

1   Anterior cruciate ligament injury
2   Chondromalacia patellae
3   Hoffa's syndrome
4   Lateral collateral ligament injury
5   Medial collateral ligament injury
6   Meniscal injury
7   Patella dislocation
8   Posterior cruciate ligament injury
9   Tibial plateau fracture

For each of the following cases, select the single most appropriate diagnosis from the options listed. Each option may be used once, more than once, or not at all.

A   A 24-year-old man sustains a twisting injury to his knee, with his body turning outwards (the tibia rotates inwards) as he falls while climbing a mountain. His binding fails to release and he feels a crack in his knee. Nothing seems to be out of place, but it swells immediately and he has to be brought down off the mountain on a stretcher. He has a positive Lachman's test.

B   An 18-year-old driver is involved in a high-energy motor vehicle accident. He sustains facial injuries from the windscreen and a fractured sternum from the steering wheel, and his right knee is painful and swollen. Radiographs are unremarkable.

C   A 32 year-old woman who plays football on weekends complains of pain over the medial aspect of the left knee and intermittent problems with an inability to straighten her leg. She has positive McMurray's test.

D   A 20-year-old footballer is involved in a heavy tackle where another player impacts with outside of his knee. He feels pain over the inner aspect of his knee, and he has a positive valgus stress test but with a firm end point.

E   A 17-year-old long jumper injures her knee by landing with it hyperextended. She now has chronic knee pain, especially when she tries to straighten it. On examination she has tenderness to palpation over the anterior fat pad.

F   A 16-year-old rugby player is tackled and feels severe pain in the knee. He notices something out of place in this knee. However, as he rolls over to try to stand up, whatever it was clicks back into place.

Answers to multiple choice questions

→ Tendon disease

1. D

Tendons are made up of tightly packed type-1 collagen bundles or fascicles that are contained with endotenon and then in turn epitenon. Tendons heal by fibroblasts laying down new collagen. As a tendon heals following injury there is a period when it is significantly weaker, particularly for 7 to 10 days after injury, before the strength recovers over the first month, but does not approach near to normal until 6 months. Inflammation of the membrane

Table 34.1 Classification of ligament injuries

Grade	Description
0	Normal ligament
1	No increase in joint laxity but tenderness around ligament
2	Increased joint laxity (partial disruption of fibres), soft clinical end point
3	Marked increase in joint laxity (complete disruption), no clinical end point

Source: Adapted from Table 41.3 in: Williams, N., Bulstrode, C., O'Connell, PR. (Eds.), *Bailey & Love's Short Practice of Surgery,* 26th ed., 2013.

surrounding the tendon (paratendinitis) routinely has a good prognosis following a period of analgesia and rest. Tendinosis (degeneration of the tendon itself) can be completely asymptomatic before it presents with failure.

➡ Ligaments

2. E

When classifying ligament injuries it is essential to compare the degree of laxity of the contralateral ligament, as this varies from patient to patient. Ligament injuries can be classified according to **Table 34.1**.

➡ Bursae

3. A

Bursae are naturally occurring fluid-filled structures found under areas of load, aiming to reduce friction where possible. Bursae are lined with synovium but do not routinely connect with the joint beneath. They can become painful, inflamed and infected, e.g., olecranon bursitis **(Figure 34.2)**, and so have a nerve supply.

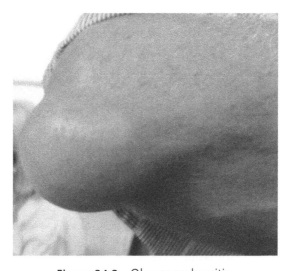

Figure 34.2 Olecranon bursitis.

Stress fractures

4. D

Stress fractures are frequently associated with low-intensity, low-load sports that involve a large number of repetitions. The pain is often not well localised and particularly incomplete fractures are difficult to see on radiographs. However, MRI is a very useful adjunct in diagnosing a stress fracture. Healing rates are often slow.

Soft tissue injuries

5. E

Most soft tissue haematomas resolve spontaneously, but if they are very large they can become infected or a cyst may form, and in rare cases the cyst may need excising. This is, however, a last resort. The anterior compartment of the thigh includes the quadriceps muscles, along with psoas major, iliacus, sartorius and pectineus. All are innervated by the femoral nerve, except for psoas (lumbar plexus); pectineus occasionally gets a branch from the obturator nerve in addition. The quadriceps muscles are detailed in **Table 34.2**.

Quadriceps tears in athletes commonly involve the rectus femoris muscle, particularly the aponeurosis. Complete quadriceps ruptures are less common. Injuries to the knee normally occur following either a direct blow or twisting mechanism to the knee. A rapid onset effusion is indicative of blood in knee (haemoarthrosis) and is associated with a cruciate rupture (e.g., anterior cruciate ligament), intra-articular fracture (e.g., tibial plateau), or patella dislocation. Isolated meniscal injuries frequently present with a slow onset effusion and possibly true locking of the knee. Damaged muscle can be replaced by cartilage and even bone (myositis ossificans).

Ankle injuries

6. C

Injuries to the ankle are common in sports, with ankle sprains one of the most common causes of morbidity. The Ottawa ankle rules can help to determine whether radiographs are required following an injury to the ankle. These include the following:

- Bony tenderness over the lateral malleolus, distal 6-cm posterior margin
- Bony tenderness over the medial malleolus, tip or distal 6-cm posterior margin
- Inability to weight bear at time of injury or on presentation

Table 34.2 The quadriceps muscles of the thigh

Muscle	Origin	Insertion	Innervation
Rectus femoris	Anterior inferior iliac spine (anterior) Superior acetabular rim (reflected)	Quadriceps tendon → patella	Femoral
Vastus lateralis	Intertrochanteric line, greater trochanter, linea aspera	Quadriceps tendon → patella	Femoral
Vastus intermedius	Anterolateral aspect of femur	Quadriceps tendon → patella	Femoral
Vastus medialis	Medial aspect of femur	Quadriceps tendon → patella	Femoral

Fractures to the ankle are routinely classified according to the AO-Weber classification, which is based on AP and lateral x-rays of the ankle. This classification helps to guide management (Table 29.3). The anatomic reduction of an ankle fracture is crucial as it is an intra-articular injury. It is suggested that if the articular fragments heal more than 2 mm out of place, there will be such high peak loads on the articular cartilage that premature osteoarthritis will result. Following anatomic reduction of any fracture, there can be no guarantee regarding function or strength in the long term. Fracture reduction is not associated with the risk of osteoporosis.

Answers to extended matching questions

→ Injuries associated with individual sports

A. 9 Tennis

Lateral epicondylitis, commonly known as tennis elbow, is common and affects up to 50% of tennis players. It is characterised by eccentric loading (repetitive supination-pronation with extended elbow), often from repetitive micro-trauma, of the common extensor origin (frequently ECRB), leading to tendinosis and inflammation. Degeneration, repair and rupture of the aponeurotic fibres can occur. Patients are tender over the lateral epicondyle of the humerus, with the pain reproduced on resisted wrist or long finger extension. Grip strength may be diminished, as this causes pain. Conservative measures are successful in the vast majority of cases and can include activity modification, nonsteroidal anti-inflammatory drugs (NSAIDS), physiotherapy, bracing and steroid injections. Surgery (common extensor origin debridement and release) is very rarely indicated and should only be considered after a prolonged trial of nonoperative measures. Medial epicondylitis, commonly known as golfer's elbow, is a similar but much less common condition that affects the common flexor origin (FCR and pronator teres frequently). It is often more difficult to manage.

B. 2 Football

Scaphoid fractures are the most common fracture of the carpus. Risk factors for a true scaphoid fracture have been found to be male gender and sports injuries, with goalkeepers most susceptible. Up to 30% to 40% of scaphoid fractures are not identified on routine primary four-view radiographs (see Chapter 29), with the clinical scaphoid fracture a diagnostic conundrum. Repeat assessment, including further imaging in the form or CT or MRI, might be required to diagnose the occult fracture. Patients are classically tender over the anatomical snuffbox, although this has very poor specificity. Treatment for undisplaced fractures routinely involves 6 to 12 weeks in a below-elbow cast. There is evidence to suggest that percutaneous screw fixation of undisplaced or minimally displaced fractures has a shorter time to return to work and sports.

C. 5 Kayaking

Compression of the posterior interosseous nerve (PIN) is associated with kayaking, amongst other things. The radial nerve passes anterior to the humeral lateral epicondyle, crossing the antecubital fossa behind brachioradialis. Once it enters the forearm it divides into the following deep and superficial branches:

- Deep branch → posterior interosseous nerve: passes between two heads of supinator, winds around the radial neck, supplies posterior forearm compartment travelling down the forearm posterior to the interosseous membrane.
- Superficial branch → superficial branch of the radial nerve: travels distally posterior to brachioradialis and provides cutaneous supply to the lateral dorsum of the hand.

Compression of the PIN is likely to be due to repetitive pronation-supination movements associated with paddling. The presentation depends on the chronicity of the problem, with weakness (or even atrophy) of the wrist and hand extensors possible. Nerve conduction studies can confirm the diagnosis and level of compression. Nonoperative treatment is first line and involves activity modification, NSAIDs, physiotherapy, splints and possibly steroid injections. Decompression of the nerve is considered after a prolonged trial of nonoperative management, with a variable outcome.

D. 7 Rugby
This patient presents with a classic jersey finger, which is an avulsion of the FDP insertion at the base of the distal phalanx. It commonly occurs when a rugby player attempts to grab an opposition player's jersey. According to the Verden zones, this is a Zone 1 (midpoint middle phalanx to fingertip) injury. The ring finger is commonly affected, and the severity of the injury can be classified according to the Leddy and Packer classification that takes into account how far back the tendon has retracted and whether there is a bony avulsion fragment. On clinical assessment, the history is one of inability to flex the DIPJ. Radiographs of the affected finger are required to exclude an associated bony avulsion. Treatment is with tendon repair +/- fixation of any osseous fragment.

Knee injuries

A. 1 Anterior cruciate ligament injury
A valgus twisting injury of the flexed knee when the foot is locked onto the ground routinely tears the anterior cruciate ligament (ACL). This is an acute intrinsic injury that is most commonly seen in males following a sports injury. Associated injuries include a tear the medial meniscus and the medial collateral ligament (triad of O'Donoghue). The ACL has a blood supply (unlike the meniscus) and so the knee swells immediately with blood (haemoarthrosis), and normally the person will not be able to continue. Patients can present chronically with a history of trauma and recurrent problems of instability when getting back to increasing levels of activity, e.g., knee giving way on changing direction.

On clinical assessment the diagnosis of a disrupted ACL is made with a positive anterior draw test or positive Lachmann's test, both of which test for abnormal subluxation of the tibia forward on the femur. The pivot shift test is another test. Radiographs of the knee to exclude a bony injury, followed by MRI are routine (Figure 34.3). Treatment is with rest, analgesia and physiotherapy. If the patient has ongoing problems with instability, ligament reconstruction using a tendon graft, e.g., hamstring, can be performed.

B. 8 Posterior cruciate ligament injury
Injuries to the posterior cruciate ligament (PCL) are less common (5%–20% knee ligament injuries) and commonly occur following a motor vehicle accident when the knee is driven back by impact with the dashboard. Missed diagnosis in the acute setting does occur. This posterior displacement of the flexed tibia on the femur ruptures the PCL. Multi-ligamentous injury can occur. Patients with a ruptured PCL have a positive anterior draw test (just like a patient with a ruptured anterior cruciate). However, the draw is forward from a posterior sag position. It is therefore the posterior sag which is diagnostic. Radiographs of the knee to exclude a bony injury followed by MRI are the investigations of choice. Surgery for athletes is often indicated.

C. 6 Meniscal injury
This woman presents with a history that is classical of true locking of the knee, most likely secondary to a meniscus tear. In this case, it is likely the medial meniscus given her area of discomfort. If the tear is bucket-handled in shape, then sometimes the bucket handle will fold over and lock in the knee joint. In the chronic setting, the patient then has to wiggle the knee to

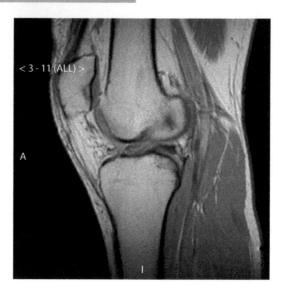

Figure 34.3 An MRI sagittal image demonstrating a rupture of the ACL.

relocate the torn fragment before she can move the knee again. The patient may have a positive McMurray's test, but this is not highly sensitive or specific, and the injury is best diagnosed by MRI or arthroscopy. In the acute setting, a torn meniscus sometimes allows a sportsperson to play on and may not swell until some hours later. For a symptomatic patient, arthroscopy with menisectomy or repair can be performed. If the meniscal tear is peripheral and amenable to repair, this is likely to give the best outcome, as peripheral tears have a good vascular supply.

D. 5 Medial collateral ligament injury
This is a common acute intrinsic injury of the knee with damage to the medial collateral ligament following a valgus force. Concomitant injury to the ACL or medial meniscus can occur. The area of tenderness is over the insertion and origin of the MCL and not the joint line. Rest with physiotherapy usually provides a good outcome.

E. 3 Hoffa's syndrome
A hyperextension injury of the knee crushes the fat pad in the front of the knee. The fat pad then becomes swollen and painful. This is called Hoffa's syndrome and usually settles spontaneously but may require arthroscopic resection of the fat pad. Examination reveals tenderness of the fat pad.

F. 7 Patella dislocation
Patella dislocation is one of the more common acute intrinsic injuries to the knee. It is most frequent in the second and third decades. Risk factors can include trochlear dysplasia, ligamentous laxity and patella alta. The patella dislocates, but then spontaneous reduction occurs (as it so often does).

The knee will be painful and swollen initially and so will be difficult to examine, but once the initial inflammation has settled the patient will be left with a patella apprehension sign. Any attempt to push the patella laterally as you passively flex the knee will be resisted by the patient, who will have a sense of discomfort and apprehension. Radiographs are important to rule out any bony injury, and there should be a low threshold for further imaging, particularly in younger patients, to determine whether there has been any damage to the articular cartilage. Conservative measures are the mainstay of treatment unless there is an acute bony pathology or recurrent problems with instability.

Multiple choice questions

→ Epidemiology

1. **Regarding the epidemiology of spinal pathology, which of the following statements are false?**
A The lifetime prevalence of lower back pain is 60%–80%.
B 80%–90% of acute low back pain episodes resolve.
C 5%–7% of 45- to 64-year-olds report back problems as a chronic illness.
D The lifetime prevalence of sciatica is 10%–15%.
E 70% of acute episodes of sciatica resolve within three months.

→ Clinical anatomy

2. **Regarding clinical spinal anatomy, which of the following statements are false?**
A Cervical lordosis is normally between 35 and 45 degrees.
B Most lumbar lordosis is between L4-S1.
C The spinal nerve roots comprise 7 cervical, 12 thoracic, 5 lumbar and 5 sacral.
D The spinal cord terminates at L1.
E The radicular artery of Adamkiewicz is the main blood supply to the lower spinal cord.

→ History

3. **Regarding the spinal patient history, which of the following is not a recognised finding in cauda equina syndrome?**
A History of malignant disease
B Unilateral or bilateral sciatica

C Saddle anaesthesia
D Lower-extremity motor weakness
E Bladder or bowel disturbance

→ Physical examination

4. **Regarding spinal physical examination, which of the following nerve roots is associated with an absent ankle jerk reflex?**
A L4
B L5
C S1
D S2
E S3

5. **Regarding spinal physical examination, which of the following is a characteristic finding of an upper motor neurone lesion?**
A Decreased tone
B Hyper-reflexia
C Fasciculation
D Down-going plantars
E Sensory loss

→ Investigations

6. **Regarding spinal investigations, which of the following statements are true?**
A Plain radiographs of the spine should be taken only if there is a history of trauma.
B Early tumour and infection can be diagnosed on plain radiographs.
C MRI is the optimal method of visualising the disc and nerve roots.
D CT is best for assessing soft tissue pathology.
E Bone scintigraphy is used to diagnose osteoporosis.

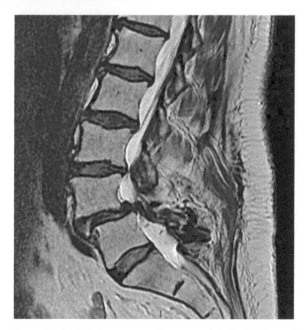

Figure 35.1 A sagittal MRI demonstrating spondylolisthesis at the L4/5 level.

→ ## Degenerative conditions of the spine

7. Figure 35.1 is a sagittal MRI that demonstrates spondylolisthesis at the L4/5 level, with associated disc pathology, facet joint arthrosis and spinal stenosis. The patient has had previous surgery to the spine. How would you classify this spondylolisthesis according to the Wiltse classification?

A Dysplastic
B Isthmic type 2A
C Degenerative
D Isthmic type 2C
E Pathological

Extended matching questions

→ ### Spine diagnoses

1 Cauda equina syndrome
2 Cervical myelopathy
3 Idiopathic scoliosis
4 Lumbar disc herniation
5 Neuromuscular scoliosis
6 Peripheral vascular disease
7 Primary spine tumour
8 Scheuermann's kyphosis
9 Spinal metastasis
10 Spinal stenosis
11 Spondylolisthesis

For each of the following cases, select the single most likely diagnosis from the options listed. Each option may be used once, more than once, or not at all.

A A 68-year-old man presents with a long-standing progressive history of lumbar back pain associated with intermittent bilateral leg pain and paraesthesia to both feet. He describes normal bowel and bladder function. His symptoms are worse when walking (5 minutes before pain comes on) but are relieved when bending forward, e.g., leaning on a trolley.

B A 70-year-old man who has smoked all his life presents with increasing back pain that is worse at night and a feeling of being generally unwell with unexplained weight loss.

C A 38-year-old man has had problems with sciatica for many years. He lifts a heavy object and subsequently develops severe back pain, bilateral leg pain and perineal numbness.

D A 40-year-old man presents with chronic lumbar back pain, with acute pain radiating down the left leg to his foot. On examination he has weakness of extensor hallucis longus on the left, with diminished sensation over the dorsum of the foot and the lateral side of the calf.

E A 13-year-old girl presents with a rib hump and a coronal curve to the spine. She has no previous past medical history of note. Abdominal reflexes are equal and normal.

Answers to multiple choice questions

⇒ Epidemiology

1. D
The chance of someone having back pain at some point in his or her life is between 60% and 80%, with more than 80%–90% of episodes resolving spontaneously within six weeks of onset without the need for aggressive investigation or treatment. However, 5%–7% of 45- to 64-year-olds report problems as a chronic illness. The lifetime prevalence of sciatica is 2%–4%, with 70% of acute episodes resolving within 3 months.

⇒ Clinical anatomy

2. C
The spine is straight in the coronal plane with the head centred over the sacrum, but in the sagittal (side) plane there is the following:

- Cervical lordosis (range 20–45 degrees)
- Thoracic kyphosis (range 20–50 degrees), which increases with age
- Lumbar lordosis (range 40–80 degrees), occurs predominantly between L4 to S1

   The thoracic kyphosis balances the cervical and lumbar lordosis. The spinal cord terminates at the level of L1. The spinal nerve roots comprise 8 cervical (7 vertebrae), 12 thoracic, 5 lumbar, 5 sacral and 1 coccygeal. The blood supply to the spinal cord is from the vertebral, deep cervical, intercostal and lumbar arteries, supplying the anterior spinal artery (majority of blood supply) and two posterior spinal arteries. The lower spinal cord is supplied by the anterior spinal artery, which is mainly supplied by the radicular artery of Adamkiewicz. Injury to this artery can lead to critical ischaemia of the cord. It is found on the left side in 80% of patients, originating anywhere from T5 to L5 (ventral roots T9–T11 commonly).

⇒ History

3. A
History of malignant disease is a red-flag symptom but is not classically associated with cauda equina syndrome (**Table 35.1**). 'Red flag' signs are possible indicators of a non-benign

Table 35.1   Red flags and classical findings of cauda equine syndrome

Red flags	Cauda equina syndrome
Age <20 years or >50 years	Low back pain
Recent significant trauma	Unilateral or bilateral sciatica or leg pain
History of malignant disease	Saddle anaesthesia
Unexplained weight loss	Lower extremity motor weakness
Systemic symptoms, e.g., fever, weight loss	Bladder or bowel disturbance
Immunosuppression, e.g., steroids	
Thoracic back pain	
Severe or progressive sensory or motor changes	
Painless retention	
Numbness in perineum or buttocks, or faecal incontinence	

Source: Adapted from Tables 35.1 and 35.3 in: Williams, N., Bulstrode, C., O'Connell, PR. (Eds.), *Bailey & Love's Short Practice of Surgery*, 26th ed., 2013.

origin and possible serious spinal pathology. 'Yellow flag' signs are psychosocial factors that potentially indicate that the back pain is not likely to be amenable to conventional surgical treatment and is more likely to be associated with long-term disability and likely psychological in origin.

→ Physical examination

4. C
The dermatome, myotome and reflex evaluation for the upper and lower limb are found in **Table 35.2.**

5. B
Characteristic findings of an upper motor neurone lesion are increased tone (spasticity), hyper-reflexia, muscles spasms, motor weakness, disuse atrophy, a positive Hoffman's sign, ankle and patellar clonus and up-going plantar response. Characteristic findings of a lower motor neurone lesion are decreased tone (flaccid), hypo-reflexia, denervation fasciculation, motor weakness, severe atrophy, sensory loss and down-going plantar response.

→ Investigations

6. C
Plain radiographs of the spine can be used as the primary investigation when there is back pain associated with 'red flag' signs. This includes trauma. Plain radiographs are not useful in the early detection of tumour or infection, as 40%–60% of bone mass destruction is required before it is detected. The best way to image the soft tissue of the spine (disc, thecal sac, nerve roots) is MRI, with CT the investigation of choice for bony pathology. Osteoporosis cannot be diagnosed reliably on radiographs or by scintigraphy, with bone densitometry being used.

→ Degenerative conditions of the spine

7. C
Although it could be argued this is a postsurgical spondylolisthesis, this patient has lumbar spinal stenosis caused by degenerative spondylolisthesis and disc pathology. Spondylolisthesis is the forward translation of one upper vertebra over the one inferior to it. A variety of

Table 35.2 The myotomes, dermatomes and reflexes of the upper and lower limb

Level	Myotome	Dermatome	Reflex
Upper Limb			
C5	Deltoid (shoulder abduction)	Lateral arm	Biceps tendon
C6	Elbow flexion or wrist extension	Lateral forearm	Brachioradialis
C7	Elbow extension/wrist flexion	Middle finger	Triceps
C8	Thumb extension/long finger flexors	Medial forearm	-
T1	Finger abduction (hand interossei)	Medial arm	-
Lower Limb			
L2	Hip flexion	Anterior thigh or groin	-
L3	Knee extension	Anterior and lateral thigh	Patellar tendon
L4	Ankle dorsiflexion	Medial leg and foot	Patellar tendon
L5	Great toe extension extensor halluces longus (EHL)	Lateral leg and dorsum of foot	-
S1	Ankle plantar flexion	Lateral foot and little foe	Achilles tendon

Source: Adapted from Table 35.4 and 35.5 in: Williams, N., Bulstrode, C., O'Connell, PR. (Eds.), *Bailey & Love's Short Practice of Surgery,* 26th ed., 2013.

classifications exist. The Myerding classifies spondylolisthesis according to the severity of the slip and is found in **Table 41.2.** The alternative Wiltse classification has the following six types:

1 Congenital (dysplastic): Associated with congenital deficiency at L5/S1
2 Isthmic: Associated with pars interarticulares lesion
   a. Lytic pars defect, i.e., pars fatigue fracture
   b. Elongated or attenuated pars
   c. Acute pars fracture
3 Degenerative: Facet joint segmental instability due to disc and facet joint degeneration
4 Traumatic: Acute fracture involving posterior elements (not pars)
5 Pathological: Pathological destruction associated with bone disease, e.g., metabolic or neoplastic
6 Postsurgical: Sometimes considered part of traumatic

Answers to extended matching questions

Spine diagnoses

A. 10 Spinal stenosis
The history is classical of spinal stenosis, which is the narrowing of the spinal canal, nerve root canal, or foramen caused by a combination of facet joint hypertrophy (e.g., osteophytes), disc bulge or herniation, ligament flavum hypertrophy, or facet cysts. Resultant neural compression and ischaemia leads to back, buttock and leg pain that is worse when walking. It can be congenital, e.g., achondroplasia (medial facets and short pedicles), post-trauma or

surgery, inflammatory (e.g., ankylosing spondylitis), or degenerative, with the latter normally presenting between 50 and 70 years of age.

It is essential to differentiate spinal and vascular claudication, as with both causes of pain is initiated on exercise. However, standing stationary relieves symptoms of vascular claudication (postural changes not seen), whereas not stopping but flexion (leaning forward) relieves spinal claudication. Generally, with vascular claudication patients get pain going uphill (when the leg muscles require more oxygen and the spine is flexed), while spinal claudicants get worse pain going downhill (when the spinal canal narrows in extension). Generally, patients with spinal claudication will have normal distal pulses unless they have concomitant peripheral vascular disease. Bladder symptoms can occur in some patients, although cauda equina syndrome is rare.

Diagnosis is confirmed with CT or MRI, with some quoting an AP diameter of less than 10 mm or a cross-sectional area of less than 100 mm^2. Spinal claudication only progresses in around one-third of cases, and if it does spinal decompression +/− fusion can offer symptom relief.

B. 9 Spinal metastasis

Most tumours of the spine are metastases (98%), with the most common being breast (21%), and lung (14%). Prostate, renal, gastrointestinal and thyroid are all under 10%.

Red flags are useful in identifying high-risk patients. The vast majority of patients present with progressive pain, with spinal cord compression less common. Routine investigations include bloods (FBC, UEs, LFTs, CRP, ESR, PSA, TFTs), plain radiographs (chest and spine; absent pedicles, vertebral erosion or collapse), CT, bone scan and bone biopsy, e.g., open or CT-guided. Whole-spine MRI is used to detect metastases and neurological compromise.

Treatment includes analgesia, steroids, bisphosphonates, radiotherapy, chemotherapy and potentially surgery, e.g., for spinal cord decompression – stabilisation and postoperative radiotherapy.

C. 1 Cauda equina syndrome

In this case, a cauda equine syndrome (central lumbar disc prolapse or herniation) has to be excluded. It is unlikely to be occult malignancy or an aneurysm, as the patient is too young and transverse myelitis is not usually painful. It is rare (2%–6% of all lumbar disc herniations), more common in men and routinely seen between 20 and 45 years of age. The most common cause is a large central disc prolapse at the L4/5 level.

There are no completely reliable signs of central disc prolapse, but saddle anaesthesia and loss of anal tone (faecal incontinence) are important (**Table 35.1**). Bladder changes include painless retention initially followed by overflow incontinence. Absence of pain does not exclude the diagnosis nor do unilateral signs. They are commonly associated with a single nerve root trapped in the lateral foramen (a paracentral or lateral disc protrusion).

Urgent MRI confirms the diagnosis. There is evidence that if surgical decompression is carried out within 24 hours of the loss of bowel or bladder control, the chance of recovery is better and so an immediate referral to a spine surgeon or unit is recommended.

D. 4 Lumbar disc herniation

Symptomatic lumbar disc herniation is rare (2%–5% of the population), more common in males, routinely seen between 30 and 50 years of age, and more than 90% occur at the L5/S1 and L4/L5 levels (**Figure 35.2**). Other risk factors include heavy manual work or lifting, occupation, socioeconomic deprivation, and smoking.

Patients often present with back pain followed by unilateral radicular leg pain. A spectrum of neurological signs can be found including paraesthesia, motor weakness, absent reflexes, and a positive straight leg-raise test. In this case, the pain radiates down to

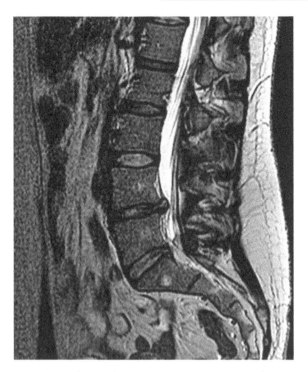

Figure 35.2   A sagittal MRI demonstrating a posterior disc protrusion at the L4-L5 level, which on further views was indenting the thecal sac and compressing the left L5 nerve root.

the foot, suggesting that it is radicular rather than referred, so facet joint arthritis and discitis or infection are unlikely to be the cause. The motor supply to extensor hallucis longus is from L5 **(Table 35.2)**, and the dermatomal distribution of L5 is the dorsum of the foot and lateral side of the calf. This will be caused by a posterolateral or paracentral disc herniation at L4/L5 or a far-lateral or extra-foraminal herniation at L5/S1. MRI confirms the diagnosis.

Conservative management (physiotherapy, analgesia) results in symptoms settling within three months for 70%–90% of patients. Nerve root steroid injections may be helpful. For cases where the symptoms persist, micro-discectomy is employed.

E. 3 Idiopathic scoliosis
The patient's age, gender, and clinical findings are consistent with adolescent idiopathic scoliosis. A coronal curve is a scoliosis, whereas a sagittal deformity can be a lordosis or kyphosis. Normal abdominal reflexes suggest that a neuromuscular scoliosis is unlikely. Lung function is commonly affected in neuromuscular or early-onset scoliosis but is rarely affected in idiopathic adolescent scoliosis. Risk factors for progression of the curve include females, how much more growth is anticipated, and the rate at which it is occurring, along with curve type (thoracic worse than lumbar, double worse than single) and size. Curves normally stabilise at skeletal maturity.

The severity of a scoliosis curve is measured with Cobb's angle on standard full PA and lateral standing views of the spine, with a right thoracic curve most common. Cobb's angle (>10 degrees diagnostic) measures the maximum angle of the spine curvature on the PA view **(Figure 35.3)**. The Lenke classification is more comprehensive and aids to guide

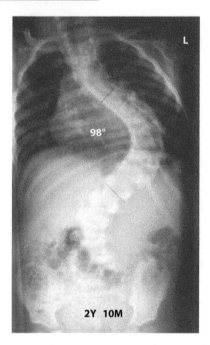

Figure 35.3 An AP standing spine view with the Cobb angle measuring 98 degrees. (From Williams, N., Bulstrode, C., O'Connell, PR. (Eds.), *Bailey & Love's Short Practice of Surgery*, 26th ed., 2013.)

treatment. Risser's staging is a method to determine skeletal maturity from the closure of epiphyseal growth plates in the pelvis and therefore predicts how much more growth (and deformity) potential there is in the skeleton. MRI is used to exclude intra-spinal anomalies, e.g., Arnold-Chiari malformation, syrinx.

Treatment is determined by the size of the curve and anticipated progression of the curve. For a Cobb angle of <25 degrees, observation with serial radiographs is recommended. Bracing aims to limit curve progression but will not correct the curve, thus the use is limited to skeletally immature patients with flexible curves between 25 and 45 degrees. For angles >40–45 degrees or trunk imbalance, surgery with continuous electrical spinal cord monitoring is indicated. Options include the following:

- Posterior instrumented spinal fusion (most common)
- Anterior instrumented spinal fusion
- Combined

36 Upper limb

Andrew D Duckworth

Multiple choice questions

→ ## Anatomy

1. Regarding anatomy of the shoulder, which of the following is not a muscle of the rotator cuff?

A Infraspinatus
B Subscapularis
C Supraspinatus
D Teres major
E Teres minor

2. Regarding anatomy of the hand, which of the following muscles would you find within the first extensor compartment?

A Extensor pollicis brevis
B Extensor carpi radialis brevis
C Extensor pollicis longus
D Extensor carpi ulnaris
E Extensor digiti minimi

→ ## Shoulder pathology, assessment and management

3. Regarding adhesive capsulitis of the shoulder, the loss of which of the following shoulder movements is pathognomonic?

A Abduction
B Flexion
C Extension
D Internal rotation
E External rotation

4. Regarding shoulder replacement surgery, which of the following are recognised benefits or options of the procedure?

A Pain relief is always guaranteed.
B Range of movement will improve dramatically.
C Deficiency to the rotator cuff is not important.

D Shoulder arthrodesis gives a much inferior range of movement.
E A partial shoulder replacement can be an option.

→ ## Elbow pathology, assessment and management

5. Regarding compression of nerves around the elbow, which nerve is associated with weakness of finger abduction?

A Anterior interossoues nerve
B Median nerve
C Ulnar nerve
D Posterior interosseous nerve
E Musculocutaneous nerve

→ ## Hand pathology, assessment and management

6. Regarding the general principles of managing hand pathology, which of the following is false?

A Avoid swelling and stiffness.
B Edinburgh position of safety is MCPJ extension, PIPJ and DIPJ flexion at 90°.
C Elevation aids with swelling.
D Movement prevents stiffness.
E Splints aim to prevent contractures.

7. Regarding rheumatoid arthritis of the hand, which of the following is not a recognised manifestation of the disease?

A Boutonnière deformity
B Extensor tendon rupture
C Prominent ulnar head
D Radial deviation of the metacarpopha- langeal (MCP) joints
E Swan neck deformity

Extended matching questions

→ ## Shoulder diagnoses

1 Acute rotator cuff tear
2 Calcific tendinitis
3 Chronic rotator cuff tear
4 Frozen shoulder
5 Osteoarthritis
6 Rheumatoid arthritis
7 Rotator cuff impingement

For each of the following cases, select the single most likely diagnosis from the options listed. Each option may be used once, more than once, or not at all.

A A 38-year-old painter and decorator presents with gradual onset of pain in both shoulders, left worse than right. This is especially severe when he is trying to paint ceilings. On examination, pain is experienced at between 60 and 100 degrees of abduction. Shoulder radiographs are normal.

B A 68-year-old woman presents with a painless but progressively weak shoulder. She can only abduct it with a trick movement hunching her shoulder. Otherwise, there seems to be very little power of abduction.

C A 52-year-old man who sustained a severe intra-articular fracture of the right shoulder as a young man now presents with increasing pain, stiffness and weakness of the shoulder.

D A 42-year-old woman presents with pain in her left shoulder, but with no history of trauma. She is tender anterolaterally and the pain is so severe that she cannot sleep. She is able to rotate the shoulder externally without much pain, but other movements are painful, especially active ones. Radiographs demonstrate a calcification between the acromion and humeral head.

→ ## Elbow diagnoses

1 Golfer's elbow
2 Loose body
3 Median nerve compression
4 Olecranon bursitis
5 Osteoarthritis
6 Radial nerve compression
7 Septic arthritis
8 Tennis elbow
9 Ulnar nerve compression

For each of the following cases, select the single most likely diagnosis from the options listed. Each option may be used once, more than once, or not at all.

A A 48-year-old woman attends with pain over the lateral side of the elbow following a weekend redecorating the house.

B A 28-year-old man who sustained a fracture to his elbow many years ago presents with pain and numbness down the medial side of the forearm into the little finger.

C A 36-year-old man presents with a red and hot lump over the posterior part of the elbow. He is systemically well, apyrexial, has a flexion arc of 100 degrees and radiographs are unremarkable.

→ Hand diagnoses

1 Boutonnière deformity
2 Carpal tunnel syndrome
3 Cubital tunnel syndrome
4 Dupuytren's disease
5 de Quervain's tenosynovitis
6 Mallet thumb
7 Pronator teres syndrome
8 Swan neck deformity
9 Trigger finger
10 Ulnar collateral ligament injury

For each of the following cases, select the single most likely diagnosis from the options listed. Each option may be used once, more than once, or not at all.

A A 46-year-old woman has a PIPJ flexion and a DIPJ hyperextension deformity of the left ring finger.

B A 52-year-old woman complains of discomfort over the lateral aspect of her right wrist and thumb. There is a positive Finkelstein's test.

C A 48-year-old man complains of being intermittently unable to extend his right ring finger, with a clicking sensation sometimes felt. There is a tender swollen nodule over the palmar aspect of the affected finger.

D A 58-year-old man with a history of chronic liver disease attends with a bilateral fixed flexion deformity of the ring and little fingers, left worse than right.

E A 47-year-old woman has a 12-week history of tingling and numbness in the hand, which is worse at night. On examination, there is wasting of the thenar eminence.

Answers to multiple choice questions

→ Anatomy

1. D

The rotator cuff includes four muscles **(Table 36.1)** that control movement and aid with stability of the glenohumeral joint. It includes the following:

• Subscapularis: Internal/medial rotation
• Supraspinatus: Abduction
• Infraspinatus: External/lateral rotation
• Teres minor: External/lateral rotation

2. A

The six extensor compartments of the wrist are as follows, from radial/lateral to ulnar/medial:

1. Abductor pollicis longus and extensor pollicis brevis

2. Extensor carpi radialis longus and extensor carpi radialis brevis

3. Extensor pollicis longus

4. Extensor indicis and Extensor digitorum communis

5. Extensor digiti minimi

6. Extensor carpi ulnaris

Table 36.1 The rotator cuff muscles of the shoulder

Muscle	Origin	Insertion	Nerve supply
Subscapularis	Subscapular fossa of scapula	Humerus lesser tuberosity	Upper and lower subscapular nerve
Supraspinatus	Supraspinous fossa of scapula	Humerus greater tuberosity – superior facet	Suprascapular nerve
Infraspinatus	Infraspinous fossa of scapula	Humerus greater tuberosity – middle facet	Suprascapular nerve
Teres minor	Lateral edge/border of scapula	Humerus greater tuberosity – inferior facet	Axillary nerve

➡ Shoulder pathology, assessment and management

3. E

Adhesive capsulitis (frozen shoulder) is an idiopathic condition that is characterised by the spontaneous onset of a stiff and painful (severe initially) shoulder. It commonly affects women in the sixth decade and is associated with minor trauma or previous surgery, comorbidities (diabetes, ischaemic heart disease, thyroid disease) and prolonged immobilisation of the shoulder. There is often an initial global reduction in passive and active shoulder movement, but loss of external rotation is pathognomonic. Imaging is routinely normal, although MRI may demonstrate contracture of the joint capsule. The mainstays of treatment are conservative measures including analgesia, steroid injections, distension arthrogram and physiotherapy. Most cases resolve within 1 to 3 years following onset. MUA or arthroscopic surgical release may be used in refractory cases.

4. E

Total shoulder arthroplasty **(Figure 36.1)** routinely provides good pain relief postoperatively; however, pain relief cannot be guaranteed with any surgery. Replacement does not routinely significantly increase the range of movement in the shoulder. Pain relief provided by a glenohumeral arthrodesis may result in a comparable or even better range of movements than a replacement, as the full range of movements available in the scapulothoracic joint can be utilised.

Prerequisites for total shoulder replacement are an intact rotator cuff and good glenoid bone stock. Rotator cuff deficiency (proximal migration of humerus, diagnosed on further imaging) makes total shoulder arthroplasty much less reliable unless the cuff can be repaired at the same time (rare), in which case hemi-arthroplasty or a reverse shoulder replacement is recommended. If the glenoid is well preserved, a hemi-arthroplasty can give good results, although pain relief is less predictable.

➡ Elbow pathology, assessment and management

5. C

The ulnar nerve arises from the brachial plexus medial cord (C8-T1). After median neuropathy, ulnar nerve compression (cubital tunnel syndrome) is the next most common compressive neuropathy of the upper limb, with the common compression sites around the elbow being the following:

- Arcade of Struthers
- Two heads of flexor carpi ulnaris (aponeurosis)
- Medial epicondyle
- Medial intermuscular septum

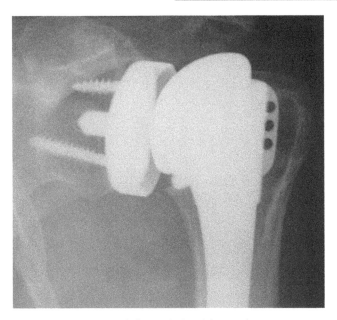

Figure 36.1 A left total shoulder replacement

There may be a background of previous elbow trauma leading to a cubitus varus or valgus deformity. Patients often present with paraesthesia in the little and ring fingers, with possibly a positive Tinel's sign over the compression site. A classic claw hand may be seen when compression of the ulnar nerve occurs at the wrist (e.g., at Guyon's canal), whereas with compression at the elbow, paradoxically (ulnar paradox) the claw is less pronounced due to the loss of innervation to the medial two digits flexor digitorum profundus. Motor findings include the following examples of wasting and weakness of the hand intrinsics:

- Hypothenar (abductor digiti minimi, flexor digiti minimi opponens digiti minimi)
- Adductor pollicis: Positive Froment's sign (see Chapter 33)
- Interossei: Abduction (dorsal) and adduction (palmar) of the fingers
- 3rd and 4th lumbricals

AP and lateral radiographs of the elbow will exclude potential bony causes, e.g., osteophytes or previous trauma (supracondylar fracture leading to cubitus varus or valgus). Diagnosis is through clinical assessment and nerve-conduction studies. Conservative measures (e.g., analgesia and activity modification) are the primary lines of treatment, with surgery involving decompression +/– transposition.

→ Hand pathology, assessment and management
6. B

Prevention and management of hand swelling and stiffness is essential to prevent permanent fibrosis and contracture leading to a loss of function. This can occur following trauma, infection, or surgery. Elevation is used to reduce swelling, particularly in the acute period. Splintage in a safe position aims to prevent contractures. The Edinburgh position of safety involves MCPJ flexion at 90°, with PIPJ and DIPJ in full extension. Early movement reduces swelling and prevents permanent stiffness.

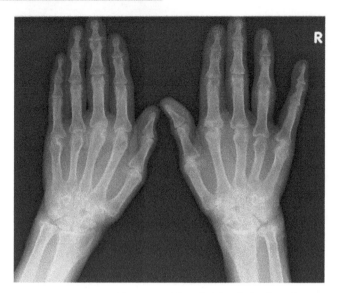

Figure 36.2 Rheumatoid arthritis of the hand

7. D

There are a large number of deformities associated with rheumatoid arthritis **(Figure 36.2)**. However, the deviation of the MCP joints is ulnar, not radial, whereas in the wrist the deviation is radial. Deformities are associated with synovial inflammation and attrition trauma, with potential abnormalities being the following:

- Extensor and flexor tendon ruptures
- MCPJ deformity: ulnar +/− volar deviation with associated subluxation/dislocation
- Wrist deformities: radial deviation, carpal supination, prominent ulna head
- Boutonnière deformity (DIPJ hyperextension and PIPJ flexion)
- Swan neck deformity (PIPJ hyperextension and MCPJ + DIPJ flexion)
- Z-thumb deformity (FPL rupture)

  Potential surgical management options include the following:

- Synovectomy: Gives good pain relief, improves function and potentially prevents tendon rupture or nerve compression.
- Ulna head excision: Reduces pain and risk of extensor tendon rupture but wrist instability can be a problem in younger patients, so replacement may be necessary.
- Wrist and small joint arthrodesis: Provides good pain relief and improves function.
- Prosthetic replacement of MCPJs.
- Tendon transfer is preferred to repair.

Answers to extended matching questions

→ Shoulder diagnoses

A. 7 Rotator cuff impingement

This case is characteristic of rotator cuff impingement, which commonly occurs as the cuff travels inferior to the acromion. The 'painful arc' is pain on active shoulder abduction, commonly between 40 and 120 degrees. Special tests include Neer, Hawkins and Jobe test (see Chapter 33). This condition can be diagnosed with an injection of local anaesthetic into the impinging area, and some patients' symptoms can settle with this in combination with physiotherapy. Subacromial decompression is the surgical option.

B. 3 Chronic rotator cuff tear

This patient presents with a painless but weak shoulder where the problem has developed over the years. This case is characteristic of a tear of the rotator cuff. These commonly occur in an older age group, with 20%–45% of 40- to 50-year-olds having asymptomatic tears, with that number rising to over 50% in the eighth decade. On examination, the characteristic finding is weakness of the affected tendons, with pain being an uncommon symptom. Radiographs might demonstrate proximal migration of the humerus or calcific tendinitis, with ultrasound or MRI being diagnostic. Management is determined by the patient and tear characteristics, with options including physiotherapy, activity modification, steroid injections and cuff repair in selected cases.

C. 5 Osteoarthritis

Glenohumeral osteoarthritis can be either primary or secondary traumatic osteoarthritis following fracture or end-stage rotator cuff disease. As with other joints, this will present with a gradual onset of pain, stiffness and weakness of the shoulder with a global reduction in the range of movement. Radiographs confirm the diagnosis, with CT used to determine the extent of any bone loss and MRI to detect any rotator cuff pathology. When conservative measures are no longer controlling symptoms, hemi/total/reverse shoulder replacements are the options. Please also see multiple choice question Answer 4.

D. 2 Calcific tendinitis

Calcific tendintis is thought to be associated with degenerative changes of rotator cuff pathology. It is seen between 20 and 50 years of age and is associated with diabetes. Severe pain and stiffness developing rapidly without any trauma can be either a frozen shoulder or calcifying tendinitis of the supraspinatus tendon. Frozen shoulder produces global pain and loss of movement, in particular external rotation. Calcific tendinitis usually does not affect external rotation to that degree but is associated with a painful arc and might have signs of impingement. Radiographs confirm the finding of a calcific deposit within the supraspinatus tendon between the acromion and the humeral head.

Conservative measures include analgesia, steroid injection, physiotherapy, or ultrasound-guided decompression of the deposit. Surgery involves arthroscopic removal of the calcific deposit +/– decompression.

→ Elbow diagnoses

A. 8 Tennis elbow

Tennis elbow (lateral epicondylitis) does not only develop after playing tennis but can start after any heavy activity where there is repetitive eccentric forced palmar flexion with pronation, which puts a specific load on to the common extensor origin. Clinical examination often reveals an area of tenderness over the humeral lateral epicondyle (common extensor origin), with pain reproduced on resisted wrist and finger extension. Nonoperative interventions are commonly successful and involve activity modification, nonsteroidal anti-inflammatory drugs (NSAIDs), physiotherapy, bracing, or steroid injections. Surgery (common extensor origin debridement and release) is very rarely indicated for prolonged failed conservative treatment. (See Chapter 34, extended matching questions, Answer A).

B. 9 Ulnar nerve compression

Please see multiple choice question Answer 5. Arthritis of the elbow can lead to irritation and compression of the ulnar nerve as it passes posterior to the elbow joint. Nerve-conduction studies should confirm the diagnosis, with decompression +/− transposition of the nerve being the definitive management.

C. 4 Olecranon bursitis

Olecranon bursitis (**Figure 34.2** in Chapter 34) is relatively common and can be diagnosed by good clinical examination. It can be associated with previous trauma or repeated minor trauma, localised infection, or comorbidities, e.g., gout. Patients present with a swelling over the extensor surface of the elbow, which can be painful, erythematous and warm (indicative of infected bursitis). Septic arthritis of the elbow is more commonly associated with hot and painful elbow joint, low-grade pyrexia and a reduced range of movement. Olecranon bursitis routinely settles with a combination of activity modification, analgesia (NSAIDs), aspiration and antibiotics if there is evidence of infection. Formal surgical drainage is occasionally warranted for a purulent collection +/− bursa excision. Chronic olecranon bursitis can be associated with calcific deposits, and bursa excision may be indicated.

→ Hand diagnoses

A. 1 Boutonnière deformity

Boutonnière deformity is associated with rheumatoid hand (but can be associated with isolated trauma, e.g., Zone 3 extensor tendon injury) and characterised by PIPJ flexion and DIPJ hyperextension (**Figure 36.3**). There is primary disruption of the extensor tendon central slip, resulting in separation and volar subluxation of the lateral bands. This ultimately results in dorsal subluxation of the head of the proximal phalanx. The resulting deformity is exacerbated and maintained through contracture of the collateral ligaments, volar plate and oblique retinacular ligament.

B. 5 de Quervain's tenosynovitis

In 1895 Swiss surgeon Fritz de Quervain originally described de Quervain's tenosynovitis – first extensor tendon compartment sheath inflammation and stenosis. Patients are commonly female and the age of onset is usually between 30 and 50 years. Some suggest an association with pregnancy, repetitive micro trauma, e.g., golf, as well as inflammatory arthropathies.

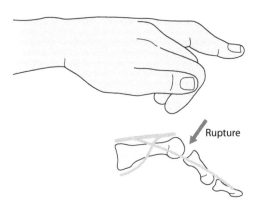

Rupture

Figure 36.3 Boutonnière deformity. (From Williams, N., Bulstrode, C., O'Connell, PR. (Eds.), *Bailey & Love's Short Practice of Surgery*, 26th ed., 2013.)

Clinical presentation is pain, tenderness and swelling over the lateral aspect of the thumb or wrist, with crepitus sometimes felt. Finkelstein's test can be positive (flex affected thumb into palm, first made around thumb, wrist ulnar deviation). Radiographs can be used to exclude other differentials, e.g., base of thumb osteoarthritis. Management includes the following:

- Conservative: Activity modification, analgesia, e.g., NSAIDs, splints, or corticosteroid injection
- Surgery: Release of first dorsal compartment

C. 9 Trigger finger

Triggering of the fingers or thumb is due to tendon sheath inflammation and fibrotic thickening, ultimately leading to a tendon-sheath size mismatch (stenosis). This causes restricted movement of the flexor tendon and the tendon becoming entrapped within the retinacular pulley, usually at the first annular (A1) pulley of the ring or middle fingers. Patients, usually females, are often between 40 and 60 years of age. Associated conditions include diabetes, rheumatoid arthritis, amyloidosis and gout. On examination, a tender nodule can be found on the flexor aspect of the affected finger or thumb, with the digit locked in flexion when passive extension is attempted. The digit usually becomes 'unlocked' with passive force, with a trigger-like pop felt (Green classification). If initial treatment with conservative measures fails (e.g., physiotherapy, steroid injection), surgery to release +/− debride the pulley can be performed.

D. 4 Dupuytren's disease

Dupuytren's contracture is an autosomal dominant condition characterised by palmar fascial nodules and cords, skin puckering with progressive fibrotic hyperplasia of the palmar and digital fascia, resulting in fixed flexion deformities of the affected fingers. It is seen commonly in people of northern European descent, males and in those who are between 40 and 60 years of age. Risk factors include smoking, trauma/postsurgery, epilepsy medication, AIDS/HIV, diabetes mellitus, hypothyroidism and alcohol cirrhosis.

The disease can be bilateral, pain is not common and the ring or little fingers are most commonly involved. Associated presentations include the following:

- Ledderhose disease: Plantar fibromatosis leading to thickening
- Peyronie's disease: Penile fibromatosis leading to curvature
- Garrod's knuckle pads: Thickened skin dorsum PIPJ

The Hueston tabletop test (unable to place open palm on table) can be used as indication for surgery, along with PIPJ flexion contracture. Management includes the following:

- Nonoperative: Collagenase therapy
- Surgery: Fasciotomy, fasciectomy, dermofasciectomy, or amputation

E. 2 Carpal tunnel syndrome

Carpal tunnel syndrome (CTS) is the most frequent upper limb compressive neuropathy. It is characterised by compression and ischaemia of the nerve as it passes underneath the flexor retinaculum at the wrist. It is commonly seen in middle-aged females. Risk factors include obesity, smoking, alcohol excess, diabetes, hypothyroidism, rheumatoid, amyloidosis, pregnancy, trauma and possibly occupation.

Patients commonly present with tingling and numbness of the radial three and half digits, which is often worse at night and relieved by shaking the hand (the 'Flick sign'). Although commonly quoted, pain is not classical. Reduced sensation over the radial three and half digits, thenar muscle atrophy and abductor pollicis brevis weakness can be found. Provocation tests include the following:

- Phalen's test (flexion of wrist until symptoms come on)
- Tinel's test

The diagnosis is made either clinically, with nerve-conduction studies, or with a combination of the two. Management includes the following:

- Nonoperative: Activity modification, night splints, steroid injections
- Operative: Open or endoscopic carpal tunnel decompression

Hip and knee

Andrew D Duckworth

Multiple choice questions

→ Hip joint – applied anatomy

1. Regarding the anatomy of the hip joint, which of the following statements are false?

A The hip joint is a ball-and-socket joint.
B The static stabilisers of the hip include the capsule.
C The dynamic stabilisers are short external rotators, iliopsoas and hip abductors.
D The primary blood supply to the femoral head is the lateral circumflex femoral artery.
E The labrum contributes to joint stability.

→ Hip joint – biomechanics

2. Regarding the biomechanics of the hip joint, which of the following statements are false?

A The hip joint reaction force is influenced by the body weight.
B The abductor muscles play a vital role in supporting the pelvis.
C Standing on one leg results in a joint reaction force of ~3 to 5 times body weight.
D Running and jumping results in a joint reaction force of ~8 to 10 times body weight.
E A stick in the ipsilateral hand helps to reduce the joint reaction force on the hip.

→ Conditions affecting the hip joint

3. Regarding avascular necrosis of the hip, which of the following is not a recognised cause?

A Alcohol excess
B Caisson disease
C Chronic liver disease
D Sickle cell disease
E Smoking

4. Regarding osteoarthritis of the hip joint, which of the following is not a recognised finding on plan radiographs?

A Joint space narrowing
B Osteophytes
C Subchondral collapse
D Subchondral cysts
E Subchondral sclerosis

→ Hip joint – surgical procedures

5. Regarding total hip replacement, which of the following is a recognised peri-operative complication?

A Compartment syndrome risk of 2%.
B Dislocation rate of 2%–5%.
C Leg length inequality of more than 10 cm.
D Mortality from any cause of 2%–5%.
E Pulmonary embolus risk of 10%.

6. Regarding surgical approaches to the hip, a Trendelenburg gait with abductor weakness could be caused by an injury to which nerve?

A Inferior gluteal nerve
B Superior gluteal nerve
C Pudendal nerve
D Sciatic nerve
E Femoral nerve

→ Knee joint – applied anatomy

7. Regarding the anatomy of the knee joint, which of the following is not a dynamic stabiliser?

A Anterior cruciate ligament.
B Biceps femoris.
C Rectus femoris.
D Semitendinosus.
E Sartorius.

→ Knee joint – surgical procedures

8. Regarding arthroscopy of the knee, which of the following is not an indication for surgery?

A Anterior cruciate ligament reconstruction.
B Diagnose and treat meniscal tear.
C Loose body removal.
D Repair a ruptured patella tendon.
E Washout for septic arthritis.

Extended matching questions

→ Conditions affecting the hip joint

1 Steinberg Stage 0
2 Steinberg Stage 1
3 Steinberg Stage 2
4 Steinberg Stage 3
5 Steinberg Stage 4
6 Steinberg Stage 5
7 Steinberg Stage 6

For each of the following cases of avascular necrosis, select the appropriate stage of Steinberg's classification from the options listed. Each option may be used once, more than once, or not at all.

A An 82-year-old woman presents with a six-month history of progressive right groin pain. She has a background of polymyalgia rheumatic and is on regular steroids. Radiographs of the pelvis reveal complete obliteration of the right hip joint space and advanced osteoarthritis of the hip.
B A 52-year-old man with a background of alcohol excess and subsequent radiographs of the pelvis demonstrates evidence of subchondral collapse (crescent sign) of the left hip.
C A 28-year-old woman with a background of sickle cell disease presents with intermittent pain to the left hip. Radiographs of the pelvis are unremarkable, but there is some signal change in the left femoral head on MRI.
D A 48-year-old woman with a background of lupus presents with pain in the right hip, and subsequent radiographs of the pelvis demonstrates evidence of flattening of the right femoral head.

→ Hip and knee joint – management

1 Arthrodesis
2 Core decompression
3 Conservative management
4 Hemi-arthroplasty
5 High tibial osteotomy
6 Hip resurfacing
7 Proximal femoral osteotomy
8 Total knee replacement
9 Total hip replacement
10 Unicompartmental knee replacement

For each of the following cases, select the single best management choice from the options listed. Each option may be used once, more than once, or not at all.

A An adolescent with Perthes' disease has a small area of collapse in the main load-bearing area of the femoral head.

B A 34-year-old man has isolated medial compartment osteoarthritis following a previous complex tibial plateau fracture. He has severe pain, but with a reasonable range of movement, and a varus deformity.

C A 49-year-old woman presents with advanced radiographic osteoarthritis of the knee, isolated to the medial compartment.

D A 78-year-old man presents with severe right groin pain, regular night and rest pain and limiting his day-to-day activities. Radiographs of the hip demonstrate moderate to severe osteoarthritis of the right hip.

E A 67-year-old woman presents with severe left knee pain affecting her mobility and quality of life. Radiographs of the knee demonstrate tricompartmental idiopathic osteoarthritis of the knee.

Answers to multiple choice questions

→ Hip joint – applied anatomy

1. D

The blood supply to the femoral head is from the retinacular branches of the medial circumflex femoral artery, with minimal contribution from the ligamentum teres. This is an important point when considering femoral neck fracture, as these arteries are intimately related to the periosteum within the joint capsule and so are disrupted in an intra-capsular fracture. Proximal femoral fractures are often classified according to disruption of the capsular blood supply to the femoral head:

- Intracapsular or sub-capital
- Extracapsular: Intertrochanteric or sub-trochanteric

The anatomical shape of the hip (ball-and-socket joint) means that the stabilisers are essential. These include the following:

1. Static stabilisers
   a. Ligaments: Iliofemoral, pubofemoral, ischiofemoral
   b. Joint capsule
   c. Acetabular labrum: Fibro-cartilaginous triangular structure that surrounds the rim of the acetabulum, except at the inferior pole (transverse ligament)

2. Dynamic stabilisers
   a. Short external rotators
   b. Iliopsoas
   c. Hip abductors

→ Hip joint – biomechanics

2. E

The hip joint reaction force is influenced by the patient's body weight and abductor muscle force. The abductor muscles provide the lever power that supports the pelvis against the fulcrum of the cup and socket of the hip joint. Both must be present and working normally for a patient to stand on one leg easily. For the following scenarios, the approximate joint reaction forces are:

- Lifting leg from bed = 1.5 x body weight
- Standing on one leg = 3-5 x body weight
- Running and jumping = 10 x body weight

Joint reaction force is reduced with a stick in the contralateral hand, as it reduces the abductor muscle force and the body weight moment arm.

Conditions affecting the hip joint

3. E

Avascular necrosis (AVN), or osteonecrosis, of the femoral head is caused by disruption of the vascular supply leading to bone necrosis. Subsequent femoral head collapse and osteoarthritis occur. It is more common in males between the ages of 35 and 50 years. Bilateral occurrence is seen in 50%–80% of cases. Causes include the following:

- Primary: Idiopathic e.g. Perthes disease
- Secondary: Trauma or infection, drugs, e.g., steroids, alcohol excess, chronic liver disease, sickle cell disease, Caisson disease (the bends), radiotherapy, chemotherapy, SLE

Smoking is not a recognised cause. Although some are initially asymptomatic, the onset of symptoms can be quite rapid, with groin pain, reduced range of movement (in particular, internal rotation) and reduced mobility. Primary investigation is with weight-bearing AP pelvis radiographs, with the classical findings being sclerosis, sub-chondral resorption or collapse (crescent sign), leading ultimately to head flattening, collapse and OA. The Steinberg modification of the Ficat classification is used, with MRI employed for early detection. In the pre-collapse stage, measures such as bisphosphonates or core decompression +/– bone grafting may be taken. When there is evidence of collapse, proximal femoral rotational osteotomy (<50% of head) or joint replacement are indicated.

4. C

Causes for osteoarthritis include the following:

- Primary: idiopathic
- Secondary: Background of trauma, septic arthritis, obesity, childhood hip disorders, e.g., DDH or Perthes disease or SUFE, AVN

There are four characteristic features of idiopathic osteoarthritis of the hip on x-ray: subchondral sclerosis and cysts, joint space narrowing and osteophyte formation (Figure 37.1). Subchondral collapse is associated with avascular necrosis.

Hip osteoarthritis is seen in 10%–25% of people over 65 years of age. The most classical presentation is of groin pain with radiation down the anterior thigh to the knee and reduced mobility. As the disease progresses, the pain goes from activity related to regular rest and night pain. A globally irritable hip with reduced range of movement is found on examination, with loss of internal rotation, leg length discrepancy (distinguish fixed flexion deformity with Thomas' test) and an antalgic gait. Blood tests are commonly normal.

Treatment includes lifestyle modification such as regular exercise and weight loss, analgesia, e.g., NSAIDs, walking aids and joint replacement.

Hip joint – surgical procedures

5. B

Primary total hip replacement is one of the most successful operations in orthopaedics, with a patient satisfaction rate of 90%–95%. When obtaining consent from a patient, it is routine

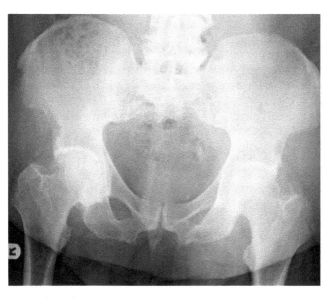

Figure 37.1 AP pelvis demonstrating the classic radiological features of osteoarthritis in the right hip.

to discuss all severe complications and any other complications with a rate of more
than 1%.

Potential intra-operative complications include neurovascular injury (sciatic nerve <1%,
femoral artery or vein <1%), femoral fracture (<1%), or retained cement. The postoperative
complications of total hip replacement are found in **Table 37.1**.
Death is a possibility for any major surgery, but the incidence is <1%. Leg-length discrepancy
does occur, but is rarely more than 2 cm, and, certainly, 10 cm would be most unlikely.
Compartment syndrome is not a routinely associated complication of total hip replacement,
although a possible but rare complication of any major surgery.

Table 37.1 Post-operative complications of total hip replacement

Complication	Rate
DVT	2%–5%
PE	<1%
Infection	1%–2%
Dislocation	2%–5%
Leg length discrepancy (>1 cm)	2%–5%
Loosening and wear	2%–5%
Heterotopic ossification	<1%
Blood loss requiring transfusion	2%–5%

Source: Adapted from Table 37.1 in: Williams, N., Bulstrode, C., O'Connell,
PR. (Eds.), *Bailey & Love's Short Practice of Surgery,* 26th ed.,
2013.

6. B

During the anterolateral approach to the hip for total hip replacement, the fibres of gluteus medius are split; with excessive splitting there may be the potential of causing damage to the superior gluteal nerve (L4-S1) that innervates gluteus medius, gluteus minimus and tensor fascia lata. Resulting loss of abductor muscle power will lead to a Trendelenburg gait. The nerve exits from the anterior sacral foramina (sacral plexus) then leaves the pelvis through the greater sciatic foramen superior to piriformis. The nerve passes ~4–5cm above the greater trochanter where it is at most risk.

Knee joint – applied anatomy

7. A

The knee is a synovial hinge joint with two articulations between the tibia and femur, and the femur and the patella. It is inherently unstable and relies heavily on the soft tissue stabilisers. These include the following:

1. Static stabilisers
    a. Ligaments
        i. Cruciates provide AP stability (ACL, PCL)
        ii. Collaterals provide valgus or varus stability (MCL, LCL)
    b. Menisci: medial and lateral
    c. Joint capsule

2. Dynamic stabilisers (muscles that cross the joint)
    a. Quadriceps (rectus femoris, vastus lateralis, vastus medialis, vastus intermedius)
    b. Hamstrings (semitendinosus, semimembranosus, biceps femoris)
    c. Sartorius

Knee joint – surgical procedures

8. D

Extra-articular problems such as a ruptured patella tendon are best treated with open repair. Knee arthroscopy is used in the diagnosis and management of cartilage defects, as well as ligamentous and meniscal injuries. It can also be used in the acute washout of a septic joint. Common indications include the following:

- Cruciate ligament reconstruction
- Diagnosis and repair or resection of meniscal tears
- Loose body removal
- Cartilage repair techniques, e.g., microfracture
- Acute washout for septic arthritis
- Synovectomy, e.g., for inflammatory arthropathy

Answers to extended matching questions

Pathological fracture risk classification

A 7 (Steinberg Stage 6)
B 4 (Steinberg Stage 3)
C 2 (Steinberg Stage 1)
D 5 (Steinberg Stage 4)

The Steinberg modification of the Ficat classification is used for avascular necrosis of the hip (Table 37.2).

Table 37.2   Steinberg's classification of femoral avascular necrosis

Stage	Description
0	No diagnostic evidence on radiographs or MRI
1	Normal radiographs, but abnormal MRI
2	Sclerosis and cysts
3	Subchondral collapse (crescent sign)
4	Femoral head flattening but normal acetabulum
5	Acetabular changes and joint space narrowing
6	Joint space obliteration and advanced degenerative changes

Source: Adapted from Table 37.2 in: Williams, N., Bulstrode, C., O'Connell, PR. (Eds.), *Bailey & Love's Short Practice of Surgery*, 26th ed., 2013.

Hip and knee joint – management

A. 7 Proximal femoral osteotomy

A patient with a local area of collapse from Perthes' disease needs that damaged area to be moved out of the load-bearing area and replaced with healthy cartilage. The method of doing this is a rotation osteotomy. Osteotomies around the hip aim to redistribute the forces and load-bearing areas to avoid areas of high-point loading. This can be done through a combination of proximal femur and acetabular osteotomies.

B. 5 High tibial osteotomy

Knee osteoarthritis is associated with varus, or less commonly valgus, deformities of the knee leading to altered load bearing and worsening disease. Osteotomies aim to realign the joint mechanics for better distribution of the load through the joint. It can do this by changing the alignment of the knee so that the bulk of the load goes through the unaffected side. The most common osteotomy around the knee is a high tibial osteotomy (open or closing wedge) for varus knee osteoarthritis. In young and active patients, a knee replacement can be avoided or delayed. If there is good range of movement, then a high tibial osteotomy will retain that range of movement while unloading the arthritic side of the joint.

C. 10 Unicompartmental knee replacement

In younger patients with intact ligaments (ACL essential), arthritis limited to the medial compartment and a varus or fixed flexion deformity of less than 15 degrees should be considered for a unicompartmental knee replacement.

D. 9 Total hip replacement

Total hip replacement provides patient satisfaction in 90%–95% of cases, with good longevity. A variety of bearing surfaces (metal on polyethylene, ceramic on polyethylene, ceramic on ceramic) and fixation techniques (uncemented versus cemented) exist.

E. 8 Total knee replacement

For conventional tricompartmental osteoarthritis of the knee, a standard total knee replacement (TKR) is the operation of choice. The aims of TKR include pain relief, mechanical realignment, balance of the collateral ligaments and normal patella-femoral tracking. Patient satisfaction is ~85%, with good longevity.

38 Foot and ankle

Andrew D Duckworth

Multiple choice questions

→ **Anatomy**

1. Regarding foot and ankle anatomy, which of the following statements are true?

A The subtalar joint is responsible for inversion and eversion of the hindfoot.

B The third metatarsal head is recessed to act as a 'keystone' in the transverse arch.

C The windlass test assesses the integrity of the flexor muscles in the sole of the foot.

D The saphenous artery contributes to the blood supply of the foot.

E The first dorsal web space of the foot is supplied by the superficial peroneal nerve.

2. Regarding compartments of the leg, which of the following structures are not found within the anterior compartment of the leg?

A Deep peroneal nerve

B Extensor hallucis longus

C Peroneus tertius

D Tibial nerve

E Tibialis anterior

→ **Pathology in the adult forefoot**

3. Regarding hallux valgus, which of the following statements are false?

A Deviation of the hallux is away from the midline.

B It is more commonly seen in men.

C There is a genetic component.

D It can be associated with pain.

E Hammering of the second toe can occur.

→ **Pathology in the adult – midfoot and hindfoot**

4. Regarding acquired pes planus, which of the following is not classically associated with the deformity?

A Tibialis posterior tendon dysfunction

B Tarsometatarsal osteoarthritis

C Charcot–Marie Tooth

D Hindfoot osteoarthritis

E Tarsal coalition

5. Regarding arthritis of the ankle (tibiotalar joint) and hindfoot, which of the following statements are false?

A Ankle replacement is indicated in low-demand patients with mild to moderate deformity.

B Arthrodesis is indicated in high-demand patients.

C Osteophyte removal can be effective for impingement with no significant osteoarthritis.

D For single joint hindfoot arthritis, triple fusion is still the treatment of choice.

E Knee deformities should be assessed and treated prior to surgery for foot or ankle problems.

Extended matching questions

→ **Foot and ankle diagnoses 1**

1 Charcot–Marie Tooth
2 Curly toes
3 Hallux rigidus
4 Hallux valgus
5 Hammer toes

6 Mallet toes
7 Physiological flatfoot
8 Tarsal coalition
9 Tight tendo Achilles

For each of the following cases, select the single most likely diagnosis from the options listed. Each option may be used once, more than once, or not at all.

A A 14-year-old boy presents with pain in the foot. On examination, there is a flatfoot deformity that does not correct when he stands up on tiptoes.

B A 6-year-old child with cerebral palsy is toe-walking and is referred for assessment and management to aid her to walk on the soles of her feet (plantigrade).

C A 38-year-old runner complains of increasing pain in her right big toe that she fractured many years ago. The first metatarsophalangeal joint is red dorsally and has a very limited range of painful movement. The patient wants to be able to continue running.

D A 9-year-old boy with a family history of a progressive neurological disorder affecting the lower limbs presents with problems in his feet. The arches are very high and the toes bent up so that they rub on his shoes.

→ Foot and ankle diagnoses 2

1 Fracture of the second metatarsal
2 Freiberg's disease
3 Hallux rigidus
4 Heel bumps
5 Metatarsalgia
6 Morton's neuroma
7 Osteomyelitis
8 Stress fracture
9 Turf toe
10 Ulcer

A A 15-year-old girl presents with pain at the base of the second toe. Radiographs demonstrate an abnormal second metatarsal head with flattening.

B A 21-year-old woman complains of increasing pain and numbness in her foot localised around the base of the second, third and fourth toes.

C An 18-year-old cricketer develops pain and swelling around the MTPJ of his big toe after a long period of fast bowling. He now has difficulty pushing off on that foot.

D A 23-year-old long-distance runner spontaneously develops a pain over the head of her second metatarsal. Radiographs reveal an undisplaced fracture across the neck of the second metatarsal.

E A 58-year-old man with insulin dependent diabetes presents with chronic erythema and discharge over an ulcerated area located over the first MTPJ of his left foot. CRP is 60 and ESR is 75. Radiographs reveal a destruction of the head of the first metatarsal.

Answers to multiple choice questions

→ Anatomy

1. A
Dorsiflexion and plantar flexion occur almost exclusively at the ankle (tibiotalar) joint, while inversion and eversion occur at the subtalar joint. The subtalar joint along with the

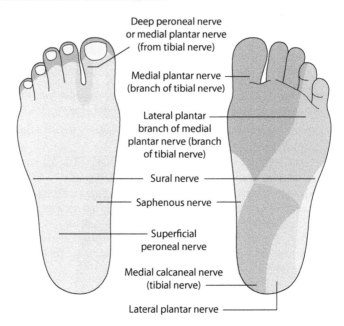

Deep peroneal nerve
or medial plantar nerve
(from tibial nerve)

Medial plantar nerve
(branch of tibial nerve)

Lateral plantar
branch of medial
plantar nerve (branch
of tibial nerve)

Sural nerve

Saphenous nerve

Superficial
peroneal nerve

Medial calcaneal nerve
(tibial nerve)

Lateral plantar nerve

Figure 38.1   The cutaneous nerve supply to the foot. (From Figure 38.1 in: Williams, N., Bulstrode, C., O'Connell, PR. (Eds.), *Bailey & Love's Short Practice of Surgery*, 26th ed., 2013.)

talonavicular and calcanecuboid joints make up the triple-joint complex. The talus is narrower posteriorly, allowing increased rotatory mobility to the plantar flexed foot. In dorsiflexion, the talus jams tightly in the mortice, externally rotating the fibula and foot. The midfoot has a longitudinal and a transverse arch. The second (not the third) metatarsal head is recessed to act as a keystone to this transverse arch. When the second tarsometatarsal joint is injured (Lisfranc), there is subsequent dysfunction of the transverse arch producing and an acquired flat-foot appearance. The 'windlass' test consists of asking the patient to stand on tiptoe. This tightens the plantar fascia (not the muscles), and if this and the arch of the foot are intact, the longitudinal arch becomes more pronounced. The blood supply to the foot is from the anterior and posterior tibial arteries and the peroneal artery. The skin on dorsum of the foot is supplied by the superficial peroneal nerve, but the first dorsal web space is supplied by the deep peroneal nerve **(Figure 38.1)**.

2. D

The tibial nerve is found in the deep posterior compartment of the leg, with all the other structures located in the anterior compartment **(Table 38.1)**. The lower leg contains four compartments contained within fascia and separated by interosseous membranes.

⇒ Pathology in the adult – forefoot

3. B

Hallux valgus is characterised by lateral deviation and rotation of the hallux away from the midline, with an associated medial deviation of the first metatarsal. Bilateral involvement is common and more frequently affects women. Risk factors include a genetic predisposition, pes planus, rheumatoid, cerebral palsy, ligamentous laxity and high-heeled or narrow shoes. Patients present with pain, swelling and deformity in the region of the first MTPJ. The hallux might overlap the second and third toes. The medial prominence (bunion) is irritated by

Table 38.1 The muscles and neurovascular structures within the four fascial compartments of the leg

Compartment	Muscles	Neurovascular structures
Anterior	Tibialis anterior Peroneus tertius Extensor digitorum longus Extensor hallucis longus	Anterior tibial artery Deep peroneal nerve
Deep posterior	Tibialis posterior Popliteus Flexor hallucis longus Flexor digitorum longus	Posterior tibial artery Tibial nerve
Superficial posterior	Gastrocnemius Soleus Plantaris	Sural nerve
Lateral	Peroneus brevis Peroneus longus	Superficial peroneal nerve

footwear creating a red thickened area of skin, a bursa (hypertrophy) and an osteophyte over the underlying bone. Pain can radiate across the metatarsal heads (metatarsalgia) and associated deformities may be found, e.g., hammering of the second toe, callosity over second MTPJ. Radiographs of the feet will help to determine the severity of the deformity, with the common angles measured being the following:

- Intermetatarsal angle (normal <9 degrees)
- MTP angle (normal <15 degrees)

Initially, management is with shoe modification (wide and comfortable shoes) and orthotic insoles when indicated. Surgery is indicated for ongoing symptoms despite conservative measures and is determined by the severity of the deformity. Procedures include first ray metatarsal osteotomy (e.g., Scarf), proximal phalanx osteotomy (e.g., Akin), soft-tissue releases and, in severe cases, joint arthrodesis. Complications include recurrence, AVN and (transfer) metatarsalgia.

Pathology in the adult – midfoot and hindfoot

4. C

Charcot–Marie Tooth is classically associated with a pes cavus deformity of the foot. Pathological causes for acquired club foot include the following:

- Tibialis posterior tendon dysfunction
- Hindfoot and tarsometatarsal osteoarthritis
- Seronegative and inflammatory arthropathy
- Charcot neuropathy
- Tarsal coalition
- Post-traumatic, e.g., spring ligament rupture

On clinical assessment patients have loss of the normal arch (pes planus), difficulty standing on tiptoes on the affected side, the hindfoot may not pull into varus, i.e., planovalgus

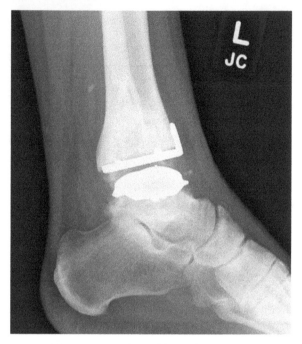

Figure 38.2 An ankle replacement.

deformity and there can be forefoot abduction (too many toes sign). Grading takes into account the degree of deformity and whether it is flexible.

5. D

Ankle replacement **(Figure 38.2)** provides a good outcome in lower-demand patients in whom there is not a severe deformity. Arthrodesis remains the operation of choice for the patient with significant deformity or high-demand patients. In an ankle where a prominent osteophyte can be seen, which is impinging (local anaesthetic injection relieves the pain), osteophyte removal might produce a significant decrease in pain and range of movement. This does not routinely work if there is significant arthritis. It used to be thought that fusion of only one joint in the hindfoot merely produced a rapid deterioration in the other joints. This is now known not to be the case, so single fusion of affected joints is a viable option for a stiff and painful hindfoot. Deformities in the knee produce highly abnormal forces in the foot, which will compromise any attempts to correct any foot pathology. It is therefore generally important to manage problems in the knee before embarking on surgery in the foot.

Answers to extended matching questions

→ Foot and ankle diagnoses 1

A. 8 Tarsal coalition

A flat foot that does not form an arch when the patient stands on tiptoes (windlass test) indicates that there is a structural abnormality such as a tarsal coalition in the foot. The bones most frequently affected are calcaneonavicular and subtalar. Clinical assessment could reveal pes planus, hindfoot valgus, forefoot abduction and calf pain secondary to peroneal spasticity. In the first instance, treatment is nonoperative as the majority are found incidentally and asymptomatic. However, if this fails, resection of the coalition or even arthrodesis may be needed.

B. 9 Tight tendo Achilles
Patients with cerebral palsy may toe-walk, partly because they often have a tight tendo Achilles, but also because the loads transmitted through to the tibia help them to stand and walk. Fixed-flexion deformities of both the hip and knee can occur. Problems might be compounded by weak or uncoordinated hip and knee extensors, so standing on tiptoes helps to prevent the knee from collapsing. If the tendo Achilles is lengthened without thinking about this, the child might be able to stand plantigrade but the knee will then collapse. It is therefore important that there is a thorough gait analysis before any surgery is undertaken.

C. 3 Hallux rigidus
Hallux rigidus is arthritis of the first MTPJ. There is commonly a history of trauma or micro trauma. Other potential causes should be considered, e.g., gout, inflammatory arthopathies. Clinical presentation is with progressive pain, swelling and stiffness over the first MTPJ, especially at toe-off. There is a reduced range of movement, particularly in dorsiflexion because of dorsal osteophyte formation. Radiographs confirm the diagnosis. Management can be with modified footwear (stiff-soled, deep toe box), but in a patient with high demands, a MTPJ fusion can be considered. When there are dorsal osteophytes but minimal evidence of arthritis, a dorsal cheilectomy may be beneficial.

D. 1 Charcot–Marie Tooth
Patients with evidence of pes cavus require a full neurological assessment, with more than 80% of cases associated with a neurological disease. One of the most common causes is Charcot–Marie–Tooth disease (HMSN – hereditary motor sensory neuropathy), which is characterised by progressive small muscle wasting of the hands and feet, calf atrophy and classical cavovarus feet. The Coleman block test can be used to determine if the hindfoot deformity is flexible or rigid. Loss of vibration sense and lower limb areflexia might be seen. Other orthopaedic manifestations include developmental dysplasia of hip (DDH) and scoliosis. Diagnosis is with nerve-conduction studies and genetic analysis. Initial treatment is with stretching exercises and orthotics. If the deformity is flexible, soft-tissue releases might correct or slow the progression of the deformity. However, if the deformity is fixed, an osseous correction, e.g., calcaneal osteotomy, or triple arthrodesis can be required.

Another cause of pes cavus deformity can be spina bifida occulta. This can leave a bar of bone or scar tissue across the spinal canal that traps the cauda equina as the teenager grows and is called a diastomatomyelia. Release of the bar does not always lead to full recovery.

Foot and ankle diagnoses 2

A. 2 Freiberg's disease
Freiberg's disease is a spontaneous osteonecrosis of the second metatarsal head, which develops in teenagers, particularly female athletes. Risk factors include a long second metatarsal. Patients present with pain, swelling and reduced movement at the second MTPJ, with symptoms worse on weight bearing. Radiographs +/– MRI are diagnostic, with the Smillie classification used. Conservative measures are often successful and involve activity and shoe modification, NSAIDs and rest. Surgery (e.g., arthrotomy and debridement) is rarely indicated.

B. 6 Morton's neuroma
This is a compressive neuropathy of the interdigital nerves, which are trapped between the metatarsal heads. It is known as Morton's neuroma and commonly affects females with some suggesting the transverse pressure (repeated micro trauma) from tight shoes to be a

predisposing factor. The third and fourth space is most commonly affected, followed by the second or third. Patients complain of pain and paraesthesia in the affected web spaces. On squeezing the metatarsal heads together, pain may be elicited consistent with metatarsalgia, but a click (Mulder's click) might be provoked when it is consistent with a neuroma. Diagnosis is confirmed with ultrasound. Conservative measures are the mainstay of treatment and include modified footwear, orthotics and steroid injections. Surgical excision of the neuroma can be performed, often successfully, if nonoperative measures prove unsuccessful. The symptoms should improve, but the patient will be left with a numb interdigital cleft.

C. 9 Turf toe

This is a tear of the proximal phalanx capsule due to forcible hyperextension of the big toe. It is known as turf toe. Stress and sesamoid fractures can occur concomitantly. Treatment is with rest, analgesia and modified footwear. Surgery is rarely indicated. Hallux rigidus can be a late complication.

D. 8 Stress fracture

The presentation is classical of a stress or 'march' fracture and is best managed with rest from the predisposing cause.

E. 7 Osteomyelitis

Diabetic patients are prone to infection due to peripheral vascular disease (poor blood supply and nutrition of tissues), peripheral neuropathy and general immunosuppression. Diabetic ulcers require prompt treatment, as infection can spread to bone. This patient has raised inflammatory markers and radiographic changes consistent with osteomyelitis. Debridement and microbiology-targeted high-dose intravenous antibiotics are required. Gram-positive cocci, e.g., *Staphylococcus aureus*, are the common causative organisms, although gram-negative organisms and anaerobes are seen with chronic infections.

The Charcot joint (neuropathic joint destruction due loss of protective sensation) is seen in diabetic patients. The foot and ankle are commonly affected. The pain is minimal, but the foot or ankle is swollen and radiographs reveal joint destruction out of all proportion to what the minimal pain would suggest. Biopsy and MRI can differentiate a Charcot joint from infection. The three stages are the following:

1 Fragmentation
2 Coalescence
3 Bone consolidation

The Charcot foot needs supportive treatment, aiming to prevent deformity and ulceration, e.g., with total contact casting. Arthrodesis provides stability but is not without complication. Amputation can be needed.

Musculoskeletal tumours

Andrew D Duckworth

Multiple choice questions

→ **General principles**

1. Regarding malignant bone tumours, which of the following is the most common primary bone malignancy?
   A Chondrosarcoma
   B Ewing's sarcoma
   C Metastases
   D Multiple myeloma
   E Osteosarcoma

→ **Metastases**

2. Regarding bone metastases, which of the following is a common primary site?
   A Brain
   B Breast
   C Colonic
   D Gastric
   E Pancreatic

→ **Osteogenic and chondrogenic tumours**

3. Regarding osteogenic and chondrogenic tumours, which of the following is associated with Ollier's disease?
   A Chondroblastoma
   B Chondrosarcoma
   C Enchondroma
   D Osteoid osteoma
   E Osteosarcoma

→ **Bone tumour classification**

4. Regarding the Enneking staging system for malignant bone tumours, what stage is a high-grade extra compartmental osteosarcoma?
   A IA
   B IB
   C IIA
   D IIB
   E III

→ **Soft tissue tumours**

5. Regarding soft tissue tumours, which of the following is not a common warning symptom or sign?
   A Increasing in size
   B Larger than 5 cm
   C Pain
   D Recurrence of previous excision
   E Superficial to the fascia

→ **Treatment**

6. Regarding the classification of surgical resection margins, which of the following defines a resection through the reactive zone of the tumour?
   A Biopsy
   B Intralesional
   C Marginal
   D Radical
   E Wide

Extended matching questions

→ Musculoskeletal tumour diagnoses

   1 Chondrosarcoma
   2 Ewing's sarcoma
   3 Fibrous dysplasia
   4 Giant cell tumour

5 Metastasis
6 Multiple myeloma
7 Osteochondroma
8 Osteoid osteoma
9 Osteosarcoma

For each of the following cases, select the single most likely diagnosis from the options listed. Each option may be used once, more than once, or not at all.

A   A 68-year-old woman presents with a painful left hip with no history of trauma and radiographs demonstrate a pathological fracture through a lytic lesion in the left proximal femur. Subsequent staging investigations show multiple lesions in the spine.

B   A 16-year-old boy finds a prominent hard lump on the back of his knee, which restricts flexion but has not changed significantly in size over the past 6 to 12 months. Radiographs reveal a pedunculated projection from the bone.

C   A 13-year-old boy presents with a history of pain and localised swelling of his left humerus, with subsequent radiographs demonstrating an 'onion skin' periosteal reaction.

D   A 66-year-old woman is found to have multiple lytic lesions in her skeleton. Urine protein electrophoresis was positive for Bence-Jones proteins.

E   A 32-year-old woman presents with pain and reduced range of movement around her right wrist. Radiographs reveal a single lytic lesion of the distal radius, with subsequent biopsy demonstrating large multinucleate osteoclast-like cells.

F   A 17-year-old boy presents complaining of severe pain in the right leg. The pain is worse at night but lessens with ibuprofen. Radiographs reveal a 1-cm radiolucent nidus surrounded by a dense cortical reaction in the right tibial diaphysis.

➜ Pathological fracture risk classification

1   Mirels score 3
2   Mirels score 4
3   Mirels score 5
4   Mirels score 6
5   Mirels score 7
6   Mirels score 8
7   Mirels score 9
8   Mirels score 10
9   Mirels score 11
10 Mirels score 12

For each of the following cases, select the Mirels score from the options listed. Each option may be used once, more than once, or not at all.

A   A 45-year-old man presents with a pathological lesion of the humerus, with malignant melanoma the known primary. He has moderate pain and a lytic-type lesion, which is 30% of the cortical thickness.

B   A 62-year-old man presents with a pathological lesion of the shaft of the femur, with renal cell carcinoma the known primary. He has moderate pain and a lytic-type lesion, which is 50% of the cortical thickness.

C   A 52-year-old woman presents with a pathological lesion of the proximal femur, with breast carcinoma the known primary. She has severe pain and a lytic-type lesion, which is 80% of the cortical thickness.

D   A 72-year-old man presents with a pathological lesion of the shaft of the humerus, with prostate carcinoma the known primary. He has mild pain and a mixed-type lesion, which involves 50% of the cortical thickness.

Answers to multiple choice questions

→ General principles

1. D

Metastases are the most common malignant bone tumours, but multiple myeloma is the most common primary malignant bone tumour. It is common after the fifth decade and in males. It is defined by the neoplastic proliferation of plasma cells in the bone marrow, resulting in solitary (plasmacytoma) or multicentric (multiple myeloma) skeletal lesions. There are major and minor criteria for the diagnosis. The prognosis is varied with median survival being three years. Osteosarcoma is the most common malignant primary bone sarcoma, with a bimodal incidence distribution (adolescents, e.g., second decade and elderly patients associated with Paget's disease). Chondrosarcoma and Ewing's sarcoma are less commonly seen.

→ Metastases

2. B

After the lung and liver, bone is the third most common site for metastases. Patients can present with symptoms and signs from the primary lesion, e.g., shortness of breath or cough in patients with primary lung cancer, along with symptoms and signs associated with bony metastases, e.g., pain. Patients can present with metabolic disturbance associated with hypercalcaemia (e.g., confusion, polyuria, muscle weakness). The most common sites are the spine (thoracic common), which can lead to neurological compromise associated with spinal cord compression, the proximal femur and proximal humerus (which can cause bone pain or pathological fracture). Haematogenous spread is the common route, with cells spreading via Batson's vertebral venous plexus (no valves allowing retrograde spread to spine, pelvis and long bones). For more than 90% of bony metastases, the primary lesion is from the following:

- Breast
- Lung
- Renal → Lytic lesions common
- Thyroid
- Prostate → Sclerotic lesions common

Routine investigations include bloods, plain radiographs, CT, bone scan and bone biopsy, when indicated. MRI is used to detect neurological compromise. Management includes pain relief, bisphosphonates, radiotherapy, chemotherapy and potentially surgery, e.g., intramedullary nailing to stabilise an actual or impending pathological fracture, spinal cord decompression. Pre-operative embolisation of the lesion is indicated for potentially highly vascular lesions, e.g., renal or thyroid metastases.

→ Osteogenic and chondrogenic tumours

3. C

Enchondroma is a common benign hyaline cartilaginous tumour found in the medullary cavity of predominantly the hands (most common bone tumour of the hand), feet and long bones. It is seen in both men and women between 20 and 50 years of age. Although enchondroma can be associated with pain, swelling, deformity and pathological fracture, many are asymptomatic incidental findings. Radiographs often demonstrate scalloped lucent or lytic lesions located in the bone metaphysis or diaphysis, with patchy calcification **(Figure 39.1)**. Solitary lesions are defined as an Enneking benign lesions stage 1 – latent. The following two multiple forms are known:

1 Ollier's disease: Multiple enchondromas, skeletal dysplasia, long bones affected with associated deformity (e.g., bowing, short), risk of malignant transformation 20%–30%.

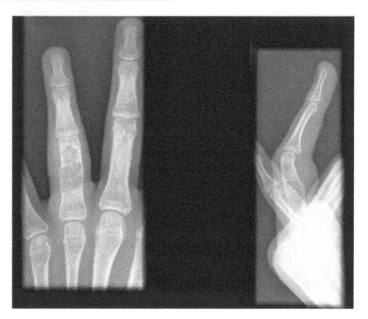

Figure 39.1 A pathological fracture of the proximal phalanx ring finger in a benign enchondroma. (From Figure 39.17 in: Williams, N., Bulstrode, C., O'Connell, PR. (Eds.), *Bailey & Love's Short Practice of Surgery,* 26th ed., 2013.)

2 Maffucci syndrome: Multiple enchondromas, soft-tissue angiomas, risk of malignant transformation is reported to be up to 100%.

→ Bone tumour classification

4. D

The following are the two Enneking classifications for bone tumours:

1. Benign

- Latent: Often asymptomatic, e.g., osteochondroma, enchondroma.
- Active: Mild symptoms and grow slowly, e.g., aneurismal bone cyst.
- Aggressive: Symptomatic and often grow rapidly, e.g., giant cell tumour.

2. Malignant: Based on the grade, whether the bone cortex has been breached (extra compartmental) and presence of metastases **(Table 39.1)**. Many bone tumours present as an Enneking stage IIB.

→ Soft tissue tumours

5. E

Soft-tissue tumours can be benign (e.g., lipoma) or malignant (e.g., liposarcoma). Soft-tissue tumour warning signs are the following:

- Increasing in size
- Larger than 5 cm
- Painful
- Recurrence of previous excision
- Deep to the fascia

Table 39.1   The Enneking staging for malignant bone tumours

Stage	Grade	Compartment
IA	Low grade	Intra compartmental
IB	Low grade	Extra compartmental
IIA	High grade	Intra compartmental
IIB	High grade	Extra compartmental
III	Metastases present	

Source: Adapted from Table 39.4 in: Williams, N., Bulstrode, C., O'Connell, PR. (Eds.), *Bailey & Love's Short Practice of Surgery*, 26th ed., 2013.

Table 39.2   Classification of surgical resection margins

Classification	Detail
Intralesional	Resection through the lesion
Marginal	Resection through the reactive zone of the tumour
Wide	Resection outside the reactive zone of the tumour
Radical	Excision of the whole affected compartment

Source: Table 39.7 in: Williams, N., Bulstrode, C., O'Connell, PR. (Eds.), *Bailey & Love's Short Practice of Surgery*, 26th ed., 2013.

Treatment

6. C
Following surgical excision of a tumour, the resection margins are classified to determine the degree of resection (**Table 39.2**).

Answers to extended matching questions

Musculoskeletal tumour diagnoses

A. 5 Metastasis
A pathological fracture in an elderly patient through a lytic lesion is most likely to be a metastasis, particularly with further lesions found within the spine. Metastases are far more common than primary bone tumours.

B. 7 Osteochondroma
This lump is not growing and therefore is likely to be benign. It appears to be an outgrowth from the bone but on radiographs is almost completely invisible. This means that it is mainly a cartilage cap on a bone stalk with a classic 'mushroom' appearance. This is characteristic of an osteochondroma, which is a common benign chondrogenic tumour frequently found in children, adolescents and young adults. Common sites are the metaphyses of the proximal and distal femur, proximal tibia and proximal humerus. Multiple hereditary exostosis (MHE) is an autosomal dominant multiple form associated with mutation in the *EXT* gene. Many solitary lesions are asymptomatic, with a palpable mass possible or less commonly

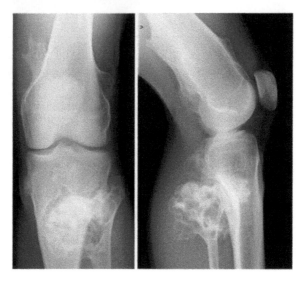

Figure 39.2   Multiple hereditary exostosis of the knee.

mechanical or neurovascular symptoms or signs due to irritation of the surrounding soft-tissue structures. MHE is associated with limb deformities, e.g., bowed forearm and early onset osteoarthritis **(Figure 39.2)**. Malignant transformation (chondrosarcoma) is rare with solitary lesions but can occur in 5%–10% in MHE. Management is with excision if symptomatic.

C. 2 Ewing's sarcoma
Ewing's sarcoma is a rare malignant small round cell sarcoma of bone commonly found in males in the second decade of life (5 to 25 years old). Genetic translocation is (t 11;22). Site is usually the diaphysis of long bones, e.g., femur, pelvis, or spine. Clinical presentation is often with a painful and tender mass, with or without possibly systemic upset, e.g., pyrexia, anaemia and raised inflammatory markers. Presentation can mimic infection. Radiographs reveal osseous destruction (moth-eaten), soft-tissue swelling (particularly evident on MRI that is required to determine extent of soft-tissue involvement) and a characteristic 'onion-skin' periosteal reaction. CT is required for staging, with lung metastases seen. Management is with chemotherapy and surgical resection.

D. 6 Multiple myeloma
After metastases, the next most common lesion in the skeleton is plasmacytoma (solitary), which is called multiple myeloma when there are many lesions. These consist of lymphoid tissue. Multiple myeloma is caused by the proliferation of plasma cells, and presentation can mimic widespread metastases. Investigations include blood tests for anaemia, raised ESR, hypercalcaemia and renal failure. Blood and urine protein electrophoresis demonstrate raised levels of immunoglobulin, and in the urine this is seen as Bence-Jones protein. Radiographs reveal multiple punched-out lesions. Bone scans can be cold. Chemotherapy is the mainstay of management, along with the following symptom controls:

- Bone pain +/− fracture: Bisphosphonates, radiotherapy, fracture stabilisation
- Anaemia: EPO
- Renal failure: Supportive, dialysis

E. 4 Giant cell tumour

A solitary lesion full of large multinucleate osteoclast-like cells is a giant cell tumour. It is a benign tumour (it does not metastasise) but is locally quite aggressive and is defined as an Enneking benign lesions stage 3 – aggressive. They are commonly found in young adults between the ages of 20 and 50 years, with females more frequently seen. Common sites include the epiphysis of long bones, e.g., proximal tibia, distal femur, proximal humerus, distal radius. Pain and reduced range of movement of local joint is common. Radiographs demonstrate a non-sclerotic expanding eccentric lytic lesion that extends to the subchondral region. Management is with radical curettage +/− adjuvant treatment, e.g., hydrogen peroxide, plus reconstruction as required. Metastases can occur to the lung (<5% cases).

F. 8 Osteoid osteoma

Osteoid osteoma is a benign osteogenic tumour commonly found in young males between the ages of 5 and 30 years. Sites include the diaphysis of the long bones and the spine. Patients often present with quite severe pain that is not associated with activity, which is characteristically worse at night and relieved by NSAIDs, e.g., ibuprofen. Radiographs demonstrate a radiolucent nidus surrounded by a dense periosteal reaction (when nidus >1.5cm osteoblastoma). Management is with conservative measures, e.g., observation and NSAIDs. Surgery (ablation or excision) is usually reserved for refractory cases.

Pathological fracture risk classification

A 5 (Mirels score 7)
B 7 (Mirels score 9)
C 10 (Mirels score 12)
D 4 (Mirels score 6)

The Mirels scoring system is used to stratify the risk of pathological fracture and involves the following four categories scored 1–3:

• Tumour site: Upper limb, lower limb, peri-trochanteric or proximal femur
• Pain: Mild, moderate, functional or severe
• Lesion: Blastic, mixed, lytic
• Size: <1/3 of cortical thickness, 1/3–2/3 cortical thickness, >2/3 cortical thickness

For a score of ≤7, the risk of fracture is less than 5%, so prophylactic fixation is not considered necessary, with observation +/− radiotherapy as indicated. For a score of 8, clinical judgement is recommended as the risk of fracture is ~15%–30%. For a score ≥9, prophylactic fixation is recommended as the risk of fracture ranges from 30%–100%.

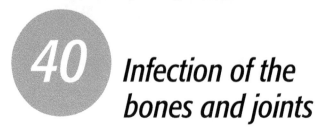

40 Infection of the bones and joints

Andrew D Duckworth

Multiple choice questions

→ ## General principles

1. Regarding bone and joint infection, which of the following is not a Gram-positive organism?

A *Staphylococcus aureus*
B Coagulase-negative staphylococci
C *Haemophilus influenzae*
D Streptococci pneumonia
E Streptococci viridans

2. Regarding acute bone and joint infections, which of the following is not routinely part of the investigative work up?

A Bloods including CRP and ESR
B Radiographs of affected bone or joint
C Ultrasound
D MRI
E Bone scan

→ ## Native joint septic arthritis

3. Regarding native joint septic arthritis, which of the following is not a recognised risk factor?

A Bacteraemia
B Intravenous drug abuse
C Nonsteroidal anti-inflammatory drugs (NSAIDs)
D Rheumatoid arthritis
E Steroids

→ ## Implant-related infection

4. Regarding implant related infection, which of the following statements is false?

A Loose implants require removal.
B In the presence of infection, well-fixed prostheses should still always be removed.

C Multiple microbiological samples are taken at the time of revision surgery.
D Revision can be a one-stage or two-stage procedure.
E Long-term antibiotics are sometimes required in patients unfit for revision surgery.

→ ## Acute osteomyelitis

5. Regarding acute osteomyelitis, which of the following statements is true?

A In young children, refusal to weight bear alone is not consistent with osteomyelitis.
B *Haemophilus influenzae* is the most common causative organism in children.
C Inflammatory markers are routinely normal.
D Radiographic changes can take over 1 week to develop.
E In the acute phase, surgery is usually required.

→ ## Chronic osteomyelitis

6. Regarding chronic osteomyelitis, infection confined to the cortical bone is denoted by which stage of osteomyelitis according to the Cierny and Mader classification?

A Stage 1
B Stage 2
C Stage 3
D Stage 4
E Stage 5

Extended matching questions

→ Bone and joint infection diagnoses

1 Charcot joint
2 Diabetic ulcer
3 Gout
4 Marjolin's ulcer
5 Osteomyelitis
6 Perthes disease
7 Pseudogout
8 Re-fracture
9 Septic arthritis
10 Transient synovitis
11 Tuberculosis

For each of the following cases, select the single most likely diagnosis from the options listed. Each option may be used once, more than once, or not at all.

A A 19-year-old man presents with a swollen and painful right knee. On examination he is pyrexial, and the knee has a large effusion and is red and hot to touch. The knee is held in the 'position of comfort' and is very painful to move. He also complains of pain on passing urine.

B A 64-year-old woman presents with increasing pain, swelling and redness to her left knee. On clinical assessment there is tenderness, swelling and erythema over the knee but with a moderate range of movement. The patient is apyrexial. Microscopy of the knee aspirate reveals positively birefringent rhomboid crystals.

C A 38-year-old man originally from the Indian subcontinent presents with persistent back pain that wakes him at night, and he complains of night sweats. Magnetic resonance imaging (MRI) shows a fluid-filled lesion surrounding the L3 vertebra.

D A 50-year-old man has had chronic problems with a large discharging sinus over his leg following a complex fracture of his tibia several years ago **(Figure 40.1)**. The sinus has recently changed in appearance and subsequent biopsy reveals a squamous cell carcinoma.

E A 4-year-old girl presents with a limp and no prior history of trauma. On clinical assessment there is a mild decreased range of movement, with pain in the right hip. The patient has borderline pyrexia of 37.8. CRP is 15 and ESR is 10. Subsequent ultrasound reveals a moderate hip effusion, with microbiological analysis of the aspirate revealing no organisms.

Answers to multiple choice questions

→ General principles

1. C

Gram-positive organisms, in particular *Staphylococcus aureus*, are the most common cause of bone and joint infection. Although common in prosthetic infection too, a wide range of organisms are seen, e.g., coagulase-negative staphylococci – a normal skin commensal. **Table 40.1** lists the common organisms by type. Identification of the causative organism is a key aspect in the treatment of both native and prosthetic joint infection. In some cases, a combination of organisms may be responsible. If generic antibiotics are started prior to microbiological samples being collected, no growth from cultures might be the result (false negative) and the diagnosis is made on clinical grounds. This should be avoided where

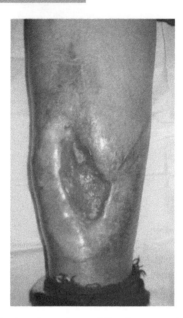

Figure 40.1 Chronic discharging ulcer of the leg associated with osteomyelitis. (From Figure 40.7 in: Williams, N., Bulstrode, C., O'Connell, PR. (Eds.), *Bailey & Love's Short Practice of Surgery,* 26th ed., 2013.)

Table 40.1 Common causative organisms for bone and joint infection

Type	Organisms	Common scenario
Gram positive	*Staphylococcus aureus*	Most common for all case types
	Coagulase-negative staphylococci	Implant related infection (chronic)
	Staphylococcus epidermidis	
	Streptococci pneumonia	
	Beta-haemolytic streptococci	
	Streptococci viridians	Implant related infection
Gram negative	*Enterobacteriaceae*	
	E. coli	Extremes of age
	Klebsiella	
	Salmonella	Sickle cell patients
	Pseudomonas	
	Haemophilus	Non-immunised children
	Neisseria	
	Neisseria meningitides	
	Neisseria gonorrhoea	Sexually transmitted infections
Others	Anaerobes	
	Fungi	Immunocompromised patients
	Mycobacteria	
	Mycobacterium tuberculosis	
	Atypical mycobacteria	

Source: Adapted from Table 40.1 in: Williams, N., Bulstrode, C., O'Connell, PR. (Eds.), *Bailey & Love's Short Practice of Surgery,* 26th ed., 2013.

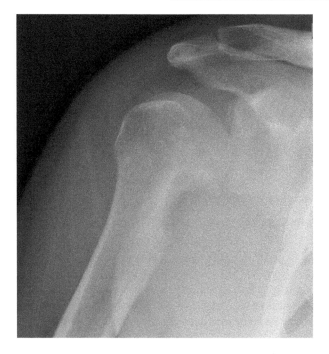

Figure 40.2   Chronic osteomyelitis of the proximal humerus.

possible, although in the presence of septic shock empirical antibiotics should be started without delay. In these cases, blood cultures and local aspiration of pus may be possible prior to administration.

2. E

The diagnosis of infection is routinely made clinically, with bloods and imaging used to confirm the diagnosis. Blood tests, in particular inflammatory markers C-reactive protein (acute marker) and erythrocyte sedimentation rate (chronic marker), are nonspecific tests for infection. Radiographs of a native joint or bone will detect only significant bone destruction **(Figure 40.2)** and in the early stages will likely be normal. For prosthetic infection, however, progressive loosening around the implants can be a marker. Ultrasound can confirm whether there is a soft-tissue collection or joint effusion, with guided aspiration or biopsy possible. CT can confirm the presence of an infected nonunion following fracture and sequestra. MRI is highly sensitive and specific and is seen by some as the gold standard. Isotope bone scan is not part of the routine work for acute infection as it is very nonspecific. However, it can be used in the diagnosis of chronic prosthetic joint infections.

Native joint septic arthritis

3. C

Bacterial infection of a native joint is an orthopaedic emergency as it can result in life-threatening sepsis, as well as joint destruction. The estimated incidence is 4–10/100,000 population in Western Europe. Risk factors include the following:

- Extremes of age
- Socioeconomic deprivation

- Co-existing joint disease, e.g., rheumatoid arthritis
- IV drug abuse
- Immunosuppression
- Diabetes
- HIV
- Drugs, e.g., steroids
- Bacteraemia: Can lead to haematogenous spread to native joints, particularly with a *Staphylococcus aureus* bacteraemia

Most NSAIDs inhibit cyclooxygenase-1 and cyclooxygenase-2. COX-2 is primarily responsible for inflammation through the production of prostaglandins. Although NSAIDs have been implicated in delayed nonunion following fracture, they are not commonly associated with bone and joint infection.

→ Implant-related infection

4. B

Infection following primary hip and knee arthroplasty is now regularly quoted to be less than 1%. Risk factors are similar to those for native joint infection, but also include obesity, skin disease e.g., psoriasis, multiple comorbidities, revision surgery and peri-operative wound infections. In the presence of infection, well-fixed prostheses can be retained but loose implants require removal. Revision surgery can be either of the following:

1 Single-stage revision: Thorough debridement of infected tissue and removal of infected or loose prosthesis, microbiological samples taken and re-implantation of prosthesis.
2 Two-stage revision: Thorough debridement of infected tissue and removal of infected or loose prosthesis, microbiological samples taken and return at a later stage to re-implant prosthesis following a course of antibiotics to eradicate the infection.

Multiple microbiological samples should always be taken (some say a minimum of six) to increase the chance of identifying the causative organism. For patients who are not medically fit or have infection refractory to attempts at eradication, long-term antibiotic therapy is an option.

→ Acute osteomyelitis

5. D

Acute osteomyelitis is infection of the bone and presents with a short history of limb pain, swelling, loss of function and possibly erythema, with associated systemic upset. In young children, where it is commonly located at the metaphysis adjacent to the epiphyseal plate, the only symptoms might be the inability to bear weight along with systemic upset including fever. Routine investigations will often demonstrate a raised WCC and CRP, although ESR may be normal in the acute phase. Blood cultures can aid in identifying the causative organism. Radiographic changes can take over 1 week to detect changes within the bone; MRI can be employed to detect early changes such as bone oedema and periosteal reaction or elevation. In young children who might require a general anaesthetic to undergo a MRI, USS may be used in the first instance. When detected early (2 to 3 days of onset), the primary treatment is with high-dose empirical intravenous antibiotics. This is based on the assumption that there is no dead bone and no concomitant septic arthritis. Rest and analgesia are often required in the initial stages. A delay in the diagnosis and management might require surgery to eradicate the infection.

Table 40.2   The Cierny and Mader classification for chronic osteomyelitis

Stage	Description
1 – Medullary	Cancellous bone (endosteal nidus) Excision using intramedullary technique, e.g., reaming or cortical window Bone grafting often not required with defect filled, e.g., antibiotic cement Structural stability unaffected post procedure
2 – Superficial	Cortical bone Debridement and excision but formal stabilisation not required Bone grafting +/− antibiotic beads Soft tissue involved, e.g., skin ulceration, excision possible +/− coverage
3 – Localised	Defined area of full thickness cortical bone death (sequestrum) Radical debridement and excision Stabilisation required (staged procedures possible) Bone grafting +/− antibiotic beads Soft-tissue involvement and coverage often difficult
4 – Diffuse	Large area (circumferential) of cortical bone involvement and soft tissue Includes all infected nonunions Segmental debridement and excision Stabilization, new bone and soft-tissue cover required, e.g., Ilizarov method

Chronic osteomyelitis

6. B

Chronic osteomyelitis is a persistent serious infection of the bone that can be long-standing and very difficult to eradicate. The pathological process involves inflammation and infection of the bone, resulting periosteum elevation, and eventual bone death due to cortex infarction (sequestrum). New bone formation (involucrum) is a consequence of this.

The Cierny and Mader classification has four stages (**Table 40.2**) and aims to define the nature and extent of the infection. It also categorises the general condition of the patient or host as follows:

A Normal with no concurrent disease or compromise to immune status
B Compromised host with a degree of reduced immunity
C Severe comorbidity preventing adequate treatment of infection, e.g., complications of surgery could be worse than long-standing chronic infection

The combined classification has been found to be prognostic following surgery and a prolonged course of antibiotics to treat the infection.

Answers to extended matching questions

Bone and joint infection diagnoses

A. 9 Septic arthritis

The history and examination are consistent with septic arthritis of a native joint. The likely causative organism in this patient is *Neisseria gonorrhoeae*, which is seen frequently in sexually active young adults. Associated symptoms include urogenital symptoms and signs, polyarthralgia, tenosynovitis and possibly a pustular-type rash.

B. 7 Pseudogout

Gout and pseudogout are characterised by crystal deposition in the joint. In the acute phase, the presentation can mimic septic arthritis. Gout is the deposition of urate crystals, whilst pseudogout produces calcium pyrophosphate crystals. The crystals can be distinguished microscopically by the fact that pyrophosphate crystals are positively birefringent, while urate crystals are negatively birefringent. The hallux MTPJ accounts for almost 50% of the presenting cases of gout. However, pseudogout predominantly affects the large joints, e.g., knee. Radiographs of the affected joint might reveal a background of osteoarthritis and calcium deposition within the joint.

C. 11 Tuberculosis

Tuberculous arthritis and osteomyelitis are rare in people from the United Kingdom, but are still problematic in developing areas of the world. It is also seen in immunocompromised patients. The thoracic spine is the most commonly affected osseous site and can be vertebral osteomyelitis, discitis, or a paraspinal abscess. Pain that wakes a patient at night and night sweats are caused by tumour or infection until proved otherwise. The fluid collection on MRI suggests infection (a cold abscess) and the patient's origin and location in the spine all support the possible diagnosis of tuberculosis. Diagnosis is through positive microbiology aspiration or biopsy. The common organism is *Mycobacterium tuberculosis*. Anti-tuberculosis drugs (e.g., rifampicin, isoniazid, pyrazanamide) are the primary treatment. Spinal orthotics can help to control pain and limit deformity. Surgery is a large undertaking and often involves thorough debridement and spinal stabilisation. Chronic infection is associated with sinus formation, kyphotic deformity and neurological deficits (Pott's paraplegia).

D. 4 Marjolin's ulcer

The history is consistent with a chronic osteomyelitis, likely following an open tibial fracture. A rare complication of a long-standing sinus is the development of a Marjolin's ulcer. This is an aggressive type of squamous cell carcinoma associated with chronic skin changes. Surgical wide excision is often required and even amputation, if indicated. Recurrence ranges from 20%–50%.

E. 10 Transient synovitis

The limping child with an irritable hip and systemic upset remains a diagnostic conundrum between septic arthritis and transient synovitis of the hip. Transient synovitis is self-limiting, with often no definitive cause identified. Patients sometimes have a history of recent trauma or viral illness. Mild pyrexia can occur and inflammatory markers may be marginally raised. However, a significant rise in WCC, CRP, or ESR mean a diagnosis of septic arthritis is more likely and must be excluded. Ultrasound may reveal an effusion, but no organism seen on aspirate is reassuring. Bed rest, analgesia (NSAIDs) and monitoring will result in most cases resolving within 2 to 3 weeks.

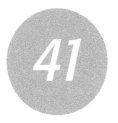

41 Paediatric orthopaedics

Andrew D Duckworth

Multiple choice questions

→ ## General paediatric orthopaedics

1. Which of the following statements are false regarding development and normal variants seen in paediatric orthopaedics?

A Limb bud embryogenesis commences at 4 weeks after fertilisation.

B An in-toeing gait is associated with a negative foot progression angle.

C In-toeing can be caused by persistent femoral neck retroversion.

D All children start with bowlegs and progress to knock-knees by 2 to 3 years of age.

E Children under the age of 3 years commonly have flat feet.

→ ## Congenital and developmental skeletal abnormalities

2. In relation to congenital and developmental skeletal abnormalities, which of the following statements are false?

A Fibular hemimelia is a transverse failure of formation of parts.

B Congenital constriction band syndrome often affects the hands and feet.

C Gigantism is an example of an overgrowth malformation.

D Achondroplasia is associated with a defect in the *FGFR3* gene.

E Reduced intake of vitamin D and calcium is associated with rickets.

→ ## Abnormalities of the hip (Developmental dysplasia of the hip [DDH])

3. In relation to DDH, which of the following statements are false?

A It is more common in boys than in girls.

B It is associated with a breech presentation.

C It is more common in first born.

D It can be assessed clinically using Ortolani and Barlow examination manoeuvres.

E Ultrasonography is the best diagnostic tool in the neonate.

→ ## Abnormalities of the hip (Perthes)

4. In relation to Legg-Calvé-Perthes' disease, which of the following statements are false?

A Perthes' disease is an idiopathic avascular necrosis (AVN) of the proximal femoral epiphysis.

B It commonly affects boys.

C Low birth weight is a risk factor.

D Sickle cell disease could lead to a similar presentation.

E Age of onset does not influence prognosis.

→ ## Abnormalities of the hip (slipped upper femoral epiphysis [SUFE])

5. In relation to slipped upper femoral epiphysis, which of the following statements are true?

A The peak age of onset is 6 years.

B Pain in the knee is uncommon.

C Hypothyroidism is a risk factor for SUFE.

D A mild slip is when <50% of the metaphysis is uncovered.

E Anatomical reduction and pinning is the optimal treatment.

Abnormalities of the foot and ankle (clubfoot)

6. In relation to congenital taclipes equinovarus (CTEV), which of the following statements are false?

A It is more common in boys.

B Spina bifida is associated with CTEV.

C Deformity is characterised by hindfoot equinus or varus and forefoot abduction or supination.

D Pirani scoring system is used to assess the severity of CTEV and guide prognosis.

E The Ponseti method for correcting deformity is successful in over ~90% cases.

Spinal deformities and back pain

7. A child presents with chronic lower back pain and subsequent x-rays reveal a spondylolisthesis of L5/S1, with a 60% slip. What is the Grade of this patient's slip?

A 1

B 2

C 3

D 4

E 5

Extended matching questions

Abnormalities of the knee and leg

1 Blount's disease
2 Chondromalacia patellae
3 Discoid meniscus
4 Osgood–Schlatter disease
5 Osteochondritis dissecans
6 Pseudoarthrosis of the tibia

For each of the following cases, select the single most appropriate diagnosis from the options listed. Each option may be used once, more than once, or not at all.

A A young man complains of clunking and locking of the knee. MRI shows that a fragment of the femoral condyle has broken off and is jamming in the joint.

B A child has a knee that clunks and locks. An MRI shows an abnormal lateral meniscus, which is a solid disc rather than a crescent.

C A child presents with a painful lump over the tibial tubercle.

D A teenage girl has pain that appears to arise from patellofemoral maltracking.

E A West Indian child presents with varus bowing of the tibia.

Abnormalities of the upper limb

1 Camptodactyly
2 Clinodactyly
3 Congenital radial head dislocation
4 Radial club hand
5 Radioulnar synostosis
6 Syndactyly
7 Trigger thumb

For each of the following cases, select the single most appropriate diagnosis from the options listed. Each option may be used once, more than once, or not at all.

A A child presents with a fixed-flexion deformity of the proximal interphalangeal joint of the little finger.

B A child with known cardiorespiratory problems since birth presents with a deformity to the forearm and an absent thumb.

C A child with Down's syndrome is found to have a congenital curvature of the little finger in the radioulnar plane.

D A 4-year-old child complains of an inability to rotate his forearm. His mother tells you that she had a similar problem when she was a child.

E A mother presents with her 6-month-old girl and says that she appears unable to extend her thumb and has a lump over the palmar aspect of the thumb.

Spinal deformities and neuromuscular conditions

1 Brachial plexus injury
2 Cerebral palsy
3 Congenital abnormality of a vertebra
4 Idiopathic scoliosis
5 Leg-length inequality
6 Muscular dystrophy
7 Polio
8 Scheuermann's disease
9 Spina bifida
10 Spondylolisthesis
11 Torticollis

For each of the following cases, select the single most appropriate diagnosis from the options listed. Each option may be used once, more than once, or not at all.

A A child who had a febrile illness now has marked motor weakness and wasting in the lower legs but no sensory loss.

B A teenager presents with a curve of the spine, which produces a rib hump when he tips forward to touch his toes.

C A teenager starts to develop sloping shoulders and a prominent thoracic kyphosis.

D A child is born with the head fixed to one side, due to a contracture of the sternocleidomastoid.

E After a difficult breech birth, a child is noted to have a flaccid arm.

Answers to multiple choice questions

General paediatric orthopaedics

1. C

An in-toeing gait is defined by a negative foot progression angle and common causes or locations are persisting femoral neck anteversion, internal tibial torsion and metatarsus varus (**Table 41.1**). Most of these conditions correct themselves as the child grows.

Limb bud embryogenesis starts very early (around week 4) and is complete by week 8 (all within the first trimester). This is the same time as some internal organs, such as the heart, are forming. This means that certain limb bud abnormalities are associated with specific

Table 41.1 Causes of a persistent in-toeing gait

Site	Cause	Details
Proximal femur	Femoral neck anteversion	Neonate femur anteverted, corrects with growth
		Associated with excessive hip internal rotation
		Can develop compensatory external tibial torsion
		Persistent clinical problems 12–13 years old →
		Proximal femoral osteotomy
Tibia	Internal tibial torsion	Associated with physiological tibia vara
		Assessed by foot or thigh angle
		Corrects with growth, usually by age 4 years
Foot	Metatarsus varus	Often clinically correctable or flexible
		Corrects with growth, 90% by 2 to 4 years
		If rigid → stretches, corrective splints, or shoes

Source: Adapted from Table 41.1 in: Williams, N., Bulstrode, C., O'Connell, PR. (Eds.), *Bailey & Love's Short Practice of Surgery,* 26th ed., 2013.

cardiac abnormalities because both are the result of the same insult to the embryo at that critical time. Children start with bowlegs and become knock-kneed by 2 to 3 years of age, and then stabilise at 7° valgus by 7 years old. Pathological causes for persistent deformity are rickets, skeletal dysplasia, or trauma. Children under the age of 3 years commonly have flat feet until the development of the medial longitudinal arch. Flat feet are associated with a valgus heel, i.e., planovalgus foot. There are two types of persistent flat feet – flexible (tiptoe arch = restores, heel corrects into varus) and rigid (does not correct on tiptoe). Flexible flat feet do not routinely require intervention. Rigid flat feet are associated with inflammatory conditions or tarsal coalition and are likely to require intervention.

Congenital and developmental skeletal abnormalities

2. A

Fibular hemimelia is a longitudinal, not transverse, failure of formation of parts. Gigantism and macrodactyly are examples of overgrowth. Congenital constriction band syndrome does routinely affect the hands and feet of children, with associated poor digit formation. Achondroplasia is a generalised skeletal dysplasia caused by an abnormality of enchondral bone formation and is associated with a defect of the fibroblast *growth factor receptor 3* gene. Clinical manifestations include disproportionate dwarfism (limbs shorter than trunk), underdeveloped foramen magnum, varus deformity of the distal tibia and spinal stenosis. Rickets is characterised by failure of mineralisation of growing bone. The most common cause is nutritional, i.e., vitamin D deficiency. Other causes include environmental (reduced sunlight exposure), genetic (hypophosphataemic rickets), renal (chronic renal failure), GI (Crohn's) and drugs (bisphosphonates). Patients can present with bone pain or deformity and failure to thrive or developmental delay.

Abnormalities of the hip (DDH)

3. A

Developmental dysplasia of the hip is approximately five times more common in girls, the left hip (4:1) and is bilateral in 10%–30%. It is thought to present in ≤20% of breech deliveries (particularly extended breech). It is more common in the first born, with a strong genetic component (strong family history, population prevalence, e.g., North American Inuit) suspected. It is associated with other congenital abnormalities including spina bifida, clubfoot,

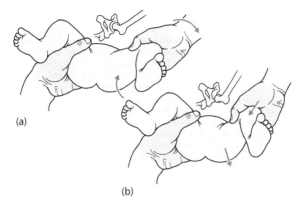

(a)

(b)

Figure 41.1   Ortolani (a) and Barlow (b) tests for DDH. (From Figure 41.10 in: Williams, N., Bulstrode, C., O'Connell, PR. (Eds.), *Bailey & Love's Short Practice of Surgery,* 26th ed., 2013.)

Down syndrome and arthrogryposis. Newborn baby checks at birth and 6 weeks should assess for hip instability. The two classical clinical tests are **(Figure 41.1)** the following:

- Ortolani's test **(Figure 41.1a)** is reducing the dislocated hip: Baby is supine with hips and knees flexed to approximately 90 degrees, thumbs over inner thighs and fingers over greater trochanters, hips are carefully abducted and the test is positive if a palpable or audible clunk is felt or heard as the femoral head reduces.
- Barlow's test **(Figure 41.1b)** is dislocating the reduced hip: Baby is supine with hips and knees flexed to approximately 90 degrees in adduction, femurs are pushed toward the couch and the test is positive if the femoral head subluxes or dislocates.

Ultrasound is used in the diagnosis and monitoring treatment for the neonate as neither the femoral head nor the acetabulum can be visualised on x-ray at birth, as they have not yet ossified (<6 months).

Abnormalities of the hip (Perthes)

4. E

Legg-Calvé-Perthes' is an idiopathic AVN of the proximal femoral epiphysis. It is of unknown aetiology, although low birth weight, delayed bone age, low socioeconomic status and secondhand smoking have been implicated. The presentation can mimic other causes of AVN of the femoral head, e.g., sickle cell disease, infection, steroids and hypothyroidism. The incidence is approximately 1 in 12,000 and affects boys (4:1) predominantly between the ages of 4 and 8 years. Diagnosis is made using x-rays (AP and frog lateral) +/− further imaging (e.g., MRI), with the Herring lateral pillar classification (A = no loss of lateral pillar, B = <50% loss of lateral pillar, C = >50% loss of lateral pillar) commonly used. Treatment depends on the age of onset, timing of presentation and severity of disease. The prognosis is improved with a younger age of onset, as there is greater remodelling potential.

Abnormalities of the hip (SUFE)

5. C

SUFE is characterised by a 'stress fracture' through the physis of the proximal femur resulting in epiphyseal posterior-inferior displacement. The overall incidence is ~5/100,000 population. The peak age of onset is related to the onset of puberty (~10–14 years); hence, it is seen at an earlier age in girls. Boys are more frequently affected (3:1), with ~25% of cases bilateral, and

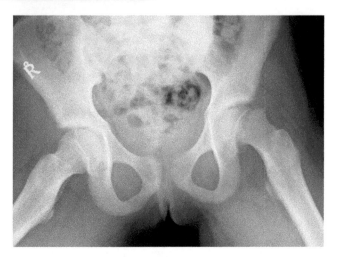

Figure 41.2   A SUFE of the left hip.

only one in four presenting concomitantly. Knee pain (along with a shortened and externally rotated leg) is a common presentation as Hilton's law states that the nerve supply to a joint is the same as the muscles acting over it. Risk factors include endocrine (growth or gonadal) disorders, e.g., hypothyroidism, renal failure, previous radiotherapy (local or pituitary), delayed puberty and obesity.

AP and frog leg lateral radiographs are essential in the diagnosis (**Figure 41.2**). Classification can be made according to the chronicity (acute, acute on chronic, chronic), the weight-bearing status with or without crutches (Loder – stable or unstable), or severity of the slip (<33% mild, 33%–66% moderate, >66% severe). For mild and moderate slips, pinning in situ is recommended. For severe slips, a femoral osteotomy might be required. Attempt is not routinely made to reduce the slip, as it is a major risk of damaging the blood supply to the femoral head leading to AVN. Therefore, in all but the most acute slips, the head is fixed in its slipped position using a single screw. As the contralateral hip is commonly involved, some surgeons will choose to pin this prophylactically before it has a chance to slip.

→ Abnormalities of the foot and ankle (clubfoot)

6. C

CTEV has a reported incidence of 1–6/1000 births, with higher incidences reported amongst certain races and the developing world. It is more frequently found in boys (2–3:1) and is bilateral in ~50% of cases. Most cases are idiopathic or might be postural. Other cases can be associated with neuromuscular (spina bifida, arthrogryposis) or syndromic (trisomy 15) disorders. The classical deformity is with the hindfoot in equinus and varus, with the forefoot in adduction and supination relative to the hindfoot. A variety of classification of scoring systems exist, with the Pirani scoring system used to determine prognosis according to the position of the foot (hind and midfoot contracture scores). The Ponseti method uses a series of manoeuvres, casting and then foot abduction orthoses to correct the deformity over time. It is a popular method with quoted success rates at 90%–95%.

Table 41.2 Classification of spondylolisthesis according to the slip severity

Grade	Description
1	<25%
2	25%–50%
3	51%–75%
4	75%–100%
5	>100% = spondyloptosis (complete translation)

Source: Adapted from Table 41.13 in: Williams, N., Bulstrode, C., O'Connell, PR. (Eds.), *Bailey & Love's Short Practice of Surgery,* 26th ed., 2013.

⟶ Spinal deformities and back pain

7. C
Spondylolisthesis is defined by the anterior translation of one upper vertebra over the one inferior to it. It is often seen as the final stage of a continuum that begins with a stress reaction within the pars interarticularis, a pars defect (spondylolysis) and then finally a spondylolisthesis. It is a common cause for lower back pain in the paediatric population and most frequently found at the L5/S1 level. A variety of classifications exist, with the six types most commonly described as follows:

1 Congenital (dysplastic)
2 Isthmic (pars weak/elongated/fractured)
3 Degenerative
4 Traumatic
5 Post-surgical
6 Pathological/neoplastic

The Myerding classifies spondylolisthesis according to the severity of the slip (**Table 41.2**). Management is determined by the severity of symptoms, in particular the presence of neurology, which is often associated with the severity of the slip.

Answers to extended matching questions

⟶ Abnormalities of the knee and leg

A. 5 Osteochondritis dissecans
Fragments of the femoral condyle can be lost in a condition called osteochondritis dissecans. These loose fragments can jam in the joint and cause locking.

B. 3 Discoid meniscus
A second possibility for a clunking, locking knee is the congenital abnormality of the lateral meniscus called discoid meniscus. In these cases, the cartilage is not a crescent but has a solid centre-like a disc. This meniscus is susceptible to tears and then causes locking in the knee.

C. 4 Osgood–Schlatter disease
A painful lump over the tibial tubercle in an adolescent is Osgood–Schlatter disease, an inflammation of the epiphysis under the tibial tubercle. It usually settles spontaneously.

D. 2 Chondromalacia patellae
Pain and possible maltracking of the patella is called chondromalacia patellae. It is most painful when going up and down stairs and after sitting still for a long period.

E. 1 Blount's disease

Varus bowing in a West Indian child might be caused by rickets. However, this case is more likely to be Blount's disease, which is an abnormality of growth of the proximal tibial epiphysis.

→ Abnormalities of the upper limb

A. 1 Camptodactyly

Camptodactyly is rare (prevalence <1%) and characterised by a fixed-flexion deformity that usually affects the proximal interphalangeal joint of the little finger. Splinting and physiotherapy are the primary treatment, with surgery reserved for progressive severe cases that cause functional disability.

B. 4 Radial club hand

Radial club hand or radial deficiency is defined as a longitudinal failure of formation of the radius. It is rare (incidence is less than 1 in 100,000) and bilateral in ~50%–70% of cases. It is associated with other developmental abnormalities, e.g., VACTERL syndrome (abnormal vertebrae, anal atresia, cardiovascular system, trachea, oesophagus atresia, tracheoesophageal fistula, renal agenesis, limb defects). The Bayne and Klug classification is used to classify it. Treatment is determined by the severity of the disease, e.g., presence of the thumb and clinical picture. Conservative measures include physiotherapy and stretching, while surgery involves hand centralisation +/– thumb reconstruction.

C. 2 Clinodactyly

Clinodactyly is characterised by a congenital curvature of the finger (middle phalanx of little finger often) in the radioulnar plane. It has an autosomal dominant inheritance and prevalence is increased in patients with Down syndrome. Most cases can be observed, with surgery (e.g., open wedging osteotomy) reserved for progressive severe cases that cause functional disability.

D. 5 Radioulnar synostosis

Congenital radioulnar synostosis is caused by failure of separation of the proximal radius and ulna. A genetic component has been noted. Patients often present at 3 to 5 years of age with a functional disability, as they are unable to supinate, and often to a lesser degree pronate, the forearm. X-rays of the affected elbow and forearm will confirm the diagnosis. Observation is routinely all that is required, with osteotomy and fusion reserved for severe cases that require a functional amount of pronation or supination.

E. 7 Trigger thumb

Congenital trigger thumb affects the interphalangeal joint of the thumb and is caused by restriction of the flexor pollicis longus tendon at the Al pulley. Patients under 1 year of age have a one in three chance of resolution, while patients over 1 year of age have less than a one in 10 chance of resolution. Treatment is with surgical release of the A1 flexor tendon pulley.

→ Spinal deformities and neuromuscular conditions

A. 7 Polio

Polio presents as a febrile illness that then goes on to permanently damage the anterior horn cells of the spinal cord, causing muscle weakness but no sensory changes. The motor signs are lower, not upper, and are not progressive.

B. 4 Idiopathic scoliosis

Idiopathic scoliosis is primarily a rotational curvature deformity of the spine, which develops in the rapidly growing spine. In this condition, the spine rotates more as the child bends forward, creating the characteristic rib hump. Scoliosis can be defined according to the age

Table 41.3   Classification of spondylolisthesis according to the slip severity

Type	Age of onset
Infantile	0–3 years
Juvenile	4–10 years
Adolescent	11–18 years
Adult	Onset at maturity

Source: Reproduced from Table 41.12 in: Williams, N., Bulstrode, C., O'Connell, PR. (Eds.), *Bailey & Love's Short Practice of Surgery,* 26th ed., 2013.

of onset **(Table 41.3)**. The Cobb angle is a radiographic measurement of deformity and aims to guide treatment (<20 degrees = observation; 25–40 degrees = bracing; >40 degrees = consider surgery).

C. 8 Scheuermann's disease

Scheuermann's kyphosis is a growth abnormality of the spine, which also develops during the adolescent growth spurt. Kyphosis exceeds the normal range of 20–50 degrees. It is characterised by ≥5 degrees of vertebral wedging at three adjacent levels with associated end-plate changes.

D. 11 Torticollis

A twisted neck is called torticollis and in this case, it is congenital and is caused by contracture and even a fibrous mass in the sternocleidomastoid muscle. It is associated with other congenital abnormalities, such as developmental dysplasia of the hip.

E. 1 Brachial plexus injury

A child with a flaccid arm after birth may have suffered injury to the brachial plexus. This is associated with a breech delivery.

Skin and subcutaneous tissue

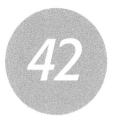

42 Skin and subcutaneous tissue

Stuart Enoch

Multiple choice questions

→ ### Anatomy

1. Which of the following statements are true regarding layers of the skin?

A The epidermis accounts for the major part of the skin.

B The lowermost layer of the epidermis contains the suprabasal keratinocytes.

C The *stratum granulosum* consists of keratohyalin granules.

D *Stratum lucidum* is present in glabrous skin of palms and soles.

E The *stratum corneum* is an effective barrier to most micro-organisms, chemicals and fluids.

2. Which of the following statements are true?

A The melanocytes originate from the neural crest.

B The skin colour of an individual is determined mainly by the number of melanocytes in the skin.

C Eccrine sweat glands secrete sweat in response to sympathetic activity.

D Apocrine sweat glands are found in the axilla and groin.

E Adnexal structures span the epidermis and dermis.

→ ### Ulcer edges

3. Which of the following descriptions of an ulcer edge denotes malignancy?

A Sloping.

B Overhanging.

C Everted.

D Punched out.

E Rolled.

→ ### Benign and pre-malignant skin conditions

4. Which of the following statements regarding Bowen's Disease are true?

A It can affect the mucous membranes.

B It usually presents as solitary lesions.

C It may be associated with pruritus.

D It is commonly associated with internal malignancies.

E It can be treated with topical corticosteroid agents.

5. Which of the following statements regarding actinic keratosis are true?

A It is a premalignant skin lesion.

B It is usually diffuse and blends with the adjacent normal skin

C It is more common in the Afro-Caribbean race.

D It can be treated using topical 5-fluorouracil cream.

E If excised surgically, it requires 8–10-mm excision margins.

6. Which of the following statements regarding keratoacanthoma are true?

A It is a form of rapidly growing solitary tumour.

B It has a predilection for sun-exposed areas.

C It is histologically similar to a squamous cell carcinoma.

D It might be associated with visceral malignant tumours.

E It might resolve spontaneously within about 4 to 6 months.

7. Which of the following statements regarding Marjolin's ulcer are true?

A It is a premalignant skin condition.

B It is an aggressive ulcerating SCC.

C It is an ischaemic ulcer in patients with chronic arterial insufficiency.

D It commonly occurs in poorly controlled diabetic patients.

E Osteomyelitis may predispose to the development of a Marjolin's ulcer.

→ Malignant melanoma

8. Which of the following are types of malignant melanoma?

A Superficial spreading

B Nodular

C Congenital melanocytic naevus

D Lentigo maligna

E Dysplastic naevus

9. Which of the following features indicate transformation of a mole into a malignant melanoma?

A Diameter >4 mms

B Ulcer with everted edges

C Colour variegation

D Itch

E Bleeding

10. Which of the following regarding malignant melanomas are true?

A Superficial spreading melanoma is the most common subtype.

B Nodular melanoma occurs in about 15%–30% of patients.

C Acral lentiginous melanoma accounts for the majority of melanomas in non-Caucasians.

D Clarke's level is more accurate and predicts the risk of metastatic disease more precisely than Breslow's thickness.

E Melanoma is most common in legs and trunk.

→ Basal and squamous cell carcinomas

11. Which of the following are true regarding basal cell carcinoma?

A Basal cell carcinoma is less common than squamous cell carcinoma.

B It is always an isolated, single, lesion.

C Pearly appearance is a recognised feature.

D The edges are usually everted.

E Fractionated radiotherapy is the first line of management.

12. Which of the following are true regarding squamous cell carcinoma?

A Excessive exposure to solar radiation is a recognised risk factor.

B The slow-growing variety of squamous cell carcinoma is usually exophytic in appearance.

C Small isolated skin ulcerations suspicious of a malignancy might be treated conservatively for 3 to 4 weeks.

D The recommended excision margin for squamous cell carcinomas is 8–10 mm.

E Once fully excised, further follow-up is not required.

→ Necrotising fasciitis

13. Which of the following statements regarding necrotising fasciitis are true?

A It is usually monomicrobial in majority of the cases.

B It always occurs in individuals with underlying immunological compromise.

C An absence of soft-tissue gas in plain x-ray safely rules out this condition.

D Pain is the most important initial feature.

E Surgery is reserved only if the condition doesn't improve with intravenous antibiotics for 5 days.

→ Neurofibroma

14. Which of the following statements are true regarding neurofibromas?

A They are solitary unencapsulated spindle cell tumours.

B Schwannomas are encapsulated by epineurium.

C von Recklinghausen's disease has an autosomal recessive inheritance.

D They never become malignant.

E Plexiform neurofibromata involve very small anatomical areas.

Extended matching questions

→ ## 1. Definitions

Diagnoses

1 Fistula
2 Sinus
3 Ulcer

Match the diagnoses with each of the following descriptions:

A An abnormal communication between two epithelial-lined surfaces. The communication or tract may be lined by granulation tissue, but in chronic cases it might be epithelialised.

B A blind-ending tract that connects a cavity lined with granulation tissue (usually an abscess) with an epithelial surface.

C A discontinuity of an epithelial surface.

→ ## 2. Infections

Diagnoses

1 Cellulitis/Lymphangitis
2 Erysipelas
3 Impetigo
4 Necrotising fasciitis
5 Purpura fulminans

Match the diagnoses with each of the following descriptions:

A A polymicrobial synergistic infection most often caused by group A beta-haemolytic *Streptococcus*.

B In this lesion there is intravascular thrombosis producing haemorrhagic skin infarction.

C This is a highly infectious skin lesion, usually affecting children, caused by *Staphylococcus* or *Streptococcus*.

D This is a generalised bacterial infection of the skin and subcutaneous tissue, usually preceded by trauma or ulceration.

E This produces a well-demarcated infection by streptococci, usually on the face.

→ ## 3. Benign skin tumours

Diagnoses

1 Basal cell papilloma
2 Compound naevus
3 Junctional naevus
4 Keratoacanthoma
5 Papillary wart

Match the diagnoses with each of the following descriptions:

A A maculopapular pigmented lesion that is most prominent at puberty. It is a junctional proliferation of naevus cells with nests and columns in the dermis.

B A deeply pigmented macular or papular lesion commonly seen in childhood. It is caused by a dermo-epidermal proliferation of naevus cells and progresses in the older person to form a compound or intradermal naevus. It has no malignant potential.

C A benign skin tumour caused by human papillomavirus (HPV), which also causes plantar warts and condylomata acuminata.

D A soft, warty lesion that is often pigmented and arises from the basal layer of the epidermal cells containing melanocytes. This is one of the most common benign skin lesions in the elderly.

E A lesion, usually found on the head, neck and face, shaped like a cup with the centre filled with a keratin plug. The lesion has a history in weeks. The aetiology is unclear but may be caused by infection of a hair follicle by a papilloma virus. Although it regresses spontaneously, it is better to excise it for a superior cosmetic outcome and also to differentiate it from squamous cell carcinoma.

4. Premalignant and malignant skin lesions

1 Basal cell carcinoma
2 Bowen's disease
3 Extramammary Paget's disease
4 Malignant melanoma (MM)
5 Squamous cell carcinoma (SCC)

Match the diagnoses with each of the following descriptions:

A This is a slow-growing, locally invasive tumour (hence also called a rodent ulcer, as it behaves like a rodent burrowing into neighbouring tissue) of a few years' duration. The edges are typically raised and rolled and occur more often on the face, head and neck.

B This occurs in the genital or perianal regions or in skin rich in apocrine glands, such as the axilla. It is a form of intraepidermal adenocarcinoma.

C This is an ulcerated skin lesion of a few months' duration, with a raised, everted edge and an indurated inflamed surrounding area. A minority might have enlarged regional lymphadenopathy from metastasis.

D There is a pigmented skin lesion on the scalp that has recently changed in colour and become itchy and started to bleed. There are a few small black spots irregularly scattered around the lesion.

E There is a slowly enlarging erythematous scaly patch on the dorsum of the right hand of an elderly male.

5. Melanoma
Diagnoses

1 Amelanotic melanoma
2 Lentigo maligna melanoma
3 Nodular melanoma

Match the diagnoses with each of the following descriptions:

A A 68-year-old woman presents to the surgical clinic with a fleshy lump over the sole of her right foot that is rapidly increasing in size. It does not appear pigmented and there are palpable lymph nodes in her groin.

B A 39-year-old woman presents to the outpatient clinic with a 4-month history of a raised, nodular, and dark pigmented lesion over her right knee. It is itchy and bleeds occasionally.

C A 72-year-old farmer presents to the outpatient clinic with a 12- to 15-year history of a brown lesion over his right cheek. He states that it has recently got bigger. On examination, the lesion is irregular in shape and measures about 8 x 10 mm; there is a darker patch within the lesion.

Answers to multiple choice questions

→ Anatomy

1. B, C, D, E
The epidermis accounts for only 5% of the total skin, while the dermis accounts for the remaining 95%. The epidermis is composed of keratinised, stratified, squamous epithelium. The dermis consists of a superficial papillary layer and a deeper reticular layer.

The epidermis of the skin is composed of stratified squamous epithelium with several distinct layers. The lowermost layer is the *stratum basale or stratum germinativum*, which contains the suprabasal keratinocytes. The next layer of cells immediately above the basal layer is the *stratum spinosum*. Above this layer is the *stratum granulosum* (granular layer), which consists of one to three layers of flattened cells containing keratohyalin granules.

Stratum lucidum is a clear layer that is present in glabrous skin of palms and soles. The outermost layer of the epidermis is called the *stratum corneum*, which is composed of multiple layers of polyhedral cells. These cells are anucleated and keratin-rich, forming the tough outer protective layer of the skin. This layer is an effective barrier to most micro-organisms, chemicals and fluids, although it is permeable to some substances (hence, topical treatments). Keratinocytes are the principal cell type within the epidermis. The basal epidermis also contains melanocytes.

2. A, C, D, E
Melanocytes originate from the neural crest and are found in the basal epidermis. Each melanocyte synthesises the pigment melanin, which protects the cell nuclei from ultraviolet radiation. The keratinocytes in the strata granulosum and spinosum contain melanin. Differences in skin colour are determined by variations in the amount and distribution of melanin within the keratinocytes (not by the number of melanocytes).

The sweat glands, eccrine and apocrine, open into pores in the hair follicles. Eccrine glands are present throughout the entire body surface, except for the lips. They secrete sweat in response to sympathetic activity such as emotion and are responsible for thermoregulation. In hyperhidrosis, where there is excessive sweating (commonly seen in the palms, axilla and lower limbs), the condition can be cured by performing a sympathectomy. Apocrine glands are found in the axillary and groin areas and become active at puberty. Persistent infection of these glands causes hydradenitis suppurativa.

Adnexal structures, such as hair follicles and sebaceous and sweat glands, span the epidermis and dermis. In injuries where the epidermis is lost, re-epithelialisation occurs from these structures.

→ Ulcer edges

3. C, E
The edges of an ulcer provide a good indication of the type of ulcer. 'Sloping edges' are classically seen with healing ulcers and such ulcers are usually shallow. Ulcers of venous origin that are progressing toward healing usually have sloping edges. 'Punched-out' is a feature of arterial or neuropathic ulcers. Ulcers where the subcutaneous tissue is affected more than the skin will have 'undermined' edges, as in tuberculosis, pyoderma gangrenosum and some forms of pressure ulcers. 'Rolled-out' edges (due to deep central crater) are classically seen

Edges or margins of ulcers

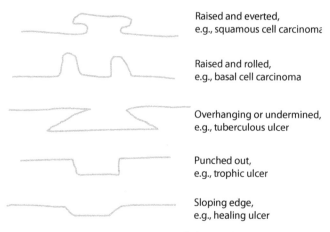

Raised and everted,
e.g., squamous cell carcinoma

Raised and rolled,
e.g., basal cell carcinoma

Overhanging or undermined,
e.g., tuberculous ulcer

Punched out,
e.g., trophic ulcer

Sloping edge,
e.g., healing ulcer

Figure 42.1 Types of ulcer edges.

in basal cell carcinomas, whilst 'everted' edges (due to edge of the ulcer growing rapidly and spilling out of the edges) are a feature of squamous cell carcinomas. **(Figure 42.1)**

Benign and premalignant skin conditions

4. A, B, C
Bowen's disease represents an intra-epithelial squamous cell carcinoma (carcinoma in situ). It can involve the skin or mucous membranes in the mouth, anus, or genitalia. Bowen's disease usually appears as a solitary, erythematous, scaly plaque. It is associated with pruritus, superficial crusting and discharge. There is only about 7% increased incidence of internal malignancies such as cancers of the bladder, bronchus, breast and oesophagus. The common modalities of treatment include surgical excision or a combination of curettage and electrodessication. Adequate excision is essential, as these lesions may subsequently become invasive squamous cell carcinomas and metastasize. Topical therapy such as 5-fluorouracil might be effective if multiple lesions are present.

5. A, D
Actinic keratosis, also known as solar keratosis, is the most common premalignant lesion. This can progress to an invasive malignancy, and the resulting cancer is mostly a squamous cell carcinoma. The lesions are discrete, well circumscribed, erythematous and maculopapular It is usually seen in older, light-complexioned individuals. They are rare in individuals with dark skin. Actinic keratosis lesions appear primarily on sun-damaged or exposed skin and are frequently multiple. Curettage, electrodessication, cryotherapy with liquid nitrogen and topical 5-fluorouracil are accepted forms of treatment. Squamous cell carcinomas that arise from actinic keratoses rarely metastasize, suggesting that surgical resection should be conservative with narrow margins (about 2 mm margin will suffice).

6. A, B, C, D, E
Keratoacanthoma **(Figure 42.2)**, described by Hutchinson in 1889, is usually a rapidly growing solitary tumour with a predilection for sun-exposed areas. It usually grows rapidly over 4 to 8 weeks and can spontaneously involute, usually within 4 to 6 months. It is histologically similar to SCC (hence the term 'self-healing epitheliomas'). Patients with multiple keratoacanthomas or with sebaceous differentiation should be evaluated for Muir-Torre syndrome, which is associated with visceral malignant tumours.

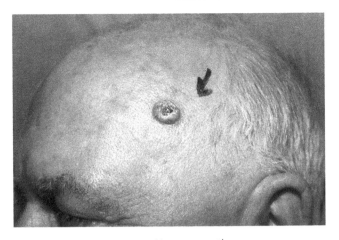

Figure 42.2 Keratoacanthoma.

7. B, E
Jean Marjolin (1828) first described an indolent ulcer arising in a burn scar. However, this term currently encompasses SCCs arising from any form of long-standing chronic ulcers or scars. Other chronic conditions such as sinuses and chronic lymphoedema can give rise to Marjolin's ulcer. Osteomyelitis also predisposes to the development of a Marjolin's ulcer.

Malignant melanoma

8. A, B, D
There are various types of melanomas, notably superficial spreading melanoma, nodular melanoma, lentigo maligna, acral lentiginous melanoma and amelanotic melanoma. Superficial spreading melanoma, nodular melanoma, and lentigo maligna melanomas constitute about 90% of all malignant melanomas. Acral lentiginous melanoma and other types together make up the remaining 10%. The congenital melanocytic nevus, a type of melanocytic nevus found in infants at birth, has a 1% incidence worldwide. They are usually circumscribed, light-brown to black-patch or plaque. It is not a type of melanoma, although the giant congenital melanocytic naevus variety has a higher risk for malignant degeneration into a melanoma. For this reason, it is acceptable to excise large congenital naevi electively. Dysplastic naevi are unusual benign moles that may resemble a melanoma. Individuals with a number of such naevi (about 10 or more) are at an increased risk of developing a melanoma. It can thus be considered as a premalignant condition (not a melanoma) that warrants regular examination and follow-up. If in doubt, an excision biopsy is warranted.

9. C, D, E
The following features (**A, B, C, D, E**) indicate a malignant transformation of a mole into a melanoma: **A**symmetry; **B**leeding; **C**olour variegation; **D**iameter expanding or greater than 6 mm; **E**levation (nodular); halo; irregular borders and itching; ulceration; and satellite lesions. Ulcer with everted edges is a feature of squamous cell carcinoma.

10. A, B, C, E
Superficial spreading melanoma is the most common subtype, accounting for about 70% of all cases. Nodular melanoma, the second most common subtype, occurs in 15%–30% of patients. As with superficial spreading melanomas, legs and trunk are the most frequent sites of occurrence. Acral lentiginous melanomas are the least common subtype, representing 2%–8% of melanoma in Caucasians, although they do account for about 50%–90% of melanoma in non-Caucasians. It typically occurs on the palms or soles, or beneath the

nail plate (subungual variant). Breslow's method is more accurate than the Clarke's level and predicts the risk of metastatic disease more precisely. Breslow thickness avoids the confounding effect of the variable thickness of the reticular dermis.

Basal and squamous cell carcinomas

11. C

Basal cell carcinoma (BCC) is the most common cutaneous malignancy in humans. It may be single or multiple and commonly occurs in sun-exposed areas of the elderly. The pearly appearance is a well-recognised feature of BCC, and it is more apparent on lightly stretched skin. It may be covered with surface telangiectasia. As the tumour enlarges central ulceration occurs, resulting in the characteristic rolled-out edge. Surgical excision is the most appropriate treatment for BCC. Other recognised treatment modalities include surgical excision, fractionated radiotherapy, Mohs micrographic surgery, cryosurgery, electrodessication and curettage and topical chemotherapy with 5-flurouracil.

12. A, B, C, D

Squamous cell carcinoma, seen primarily in older patients, originates from the keratinizing or Malpighian cell layer of the epithelium. The prime etiologic factor is excessive exposure to solar radiation. In addition, chemicals, cytotoxic drugs, immunosuppressant drug treatment and chronic ulcers (e.g., Marjolin's ulcer) play a role in its development. There are two main types of SCC: (i) a slow-growing variety that is verrucous in nature and exophytic in appearance. This is locally invasive, penetrating deeper structures, and is more likely to metastasize; and (ii) a nodular and indurated type, with rapid growth and early ulceration combined with local invasiveness. Metastasis is late compared to the verrucous type. Small isolated skin ulcerations suspicious of a malignancy might be treated conservatively with a topical chemotherapeutic agent such as 5-flurouracil for 3 to 4 weeks. Any lesion that has not healed after this period must be considered as a skin cancer until proved otherwise. As a rule of thumb, an excision margin of 8–10 mm will suffice for most squamous cell carcinomas. Even if the lesion is completely excised, there is a chance for recurrence and thus patients require 3- to 4-monthly follow-up for a minimum of 2 years. The precise frequency and duration of follow-up depends on the age of the patient, site/size/type of lesion and presence or absence of metastasis.

Necrotising fasciitis

13. B, D

This condition is a polymicrobial synergistic infection in the majority of the cases caused by a variety of organisms such as coliforms, staphylococci, anaerobic streptococci and *Bacteroides* species. It occurs in patients who are immunocompromised, such as those with uncontrolled diabetes, on chemotherapy, or who have chronic renal failure or are malnourished. However, it can also occur in previous fit and healthy individuals. A plain x-ray or CT scan might show gas in the soft or subcutaneous tissue, but there are many false negatives such that absence of gas does not rule out the condition.

The typical clinical feature is pain in the wound out of proportion with the original surgical insult, spreading inflammation with subcutaneous crepitus and a malodorous discharge. When it occurs in the abdomen it is called Meleney's synergistic hospital gangrene and when the scrotum is involved it is known as Fournier's gangrene. Treatment should be prompt and aggressive in the form of broad-spectrum antibiotics, full circulatory support along with extensive excision and debridement of all dead tissue; this procedure may have to be repeated. Once the patient has recovered, the patient may need reconstructive surgery to cover the defect. Untreated or inadequately treated, the patient may succumb to multi-system organ failure.

→ Neurofibroma

14. A, B
Neurofibromas are solitary unencapsulated spindle cell tumours arising from the neural sheath. Schwannomas or neurilemomas are distinct nerve sheath tumours that are encapsulated by epineurium. Multiple neurofibromatosis occurring in von Recklinghausen's disease have an autosomal dominant inheritance pattern with variable penetrance. They carry a risk of malignant transformation. Plexiform neurofibromata might involve large anatomical areas and can cause gross deformity of the underlying skeleton, in particular of the craniofacial region.

Answers to extended matching questions

→ 1. Definitions

1. A Fistula
A fistula is an abnormal communication lined by granulation tissue between two epithelial-lined surfaces. These may be congenital, as in tracheo-oesophageal or rectourethral fistulae, or acquired, as in enterocolic, colovesical, enteroenteric fistulae.

2. B Sinus
A sinus is a blind tract connecting a cavity with an epithelial surface. The cavity is usually an abscess. It might be classified as congenital, as in a remnant of a thyroglossal tract that becomes a cyst that gets infected and bursts, which, although called a 'fistula', is strictly a sinus. Acquired causes are a retained foreign body, specific chronic infection, inflammation and malignancy.

3. C Ulcer
An ulcer is a discontinuity of an epithelial surface characterised by gradual destruction with a base that may be necrotic, granulating, or malignant. These can be classified as specific, nonspecific and malignant.

→ 2. Infections

1. D Cellulitis/Lymphangitis
Cellulitis/lymphangitis is a generalised bacterial infection of the skin and subcutaneous tissue associated with trauma or ulceration. The patient has fever with a red, swollen, tender area with overlying reddish streaks of lymphangitis; *Streptococcus* is the commonest causative organism. Treatment is the prompt administration of appropriate intravenous antibiotics with rest and elevation to the affected part.

2. E Erysipelas
Erysipelas is a well-localised streptococcal infection of the superficial lymphatics, usually associated with trauma to the skin of the face. The area is red and oedematous, and the patient has fever with leucocytosis. The appropriate broad-spectrum antibiotic is the treatment of choice.

3. C Impetigo
Impetigo is a very infectious superficial skin lesion, usually affecting children. The infection produces blisters that rupture and join up and is covered by honey-coloured crust. Treatment is washing of the area and application of topical or broad-spectrum oral antibiotics.

4. A Necrotising fasciitis

Necrotising fasciitis used to be called synergistic gangrene. It results from polymicrobial infection, most commonly group A beta-haemolytic *Streptococcus* along with *E. coli*, *Pseudomonas*, *Proteus*, *Bacteroides*, or *Clostridium*. The majority occur following trauma or infection, particularly in a smoker or diabetic. The typical signs are oedema beyond the skin erythema, woody-hard induration of the subcutaneous tissue, inability to distinguish between fascial planes and muscle groups, soft-tissue crepitus and severe pain. This must be treated very promptly with resuscitation, antibiotics and surgical debridement; otherwise the patient may go into septic shock.

5. B Purpura fulminans

Purpura fulminans is a rare condition, usually occurring in children, where intravascular thrombosis produces haemorrhagic skin infarction. It can rapidly progress to septic shock. There are three types, and they are acute infectious purpura fulminans caused by both acute bacterial or viral infection and which may result in extensive tissue loss requiring limb amputation; neonatal purpura fulminans; and idiopathic purpura fulminans.

3. Benign skin tumours

1. D Basal cell papilloma

Basal cell papillomas (also called seborrhoeic keratoses or senile warts) are benign lesions found in the elderly as part of the ageing process. Some individuals have an inherited tendency (in an autosomal dominant pattern) to develop a large number of these lesions. It is not generally caused by exposure to the sun, although they can follow sunburn or dermatitis. It looks as flat-topped or warty-looking lesions, with a 'stuck on' appearance to the skin and having a well-circumscribed border. They are usually deeply pigmented although some may be paler in colour.

2. A Compound naevus

Compound nevus is a mixture of junctional and intradermal proliferation. They usually arise from a flat (junctional) naevus that exists earlier in life and might have a raised central portion of deeper pigmentation with surrounding tan-brown macular pigmentation. They are usually of a round or oval shape and roughly 2–7 mm in diameter. Compound naevi are considered to be benign neoplasms of melanocytes if they arise in later life. Their name is derived from the fact that they contain junctional melanocytes (responsible for their pigmentation) and intradermal melanocytes (responsible for the elevation of the lesion).

3. B Junctional naevus

Junctional naevus is a form of melanocytic naevus (or mole) where the accumulation of melanocytes is located predominantly at the dermo-epidermal junction. They are often quite darkly pigmented, macular, or very thinly popular and with minimal elevation above the level of the skin. They are most often uniform in colour and range <7 mm or so in diameter. With advancing age, they may progress to form a compound or intradermal naevus.

4. E Keratoacanthoma

Keratoacanthoma is a common low-grade skin tumour (in situ tumour) originating from the neck of a hair follicle. However, some pathologists label keratoacanthoma as a 'well-differentiated squamous cell carcinoma, keratoacanthoma variant', because about 5%–6% of keratoacanthoma might manifest itself as squamous cell carcinoma if left untreated. It is commonly found on sun-exposed skin, and often is seen on the face, forearms and hands. The defining characteristic of a keratoacanthoma is its dome-shaped and symmetrical appearance, surrounded by a smooth wall of inflamed skin capped with keratin scales. It has a characteristic growth pattern: A period of rapid growth for 8 to 12 weeks, then a plateau phase for a few months, followed by regression over the next 12 to 16 weeks. If in doubt (i.e., if a distinction cannot be clinically made between a keratoacanthoma and an SCC), then a diagnostic or excision biopsy is indicated.

5. C Papillary wart
A papillary wart (benign papillomatous tumour), derived from the epithelium, appears as white or normal skin coloured cauliflower-like projection (pedunculated or sessile appearance). These benign proliferations in the skin and mucosa are usually caused by infection with human papilloma virus. It is particularly common in childhood but may arise at any age. They are spread by direct contact or autoinoculation with a latency of weeks to years.

4. Premalignant and malignant skin lesions

1. A Basal cell carcinoma
The duration of this slow-growing lesion (rodent ulcer) is usually in years and caused by exposure to ultraviolet light. It most often occurs on the head, neck and face **(Figure 42.3)**. It has a raised, rolled edge, which might look like a pearl. Although there are several clinical types, by far the most common is the nodular and nodulocystic type, which is localised. The generalised types are superficial spreading, multifocal, or infiltrative, sometimes called geographical type. Surgical excision and primary closure, if possible, or skin grafting or use of rotational flaps by a plastic surgeon comprises the optimum treatment. Although the condition is radiosensitive, this form of treatment is rarely used because the location of the tumour precludes the use of radiotherapy to prevent damage to neighbouring vital structures, such as the lens and cartilages of the ear or nose.

2. E Bowen's disease
This is a squamous carcinoma in situ first described in 1912 by John Templeton Bowen, professor of dermatology at Harvard University. It is elevated from the skin surface, red and scaly and spreads locally **(Figure 42.4)**. A minority of these lesions may progress to SCC. Chronic exposure to sun, HPV 16 and inorganic arsenic compounds have been thought to be possible causes. When the condition occurs on the glans penis, it is called Queyrat's erythroplasia (Parisian dermatologist Auguste Queyrat described the condition in 1911, although Paget described the same disease 50 years earlier). Treatment is by topical application of 5-fluorouracil or surgical excision.

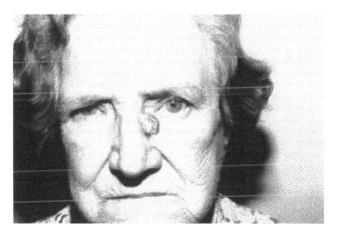

Figure 42.3   Basal cell carcinoma.

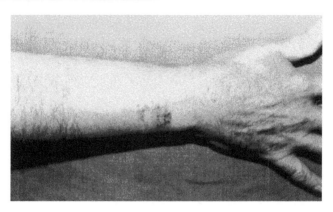

Figure 42.4   Bowen's disease.

3. B Extramammary Paget's disease

This is an intraepidermal adenocarcinoma occurring in the genital or perianal regions or axilla (extramammary Paget's disease: Sir James Paget 1814–1899, surgeon, St Bartholomew's Hospital, London). About one-quarter of them are associated with an underlying invasive neoplasm. Surgical excision is the treatment.

4. D Malignant melanoma

This is a malignant melanoma (MM) with satellite nodules **(Figure 42.5)**. It is a malignant tumour arising from the melanocytes. Therefore it can arise from any organ where melanocytes are present, such as the choroid of the eye, leptomeninges and bowel mucosa. Although it accounts for less than 5% of skin malignancy, it is responsible for more than 75% of deaths caused by skin malignancy. MM accounts for 3% of all malignancies worldwide and is the most common cancer in 20- to 39-year-olds.

Exposure to ultraviolet rays is the major cause whilst the risk factors are enhanced in xeroderma pigmentosum, family history, previous melanoma, large number of naevi, dysplastic naevi, red hair, giant congenital pigmented naevus and immunocompromised

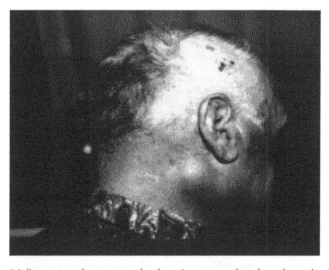

Figure 42.5   Malignant melanoma scalp showing secondary lymph nodes in the neck.

patients. The various types are superficial spreading (70%), nodular (15%), lentigo maligna melanoma (5%–10%) and acral lentiginous melanoma (2%–8%). The presenting features in a naevus suggesting MM are change in shape, size, colour, surface, itchiness and serosanguinous discharge. MM also occurs underneath the nail bed; these are usually a superficial spreading type and confirmation is by biopsy of the nail matrix. Amelanotic melanoma usually occurs in the gastrointestinal tract.

In a suspected MM regional lymph node metastasis should be sought, besides evidence of distant spread. Confirmation is done by excision biopsy with a 2-mm margin of skin and subdermal fat. Histology is reported according to the Breslow thickness (Alexander Breslow, 1928–1980, American pathologist). This is a guide to further definitive treatment and indicates prognosis. Radical regional lymph node dissection is done when there is metastasis.

Clinically, impalpable lymph nodes might have microscopic metastasis, particularly in those where the Breslow thickness is more than 1 mm. Therefore, in such patients, sentinel lymph node biopsy (SLNB) should be offered and in node-positive patients block dissection is carried out. Of those with SLNB-positive disease, 70%–80% will have no other involved regional nodes. In those with clinically involved nodes, 70%–85% will have occult distant metastases, such as in the lung or liver.

5. C Squamous cell carcinoma

Squamous cell carcinoma (SCC), the second most common form of skin cancer, arises from the keratinising cells of the epidermis or its appendages and usually affects the elderly **(Figure 42.6)**. The usual causes are prolonged exposure to sun, chronic inflammation, scars or burns and immunosuppression. The duration is usually in months. The lesion is an ulcer with a raised everted edge with the surrounding area red and indurated. Regional lymphadenopathy is more often due to infection as only 2% metastasise.

The histology of the excised lesion should include the pathological pattern, cellular morphology, Broders' grade (Albert Compton Broders, 1885–1964, American pathologist), depth of invasion, presence of any perineural or vascular invasion and vertical and circumferential excision margin clearance. Depending upon the size and the location, the surgical management should be a multidisciplinary team effort between the plastic surgeon, radiation oncologist and pathologist.

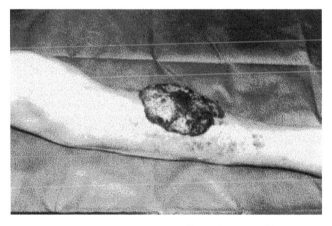

Figure 42.6 Squamous cell carcinoma of leg.

→ ## 5. Melanoma

1. A Amelanotic melanoma

Amelanotic melanoma is a variant of melanoma in which the cells do not make melanin. Classically, the lesions are pink or red appearing as erythematous papules or nodules. Patients frequently present with advanced disease and lymph node involvement.

2. B Nodular melanoma

Nodular melanomas form the second most common subtype of all melanomas. They might occur over any part of the body but are more common over the legs and trunk. They are raised and dark pigmented, and they bleed or ulcerate. Histologically, the cells are predominantly in the vertical growth phase. Lymphatic involvement occurs early.

3. C Lentigo maligna

Lentigo maligna melanoma (Hutchinson's melanotic freckle) commonly arises over the sun-damaged skin of the face. It is the least malignant variety and presents as an irregular brown patch. The precursor in situ lesion, lentigo maligna, is usually present for many years before progressing to malignancy. Malignant degeneration is characterised by thickening and the development of a discrete tumour nodule within the lesion.

43 Elective neurosurgery

Harry Bulstrode

Multiple choice questions

→ Hydrocephalus – anatomy and physiology

1. **Select the correct statement from the following list. CSF is produced in adults:**

A at a rate of ~20 mL/hour by the choroid plexus.

B at a rate of ~20 mL/hour by the arachnoid villi.

C at a rate of ~150 mL/hour from the walls of the ventricle.

D at a rate of ~150 mL/hour by the arachnoid villi.

E at a rate of ~150 mL/hour by the choroid plexus.

2. **Select the correct statement from the following list. In the normal human brain, CSF flows:**

A from the lateral ventricles through the foramen of Monro to the third ventricle, then through the cerebral aqueduct to the fourth ventricle.

B from the lateral ventricles via the foramina of Magendie and Luschka to the third ventricle, then through the cerebral aqueduct to the fourth ventricle.

C from the subarachnoid space via the cerebral aqueduct to the lateral ventricles, and then via the foramen of Monro to the third ventricle.

D from the lateral ventricles through the foramen of Monro to the third ventricle, then via the interpeduncular cistern to the subarachnoid space.

E from the third ventricle to the fourth ventricle via the foramen of Monro, then to the subarachnoid space through the foramina of Magendie and Luschka.

→ Neuro-oncology

3. **Which of the following disorders is not associated with increased incidence of primary brain tumour?**

A Neurofibromatosis Type I (NFI mutation).

B Li-Fraumeni syndrome (p53 mutation).

C Multiple endocrine neoplasia Type II.

D Cowden's disease (PTEN mutation).

E Hereditary non-polyposis colon cancer.

→ Complications of neurosurgery

4. **Which of the following is a commonly encountered complication of cranial neurosurgery?**

A Cryptococcal brain abscess

B *N. meningitides* meningitis

C *H. influenzae* meningitis

D Tuberculous abscess

E Staphylococcal subdural empyema

5. **Which of the following conditions is generally managed by operative neurosurgery at diagnosis?**

A Pituitary prolactinoma

B Multiple cerebral metastases

C Trigeminal neuralgia

D Myelomeningocoele

E Arachnoid cyst

Extended matching questions

1. **Match to the clinical descriptions the following problems arising in patients with ventriculoperitoneal shunts in situ:**

1 Acute shunt blockage
2 Low pressure headache
3 Pathology unrelated to the shunt
4 Shunt infection
5 Subdural haematoma

→ Presentations

A Recurrent unilateral headache heralded by a localised flickering visual disturbance and associated with nausea and photophobia.
B Progression over hours of headache, worse on coughing or lying down, then vomiting and lethargy. No evidence of papilloedema.
C Persistent headache since shunt insertion, worse on standing.
D Worsening headaches since alteration of programmable shunt setttings 3 weeks previously. Progressive right arm and leg weakness.
E Fever, headache and vomiting, with neck stiffness and photophobia on examination.

2. **Match the following presentations with a likely clinical diagnosis from the list:**

1 Bacterial meningitis
2 Brain abscess
3 Brain tumour
4 Intracerebral haemorrhage
5 Subarachnoid haemorrhage

→ Presentations

A 30-year-old female – sudden onset severe headache during intercourse. Fever and meningism on examination.
B 25-year-old male – chronic otitis media; progressive headache and malaise, then confusion and right arm weakness.
C 55-year-old male – sudden onset headache with right arm and leg weakness, then deteriorating consciousness level.
D 65-year-old male – headaches worse in the morning for some weeks, presents with right arm weakness.
E 18-year-old male – progressive headache with fever, meningism and reduced consciousness level.

3. **The following conditions are causes of disordered of CSF flow:**

1 Communicating hydrocephalus
2 Hydrocephalus ex vacuo
3 Idiopathic intracranial hypertension
4 Normal pressure hydrocephalus
5 Obstructive hydrocephalus

→ Presentations

A An obese young woman complains of headache and blurred vision, with florid papilloedema evident on examination. Head imaging is unremarkable.
B During treatment for bacterial meningitis, an infant is noted to have a rapidly enlarging head circumference and bulging fontanelle.

C A 78-year old gentleman, presenting with progressive cognitive decline and reduced mobility, has large ventricles on CT. CSF drainage results in no improvement in his walking.

D A 75-year old gentleman has early dementia with associated incontinence. Lumbar infusion testing demonstrates reduced brain compliance, and his gait is markedly improved 24 hours after CSF drainage.

E A patient presents obtunded with a short history of headache, vomiting and blurred vision. CT demonstrates a large pineal region tumour.

4. **Match the clinical scenarios that follow to the most likely underlying brain tumour pathology:**

1 Frontal meningioma
2 Medulloblastoma
3 Parietal lobe metastasis
4 Pituitary adenoma
5 Temporal lobe low-grade glioma

➡ Presentations

A A 30-year-old man with no medical history presents with two episodes of focal seizure.

B An 8-year-old boy presents with some weeks of poor balance and clumsiness, followed by acute deterioration with headache, vomiting and drowsiness.

C A 40-year-old woman presents with sudden severe headache and blurred vision, and has a right VIth nerve palsy on examination.

D A 50-year-old woman is admitted after suffering a minor road-traffic accident. She is found to have a right-sided inattention.

E A 60-year-old man lives alone and has become increasingly reclusive over several years. He is unsteady on his feet and expresses paranoid ideation.

Answers to multiple choice questions

1. A
CSF is produced in adults at a rate of ~20 mL/hour by the choroid plexus, so that the total CSF volume of 150 mL is replaced three times per day.

2. A
CSF is generated in the choroid plexus, and flows from the lateral ventricles through the foramen of Monro to the third ventricle, then through the cerebral aqueduct to the fourth ventricle. It exits the ventricular system to the subarachnoid space through the midline foramen of Magendie and paired lateral foramina of Luschka (**Figure 43.1**).

3. C
MEN Type II. The mutations listed each affect a tumor suppressor gene. Somatic mutations in P53, PTEN and NF1 are frequent in gliomas in general, and syndromes involving germline mutation in these genes predispose to these and other tumours. HNPCC is associated with a number of distinct gene mutations affecting DNA mismatch repair, and collectively these mutations also confer increased risk of glioma. Certain menin gene mutations confer risk of risk of pituitary adenoma (MEN Type I- pituitary, parathyroid, pancreas). MEN Type II is associated with medullary thyroid cancer, phaeochromocytoma and parathyroid tumours.

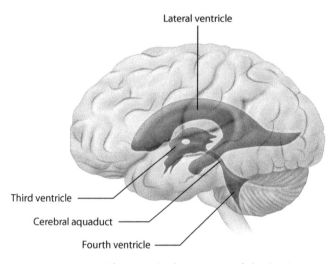

Figure 43.1 The ventricular system of the brain.

4. E

Fluid in the subdural space is a typical finding after craniotomy. Infection by the spectrum of organisms implicated in postsurgical meningitis, including *Staphylococcus aureus*, Enterobacteriaceae, Pseudomonas and Pneumococci, is a recognized complication, and these organisms are also typical in postsurgical abscess. *N. meningitides* and *H. influenzae* are found in spontaneous bacterial meningitis, and cryptococcal and tuberculous abscesses are the result of haematogenous spread.

5. D

Myelomeningocoele is a neural tube defect comprising herniating meninges, often containing neural elements. There is a high risk of meningitis, especially if the sac has ruptured, and early surgery is preferred to close the defect prior to surface bacterial colonization.

Prolactinomas **(Figure 43.2a)** are typically managed medically using dopamine antagonists, except in cases of rapid visual deterioration. Surgical resection of metastases is generally limited to solitary lesions in patients with well-controlled systemic disease and good functional status.

Trigeminal neuralgia is managed pharmacologically in the first instance; surgical microvascular decompression is the gold standard for treatment of refractory primary neuralgia.

Arachnoid cysts **(Figure 43.2b)** are usually an incidental finding, so that often follow-up imaging only to exclude enlargement is required.

Answers to extended matching questions

➡ ## Scenario 1

1. B Acute shunt blockage

Headache, nausea and lethargy point to raised intracranial pressure. Papilloedema is slow to develop and might be altogether absent in acute shunt blockage. Shunt infection or the combination of infection and blockage should also be considered.

2. C Low pressure headache

Shunt overdrainage accounts for significant morbidity, with postural headaches reflecting the siphon effect of the distal peritoneal shunt catheter when the patient is standing. ICP monitoring might be useful to confirm a correlation between low pressure and headache.

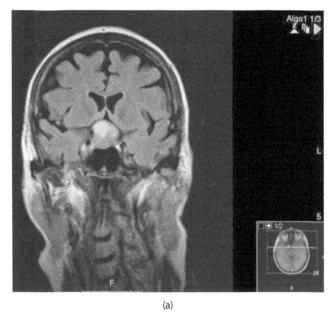

(a)

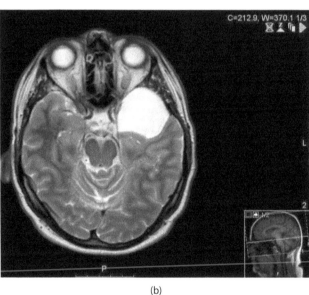

(b)

Figure 43.2   (a) Coronal T2 FLAIR MRI demonstrates a pituitary lesion character-istic of macroadenoma. (b) T2 MRI demonstrates a CSF-density collection at the left temporal pole, an arachnoid cyst.

3. A Pathology unrelated to the shunt
Headaches are common, irrespective of the presence of a VP shunt; in this case, the unilateral pain and aura are suggestive of migraine.

4. E Shunt infection
Fever and meningism imply shunt infection unless the CSF provides evidence to the contrary.

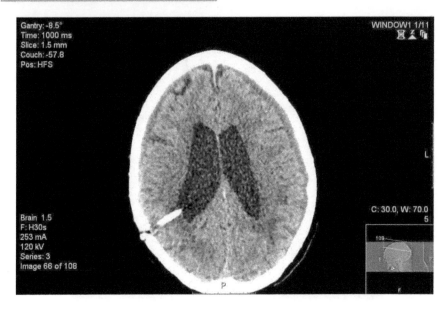

Figure 43.3 CT demonstrates a shunt tip entering the right lateral ventricle. There are low-density collections (representing chronic subdural haematoma) overlying both hemispheres. This is likely to represent a complication of shunt overdrainage.

5. D Subdural haematoma
Subdural haematoma is a potential complication of shunt overdrainage especially in the elderly **(Figure 43.3)**.

⇨ Scenario 2

1. E Bacterial meningitis
This is a typical presentation for a spontaneous bacterial meningitis, typically caused by *S. pneumonia, H. influenzae,* or *N. meningitides.*

2. B Brain abscess
Brain abscess can present with fever, focal neurological deficit and raised ICP. This presentation should prompt urgent investigation **(Figure 43.4)**. Local spread from an infected middle ear is common.

3. D Brain tumour
Focal neurological deficit, seizure and raised ICP are the classic triad of presenting features. Headache is not typically the main complaint at presentation.

4. C Intracerebral haemorrhage
ICH typically presents with progressive focal deficit as the accumulating blood dissects and impinges on eloquent tissue. Larger volume bleeds can then lead to raised ICP as compensation is exhausted.

5. A Subarachnoid haemorrhage
Thunderclap headache with an onset that can be pinpointed in time is classical for subarachnoid haemorrhage. Ongoing fever and meningism stemming from meningeal irritation by blood are very compatible with this diagnosis.

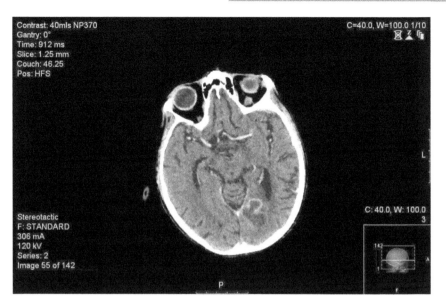

Figure 43.4   Post-contrast CT demonstrating a left occipital brain abscess (tumour is also a differential for this CT appearance).

Scenario 3

1. B Communicating hydrocephalus
Acute bacterial meningitis causes accumulation of protein and cellular debris in the CSF, and this can compromise reabsorption at the arachnoid villi. Obstruction of CSF flow by accumulation of these constituents is also seen occasionally.

2. C Hydrocephalus ex vacuo
Ventriculomegaly in the context of cognitive decline is most commonly secondary to brain atrophy, 'hydrocephalus ex vacuo.' Lumbar infusion and lumbar drainage testing can be helpful where there is clinical doubt. Failure to improve after CSF drainage makes normal pressure hydrocephalus (NPH) unlikely.

3. A Idiopathic intracranial hypertension
Progressive headache and visual disturbance over months in a young obese female is strongly suggestive of IIH. The condition is also known as pseudotumuor cerebri, and head imaging by MRI to exclude a space-occupying lesion is mandatory prior to lumbar puncture to confirm the diagnosis.

4. D Normal pressure hydrocephalus
The classic triad of cognitive decline, urine incontinence and gait disturbance, together with a clinical response to CSF drainage, suggests a diagnosis of NPH and predicts a good response to long-term CSF diversion using a shunt.

5. E Obstructive hydrocephalus
Space-occupying lesions, especially within the ventricles or in proximity to the cerebral aqueduct, can produce mass effect resulting in an obstructive hydrocephalus.

Scenario 4

1. E Frontal meningioma
Frontal lesions are associated with personality change, cognitive deficit and disturbance of gait and sphincter control. The insidious nature of the presentation is suggestive of a low-grade lesion such as meningioma (Figure 43.5).

2. B Medulloblastoma
The boy's presentation is suggestive of posterior fossa pathology, with cerebellar dysfunction progressing to evidence of acute hydrocephalus, which is likely to require immediate CSF diversion. Medulloblastoma, a posterior fossa tumour, is among the most common solid organ tumours in this age group (Figure 43.6).

3. D Parietal lobe metastasis
Parietal lobe lesions can produce subtle deficits including sensory attention. Dominant lobe lesions can result in Gerstmann's syndrome (acalculia, agraphia, left-right disorientation and finger agnosia).

4. C Pituitary adenoma
The patient's presentation is suggestive of pituitary apoplexy, the clinical manifestation of acute haemorrhage or infarction within a pituitary tumour.

5. A Temporal lobe low-grade glioma
Seizure activity is a common presentation of low-grade glioma, especially in the temporal lobe. The patient's age and absence of comorbidity are less suggestive of metastasis or meningioma.

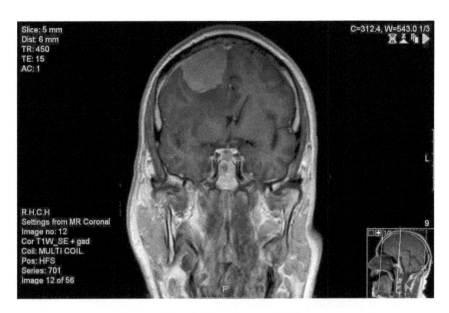

Figure 43.5 Coronal T1-weighted MRI after gadolinium contrast demonstrates right convexity meningioma. The lesion is durally based and distinct from brain tissue.

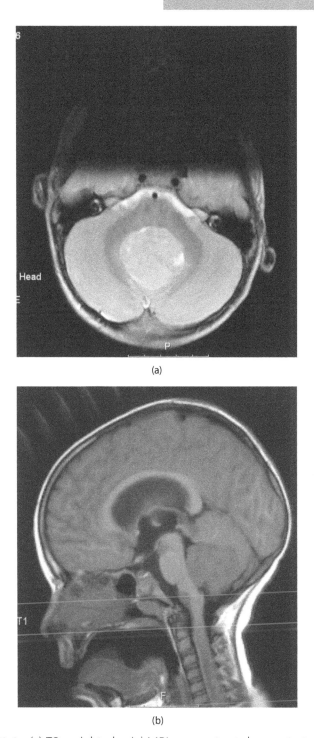

(a)

(b)

Figure 43.6 (a) T2 weighted axial MRI pre-contrast demonstrates a large posterior fossa mass occluding this infant's fourth ventricle. This represents a medulloblastoma. (b) T1 weighted sagittal view with evidence of triventricular hydrocephalus and obstruction of the aqueduct or fourth ventricle.

44 The eye and orbit

Brian W Fleck

Multiple choice questions

Tears

1. How do tears produced in the lacrimal gland enter the conjunctival sac?

A Through the nasolacrimal duct.
B Through the lacrimal duct.
C Through the 10–15 lacrimal gland ducts.
D Through the meibomian orifices.
E Through the ducts of Moll.

Spread of infection

2. What is a potential route of spread of infection from the eyelid skin to the intracranial cavity?

A Orbital lymphatics.
B Ophthalmic veins.
C Subperiosteal potential spaces.
D Facial artery.
E Perineura of branches of the trigeminal nerve.

Meibomian cysts

3. What does a meibomian cyst consist of?

A A meibomian eyelash follicle infection.
B A sebaceous ('meibomian') cyst of the eyelid margin skin.
C A meibomian sweat gland inclusion cyst.
D Chronic granulomatous inflammation of a meibomian gland.
E An epidermoid cyst of embryonic meibomian structures.

4. How are persistent meibomian cysts treated?

A Incision and curettage from the conjunctival surface.
B Incision and curettage from the eyelid margin surface.
C Incision and insertion of a small pack.
D Long-term oral antibiotic therapy.
E Excision biopsy.

Basal cell carcinoma

5. How should a recent-onset suspected basal cell carcinoma of the eyelid skin be treated?

A Photograph and clinical follow-up.
B Liquid nitrogen cryotherapy.
C Curettage.
D Excision biopsy.
E Radiotherapy.

Infection of the tear sac

6. What is the typical cause of acute infection of the tear sac (acute dacryocystitis)?

A Spread of infection from the ethmoid sinus.
B Nasolacrimal duct obstruction.
C Spread of infection from the maxillary sinus.
D Spread of infection from the nasal mucosa.
E Viral infection of the lacrimal gland.

Dysthyroid exophthalmos

7. In acute dysthyroid exophthalmos, when should urgent orbital decompression surgery be considered?

A Diplopia is present.
B Raised intraocular pressure is present.
C Fat prolapse into the eyelids is present.
D Eyelid oedema is present.
E Compressive optic neuropathy is present.

Retinoblastoma

8. **How does retinoblastoma, a malignant tumour of the retina, commonly present in young children?**

A Reduced vision.
B Pain.
C A swollen eye.
D A white pupil reflex.
E Regional lymphadenopathy.

Ocular tumour

9. **What is the most common ocular tumour in adults?**

A Lung carcinoma metastases to the retina.
B Choroidal malignant melanoma.
C Choroidal sarcoma.
D Retinal glioma.
E Choroidal epithelioma.

Herpes simplex infection of the cornea

10. **How is herpes simplex infection of the cornea typically diagnosed?**

A Viral culture of cases of conjunctivitis.
B The presence of typical herpetic vesicles on the eyelid skin.
C The presence of a branching pattern of epithelial fluorescein staining.
D The presence of a herpetic vesicle of the corneal epithelium on fluorescein staining.
E The presence of an inflamed 'phlycten' lump at the junction of the cornea and sclera.

Fracture of the orbit

11. **How is a 'blow-out' fracture of the orbit typically seen on radiography?**

A Fracture of the ethmoid lamina papyraceum.
B Blood in the ethmoid sinus.
C Blood in the maxillary antrum.
D Air in the orbit.
E Soft-tissue prolapse in the maxillary antrum.

Hyphaema

12. **What does the finding of hyphaema following blunt trauma indicate?**

A That the anterior chamber should be washed out promptly to prevent corneal staining.
B That thrombolytic treatment should be given immediately to prevent the development of glaucoma.
C That strict bedrest, with bandaging of the affected eye, should be instituted immediately to prevent secondary haemorrhage.
D That associated intracranial haemorrhage is likely and that a cranial CT scan should be ordered immediately.
E That the eye should be carefully examined for associated injuries, especially of the retina.

Irregular pupil

13. **A front-seat passenger in a road-traffic accident presents with facial lacerations and an irregular pupil in one eye. What is the most likely cause of the irregular pupil?**

A A perforating injury of the globe, with some iris prolapse.
B Blunt trauma to the pupil sphincter.
C A partial third cranial nerve injury.
D Traumatic Horner's syndrome.
E Distortion of the anterior lens capsule due to traumatic cataract development.

Intraocular foreign body

14. **When an intraocular foreign body due to a hammer-and-chisel injury is suspected, which of the following imaging techniques should not be ordered?**

A Plain radiograph of the eye and orbit.
B Ultrasound examination of the eye.
C Magnetic resonance imaging (MRI) scan of the eye and orbit.
D Computed tomography (CT) scan of the eye and orbit.
E Optical tomography of the eye.

→ Tissue burns with ischaemic necrosis

15. **Which of the following are most likely to cause severe tissue burns with ischaemic necrosis?**

A Acid chemicals.
B Alkaline chemicals.
C Ultraviolet radiation.
D Thermal energy.
E Ionising radiation.

→ Herpes simplex corneal infection

16. **Which of the following topical treatments are contraindicated for herpes simplex corneal infection?**

A Aciclovir ointment.
B Atropine eye drops.
C Steroid eye drops.
D Chloramphenicol eye drops.
E Nonsteroidal anti-inflammatory eye drops.

→ Painful, red eye

17. **Which of the following may cause a painful red eye accompanied by vomiting?**

A Conjunctivitis.
B Iritis.
C Acute glaucoma.
D Episcleritis.
E Keratitis.

→ Investigation of loss of vision

18. **Which of the following suspected diagnoses requires immediate measurement of erythrocyte sedimentation rate (ESR) and C-reactive protein (CRP) level?**

A Retinal detachment.
B Central retinal vein occlusion.
C Posterior vitreous detachment.
D Cranial arteritis.
E Macular degeneration.

→ Surgical techniques

19. **What does LASIK refer to?**

A Laser in situ keratomileusis.
B Laser-assisted interstitial keratectomy.
C Long-acting stromal inhibition keratotomy.
D Laser epithelial keratomileusis.
E Lateral segment interstitial keratotomy.

20. **Following cataract surgery, how might thickened posterior lens capsule tissue be cut?**

A Ruby laser capsulotomy.
B Photodisruptive YAG (yttrium aluminium garnet) laser capsulotomy.
C Photoablative argon laser capsulotomy.
D Photodisruptive eximer laser capsulotomy.
E Diode laser capsulotomy.

21. **What is removed in the operation of eyeball evisceration?**

A The intact eyeball, along with short portions of the extraocular muscles.
B The complete contents of the orbit, within the orbital periosteum.
C The vitreous body of the eye.
D The crystalline lens and the vitreous body of the eye.
E The cornea and contents of the eye within the sclera.

22. **What is used in incision and curettage of a meibomian cyst?**

A A skin incision tangential to the lid margin.
B A skin incision radial to the lid margin.
C A tarsal conjunctiva incision tangential to the lid margin.
D A tarsal conjunctiva incision radial to the lid margin.
E An eyelid crease skin incision.

Extended matching questions

→ Initial investigations

A Arrange plain skull x-rays.
B Measure blood pressure, random blood glucose and full blood count.
C No investigations. Contact the duty ophthalmologist.
D Arrange urgent CT scan of the orbits.
E Send blood for ESR and CRP.
F Arrange urgent abdominal ultrasound.
G Send blood for connective tissue diseases screen.
H Discuss urgent MR angiogram with the duty neuroradiologist.
I Request urgent measurement of ophthalmic artery perfusion using Doppler ultrasound.
J Measure blood pressure, random blood glucose and request carotid duplex ultrasound.

Choose the correct action to be taken by the A&E doctor with each of the following scenarios:

1 An 83-year-old woman presents with sudden loss of vision on the right eye, and gives a 3-week history of scalp tenderness. On ophthalmoscopy the right optic disc is pale and oedematous. You suspect cranial arteritis. What initial investigation(s) would you arrange?

2 A 63-year-old male presents with an acute-onset, complete right third cranial nerve palsy and headache. You are concerned about a possible intracranial aneurysm. What initial investigation(s) would you arrange?

3 A 67-year-old female presents with a painful left eye and vomiting. The symptoms have been present for 18 hours. The eye is red, the cornea is hazy, the pupil is large and does not react and the eye feels hard to palpation. What initial investigation(s) would you arrange?

4 A 70-year-old female presents with acute loss of vision in the right eye. On ophthalmoscopy there are numerous retinal haemorrhages in the eye, and a central retinal vein occlusion is suspected. What initial investigation(s) would you arrange?

5 A 70-year-old male presents with acute loss of vision in the left eye. On ophthalmoscopy the retina is pale, with a cherry red spot at the fovea. You suspect a central retinal artery occlusion. What initial investigation(s) would you arrange?

→ Eyelid lumps

A Squamous cell carcinoma
B Lacrimal sac mucocele
C Molluscum contagiosum
D Lacrimal gland tumour
E Sebaceous cyst
F Dermoid cyst
G Preseptal cellulitis
H Meibomian cyst
I Cyst of Moll
J Basal cell carcinoma

Choose the correct diagnosis for each of the scenarios that follow:

1 A 2-year-old child presents with acute swelling and redness of the eyelids of the left eye. The underlying eye and orbit appear normal.

2 A 16-year-old male presents with a slightly red, firm lump deep to the skin of the left lower eyelid. It has been present for several months and remains unchanged in size. It is not painful.

3 A 72-year-old female presents with a tense, fluctuant swelling just medial to the medial canthus of the left eye.

4 A 9-year-old girl presents with a small firm lump at the margin of the left upper eyelid. The left eye has been intermittently red and irritable for 6 weeks.

5 A 70-year-old male presents with a slowly enlarging pearl-coloured, firm, smooth lump on the skin of the right lower eyelid. The lump has a small central crater that tends to bleed at times.

Causes of red eye

A Acute angle closure glaucoma
B Allergic conjunctivitis
C Subconjunctival haemorrhage
D Uveitis
E Scleritis
F Bacterial conjunctivitis
G Adenovirus conjunctivitis
H Bacterial keratitis
I Scleritis
J Herpes simplex keratitis

Choose the correct diagnosis for each of the scenarios that follow:

1 A 23-year-old male presents with pain and photophobia of the right eye. On examination the vision is slightly reduced, there is pink coloration around the edge of the cornea and the pupil is small and irregular.

2 A 33-year-old female presents with an irritable right eye. The vision is slightly blurred and the eye is slightly red. When fluorescein dye is instilled, there is an area of branching-shaped staining of the corneal epithelium.

3 A 63-year-old female presents with a bright red discoloration of the temporal part of the sclera of the right eye. Her vision is normal and she has no discomfort.

4 A 12-year-old girl presents with red, sticky eyes. On awakening in the morning, the eyelids are crusted and stuck together. Her vision remains normal.

5 A 55-year-old female presents with moderately severe pain in the right eye. On examination the temporal and superior sclera is a deep red colour, with some overlying oedema.

Management of ocular trauma

A Instil antibiotic ointment and place an eyepad over the eye.
B Commence prophylactic intravenous antibiotics and perform a temporary tarsorrhaphy.
C Instil local anaesthetic and perform irrigation of the cornea and the conjunctival sac with saline.
D Arrange plain x-ray or CT scan of the eyes.
E Arrange ultrasound examination of the orbits.
F Arrange a CT scan of the facial and orbital bones, to include coronal views.
G Arrange an MRI scan of the eyes and orbits.
H Arrange examination under anaesthetic and surgical repair as required.
I Take a corneal scrape for bacterial culture.
J Irrigate the cornea and conjunctiva with weak acetic acid, until the pH is neutral.

Choose the correct management actions for each of the scenarios that follow:

1 A 23-year-old male was punched in the right eye. There is some bruising of the eyelids, but the eye is intact. However, he complains of double vision and has restricted eye movement on attempted upward gaze.

2 A 48-year-old male was grinding metal and presents with a metal foreign body adherent to the cornea. You instil local anaesthetic, and remove the foreign body with a needle.

3 A 36-year-old male was hammering a metal block with a chisel. He was not wearing eye protection. His right eye suddenly became painful, with blurred vision. There is a small conjunctival laceration just lateral to the cornea, with associated subconjunctival haemorrhage.

4 A 33-year-old male was washing out a glass container that contained alkaline liquid. Some of the liquid splashed into his right eye and the eye is now very painful.

5 A 55-year-old man was punched in the right eye during a fight. The vision is reduced and there is a large volume of subconjunctival haemorrhage. The pupil is distorted, the anterior chamber is shallow and you think there might be some prolapsed iris tissue.

Answers to multiple choice questions

⇒ Tears

1. C

The lacrimal gland lies under the upper, outer orbital rim and opens into the upper conjunctival fornix through 10–15 ducts. Trauma, surgery, or inflammatory scarring in this area can result in a dry eye.

⇒ Spread of infection

2. C

The orbit contains branches of the ophthalmic veins, which anastomose anteriorly with the face and posteriorly with the cranial cavity. These channels can provide a route for the spread of sepsis.

⇒ Meibomian cysts

3. D

The meibomian glands are situated within the tarsal plates and open at the eyelid margin. Retention cysts of the meibomian glands result in the accumulation of granulomatous reaction around meibomian lipid secretions. A meibomian cyst is a chronic granulomatous inflammation of a meibomian gland.

4. A

Meibomian cysts often resolve spontaneously over a period of months. However, persistent meibomian cysts can be treated by incision and curettage from the conjunctival surface. Atypical or recurrent cysts should be biopsied.

⇒ Basal cell carcinoma

5. D

Recent-onset basal cell carcinoma may be treated by excision biopsy, with histological confirmation that the excision has been complete. More extensive lesions might require treatment with Mohs' micrographic surgical excision.

→ Infection of the tear sac

6. B

Obstruction of the nasolacrimal duct might lead to formation of a mucocele within the tear sac. If this becomes infected, acute dacryocystitis occurs. Following initial antibiotic treatment, a dacryocystorhinostomy bypass operation should be performed.

→ Dysthyroid exophthalmos

7. E

Orbital decompression surgery might be needed when compression of the optic nerve results in reduced vision. Systemic glucocorticoid therapy might be used to provide temporary control, pending surgery.

→ Retinoblastoma

8. D

These tumours are often calcified and frequently present with the appearance of a white pupil reflex. They might also present with a squint, and all children with a squint should have a careful fundus examination performed.

→ Ocular tumour

9. B

Malignant melanoma of the uvea (iris, ciliary body, choroid) is the most common tumour in adults. It most often arises in the choroid, and the prognosis is less good for choroid lesions than for the iris. Treatment by brachytherapy or proton-beam irradiation can be performed to preserve the eye, but enucleation is needed in some cases. The most common site of metastasis is the liver.

→ Herpes simplex infection of the cornea

10. C

Fluorescein staining of the corneal epithelium, viewed in blue light, demonstrates any epithelial disturbance. Herpes simplex infection causes a typical branching ('dendritic') pattern of staining.

→ Fracture of the orbit

11. E

The floor of the orbit is the weakest point when the orbital pressure is acutely elevated by blunt trauma. This results in a 'blow-out' fracture, with downward prolapse or the inferior orbital tissue. Reduced upward eye movement results.

→ Hyphaema

12. E

Hyphaema refers to blood in the anterior chamber following blunt trauma. Hyphaema can be followed by secondary haemorrhage, with related raised intraocular pressure. However, associated injuries to other structures of the eye, especially the retina, may be present.

→ Irregular pupil

13. A

Perforating eye injuries are less common when seat belts are worn. Perforating injuries of the cornea and adjacent sclera result in areas of iris prolapse. The pupil becomes distorted, due to displacement of the iris. The eye should not be examined extensively, but should be protected with a shield, pending examination under anaesthetic and primary surgical repair.

Intraocular foreign body

14. C
Intraocular foreign bodies are often composed of ferrous metal in this situation. A magnetic field will result in movement of the foreign body within the eye, with resulting iatrogenic trauma.

Tissue burns with ischaemic necrosis

15. B
Alkaline chemicals penetrate tissues quickly and can cause extensive ischaemia and necrosis. Immediate irrigation is required and should be continued until a neutral pH is obtained.

Herpes simplex corneal infection

16. C
Herpes simplex corneal infections show a characteristic branching ('dendritic') pattern when stained with fluorescein dye. They should be treated with topical antiviral preparations such as aciclovir ointment. Steroid eye drops cause marked worsening of the infection, which might result in severe corneal scarring.

Painful, red eye

17. C
Acute elevation of intraocular pressure results in an oedematous cornea and hard eye on palpation. The severe, visceral pain that accompanies acute glaucoma may cause vomiting, and the condition might be mistaken for an acute abdominal diagnosis.

Inflammatory markers

18. D
The ESR and CRP are often very elevated in cranial arteritis. Prompt diagnosis, leading to prompt therapy with glucocorticoids, can prevent blindness due to bilateral arteritic anterior ischaemic optic neuropathy.

Surgical techniques

19. A
A superficial corneal flap is cut, and a layer of corneal stroma is ablated with an eximer laser. The flap is then repositioned.

20. B
Short pulses of YAG laser energy produce photodisruption, with no thermal effect. Tissue such as the posterior lens capsule, iris and vitreous bands might be divided.

21. B
Evisceration refers to removal of all tissue within the sclera. The cornea is excised, and all intraocular tissue is removed with a curette. All fragments of the uveal tract (iris, ciliary body and choroid) are removed.

22. D
The incision is made on the inner surface of the eyelid to avoid a visible scar. The incision is radial to the lid margin, in line with the affected meibomian gland, to avoid cicatricial shortening of the tarsal plate.

Answers to extended matching questions

→ Initial investigations

1. E Send blood for ESR and CRP
A high index of suspicion should be maintained for cranial arteritis. The ESR and CRP are usually elevated. Prompt treatment with glucocorticoids might prevent bilateral blindness.

2. H Discuss urgent MR angiogram with the duty neuroradiologist
The combination of acute third cranial nerve palsy and pain is suggestive of an intracranial aneurysm. Prompt treatment might prevent catastrophic subarachnoid haemorrhage.

3. C Contact the duty ophthalmologist
Acute angle closure glaucoma causes severe pain, which may result in vomiting and be mistaken for an acute abdominal pathology.

4. B Measure blood pressure, random blood glucose and full blood count
Underlying causes for central retinal vein occlusions include hypertension, diabetes and hyperviscosity syndromes (and glaucoma). These should be treated, if detected, and the patient should be referred for a 'soon' ophthalmology outpatient appointment.

5. J Measure blood pressure, random blood glucose and request carotid duplex ultrasound
In addition to asking if the patient smokes, causes of arteriosclerosis should be sought. Therapy is based on reduction of cardiovascular risk factors, aspirin and assessment for possible carotid endarterectomy surgery.

→ Eyelid lumps

1. G Preseptal cellulitis
Cellulitis of the eyelids is often due to underlying sinus disease. Aggressive antibiotic treatment is necessary.

2. H Meibomian cyst
Meibomian cysts are retention cysts of the meibomian glands and contain sebaceous material. They slowly resolve spontaneously but may be incised on the inner aspect of the eyelid and curetted, if desired.

3. B Lacrimal sac mucocele
A mucocele of the lacrimal sac occurs when proximal and distal outflow from the sac are occluded. Recurrent infection may occur, and the definitive treatment consists of dacryocystorhinostomy surgery.

4. C Molluscum contagiosum
Viruses shed from molluscum contagiosum lesions cause a recurring viral conjunctivitis. The lesion can be curetted, excised, or treated with cryotherapy.

5. J Basal cell carcinoma
Basal cell carcinomas are a common form of eyelid skin neoplasia. They are locally invasive and must be fully excised with a generous margin.

→ Causes of red eye

1. D Uveitis
Anterior uveitis, in which the iris is inflamed, results in spasm of the pupil sphincter muscle and adhesions between the iris and the lens. Deposits of inflammatory cells can be seen on the inner surface of the cornea. Treatment is with pupil-dilating eye drops and steroid eye drops.

2. J Herpes simplex keratitis

Herpes simplex infection of the corneal epithelium typically causes a branching-patterned disturbance of the corneal epithelium. Treatment is with aciclovir ointment. Steroid treatment must be avoided, as this will cause severe worsening of the condition and permanent scarring.

3. C Subconjunctival haemorrhage

Subconjunctival haemorrhages look dramatic but are of no functional significance. They might occur following straining, coughing, sneezing, or minor trauma. They are said to be associated with hypertension. However, typically no underlying cause is evident.

4. F Bacterial conjunctivitis

Bacterial conjunctivitis is a common, self-limiting condition. Typically, there is a purulent exudation. Antibiotic eye drops slightly shorten the duration of the infection, but are unnecessary, as the condition is self-limiting.

5. E Scleritis

Scleritis is a form of connective tissue inflammation frequently associated with rheumatoid arthritis. The inflammation may be controlled with nonsteroidal anti-inflammatory drugs, but in more severe cases, glucocorticoids are needed.

→ Management of ocular trauma

1. F Arrange a CT scan of the facial and orbital bones, to include coronal views

The clinical features are typical of 'blow-out' fracture of the floor of the orbit, with entrapment of soft tissue attached to the inferior rectus muscle. The fracture, and soft tissue prolapsed into the maxillary antrum, will be demonstrated with coronal CT scan views of the orbital floor.

2. A Instil antibiotic ointment and place an eyepad over the eye

After removal of a corneal foreign body, there is risk of infection and the eye is painful. Antibiotic ointment and an eyepad are generally used in this circumstance. This treatment is also appropriate for a corneal abrasion.

3. D Arrange plain x-ray or CT scan of the eyes

There is a high likelihood of the presence of a metallic intraocular foreign body in this circumstance. Even very small radio-opaque foreign bodies might be demonstrated with a plain x-ray or CT scan. Ultrasound examination can be done very gently, but there is a risk of causing further injury by pressing on the eye. MRI scanning is absolutely contraindicated, as magnetic force will cause movement of an intraocular ferrous foreign body, with further injury.

4. C Instil local anaesthetic and perform irrigation of the cornea and the conjunctival sac with saline

A large volume of saline should be used to irrigate the eye, until all traces of alkaline chemical have been removed. Alkaline substances are much more damaging than other chemicals, as they denature proteins and penetrate deeply into the tissue.

5. H Arrange examination under anaesthetic and surgical repair as required

It is very likely that the eye has been ruptured. Attempts to examine the eye in further detail might result in further injury. A more complete examination should be performed under anaesthetic. The injury should be explored and a primary repair performed.

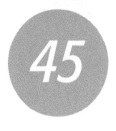

45 Cleft lip and palate: Developmental abnormalities of the face, mouth and jaws

KS Krishna Kumar, Pratap Nadar and Ajit Kumar Pati

Multiple choice questions

→ Anatomy of cleft palate

1. **In cleft palate anatomy, which of the following are true?**

A Primary palate is anterior to incisive foramen.

B The maxillary complex in cleft palate patients has normal growth potential.

C In cleft palate the muscles are oriented transversely.

D Bifid uvula is present.

E Notched posterior hard palate is present.

F Levator palatini is the most important muscle for velopharyngeal closure.

→ Cleft palate – general

2. **Which of the following statements about cleft palate are true?**

A The incidence of cleft lip and palate is one in 6000 live births.

B The incidence of cleft palate is one in 1000 live births.

C The typical distribution of cleft lip alone is 35%.

D The typical distribution of isolated cleft palate is 40%.

E Cleft palate alone is more common in males

→ Orofacial congenital abnormalities

3. **Which of the following statements regarding congenital abnormalities of cleft lip and palate are true?**

A The most common congenital abnormalities of the orofacial structures are cleft lips, alveolus and palate.

B They are also an associated feature in more than 300 recognised syndromes.

C There is an increased incidence in the black population.

D Genetics and the environment both play a part in causation.

E Family history with a first-degree relative affected increases the risk to one in 100 live births.

→ Causes and syndromes

4. **Which of the following statements regarding causal factors of cleft lip and palate are true?**

A Environmental factors are less important for cleft palates than for cleft lip/palate.

B Environmental maternal epilepsy is one factor not associated with clefts.

C Down syndrome can be associated with clefts.

D Apert's and Treacher–Collins syndromes are not associated with clefts.

E An isolated cleft palate is more commonly associated with a syndrome than cleft lip alone.

→ Pierre Robin syndrome

5. **Which of the following statements are true?**

A Pierre Robin syndrome is the most common syndrome associated with clefts.

B Pierre Robin syndrome includes glossoptosis.

C Retrognathia is not a feature of Pierre Robin syndrome.

D Pierre Robin syndrome is named after the first patient in whom the condition was described in 1729.

E Pierre Robin syndrome is associated with early respiratory and feeding difficulties.

Muscle and structural considerations

6. Which of the following statements are true?

A In cleft lip there is disruption of the two groups of muscles of the upper lip and nasolabial region.

B In bilateral cleft lip, the disruption is associated with a prolabium.

C Prolabial tissue contains muscle tissue.

D The secondary palate is defined as the structures anterior to the incisive foramen.

E Cleft palate results owing to failure of fusion of the two palatine shelves.

Further anatomical consideration

7. Which of the following statements are true?

A In a complete cleft palate, the nasal septum and vomer are completely separated from the palatine processes.

B In a cleft of the soft palate, the muscle fibres are oriented wrongly but insert into the posterior edge of the hard palate.

C In a submucous soft-palate cleft, the mucosa is not intact.

D The LAHSHAL system of classification describes the features of a cleft.

E Using the LAHSHAL classification, the incomplete right unilateral cleft lip and incomplete cleft of soft palate extending onto the hard palate are represented by lahSh.

Use of scans in clefts. Respiratory and nutritional considerations

8. Which of the following statements are true?

A Antenatal scans are useful in the early diagnosis of cleft palates.

B As a result of scan results, the parents-to-be should get appropriate support and counselling.

C Diagnosis by scan of a cleft can be made before 15 weeks of gestation.

D Most babies born with a cleft lip and palate feed well and thrive.

E Major respiratory problems occur exclusively in Pierre Robin syndrome.

Pierre Robin syndrome problems and muscle structure in clefts

9. Which of the following statements are true?

A Labioglossopexy is not a procedure used in Pierre Robin syndrome problems.

B Hypoxia is more likely to occur in the awake Pierre Robin baby than during sleep.

C In cleft surgery, the emphasis is repair of the muscles.

D There are four muscles of the soft palate.

E Tensor palati is a soft palate muscle.

Repair of cleft lip and palate

10. In cleft palate repair, which of the following statements are true?

A Adult cases are less problematic because of larger area to work.

B Future facial growth depends upon the nature of surgery.

C Minimal dissection to detach the abnormal soft palate muscles decreases facial growth abnormality.

D Speech results are better if palate repair is done early.

E Facial growth is better if palate repair is done early.

F Primary goal of palate repair is to prevent nasal regurgitation of food material.

G Pushback techniques of palate lengthening are adequate for proper speech development.

11. Which of the following statements are true?

A Restoration of normal anatomy does not encourage normal facial growth in cleft surgery.

B Cleft lip repair is usually performed between 3 and 6 months of age.

C Cleft palate repair is frequently performed between 19 and 24 months.

D A two-stage repair of cleft palate means more tissue damage occurs.

E The Delaire method of repair of a cleft lip is the only satisfactory method for cleft lip closure.

→ Team approach in clefts and care of the ear

12. Which of the following statements are true?

A Management of clefts requires a multidisciplinary team approach.

B Long-term review is not required.

C In cleft palate, Eustachian tube dysfunction is not the cause of otitis media.

D Early (6 to 12 months) prophylactic myringotomy and grommet insertion temporarily eliminate middle ear effusion.

E Regular audiology tests should always be done during childhood.

→ Speech problems

13. Which of the following statements regarding speech problems in cleft patients are true?

A Speech problems are common in cleft palate patients.

B Assessment should be performed at 18 months.

C Speech problems are not associated with airflow.

D Velopharyngeal incompetence is associated with hyponasal speech.

E Speech problems are managed by speech and language therapy, surgery and speech training devices.

→ Dental care

14. Which of the following statements regarding dental care in cleft patients are true?

A Tooth management is not usually an issue in cleft cases.

B Orthodontic care should only be done in cases where dentition is diseased or poorly maintained.

C An abnormal number of eruption problems of teeth rarely occur in cleft patients.

D Orthodontic treatment is commonly carried out at 8–10 years and 14–18 years.

E Expansion of the maxillary arches is done at 14–18 years.

→ Revisional surgery

15. Which of the following statements are true?

A Revisional lip surgery in previously repaired cleft lips should usually be delayed for 2 years unless the original muscle repair has been judged inadequate.

B Nasal deformity confirms incomplete reconstruction of skin deformity.

C The Cupid's bow is an important cosmetic area of the soft palate.

D Alveolar bone grafts should be performed long before orthodontics are considered.

E Alveolar bone grafts are useful in closing residual fistula of the anterior palate.

→ Bone grafts

16. Which of the following statements are true?

A Alveolar bone grafts can receive an osseointegrated dental implant.

B Alveolar bone grafts cannot be used with simultaneous secondary lip revision.

C Alveolar bone grafts are obtained from the humerus and femur.

D It is useful to ensure a tooth erupts into the alveolar bone graft.

E Failure of D results in bone absorption in the long term.

→ ## Surgical repair

17. Which of the following statements are true?

A Orthognathic surgery is designed to correct poor mid-face growth.

B Elective setback of the maxilla is the method of choice to correct the mid-face problem.

C Mandibular advancement might also help.

D Orthognathic surgery does not commence until the age of 6 years.

E Major osteotomies are required in Apert's and Crouzon's syndromes, when a craniofacial team working in designated centres must be involved.

→ ## Role of nasal surgery and audit

18. Which of the following statements are true?

A Open rhinoplasty is not a procedure to be done after orthognathic surgery.

B Open rhinoplasty is indicated when there is dislocation of cartilaginous septum into the cleft nostril.

C Open rhinoplasty is also indicated when there is collapse of the lower lateral cartilage on the cleft side.

D Tip projection of the nose cannot be improved by a postauricular onlay graft.

E Meticulous recordkeeping, including speech recordings and audits, is essential in the overall care of cleft patients.

→ ## Tooth structure in cleft lip patients

19. Which of the following statements regarding tooth structure are true?

A Partial anodontia is not found in cleft lip patients.

B Removal of supernumerary teeth encourages eruption of secondary dentition.

C Genetic disorders can cause changes in structure and attrition of teeth.

D Measles does not cause defects in the structure of teeth.

E Tetracycline can cause defects in the structure of teeth.

→ ## Tooth eruption

20. Which of the following statements regarding tooth eruption are true?

A Eruption of teeth might be impaired by a dentigerous cyst.

B Eruption of teeth is not a problem in cleidocranial dysostosis.

C Management of partial anodontia is not possible.

D Management of unerupted teeth involves removal of any obstruction, including overcrowding caused by supernumerary teeth.

E The most common site for supernumerary teeth is in the mandible.

→ ## Mandible and maxilla problems

21. Which of the following statements are true?

A Dental occlusion problems can arise when there is disproportion in growth between the maxilla and mandible.

B Class II occlusion deformity is associated with over development of the mandible.

C Condylar hyperplasia is an idiopathic condition occurring between 35 and 45 years of age.

D Condylar hyperplasia causes asymmetrical growth of the jaw in both the vertical and horizontal planes.

E Facial disproportionate growth is not a feature of Treacher–Collins syndrome.

→ ## Deformities of the jaw – investigation and treatment plans

22. Which of the following statements are true?

A A bone scan is a useful investigation in condylar hyperplasia.

B Orthognathic surgery is the term given to surgical correction of deformities of the jaw.

C A combination between orthodontic and maxillofacial surgeons is important in orthognathic surgery.

D Treatment planning usually begins with orthodontic treatment at the age of 17–18 years.

E Cephalometric studies are of little value in the above planning.

23. Complications of cleft repair

An 11-year-old boy came for follow-up following a cleft lip and palate repair with regurgitation of food material per nose and speech problem. Which of the following could be the probable causes?

A Palatal fistula
B Inadequate veloplasty
C Residual alveolar cleft
D Infection
E Intrinsic muscle abnormality
F Dehiscence
G Bleeding
H Nasal cartilage abnormality
I Inadequate speech therapy
J Hypertrophic scarring
K Airway obstruction

Extended matching questions

→ ### 1. Anatomy of cleft lip

Options:

A Vertical height discrepancy
B Failure of fusion of medial and lateral nasal process
C Intrinsic maxillary bone growth retardation
D Abnormal muscle insertion also influences the cleft
E Horizontal width discrepancy
F Protruded premaxilla
G Columellar shortening
H Prolabium is devoid of any muscle
I Deformed nasal cartilage
J Cleft of alveolus
K Thinning of nasolabial and orbicularis oris muscles

Match the listed options with the characteristics that follow:

1 Unilateral complete cleft lip
2 In complete cleft lip
3 Bilateral cleft lip

→ ### 2. Principles of repair of cleft lip

Options:

A Vertical height discrepancy correction by rotational flap advancement
B Lip adhesion
C Naso alveolar moulding
D Alveolar bone grafting
E Open rhinoplasty
F Columellar lengthening
G Anterior palate repair
H Labial muscle repair
I Incomplete cleft lip repair does not require extensive labial muscle exposure

Match the listed options with the facts that follow:

1 Unilateral cleft lip repair does not include
2 Bilateral cleft lip repair includes

3. Secondary deformities

Options:

A Malaligned vermillion
B Poor nasal tip projection
C Asymmetrical cupids bow
D Maxillary retrusion
E To promote eruption of canine tooth
F Oronasal fistula
G Poor speech
H Collapse of lower lateral cartilage
I Deviated nasal septum

Match the listed deformities with the following procedures:

1 Cleft lip revision would be of benefit in which of the above conditions?
2 Rhinoplasty would be of benefit in which of the above conditions?

Answers to multiple choice questions

Anatomy of cleft palate

1. A, B, D, E, F

Embryologically, the primary palate consists of all anatomical structures anterior to the incisive foramen. The secondary palate is defined as the part of the palate behind the incisive foramen, which is divided into hard palate anteriorly and soft palate posteriorly.

The cleft of the secondary palate does not disrupt a basic growth mechanism of the upper jaw, hence the maxillary complex has normal growth potential. In normal palate, muscles are oriented transversely and meet in midline, while in cleft palate the muscle fibers are oriented in the anteroposterior direction inserting into the posterior edge of hard palate and cleft mucosa.

Bifid uvula and notched posterior hard palate are indications of submucous cleft palate through bifid uvula might be present in 2% of normal population. The levator palatini muscles of both sides form a sling and are mostly responsible for pushing the soft palate backward for velopharyngeal closure during speech (see **Figures 45.1** through **45.4**).

2. B, D

The incidence of cleft lip and palate is 1 in 600 live births and that of isolated cleft palate is 1 in 1000 live births. Cleft lip alone comprises 15% of all clefts, while cleft palate alone comprises 40%. The latter is more common in females.

Orofacial congenital abnormalities

3. A, B, D

The most common orofacial congenital abnormalities are cleft lips, alveoli and cleft palates. There are at least 300 recognised syndromes that have associated cleft problems. The black population does not have an increased cleft incidence, but it is increased in ethnic Chinese and highest among the Native American tribes of Montana, United States. Both genetic and environmental factors play a part in causation. A family history of a cleft in a first-degree relative increases the risk to 1 in 25 live births.

Normal Palate

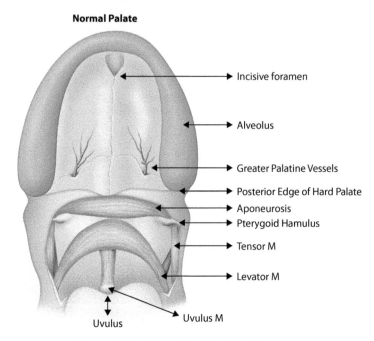

Figure 45.1   Normal palate line diagram.

Cleft Palate

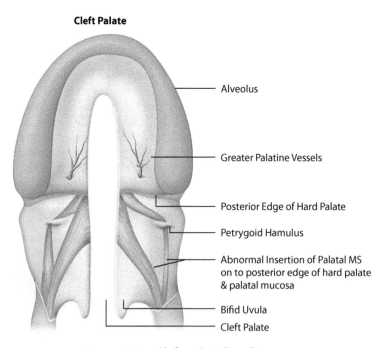

Figure 45.2   Cleft palate line diagram.

Cleft Palate Pre OP

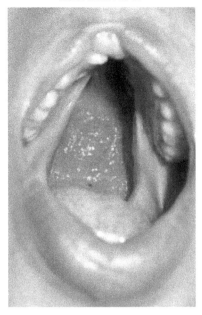

Figure 45.3   Cleft palate.

Cleft Palate Post OP

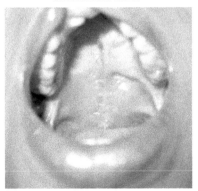

Figure 45.4   Repaired cleft palate.

⇒ Causes and syndromes

4. C, E

The environment is of greater importance in cleft palate than in cleft lip/palate. Environmental factors implicated in clefts include maternal epilepsy and drugs, including steroids, diazepam and phenytoin. Down, Apert's and Treacher–Collins syndromes can be associated with clefts, especially an isolated cleft palate.

→ ## Pierre Robin syndrome

5. A, B, E

Pierre Robin was a professor of dentistry, who described the syndrome in 1929. Glossoptosis and retrognathia in this syndrome contribute to early respiratory and feeding problems. It is the most common syndrome associated with clefts.

→ ## Muscle and structural considerations

6. A, B, E

Cleft lip is caused by disruption of the nasolabial and bilabial muscles, with this more profound and symmetrical in bilateral clefts. The prolabium has no muscle tissue and is associated with bilateral cleft lips. The secondary palate is found posterior to the incisive foramen, and a cleft palate is the result of failure in fusion of two palatine shelves.

→ ## Further anatomical consideration

7. A, B, D

In complete cleft palate, the nasal septum and vomer are separated from the palatine processes. The attachment of the muscle fibres is into the posterior edge of the hard palate in a cleft of the soft palate. In submucous clefts of the soft palate, the mucosa is intact and a groove occurs as a result of muscle abnormality. Classification of clefts can simplified using the LAHSHAL system – lahSh is an incomplete right unilateral cleft lip and alveolus with a complete cleft soft palate extending partly onto the hard palate (see **Figure 45.2**).

→ ## Use of scans in clefts and respiratory and nutritional considerations

8. B, D, E

Antenatal scans are of use in diagnosing cleft lips but they are of no value in the diagnosis of cleft palates. Appropriate counselling should be given to prospective parents when the diagnosis has been made. Ultrasonic scans and diagnosis of cleft lips can be made after 18 weeks' gestation but not before. Feeding and thriving in cleft lip and palate babies are usually normal. Major respiratory problems can occur in the Pierre Robin syndrome.

→ ## Pierre Robin syndrome problems and muscle structure in clefts

9. C, E

A technique that might be useful in preventing respiratory complications in Pierre Robin cases is labioglossopexy. In that syndrome, hypoxia occurs while asleep, not awake. Repair of muscle is the crucial thing in cleft repairs. There are five muscles that control activity in the soft palate, one of which is the tensor palati muscle.

→ ## Principles of cleft palate repair

10. B, C, D

Primary goal of cleft palate repair is proper development of speech, tension free closure of cleft and prevention of ear problems. Through speech results are better if palate repair is done early, i.e., before beginning of language learning, ideally by 12 months, simultaneous facial growth disturbance because of post-op scarring should also be considered. But speech is the most important goal and should be given priority (see **Figures 45.3** and **45.4**).

Dissection should be limited to adequate mobilisation of mucoperiosteal flaps to ensure tension-free closure. Freeing up of all the abnormal muscular attachments and achieving an adequate pushback is of utmost importance to have a good speech. The muscle pushback is achieved by the Intravelar veloplasty principle of Sommerlad or the double opposing Z-plasty principle of Furlow.

Cleft palate repair obtains tension-free complete nasal and oral closure from front to back and detachment of abnormal insertions of levator and tensor muscles with re-establishment of muscle sling with adequate pushback of soft palate, which helps in proper speech.

Adult cases are more problematic because of more bleeding.

11. B

It is important in cleft surgery to encourage normal facial growth by restoring normal anatomy. Cleft lip repair is done at the age of 3 to 6 months, while cleft palates are repaired at 6 months. When there are combined cleft lip and palates, usually there are two operations, the second being the repair of the hard palate with or without lip revision at 15–18 months. A two-stage repair of palatal clefts is sensible as well as being less destructive than a single-stage one. There are several techniques available for cleft repairs, and the Millard methods have become popular in recent years.

Team approach in clefts and care of the ear

12. A, D, E

A multidisciplinary team approach is essential in the management of clefts as is long-term review including audit of results. Otitis media is associated with cleft palate and Eustachian tube problems. Elective myringotomy and insertion of grommets at 6–12 months can eliminate middle-ear effusion. Audiology tests should always be done throughout childhood to check on potential hearing problems.

Speech problems

13. A, B, E

Speech problems are commonly found in cleft patients and are associated with airflow problems. They are assessed at the age of 18 months. Velopharyngeal incompetence is associated with hypernasal speech. The management of speech problems involves surgery, therapists and speech training devices.

Dental care

14. D

Problems with teeth are common in cleft patients – orthodontic care is used to prevent disease and abnormal dentition, including eruption problems or abnormal numbers of teeth. It is done at 8–10 and 14–18 years of age. Expansion of the maxilla is done earlier than 14–18 years; this is when surgery to correct a malpositioned or retrusive maxilla by osteotomy is performed.

Revisional surgery

15. A, E

Any revision of previously repaired cleft lips is considered after 2 years. Nasal cleft deformities are the result of incomplete reconstruction of the nasolabial muscle ring. The Cupid's bow is an important cosmetic feature of the upper-lip repair – and the normal lip. Alveolar bone grafts are done as a rule, though not always, after a period of orthodontics and can be useful in closing a fistula of the anterior palate.

Bone grafts

16. A, D, E

Alveolar bone graft can receive an osseointegrated dental implant and can be performed at the same time as secondary lip revision. Bone for grafting is obtained from the iliac crest or tibia. It is useful to get any teeth to erupt into the graft, and failure for this to happen will result in bone absorption in the long term.

Surgical repair

17. A, E

Orthognathic surgery is used to correct poor mid-face growth problems. The mandible is set back while the maxilla is set forward when mid-face retrusion exists. This type of surgery is not performed at the age of 5 years but is best done before the canine tooth erupts – between 8 and 11 years. Major osteotomies in Apert's or Crouzon's syndromes are operated on by specialised craniofacial surgeons in designated centres.

→ Role of nasal surgery and audit

18. C, E

Open rhinoplasty is usually performed after orthognathic surgery has corrected facial structure and deformities. It is done when there is dislocation of the central septum into the non-cleft nostril, or there is collapse of the lower lateral cartilage on the cleft side. Tip projection is done by using cartilage onlay graft material, which can be obtained from the ear – by a postauricular or a preauricular approach. Meticulous recordkeeping and audit and analysis over many years are essential in the overall management of cleft patients.

→ Tooth structure in cleft lip patients

19. B, C, E

Partial anodontia can be found in clefts, and removal of supernumerary teeth will encourage the eruption of secondary dentition. Genetic disorders can cause changes in the structure and attrition of teeth. Diseases, such as measles, and drugs, such as tetracycline, can also cause disorders of teeth.

→ Tooth eruption

20. A, D

Dentigerous cysts can cause non-eruption of teeth, and this is also a feature of cleidocranial dysostosis. The management of partial anodontia is possible and management of unerupted teeth by removal of any obstruction, including supernumerary teeth, is very helpful. The most common site of supernumerary teeth is in the maxilla and not the mandible.

→ Mandible and maxilla problems

21. A, D

Dental occlusion disparity causes growth problems for the mandible and maxilla. In class II dental occlusion, the mandibular teeth are placed posterior to the maxillary teeth. Condylar hyperplasia occurs in the 15–30 year age group and causes abnormal growth of the jaw in vertical and horizontal planes. Treacher–Collins syndrome is associated with facial growth disparity.

→ Deformities of the jaw – investigation and treatment plans

22. A, B, C

A bone scan is a useful method of examination in cases of condylar hyperplasia. The correction of jaw deformities is orthognatics surgery, and the combination of orthodontics and maxillofacial surgery is important in orthognathic surgery. Orthodontic care should be done earlier than the age of 17–18 years of age. Cephalometric investigations are helpful and important in abnormalities of facial growth.

→ Complications of cleft lip repair

23. A, B, C, I

Complications of cleft lip and palate repair can be immediate, early and late. **Immediate complications** are usually bleeding (usually treated with ice-cold fluids and pressure, but may need re-exploration) and nasal obstruction, especially in bilateral lip and nose repair.

Early complication can be bleeding, respiratory difficulty, infection, wound dehiscence and loss of prolabial flap in case of bilateral cleft.

Late Complication

Palatal repair
Palatal fistula usually occurs at the junction of hard and soft palates in wide defect or at the junction of primary and secondary palate in pushback techniques.

Lip repair
Hypertrophic scarring, lip contraction and notching.

Early complication of cleft lip repair

D, E, G, K
Cleft lip repair can be complicated by bleeding, infection, or wound dehiscence, which is more common in bilateral cleft lip repair than unilateral cases. However, the most serious complication of bilateral repair is airway obstruction. Infection is essentially a stitch abscess. Ischemic loss of premaxilla is an uncommon complication.

Answers to extended matching questions

Anatomy of cleft lip

1. A Vertical height discrepancy   B   Failure of fusion of medial and lateral nasal process   C   Intrinsic maxillary bone growth retardation   D   Abnormal muscle insertion also influences the cleft   G   Columellar shortening   I   Deformed nasal cartilage   J   Cleft of alveolus   K   Thinning of nasolabial and orbicularis oris muscles

Normal upper lip is characterized by a Cupid's bow, two philtral ridges, a well-defined white roll (junction between skin and lip mucosa), red line (junction between wet and dry vermilion), nasal columella in the mid-line with symmetrical ala on both sides. Unilateral cleft lip deformity is due to failure of fusion of medial and lateral nasal process, with disruption and abnormal insertion of nasolabial and orbicularis oris on one side. Clefting usually occurs along the phitral ridges. This results in an asymmetrical deformity in form of loss of Cupid's bow, lip vertical height shortening on cleft side, columellar shortening and deformities of external nasal cartilages and nasal septum and premaxilla (see **Figures 45.5** through **45.7**).

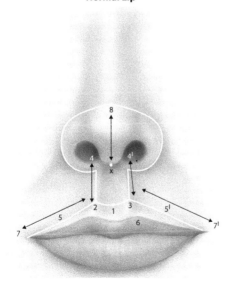

Normal Lip

1. Lowest point of cupid's bow
2. Highest point of cipid's bow right side
3. Highest point of cupid bow left side
4. Collumellar base right side
4^l. Collumellar base left side
5, 5^l White line
6. Red line
7. Oral commisure right side
7^l Oral commisure left side
8. Tip of the nose
X. Mid point of columella

2–4 & 3–4^l. Philitral ridge - Lip height
2–7 & 3–7^l. Lip length
X–8. Nasal Height

Figure 45.5   Normal lip line diagram.

Cleft lip

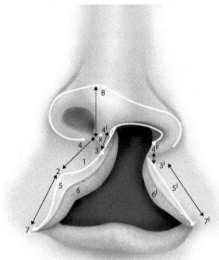

1. Lowest point of cupid's bow
2. Highest point of cipid's bow right side
3. Highest point of cupid's bow non cleft side
3^l. Point where white line fades on cleft side
4. Columellar base non cleft side
4^l. Columellar base cleft side
4^{ll}. Alar base cleft side
$5, 5^1$. White line
6. Red line
7. Oral commisure right side
7^l Oral commisure left side
8. Tip of the nose
X. Mid point of columella

2–4 . Lip height non cleft side
2–7 & 3^l–7^l. Lip length
X-8. Nasal Height

Vertical height discrepancy = Difference of the length between points 2–4 & 3–4 = 3^l – 4^{ll}

Figure 45.6 Cleft lip line diagram.

Cleft Lip Pre OP

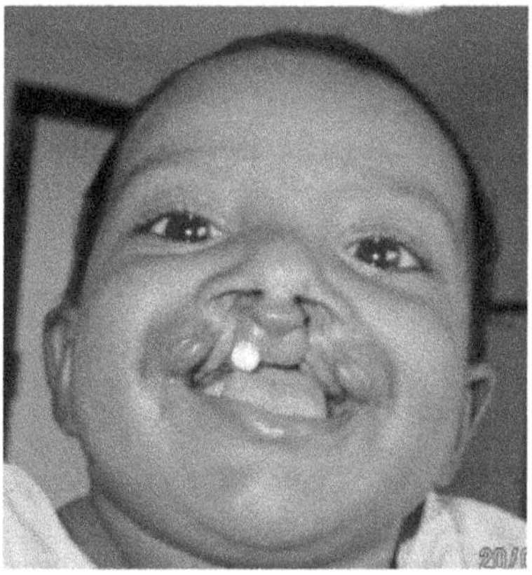

Figure 45.7 Bilateral cleft lip.

2. **A   Vertical height discrepancy   B   Failure of fusion of medial and lateral nasal process   C   Intrinsic maxillary bone growth retardation   D   Abnormal muscle insertion also influences the cleft   K   Thinning of nasolabial and orbicularis oris muscles**

In case of incomplete cleft lip, there is a rim of tissue with varying amounts of muscle, on the nasal sill. Bony and muscle anatomical abnormality associated with incomplete cleft lip is similar to a complete cleft but of a lesser degree (see **Figures 45.1, 45.2, 45.7 and 45.8**).

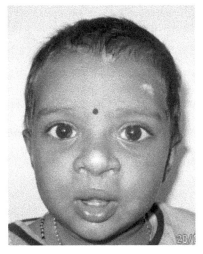

Figure 45.8 Repaired bilateral cleft lip.

3. A   Vertical height discrepancy   C   Intrinsic maxillary bone growth retardation   D   Abnormal muscle insertion also influences the cleft   E   Horizontal width discrepancy   F   Protruded premaxilla   G   Columellar shortening   I   Deformed nasal cartilage   J   Cleft of alveolus   K   Thinning of nasolabial and orbicularis oris muscles

Bilateral cleft lip is symmetrical clefting along the philtral ridges on both sides extending to the alveolus, resulting in a protruded premaxilla and prolabium, which is devoid of any muscle. In bilateral cleft the deformity is more severe, and the bony, cartilaginous and muscular abnormalities are more profound, which is to be kept in mind during surgical planning.

2. Principles of repair of cleft lip

1. Incomplete cleft lip repair does not require extensive labial muscle exposure

In cleft lip repair, the ideal goal is to correct the vertical height discrepancy between the cleft and non-cleft side, approximate cleft edges with recreation of Cupid's bow in balanced position, removal of abnormal muscle and insertion and alignment resulting in pouting of lip, and matching of red line and white line. This is usually achieved by one of the modifications of the rotation advancement technique of Millard, or by one of the variants of the triangular wedge technique.

Ideally nasal correction should be done along with the primary lip repair achieving a matched alar base and alar flare, equal columella and tip height on both sides. Lip adhesion and naso alveolar molding are more commonly indicated in bilateral cleft lip cases but can be very rarely used for wide unilateral cleft lip defect with significant alveolar arch collapse.

Even in incomplete cases, full muscular exposure and restoration is required. Anterior palate should be repaired along with lip repair in case of complete clefts. Alveolar bone grafting may be required in later stages.

2. A   Vertical height discrepancy correction by rotational flap advancement   B   Lip adhesion   C   Naso alveolar moulding   D   Alveolar bone grafting   E   Open rhinoplasty   F   Columellar lengthening   G   Anterior palate repair   H   Labial muscle repair

In bilateral cleft repair, the severity of deformity must be considered prior to surgical planning. Often lip adhesion and nasoalveolar molding are required to align the severely protruded premaxilla along the lateral alveolar arches, which facilitates the muscular sling reconstruction on later stage. Lip adhesion is done without violating the important anatomical landmarks and might be useful in final definitive repair.

In normal palate muscles are oriented transversely and meet in midline, while in cleft palate the muscle fibers are oriented in the anteroposterior direction inserting into the posterior edge of hard palate and cleft mucosa.

Bifid uvula and notched posterior hard palate are indications of submucous cleft palate, though bifid uvula may be present in 2% of normal population. The levator palatini muscles of both sides form a sling and are mostly responsible for pushing the soft palate backward for velopharyngeal closure during speech.

3. Secondary deformities

1. A   Malaligned vermillion   C   Asymmetrical cupids bow

Malaligned vermillion occurs due to poor alignment during initial lip repair. Asymmetrical Cupid's bow occurs due to poor alignment, notching due to poor muscle repair and repeated scar revision can produce a short lip. Hypertrophic scars can occur in lip. Lip revision in the form of 'z' plasty and 'w' plasty can be used in minor discrepancies. In major discrepancies, a formal repair is recommended.

For maxillary retrusion, orthognathic surgery is indicated. Alveolar bone grafting promotes eruption of canine tooth. Oronasal fistula occurs in palate surgeries and would benefit from fistula closure using local flaps. Poor speech is frequently due to poor muscle repair or velopharyngeal incompetence and would benefit from re-repair of muscle or pharyngoplasty.

2. B   Poor nasal tip projection   H   Collapse of lower lateral cartilage   I   Deviated nasal septum

Following revisional cleft lip and palate surgery, orthognathic surgery and alveolar bone grafting, many patients still require definitive nasal correction. The principal deformity is collapse of the lower lateral cartilages on the cleft side, together with a dislocation of the cartilaginous septum with the non-cleft nostril. Rhinoplasty is done to relocate alar cartilages, correct septal deformity and improve nasal tip projection.

46 The nose and paranasal sinuses

Shamim Toma and Iain J Nixon

Multiple choice questions

→ Nasal anatomy

1. Which of the following statements are true?

A Kiesselbach's plexus is located on the posterior nasal septum.

B The nose and paranasal sinuses receive blood supply from both the external and internal carotid artery.

C The upper and lower lateral cartilages form the cartilaginous nasal septum.

D The sphenoid sinus ostium opens onto the lateral nasal wall.

E Intracranial complications may result from spread of nasal sepsis via the ophthalmic vein.

→ Nasal trauma

2. Which of the following statements are true?

A The reduction of a nasal fracture should be performed within the first week of injury.

B Septal haematomas do not require drainage.

C Septal deviation following trauma requires a formal septoplasty.

D Clear rhinorrhoea following violent frontal nasal trauma should raise concerns of a CFS leak.

E Catastrophic haemorrhage following nasal trauma is usually due to trauma to the posterior ethmoidal artery.

→ Septal perforation

3. Which of the following statements are true?

A A septal button prosthesis is used in the management of perforations.

B Septal perforations are usually treated successfully with surgical closure.

C Septal perforations usually heal spontaneously.

D Septal perforations may be associated with autoimmune conditions.

E Nasal obstruction is not a symptom associated with a septal perforation.

→ Nasal polyps

4. Which of the following statements are true?

A Nasal polyps are a sign of cystic fibrosis in 10% of children with nasal polyps.

B Nasal polyps arising from the ethmoid sinuses are of the antrochoanal type.

C Nasal polyps rarely present with nasal obstruction.

D Nasal polyps are characteristically painful when palpated with a probe.

E Oral steroids are never used in the treatment of simple nasal polyps.

→ Epistaxis

5. Which of the following statements is true?

A Nose picking is one of the most common causes of epistaxis.

B Juvenile angiofibroma affects adolescent girls.

C Elderly people bleed from the posterior part of the nose.

D Oestrogen is used in the management of epistaxis due to Osler's disease.

E Ligation of the common carotid artery is used to secure haemostasis in uncontrolled life threatening epistaxis.

→ Sinusitis

6. Which of the following statements are true?

A Aerobic infection is more commonly due to dental sepsis.

B MRI is the imaging modality of choice for frontoethmoiditis.

C Antral lavage is a useful diagnostic procedure performed via the inferior meatus.

D The most common causative pathogen in acute sinusitis is *Staphylococcus aureus*.

E Cavernous sinus thrombosis is not a complication of frontoethmoidal sinusitis.

Extended matching questions

→ Diagnoses

1 Adenocarcinoma ethmoid sinus
2 Inflammatory nasal polyps
3 Juvenile angiofibroma
4 Maxillary sinusitis
5 Periorbital cellulitis

Match the diagnoses with the clinical scenarios that follow:

→ Clinical scenarios

A A 53-year-old man presents with long-standing bilateral nasal obstruction, poor sense of smell and clear nasal discharge.

B A 16-year-old boy presents with left-sided nasal obstruction and recurrent sided epistaxis. A CT scan reveals a mass causing anterior bowing of the posterior maxillary wall.

C A 3-year-old presents with raised temperature and right eye swelling following an URTI.

D A 35-year-old woman presents with recent onset headache, nasal obstruction and unilateral upper dental pain.

E A 68-year-old retired wood worker presents with epistaxis, right-sided nasal obstruction.

Answers to multiple choice questions

→ Nasal anatomy

1. B,E

The nasal cavity and sinuses receive their blood supply via both the external and internal carotid arteries. The external carotid artery supplies the interior of the nose via the maxillary and sphenopalatine arteries. Any of these arteries may be ligated in the surgical management of epistaxis, although the endoscopic approach to the nose now facilitates a minimally invasive approach to the sphenopalatine artery as first-line therapy. The greater palatine artery (terminal branch of the maxillary artery) supplies the anterior inferior septum. The anterior and posterior ethmoidal arteries are branches of the internal carotid artery. Together, this complex arterial supply forms Kiesselbach's plexus on the anterior part of the nasal

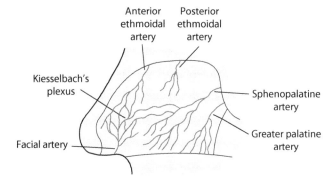

Figure 46.1   Arterial blood supply to the left side of the nose.

septum. Venous drainage is via the ophthalmic and facial veins. Intracranial sepsis might result from spread of infection in the nose via the ophthalmic veins and communication with the cavernous sinus.

The septum consists of the anterior quadrilateral cartilage, bony perpendicular plate of the ethmoid and vomer. The upper and lower lateral cartilages form the outer nasal skeleton, together with the nasal bones and frontal process of the maxilla. All of the ostea of the nasal sinuses open onto the lateral nasal wall except the sphenoid sinus, which is situated posterosuperiorly within the nose **(Figure 46.1)**.

Nasal trauma

2. C, D

Blunt trauma to the front of the nose may result in fractures of the nasal bones and cartilages. Catastrophic haemorrhage tends to result from a tear in the anterior ethmoidal artery. Violent trauma to the frontal area of the nose can result in fracture of the frontal and ethmoidal sinus, which might extend into the anterior cranial fossa resulting in dural tears and cerebrospinal fluid (CSF) leak. Clear rhinorrhoea should raise suspicion of a CSF leak. Suspected nasal fractures should be reviewed at 4 to 5 days when the soft-tissue swelling has reduced. Significant nasal bony deformity can be corrected by manipulation under local or general anaesthetic. This should be carried out within 3 weeks of injury, whilst the bony fragments are still mobile and soft-tissue swelling has subsided. Blunt trauma may lead to lateral deviation of the nasal septum and consequent nasal obstruction, which requires a formal septoplasty to correct. This is usually performed at least 6 months following the injury. A septal haematoma, due to haemorrhage into the sub-mucoperichondrial plane, requires urgent incision and drainage to prevent septal abscess formation with the potential for intra-cranial sepsis. In addition, the resulting cartilage necrosis leads to nasal collapse.

Septal perforations

3. A, D

A septal perforation **(Figure 46.2)** results in turbulent nasal airflow, resulting in a sensation of nasal obstruction, crust formation and epistaxis. These symptoms generally occur with larger perforations (>1 cm). Patients may report whistling on breathing with smaller perforations. Large perforations can reduce support of the nasal dorsum, resulting in a saddle-nose deformity and collapse of the middle third of the nose **(Figure 46.3)**. Septal perforations may result from iatrogenic injury (following submucosal resection [SMR] or septoplasty) or autoimmune conditions, e.g., Wegner's granulomatosis. Septal perforations rarely heal spontaneously. Surgical repair with

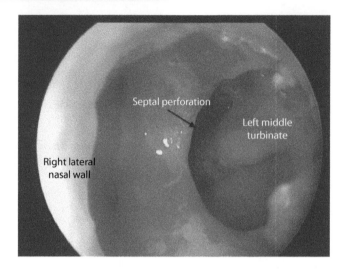

Figure 46.2 Septal perforation.

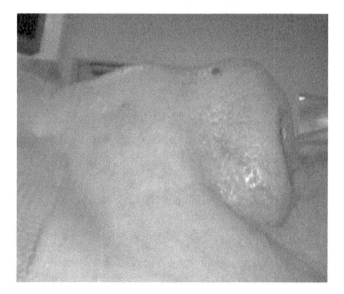

Figure 46.3 Saddle deformity of the nose.

sliding mucoperichondrial flaps or grafts utilising ear cartilage have been described, although success rates are low. Conservative treatment in the form of custom-made silastic button prosthesis can be inserted to occlude the perforation in particular for perforations larger than 1 cm diameter.

Nasal polyps

4. A
Patients with nasal polyps usually present with nasal obstruction, watery rhinorrhoea and anosmia. Nasal polyps are insensate and mobile, which aids distinction form a hypertrophied inferior turbinates on clinical examination. Antrochoanal polyps are large single polyps arising from the maxillary sinus. Nasal polyps are rare in children and should raise the suspicion

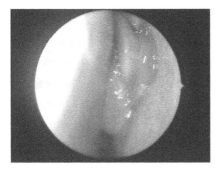

Figure 46.4 Endoscopic view of nasal polyps-left nasal cavity.

of cystic fibrosis occurring in 10% of cases. The use of a short course of systemic steroids is advocated in medical treatment of nasal polyps, reducing the size of the polyps and improving symptoms of nasal obstruction. Surgery may be required in cases of extensive nasal polyps or those refractory to medical treatment **(Figure 46.4)**.

→ Epistaxis

5. A, C, D

Nose picking is a common cause of anterior epistaxis in children and the elderly. The causes of epistaxis can be divided into local and systemic (see **Table 46.1**) In the elderly, arteriosclerosis and hypertension are the underlying causes of arterial bleeding from the posterior part of the nose.

Juvenille nasaopharyngeal angiofibroma is a benign tumour arising from the base of the medial pterygoid plate and the region of the sphenopalatine artery foramen. It is a benign vascular tumour consisting of fibrous tissue and is most common in adolescent males.

Osler Weber Rendu disease (hereditary haemorrhagic telangectsia) is an autosomal dominant disorder that leads to multifocal bleeding from thin-walled vessels deficient in muscle and elastic tissue **(Figure 46.5)**. The diagnostic criteria for HHT are as follows:

1 Recurrent and spontaneous epistaxis, which may be mild to severe.
2 Multiple telangectasias on the skin of the hands, lips, or face, or inside of the nose or mouth.

Table 46.1 Causes of epistaxis

Local	Nose picking
	Nasal trauma
	Nasal foreign bodies
	Tumours
	Infection
	Granulomatous disorders
	Juvenile angiofibroma
Systemic	Hypertension
	Warfarin therapy
	Aspirin therapy
	Haemophilia
	Von Willebrand's disease
	Leukaemia
	Haemorrhagic telangiectasia

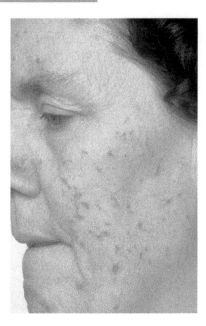

Figure 46.5 Osler's disease showing multiple telangiectasia.

3 Arteriovenous malformations or telangiectasias in the internal organs, including the lungs, brain, liver, intestines, stomach and spinal cord.
4 A family history (i.e., first-degree relative such as brother, sister, parent or child who meets these same criteria for definite HHT or has been genetically diagnosed).

Epistaxis should be managed in a stepwise manner. Initial first aid measures (sitting forward, pinching the soft part of the nose and ice packs) and resuscitation as required, cauterization of bleeding points or prominent vessels may stop the bleeding. Anterior and posterior nasal packing may be required if bleeding continues. Surgical intervention may be required if conservative measures fail to control the bleeding. Arterial ligation of: anterior and posterior ethmoid arteries, sphenopalatine artery, maxillary artery via the maxillary antrum and in severe life threatening epistaxis ligation of the *external* carotid may be required.

→ Sinusitis

6. C

Lavage of the maxillary antrum may be performed under general or local anaesthesia. It is a useful diagnostic procedure in both confirming the presence of pus and obtaining samples for microbiology. The procedure involves inserting a trocar and cannula into the maxillary antrum via the inferior meatus. The most common causative organisms in maxillary sinusitis are *Streptococcus pneumonia* and *Haemophilis influenza*. Dental sepsis more commonly results in anaerobic infection. Computer tomography scanning is the modality of choice to investigate sinus disease. Coronals, axials and saggital views should be evaluated in particular fro frontoethmoidal disese. Complications from acute ethmoidal sinusitis include periorbital cellulitis and cavernous sinus thrombosis. In such acute cases, contrast enhanced imaging including the sinuses, orbit and cranial cavity should be performed to assess the extent of disease and identify associated complications.

1. E Adenocarcinoma ethmoid sinus

Adneocarcinoma has an association with hardwood dust involved in furniture manufacture. Ethmoidal tumours often present late, as their early symptoms mimic those of chronic rhinosinusitis. Sino-nasal malignancies can cause nasal obstruction and epistaxis, progressing to diplopia and proptosis in advanced disease. CT scanning of the paranasal sinuses, neck and chest to delineate the extent of the lesion, bone erosion and for staging. MRI of the sinuses, orbit and brain is also helpful for determining invasion of the soft tissue and base of skull. Biopsy is required to confirm the diagnosis. In resectable disease, optimal treatment is surgery followed by radiation. Proximity to critical structures such as the orbital apex, carotid artery and brain result in a significant proportion of cases being considered unresectable,

2. A Inflammatory nasal polyps

Symptoms due to nasal polyps tend to present gradually over years. Nasal obstruction is the predominant symptom, however, the patient may experience anosmia, rhinorrhoea and postnasal drip. Long-standing gross nasal polyposis may eventually cause widening of the nasal bridge (hypertelorism).

Nasal polyps most commonly occur in the ethmoid sinuses and tend to be bilateral. Patients may have an underlying allergy, e.g., house dust mite or genetic predisposition, e.g., late-onset asthma, aspirin intolerance and nasal polyps known as 'Samter's triad.' The nasal polyposis in these patients tends to be extensive and a low-salicylate diet might be helpful. Treatment of nasal polyps depends on the severity of symptoms and extent of disease. Medical treatment should be trialled initially and varies from topical steroid drops or spray to a short course of oral steroids for severe symptoms. Doxycycline has also been shown to reduce polyp size and postnasal drip symptoms. For large polyps filling the nasal cavity or patients who fail medical therapy, surgical treatment with functional endoscopic sinus surgery and polypectomy should be considered. Surgery is not a cure for polyps and the aim should be to improve the nasal airway to allow instillation of topical medical therapy. Preoperative CT scanning should be performed to the relevant anatomy for surgical planning. Preoperative preparation with oral steroids has been shown to reduce intra-operative bleeding and potential surgical complications.

3. B Juvenile angiofibroma

Juvenille nasaopharyngeal angiofibroma is a benign tumour arising from the base of the medial pterygoid plate and region of the sphenopalatine artery foramen. It is a benign vascular tumour consisting of fibrous tissue. It tends to occur in adolescent males.

Symptoms include progressive nasal obstruction, recurrent severe epistaxis, hyponasal speech and unilateral glue ear, secondary to obstruction of the Eustachian tube orifice. Extension of the tumour into the ethmoidal region can cause bowing of the medial orbital wall. Investigation of such a mass will involve both CT and MRI but not biopsy, given the potential for bleeding. Preoperative embolisation of feeding vessels is used to minimise perioperative blood loss. Recurrence might recur following surgery if not completely excised.

4. D Maxillary sinusitis

Acute rhinosinusitis is defined as acute inflammation of the lining of the nose and paranasal sinuses lasting for up to 4 weeks. It is usually due to a secondary bacterial infection following a viral upper-respiratory tract infection. Maxillary sinus infection is occasionally due to dental sepsis. Clinical features include nasal congestion, mucopurulent nasal discharge and facial pain. Treatment is with oral broad-spectrum antibiotics nasal decongestants for 2 weeks. Underlying dental disease should also be treated. Patients who fail to respond to medical therapy should be considered for maxillary antral lavage, or functional endoscopic sinus surgery, to facilitate decompression of the sinus.

5. C Periorbital cellulitis

Orbital cellulitis is a sight-threatening condition and therefore a medical emergency. It is usually seen in children who present with upper-respiratory tract symptoms, pyrexia and both chemosis and erythema of the preseptal orbital tissues. Progression of infection leads to involvement of the post-septal tissues, which raises the intraorbital pressure resulting in proptosis and reduced eye movements. As the infection progresses, abscess formation might occur. A collection within the orbit increases the intraorbital pressure and might result in ischaemia of the optic nerve, leading to blindness. An urgent contrast-enhanced CT scan of the paranasal sinuses and orbits and brain should be performed. Early identification and prompt treatment is vital. Intravenous broad-spectrum antibiotics should be commenced together with nasal decongestants. If an abscess is present on CT scanning it should be drained urgently, usually via an external approach.

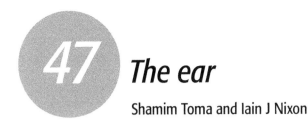

47 The ear

Shamim Toma and Iain J Nixon

Multiple choice questions

→ ## Anatomy

1. Which of the following statements are true?

A In the outer ear, two-thirds of the external ear canal is cartilaginous; the inner third is bony.

B The external and middle ear are derived from the first two branchial arches.

C The light reflex lies in the antero-superior quadrant of the tympanic membrane.

D The malleus articulates with the stapes.

E Epithelial migration occurs outwards from the tympanic membrane along the ear canal.

→ ## Anatomy

2. Which of the following statements are true?

A The cochlea contains endolymph, which has a high concentration of sodium and communicates with CSF.

B The cochlea contains perilymph, which has a high concentration of potassium and communicates with CSF.

C Each inner hair cell responds to a particular frequency of vibration.

D The three semicircular canals are arranged at right angles to each other.

E The utricle and saccule detect angular head movement.

→ ## Anatomy – sensory nerve supply

3. Which of the following statements are true?

A Cranial nerve V supplies the external ear.

B Cranial nerve VII supplies the external ear.

C Cranial nerve VIII supplies the external ear.

D Cranial nerve IX supplies the external ear.

E Cranial nerve X supplies the external ear.

→ ## Examination assessment of the ear

4. Which of the following statements are true?

A Weber's test can distinguish a conductive hearing loss from a sensorineural hearing loss.

B A 512 Hz tuning fork is used to conduct Rinne's test.

C Computed tomography (CT) is the radiological investigation of choice for identification of lesions of the VIIIth (auditory) cranial nerve.

D Magnetic resonance imaging (MRI) is the radiological investigation of choice for identification of lesions of the VIIIth (auditory) cranial nerve.

E MRI is the investigation of choice for imaging bone erosion and cholesteatoma.

→ ## Conditions of the external ear

5. Which of the following statements are true?

A A pinna haematoma occurs when blood collects between the skin and perichondrium.

B Pinna haematoma should be treated with urgent incision and drainage.

C Otitis externa is commonly caused by streptococcal infection.

D Otitis externa can be distinguished from otitis media by pain on movement of the pinna.

E Otitis externa is best treated initially with oral antibiotics.

→ **Conditions of the external ear**

6. Which of the following statements is true?

A Necrotising otitis externa should be suspected in elderly diabetics.

B Necrotising otitis externa spares cranial nerve VII.

C Necrotising otitis externa is caused by a pseudomonal infection.

D Malignant lesions of the external ear are best treated with chemotherapy.

E Malignant lesions of the external ear metastasise first to the submandibular region.

→ **Conditions of the middle ear**

7. Which of the following statements are true?

A Suppurative otitis media is most common in adults.

B Suppurative otitis media is usually caused by *Streptococcus pneumonia.*

C Suppurative otitis media is most painful immediately following rupture of the tympanic membrane.

D Oral antibiotics are the initial treatment of mastoiditis.

E Mastoiditis may lead to intracranial infection.

→ **Conditions of the middle ear**

8. Which of the following statements are true?

A Otitis media with effusion (OME) presents with otalgia.

B OME is due to Eustachian tube dysfunction.

C OME is more common in adults.

D Persistent unilateral OME might be due to a malignancy.

E A 'watch and wait' policy in children results in improvement of 50% over 6 weeks.

→ **Conditions of the middle ear**

9. Which of the following statements are true?

A Tubotympanic chronic suppurative otitis media is more commonly associated with intracranial complications.

B Atticoantral chronic suppurative otitis media is more commonly associated with intracranial complications.

C Cholesteatoma is a benign ear condition that is self-limiting.

D Cholesteatoma is a benign ear condition that is locally destructive.

E Cholesteatoma is a malignant ear condition that is locally destructive.

→ **Hearing loss**

10. Which of the following statements are true?

A Noise-induced hearing loss is greatest at 4000Hz.

B Presbycusis usually affects low frequencies.

C Presbycusis usually affects the high frequencies.

D Presbycusis tends to affect adolescents.

E Aminoglycosides are not ototoxic.

Extended matching questions

→ **1. Middle ear anatomy**

Structure:

1 Eustachian tube opening
2 Facial nerve
3 Long process of incus
4 Malleus
5 Rim of tympanic membrane

6 Round window niche
7 Stapes crura
8 Stapedius muscle

Match the structures with the anatomical structures labelled that follow:

A Long process of incus
B Stapes crura
C Stapedius muscle
D Round window niche
E Malleus
F Facial nerve
G A rim of tympanic membrane
H Eustachian tube

2. Conditions of the inner ear

Diagnoses

1 Acoustic neuroma
2 Acute vestibular failure
3 Bells Palsy
4 Benign paroxysmal positional vertigo (BPPV)
5 Meniere's disease

Match the clinical scenarios that follow with the most likely diagnosis.

Clinical scenarios

A A 53-year-old woman presents with a sudden onset unilateral facial paralysis. There is a history of a preceding upper-respiratory tract infection.
B A 40-year-old woman presents with intermittent episodes of vertigo associated with loud tinnitus and reduced hearing. The episodes last for several hours.
C A 58-year-old man presents with a 3-month history of unilateral tinnitus and a progressive sensorineural hearing loss.
D A 60-year-old woman presents with a vertigo lasting a few seconds on turning on her right in bed.
E A 31-year-old man presents with mild intermittent vertigo precipitated by sudden head movements. There is a history of an episode of severe vertigo for 48 hours associated with vomiting 6 months ago.

Answers to multiple choice questions

Anatomy

1. A, B, E

The external and middle ear develop from the first two branchial arches. First and second arch anomalies can result in microtia (a malformed rudimentary auricle), pre-auricular sinuses, atresia of the external auditory canal and malformations of the ossicles resulting in a conductive hearing loss. The external ear canal is 3 cm in length: the lateral two-thirds is cartilaginous and the medial third is bony. The tympanic membrane has three layers: outer skin, middle collagenous and inner mucosal layer. The outer epithelial layer migrates laterally from the tympanic membrane out of the ear canal. Therefore, most people's ears are self-cleaning. When the migration is misdirected, e.g., secondary to retraction of the tympanic membrane, epithelial debris accumulates. This debris forms a keratinous cyst, which is commonly infected and is described as a cholesteatoma (**see Answer 9**). The light reflex (if present) can be seen in the antero-inferior quadrant of the tympanic membrane. The malleus articulates with the incus, which articulates with the stapes.

Anatomy

2. C, D

The cochlea is a bony spiral containing the scala vestibule, scala tympani and scala media. Different areas of the cochlea are frequency-specific, i.e., tonotopic representation. The scala vestibuli contains perilymph and opens close to the oval window. The scala tympani, which also contains perilymph, is a blind-ending tube terminating at the round window. The scala media, also known as the cochlea duct, contains endolymph. The scala vestibuli (perilymph) and the scala media (endolymph) are separated by Reissner's membrane (**Figure 47.1**). The perilymph is in communication with the CSF and has a high sodium concentration. The endolymph has a high concentration of potassium, similar to intracellular fluid. The hair cells are present on the Basilar membrane that separates the scala media from the scala tympani. There are inner and outer hair cells in the cochlea. Each inner hair cell is sensitive to a particular frequency that causes depolarisation and generation of action potentials in the auditory nerve. The vestibular labyrinth consists of five distinct organs – three semicircular canals (superior, lateral and posterior), utricle and saccule (otolith organs). The three semicircular canals are arranged in the three planes of space at right angles to each other. The semicircular canals detect angular acceleration, whereas the otolith organs detect linear acceleration.

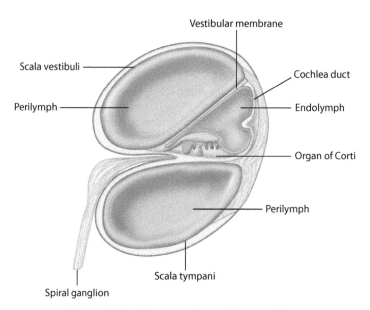

Figure 47.1 Cross-section of the cochlea.

Anatomy

3. A, B, D, E

Sensation to the external ear is complex. Cranial nerves V, VII, IX and X with branches of C2, 3 all give sensory supply to the external ear. The middle ear mucosa is supplied by the glossopharyngeal nerve (IX). The importance of this rich and complex sensory innervation is that referred otalgia is common and may originate from the normal distribution of any of these nerves. Sensory supply to the larynx is via the superior laryngeal nerve, from the vagus nerve, (X). Therefore, referred otalgia may be caused by laryngeal cancer. Ramsay Hunt syndrome is the presence of vesicles within the ear canal in association with herpes zoster infection of cranial nerve VII. The clinical picture in this syndrome is explained by the sensory innervation of the external ear.

Assessment of the ear

4. B, D

Tuning fork tests are a basic hearing screening tool that can be used in general examination of the ear. Weber's test uses bone conduction only. A resonating tuning fork is placed in the midline of the patient's forehead and he or she is asked if he or she can hear it in the midline or toward one ear. Patients with normal hearing or bilateral and equal hearing loss will report the sound centrally. Patients with a unilateral conductive hearing loss will lateralise the sound to the poorer-hearing ear. Patients with a sensorineural hearing loss will lateralise the sound to the better-hearing ear. Rinne's test compares air conduction and bone conduction. A 512-Hz tuning fork is used for this test. The tuning fork is made to resonate and its base placed on the mastoid process of the ear and the patient is asked if he or she can hear it. Gentle pressure is applied by the examiner's hand to the opposite side of the patient's head to ensure that good contact is achieved. The patient is then asked to report when he or she can no longer hear the sound. At this point, the tines of the tuning fork are placed in line with the external auditory canal at approximately 2.5–4 cm. The patient is then asked if he or she can hear the sound. A positive response indicates the lack of a conductive hearing loss, which is present in normal-hearing ears and those with a pure sensorineural loss. A negative Rinne suggests that bone conduction is better than air conduction (a conductive hearing loss). In secondary care, tuning fork tests are used in conjunction with other audiological tests.

Pus, bone and air are demonstrated well on computed tomography (CT). CT scanning of the temporal bones is used preoperatively to identify anatomical variants. Although the diagnosis of cholesteatoma is clinical, it is useful to confirm bony erosion caused by cholesteatoma therefore confirming the diagnosis, to delineate the extent of the disease and for surgical planning. Magnetic resonance imaging (MRI) is better than CT at imaging soft tissue. It is the best method for imaging tumours of the auditory nerves but is not in routine use for assessment of the middle and external ear.

Conditions of the external ear

5. B, D

A pinna haematoma occurs when blood collects under in the sub-perichondrial plane between perchondrium and cartilage. This usually occurs following blunt trauma to the pinna, e.g., contact sports such as rugby. The cartilage receives its blood supply from the perichondrial layer. If a haematoma is not evacuated, then fibrosis will result in a permanent cauliflower ear deformity. In addition, infection of the haematoma might result in underlying cartilage necrosis and increased cosmetic deformity. It is important to exclude an associated head injury, as this takes priority over the ear trauma. Treatment is with prompt drainage under local or general anaesthesia. Adequate drainage will be achieved with a generous incision. The haematoma should be evacuated, and the wound should not be closed to prevent reaccumulation. A pressure dressing should be applied and antibiotic cover prescribed. The wound should be reviewed in 4 to 5 days.

Otitis externa is inflammation of the skin of the external auditory meatus, which may be acute or chronic. There are local risk factors for developing the condition – warm climate, water exposure (swimmer's ear), altered ear canal pH – and systemic factors – general skin disorders such as eczema and psoriasis and local trauma. Common pathogens are *Pseudomonas* and *Staphylococcus* bacteria, *Candida* and *Aspergillus*. Inflammation leads to oedema of the ear canal resulting in debris accumulation, potentiating infection. Pain is the hallmark clinical feature. Movement of the pinna elicits pain, which distinguishes it from otitis media. The skin of the ear canal is swollen, erythematous and itchy, and it will contain debris. Occasionally there is an associated cellulitis of the pinna. Initial treatment is with topical antibiotic and steroid eardrops and analgesia. Suction clearance of debris under a microscope might be required. Fungal infection requires meticulous microsuction and topical antifungal eardrops. Systemic antibiotics are rarely required for otitis externa unless there is evidence of cellulitis of the pinna.

→ Conditions of the external ear

6. A, C
Necrotising otitis externa is a rare but important condition. It presents as severe, persistent unilateral otitis externa. The patient is usually an immunocompromised individual; elderly diabetics, in particular, are susceptible. It results in osteomyelitis of the skull base and can involve cranial nerves VII, IX and X. *Pseudomonas aeruginosa* is usually the infective organism. Treatment is with a prolonged course (at least 6 weeks) of systemic antibiotics and should be closely monitored with sequential imaging. Most malignant primary tumours of the external ear are basal cell carcinomas (BCC) or squamous cell carcinomas (SCC). They tend to present as slow-growing, ulcerating and crusting lesions. SCCs metastasise to parotid or neck nodes. Tumours from the parotid gland or postnasal space might extend to invade the ear canal. Treatment is by surgical-wide excision for a BCC of 2–3 mm margin, and for SCC a 5-mm margin is desirable. Radiotherapy might be needed postoperatively or as the primary modality depending on tumour extension, and the potential for poor cosmetic result following excision.

→ Conditions of the middle ear

7. B, E
Suppurative otitis media is extremely common in childhood. The peak incidence is in the first 12 months of life. It is characterised by the purulent fluid in the middle ear, and the most common infecting organisms are *Streptococcus pneumoniae* and *Haemophilus influenza*. There is usually a preceding upper-respiratory infection, followed by hearing loss, otalgia and pyrexia. If perforation occurs, the otalgia improves. Many cases will not require treatment and are self-resolving. For severe or prolonged cases, appropriate treatment is a course of systemic antibiotics usually for 7 to 10 days. Complications of suppurative otitis media might be extracranial or intracranial. Spread of infection to the mastoid cortex (subperiosteal abscess) causes the pinna to be pushed forward, retro-auricular swelling that is fluctuant and painful. A CT scan of the brain and temporal bones should be performed to exclude intracranial sepsis. Oral antibiotics do not have a role in the initial management of mastoiditis. Urgent broad-spectrum intravenous antibiotics should be commenced. Those cases, which fail to respond to initial therapy, are candidates for incision and drainage of the abscess and insertion of a ventilation tube.

Conditions of the middle ear

8. B, D, E

Otitis media with effusion (OME) is very common in children. It is thought that Eustachian tube dysfunction that leads to negative middle ear pressure and a resultant transudation of fluid into the middle ear space. Children with OME present with delayed speech and language development and behavioural concerns. Otalgia is not a common symptom. Fifty percent of cases of OME are transient and resolve spontaneously. Clinical assessment and audiometry should be repeated following a 3-month period of 'watch and wait'. Grommets +/– adenoidectomy are indicated in bilateral persistent OME. OME is rare in adults, and a persistent effusion warrants examination +/– biopsy of the postnasal space to exclude a nasopharyngeal lesion causing obstruction of the Eustachian tube. Such patients require urgent referral to an ENT specialist.

Conditions of the middle ear

9. B, D

Chronic suppurative otitis media (CSOM) is defined as the presence of chronic otorrhoea with a tympanic membrane perforation. Tympanic membrane perforations have been classified in to tubotympanic (pars tensa) and attico-antral (attic or pars flaccida). Although tubotympanic and atticoantral CSOM may both be associated with intracranial complications due to the risk of development of cholesteatoma with attico-antral CSOM, there is an overall higher risk of developing and intracranial complications. Retraction pockets in the pars flaccida cause epithelial migration to be misdirected. A cholesteatoma is a benign keratinizing squamous sac surrounded by chronically inflamed connective tissue. Squamous debris accumulates and superimposed infection stimulates the release of lytic enzymes, which leads to bone destruction and allows expansion of the cholesteatoma. A low-grade osteomyelitis leads to a foul-smelling discharge. The close proximity of the middle ear and mastoid to the middle and posterior skull base means that intracranial infections can result from CSOM with or without cholesteatoma. Intracranial infection might result from spread of sepsis via emissary veins connecting the middle ear mucosa to the dura or through direct invasion of disease through bone **(Figure 47.2)**.

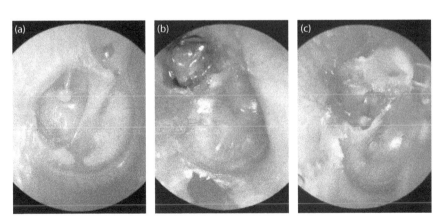

Figure 47.2 (a) Empty attic retraction pocket, right ear. (b) Attic crust covering cholesteatoma, right ear. (c) Attic erosion with cholesteatoma, right ear.

⟶ Hearing loss

10. A, C

Noise-induced hearing loss is due to damage to the inner ear caused by loud noise exposure. The damage is related to the volume of sound and its duration. It is usually a bilateral symmetrical sensorineural hearing loss with a maximal loss at 4000 Hz. In some cases, e.g., following rifle shooting, the hearing loss may be unilateral. Hearing aids might be required and ensuring health and safety measures at work are implemented is necessary to prevent noise-induced hearing loss.

Presbyacusis is age-related hearing loss affecting more men usually over the age of 60 years. It presents as a bilateral progressive sensorineural hearing loss, with no history of noise exposure. The hearing loss usually affects the higher frequencies. Hearing aids are used to treat the disability caused by this hearing loss.

Many drugs are potentially ototoxic. Aminoglycosides are commonly prescribed and can cause an irreversible hearing loss. Aminoglycosides are present in antibiotic eardrops, and their use in the presence of a perforation is controversial. However, there is little evidence to suggest that a short course in the presence of active infection causes significant damage. Patients should be counselled about this and that hearing might be affected by an untreated ear infection. Caution is advised in their use in an only-hearing ear.

Answers to extended matching questions

⟶ 1. Middle ear anatomy

Structure:

1. Eustachian tube opening-H
2. Facial nerve-F
3. Long process of incus-A
4. Malleus-E
5. Rim of tympanic membrane-G
6. Round window niche-D
7. Stapedius muscle-C
8. Stapes crura-B

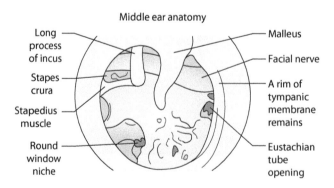

Middle ear anatomy

2. Conditions of the inner ear

1. C Acoustic neuroma

Acoustic neuromas (vestibular schwannoma) are benign slow-growing tumours of the vestibular division of the VIIIth nerve. They present with unilateral hearing loss (sensorineural), unilateral tinnitus, or both. As they expand, they can cause symptoms of raised intracranial pressure and cranial nerve palsies. Investigations include an audiogram (unilateral sensorineural hearing loss) and MRI. Treatment depends on size and symptoms. Serial monitoring of tumour growth should be performed for small lesions (<2 cm) and if there is progression, surgery should be considered early to reduce morbidity, in particular facial nerve palsy.

2. E Acute vestibular failure

Meniere's disease describes a triad of symptoms – vertigo, tinnitus and hearing loss lasting from 20 minutes to several hours. The patient may experience aural fullness (sensation of pressure in the ear before an attack), nausea and vomiting. It is more common in women, occurring usually between the ages of 35 and 40 years old. The underlying cause might be related to endolymphatic hydrops (excessive accumulation of endolymphatic fluid), which distends the endolymphatic compartment and ruptures Reissner's membrane. The hearing loss is typically sensorineural and most pronounced in the low frequencies in early stages of the disease, and high frequency as the disease becomes established. Investigations should include audiometry to assess hearing loss (though this might be normal between attacks) and MRI to exclude mass lesions at the cerebellopontine angle, which might present with similar symptoms. Medical treatment includes diuretics and betahistine. Surgical treatment is indicated when medical treatment has failed and might be intratympanic injection of gentamycin or surgical destruction of vestibular system (labyrinthectomy).

3. A Bells Palsy

Bell's palsy is a common cause of unilateral facial nerve palsy. Its exact aetiology is unknown, though it is likely due to viral infection (herpes virus), which causes swelling and subsequent ischaemia of the nerve due to compression within its bony canal. Around 85%–95% of patients make a good recovery. A thorough otoneurological examination should be performed. In those cases, which recur or fail to resolve completely, an MRI scan of the internal auditory meatus is required to exclude other causes. Evidence suggests that early treatment with high-dose steroids improves outcome. There is less evidence to support the use of antivirals. It is essential to protect the eye by taping it closed at night and prescribing lubricating eyedrops.

4. D Benign paroxysmal positional vertigo (BPPV)

BPPV is a common cause of vertigo. It is characterised by episodes of rotatory vertigo lasting for a few seconds brought on by head movement, in particular, rolling over in bed or looking up. Position testing (Dix- Hallpike) will elicit torsional nystagmus supporting the diagnosis. It is thought to result from stimulation of the posterior semicircular canal by otoconia (bony fragments). It is usually self-limiting. Epley's manoeuvre repositions the displaced otoconia and brings relief in 90% although might need to be repeated.

5. B Meniere's disease

Acute vestibular failure or labyrinthitis presents as a sudden episode of vertigo lasting for 1 to 2 days. The aetiology is suspected to be viral in origin. There may be a preceding upper-respiratory tract infection. Symptoms tend to improve over a period of weeks due to central compensation, although recurring episodes of vertigo for up to 18 months might be experienced.

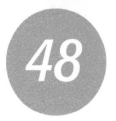

48 Pharynx, larynx and neck

Shamim Toma and Iain J Nixon

Multiple choice questions

→ ### Clinical anatomy

1. Which of the following statements is false?

A The nasopharynx contains the fossa of Rosenmüller.

B The oropharynx contains the adenoids.

C The oropharynx contains the palatine tonsils.

D The oropharynx is bounded inferiorly by the superior border of the epiglottis.

E The hypopharynx is bounded inferiorly by the cricoid cartilage.

→ ### Clinical anatomy

2. The parapharyngeal space contains all of the following except:

A Cervical sympathetic trunk.

B Internal jugular vein.

C Carotid vessels.

D Cranial nerve VII.

E Cranial nerve XII.

→ ### Clinical anatomy

3. Which of the following statements about the larynx are true?

A The cricoid cartilage is the only complete ring of cartilage in the airway.

B The sensory nerve supply to the larynx is from branches of the vagus nerve (X).

C The main motor nerve supply to the larynx is from the superior laryngeal nerve.

D Posterior cricoarytenoid is the only adductor of the vocal cords.

E Serves to protect the lower respiratory tract.

→ ### Adenoidectomy

4. Which of the following statements about adenoidectomy are true?

A Adenoid tissue forms part of Waldeyer's ring and is located in the oropharynx.

B Adenoid tissue hypertrophies with increasing age.

C Adenoidectomy may be indicated in obstructive sleep apnoea.

D Size of adenoid tissue alone is an indication for adenoidectomy.

E Adenoidectomy is indicated in some cases of persistent otitis media with effusion (OME).

→ ### Nasopharyngeal carcinoma

5. Which of the following statements are true?

A Aetiological factors include the herpes simplex virus.

B Are usually adenocarcinomas.

C Has a bimodal distribution.

D Presents with unilateral otitis media in approximately 20%.

E Primary treatment is surgery.

Sore throat

6. Which of the following statements are true?

A Peritonsillar abscess should be treated with transoral incision and drainage.

B Obstructive sleep apnoea is not an indication for tonsillectomy in children.

C Acute retropharyngeal abscess is most commonly seen in children.

D Chronic retropharyngeal abscess is most commonly due to tuberculosis.

E Infectious mononucleosis is confirmed by a positive Paul-Bunnell test.

Dysphagia

7. Which of the following statements are true?

A A pharyngeal pouch is a protrusion diverticulum through Killian's dehiscence.

B A pharyngeal pouch might present as recurrent chest infections.

C A pharyngeal pouch cannot be treated via a transoral approach.

D A pharyngeal pouch is associated with iron deficiency anaemia in some cases.

E Open excision of a pharyngeal pouch is not associated with a risk of mediastinitis.

Oropharyngeal tumours

8. Which of the following statements are true?

A Squamous cell carcinoma is associated with smoking and alcohol.

B Cervical metastases are uncommon.

C Oropharyngeal tumours present often as an occult primary.

D Treatment for early squamous cell carcinoma is with radiotherapy.

E Hodgkin's lymphoma is common in the oropharynx.

Tracheostomy

9. Which of the following is not an indication for a tracheostomy?

A Upper airway obstruction.

B Potential upper airway obstruction.

C Pneumothorax.

D Prolonged artificial ventilation.

E Protection of the lower airway.

Tracheostomy

10. Which of the following statements are true?

A Tracheostomy might be performed under local anaesthetic.

B Tracheostomy increases the work of breathing.

C Tracheostomy reduces the anatomical dead space by approximately 50%.

D Alveolar ventilation is decreased.

E Tracheostomy increases the rate of moisture exchange from the upper airway.

Hoarseness

11. Which of the following statements are true?

A Vocal cord nodules can be treated with speech and language therapy.

B Unilateral vocal cord palsy is most commonly right sided.

C Glottic tumours almost always present with voice change.

D Early-stage laryngeal cancer is usually treated with total laryngectomy and adjuvant postoperative radiotherapy.

E Radiotherapy is an acceptable alternative to surgery for early-stage laryngeal cancer.

Neck lumps

12. Which of the following statements are true?

A Branchial fistula is a second brachial cleft anomaly.

B Brachial cysts present in the neonatal period.

C Cystic hygromas characteristically transilluminate brilliantly.

D Thyroglossal duct cysts move downward on tongue protrusion.

E Surgical treatment of thyroglossal duct cysts includes excision of the central part of the hyoid bone.

Carotid body tumours

13. Which of the following statements are true?

A Carotid body tumours commonly present as a rapidly enlarging painless neck mass.

B Carotid body tumours might cause medial displacement of the tonsil.

C Carotid body tumours are more common in populations living at high altitudes.

D Pre-operative biopsy is used to confirm the diagnosis of carotid body tumours.

E Radiotherapy is the treatment of choice for carotid body tumours.

Neck dissection

14. In which of the following procedures are all lymph nodes on one side of the neck but the accessory nerve, jugular vein and sternomastoid muscle preserved?

A A radical neck dissection

B A classical neck dissection

C A selective neck dissection

D A subtotal neck dissection

E A modified radical neck dissection

Extended matching questions

Management of the patient with an acute airway

A A short course of steroids
B Cricothyroidotomy
C Early tracheostomy
D Endoscopic debridement of lesions
E Insertion of an oral airway
F Intubation until swelling subsides
G Per-oral incision and drainage
H Soft tissue neck x-ray
I Transfer to theatre with experienced anaesthetist and surgeon
J Ultrasound-guided aspiration

Choose the most appropriate management for clinical scenarios that follow:

Clinical scenarios

1 A 16-year-old stertorous with tonsillitis, Paul-Bunnel test positive, fails to improve with intravenous fluids, antibiotics and analgesia.
2 A 31-year-old who presents with a sore throat, pyrexia and trismus has swelling of the left tonsil and deviation of the uvula to the right side.
3 A 3-year-old presents with a short history of drooling, fever and stridor.
4 A 40-year-old involved in an road-traffic accident presents with bruising over the neck, stridor and hoarseness.
5 A 5-year-old presents with hoarseness and stridor on exertion due to laryngeal papillomas.

Answers to multiple choice questions

Clinical anatomy

1. B

The nasopharynx lies anterior to the first cervical vertebra and has the openings of the Eustachian tubes in its lateral wall, behind which lie the pharyngeal recesses, the fossae of

Rosenmüller. The adenoids are situated submucosally at the junction of the roof and posterior wall of the nasopharynx.

The oropharynx extends from the anterior tonsillar pillar to the posterior pharyngeal wall from the level of the hard palate to the level of the hyoid. The oropharynx contains the palatine tonsils, base of tongue, soft palate and posterior pharyngeal wall. The palatine tonsils are part of Waldeyer's ring, a complete ring of lymphoid tissue, together with the adenoids and lingual tonsils on the posterior third of the tongue.

The laryngeal inlet forms the superior boundary of the hypopharynx. Its inferior border is the lower border of the cricoid cartilage where it continues into the oesophagus. The hypopharynx is commonly divided into three areas – the paired pyriform fossae, posterior pharyngeal wall and post-cricoid area. The mucosa of these areas is, however, continuous so disease processes, such as squamous carcinoma, can easily involve more than one area and might also spread submucosally.

Clinical anatomy

2. D
The parapharyngeal space is a cone-shaped potential space, which lies one on either side, lateral to the pharynx. The base is situated at the skull base and the apex is at the greater cornu of the hyoid bone. The medial wall is formed by the visceral layer of the deep layer of deep cervical fascia, which overlies the lateral pharyngeal wall. The lateral wall is the superficial layer of deep cervical fascia, and fascia overlying the mandible, the medial pterygoid muscle and parotid gland. It contains the carotid vessels, internal jugular vein, deep cervical lymph nodes, the last four cranial nerves and the cervical sympathetic trunk. Dental and tonsil infections might track through this space to the superior mediastinum. Patients with parapharyngeal space infection present with trismus due to inflammation and spasm of the medial pterygoid muscle and drooling and hold their head in a slightly flexed position.

Clinical anatomy

3. A, B, E
The cricoid cartilage is the only complete ring in the entire airway and bounds the subglottis. This is the most common site for stenosis from prolonged endotracheal tube intubation.

The sensory nerve supply to the larynx above the vocal folds is from the superior laryngeal nerve and below the vocal folds is from the recurrent laryngeal nerve. Both these nerves are branches of the vagus nerve (X). The motor nerve supply to the larynx is from the recurrent laryngeal nerve, which is a branch of the vagus nerve and supplies all intrinsic muscles. The posterior cricoarytenoid is the only abductor the vocal folds. All other intrinsic muscles adduct the cords. As the recurrent laryngeal nerve supplies all of the intrinsic muscles of the larynx, damage to this nerve or to the vagus nerve will cause paralysis of the vocal fold resulting in hoarseness. Damage to the superior laryngeal nerve, which runs close to the superior pole of the thyroid, will cause a change in voice, which may only be detectable whilst singing.

The primary function of the larynx is to protect the lower respiratory tract. The larynx is well developed for phonation in the human and also helps control pressure during the respiratory cycle.

Adenoidectomy

4. C, E
The most common cause of an enlarged adenoid is physiological hypertrophy. The size of the adenoid alone is not an indication for removal. It is often associated with hypertrophy of the other lymphoid tissues of Waldeyer's ring. If excessive hypertrophy causes blockage

of the nasopharynx in association with tonsil hypertrophy, the upper airway might become compromised during sleep causing obstructive sleep apnoea. Adenoid tissue can be removed alone or in conjunction with a tonsillectomy.

The indications for adenoidectomy are the following:

- Obstructive sleep apnoea associated with post-nasal obstruction
- Post-nasal discharge
- Recurrent acute otitis media or prolonged serous otitis media, usually longer than 3 months' duration
- Recurrent rhinosinusitis

Nasopharyngeal carcinoma

5. C, D

Nasopharyngeal carcinomas are usually squamous cell carcinomas. The aetiology of nasopharyngeal carcinoma is multifactorial. Genetic susceptibility is a factor and certain HLA subtypes e.g., HLA-A2, Epstein–Barr virus infection and consumption of salted fish, are known to be risk factors. Nasopharyngeal carcinoma has a bimodal distribution with an increased incidence in young adults and then again in the 50–60 age group.

Clinical presentation includes early lymph node metastases (70%), in particular, retropharyngeal nodes and cervical lymphadenopathy in levels 2 or 5. Fine-needle aspiration biopsy of a neck node showing undifferentiated carcinoma requires immediate thorough examination of the nasopharynx. Symptoms related to primary disease include nasal discharge, obstruction and epistaxis, which occurs in one-third of patients. Aural symptoms of unilateral deafness as a consequence of Eustachian tube obstruction and secretory otitis media occur in approximately 20% In around 5% of patients, the nasopharynx might look normal or minimally asymmetrical but contains submucosal nasopharyngeal carcinoma. A biopsy of the nasopharynx is essential if there is suspicion of nasopharyngeal malignancy.

The primary treatment of nasopharyngeal carcinoma is radiotherapy, as the majority of the tumours are radiosensitive undifferentiated squamous cell carcinomas. Elective bilateral radiotherapy is given at the skull base and neck in all patients, even when no neck nodes are apparent, as rates of occult metastasis are high. Platinum-based chemotherapy may be given in both the adjuvant and neoadjuvant setting, particularly in high-risk cases. Due to the proximity of vital structures in the immediate vicinity of the nasopharynx, surgery is complex and often impossible. Recurrent neck disease may be an indication for neck dissection, but recurrent disease at the primary site is very challenging surgically. Although there is experience with nasopharyngectomy in the Far East, few centres in Europe or North America have significant experience of these techniques. For early disease, 3-year disease-free survival rates of more than 75% are common; however, in advanced disease the results are less good, with 3-year disease-free survival rates of 30%–50%.

Sore throat

6. A, C, D, E

Peritonsillar abscess or quinsy describes the formation of pus in the peritonsillar space. Patients experience severe pain and trismus due to inflammation around the pterygoid muscles. The tonsil and uvular are pushed medially. Intravenous broad-spectrum antibiotics, fluids and analgesia should be commenced; however, transoral incision and drainage of the pus should be carried out under local anaesthesia.

The retropharyngeal space is a potential space that lies posterior to the pharynx, bounded anteriorly by the posterior pharyngeal wall and its covering buccopharyngeal fascia and

Table 48.1 Indications for tonsillectomy

Absolute	Sleep apnoea, chronic respiratory tract obstruction, cor ulmonale
	Suspected tonsillar malignancy
Relative	Documented recurrent acute tonsillitis
	Chronic tonsillitis
	Peritonsillar abscess (quinsy)
	Tonsillar asymmetry
	Tonsillitis resulting in febrile convulsions
	Diphtheria carriers
	Systemic disease caused by β-haemolytic Streptococcus (nephritis, rheumatic fever)

posteriorly by the cervical vertebrae. It contains the retropharyngeal lymph nodes. These nodes are more developed in young children, and it is at this age that they are most likely to be involved in inflammatory processes, which, if severe, might affect swallowing and the airway as a result of swelling and suppuration of the retropharyngeal space. A retropharyngeal abscess is associated with infection of the tonsil, oropharynx, or nasopharynx. Signs and symptoms include airway compromise, dysphagia, torticollis, stiff neck and swelling of the midline of the posterior pharyngeal wall. Operative approaches to a retropharyngeal space abscess include peroral or an external approach, and a decision on approach will be based on imaging findings.

Chronic retropharyngeal abscess is now rare and most commonly the result of an extension of tuberculosis of the cervical spine, which has spread through the anterior longitudinal ligament to reach the retropharyngeal space (**Table 48.1**).

Infectious mononucleosis (or glandular fever) is caused by the Epstein–Barr virus. It is common in teenagers and young adults. Signs and symptoms are similar as for bacterial tonsillitis; however, the tonsils are typically erythematous with a creamy grey exudate and cervical or generalised lymphadenopathy is present. Occasionally, hepatosplenomegaly occurs. The diagnosis is confirmed by serological testing showing a positive Paul-Bunnell test, an absolute and relative lymphocytosis and presence of atypical monocytes in the peripheral blood.

Dysphagia

7. A, B ,D

A pharyngeal pouch is a protrusion of mucosa through Killian's dehiscence, a weak area of the posterior pharyngeal wall between the oblique fibres of the thyropharyngeus and the transverse fibres of cricopharyngeus at the lower end of the inferior constrictor muscle. (**Figure 48.1**). It is thought to be in part due to a hyperactive upper oesophageal sphincter, and is more common in men over 60 years old.

Patients might experience regurgitation of undigested food, sometimes hours after a meal, and halitosis. Occasionally, they might present with recurrent, unexplained chest infections as a result of aspiration of the contents of the pouch. As the pouch increases in size, the patients might notice gurgling noises from the neck on swallowing and the pouch may become large enough to form a visible swelling in the neck. Surgery is indicated when the symptoms are affecting the patient's quality of life, in particular, weight loss and recurrent pulmonary complications due to aspiration. A barium swallow demonstrates the pouch position and size.

Endoscopic stapling has superseded the open approach, however, both are still performed. The endoscopic technique is associated with a high symptomatic success rate, decreased operating time and length of stay and lower rates of complications such as wound infection, mediastinitis, pharyngeal fistula formation, recurrent laryngeal nerve palsy and stenosis of the upper oesophagus.

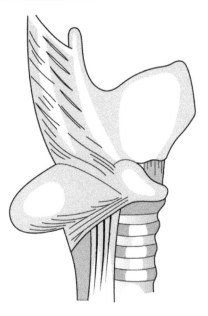

Figure 48.1 A pharyngeal pouch.

A post-cricoid web might also cause dysphagia and can be identified on a barium swallow. It is rare and is known as Patterson Brown-Kelly or Plumber–Vinson syndrome. It is linked with iron-deficiency anaemia and has malignant potential; therefore, endoscopy and biopsy should be performed.

Oropharyngeal tumours

8. A, C, D

Cigarette smoking and consumption of alcohol are significant risk factors for squamous carcinomas of the oropharynx. Cervical lymph node metastases are common due to the extensive lymphatic drainage of the oropharynx. They might be the only presenting feature with an apparent occult primary tumour. Often, the primary is from the tonsil or tongue base but undetectable. Early-stage tumours are usually treated with radiotherapy, although with improvements in surgical access provided by transoral laser and robotic techniques, surgical excision is gaining popularity. Recurrent disease following radiotherapy is usually managed surgically, and reconstruction of the oropharynx might require regionally-based myocutaneous or microvascular free flaps with microvascular anastomosis.

Hodgkin's disease and non-Hodgkin's lymphoma commonly present as lymph node enlargement in the neck. Hodgkin's disease is rare in the oropharynx, but non-Hodgkin's lymphoma accounts for 15%–20% of tumours at this site. Radiotherapy is the treatment of choice for localised non-Hodgkin's lymphoma and might give control rates as high as 75% at 5 years. For disseminated non-Hodgkin's lymphoma, systemic chemotherapy is preferred.

Tracheostomy

9. C

Tracheostomy

10. A, C

A tracheostomy bypasses the upper airway and has the following advantages:

- The anatomical dead space is reduced by approximately 50%.
- The work of breathing is reduced.
- Alveolar ventilation is increased.
- The level of sedation necessary for patient comfort isdecreased and, unlike endotracheal intubation, the patient might beable to talk and eat with a tube in place.

However, there are several disadvantages, including the following:

- Loss of heat and moisture exchange performed in the upper respiratory tract.
- Desiccation of tracheal epithelium, loss of ciliated cells and metaplasia.
- Presence of a foreign body in the trachea stimulates mucous production; where no cilia are present, this mucociliary stream is arrested.
- The increased mucus is more viscid and thick crusts may form and block the tube.
- Splinting of the larynx might prevent normal swallowing and lead to aspiration.

Hoarseness

11. A, C, E

Vocal cord nodules are bilateral whitish lesions that tend to be at the junction of the anterior one-third and posterior two-thirds of the vocal cords. They tend to occur in children and singers, and are the result of vocal abuse. Primary treatment is speech therapy. Occasionally, the nodules will need to be surgically removed using microlaryngeal surgery.

Vocal cord paralysis may be unilateral or bilateral. A unilateral left vocal fold palsy is the most common because of the long intrathoracic course of the left recurrent laryngeal nerve, which arches around the aorta, and a bronchial malignancy should be suspected. A CT scan of the skull base to diaphragm should be performed to image the nerve's course.

Squamous carcinoma is the most common malignant tumour, and it is responsible for more than 90% of tumours within the larynx. Patients almost always present with hoarseness. In early-stage disease, e.g., confined to one vocal fold; treatment with radiotherapy or carbon dioxide laser excision is associated with a 5-year disease-free survival of more than 90%. Both modalities give comparable quality of voice outcomes.

Supraglottic and glottic tumours, stages I and II, are optimally treated with radiotherapy or trans oral laser resection, with the aim of preservation of function. Advanced-stage laryngeal carcinomas (stage III/IV) might betreated with chemoradiotherapy for organ preservation or surgery. Decisions relating to the choice of therapy include the degree of cartilage invasion and safety of the airway.

Neck lumps

12. A, C, E

A branchial cyst is thought to develop from the embryological remnants of the second branchial cleft. Such cysts are lined by stratified squamous epithelium and contain thick, turbid fluid full of cholesterol crystals. The cyst usually presents in the upper neck in early or middle adulthood and is found at the junction of the upper third and middle third of the sternomastoid muscle at its anterior border. If the cyst becomes infected, it becomes erythematous and tender. Ultrasound and fine-needle aspiration aid diagnosis, and treatment is by complete excision, which is best undertaken when infection has settled. In older patients with cystic neck masses, malignancy with a cystic neck metastasis should be considered. Primary disease in the oropharynx is the most common cause.

A branchial fistula might be unilateral or bilateral and is thought to represent a persistent second branchial cleft and pouch. The external opening is nearly always situated in the lower third of the neck near the anterior border of the sternocleidomastoid, while the internal opening is usually located in the tonsillar region. Excision involves removing an ellipse of skin around the tract and dissecting it out in a cephalad direction. Further stepladder incisions might be required.

Cystic hygromas (lymphatic malformations) usually present in the neonate or in early infancy. The characteristic that distinguishes it from all other neck swellings is that it is brilliantly translucent. They tend to grow steadily with the child and can lead to disfigurement and airway obstruction and require a tracheostomy. Investigation will outline the anatomy and consistency of the cyst. The cyst might become infected. Definitive treatment is complete excision of the cyst, where possible. Injection of a sclerosing agent, for example, picibanil (OK-432), might also be an option, although in cases where multiple cysts are present, both surgery and sclerosing therapy are challenging.

Thyroglossal duct cysts are an embryological remnant of the thyroglossal duct and might occur anywhere in, or adjacent to, the midline from the tongue base to the thyroid isthmus. Rarely, a thyroglossal cyst might contain the only functioning thyroid tissue in the body. Classically, the cyst moves upward on swallowing and with tongue protrusion, due to its attachment to the hyoid bone. Thyroglossal cysts might become infected and rupture onto the skin of the neck, presenting as a discharging sinus. Treatment is excision of the tract with a core of tissue and middle third of the hyoid bone to remove the embryological tract that resulted in the cyst. This operation is known as Sistrunk's operation and reduces recurrence in comparison with excising the cyst alone.

Carotid body tumours

13. B, C

This is a rare tumour (paraganglioma) that has a higher incidence in areas where people live at high altitudes because of chronic hypoxia leading to carotid body hyperplasia. Approximately 10% of patients have a family history, and there is an association with multiple endocrine neoplasia (MEN) type 2A and 2B. There is often a long history of a slowly enlarging, painless lump at the carotid bifurcation. Approximately one-third of patients will present with a pharyngeal mass that pushes the tonsil medially and anteriorly. The mass is firm, rubbery, pulsatile, mobile from side to side but not up and down and can sometimes be emptied by firm pressure, after which it slowly refills in a pulsatile manner.

Investigations include a carotid angiogram and MRI scan. This tumour should not be biopsied due to the risk of haemorrhage.

Carotid body tumours rarely (3%) metastasize, and their overall rate of growth is slow. The need for surgical removal must be considered carefully, as complications of surgery are potentially serious. Treatment is surgical.

Neck dissection

14. E

The classical, radical neck dissection involves removal of all nodes, the sternomastoid, jugular and accessory. Selective neck dissections remove only lymphatics, but not all levels. Modified neck dissections can be classed 1–3 depending on the number of structures preserved from the nerve, vein and muscle. Subtotal is not a term applied to neck dissection.

1. A A short course of steroids

Stertor is the sound made by upper airway obstruction at a level above the larynx. The Epstein–Barr virus can cause tonsillitis, often presenting with a grey or white film over the tonsils. The tonsils can be enlarged sufficiently to threaten the airway. If they fail to respond to antibiotics, a short course of steroids should be given.

2. G Per-oral incision and drainage

This patient has a peritonsillar abscess, which can be treated with incision and drainage through the mouth. The mucosa is prepared with a local anaesthetic spray, and a scalpel blade is used to incise the abscess wall. These patients will also be managed with antibiotics, fluids and analgesia until their oral intake is sufficient. An alternative option is aspiration with a 10-mL syringe and wide-bore needle.

3. I Transfer to theatre with experienced anaesthetist and surgeon

This child should be considered to have epiglottitis. These patients should be managed in a calm environment, with nothing done to upset them, particularly no attempts to examine the throat, which can precipitate respiratory arrest. The patient should be transferred to theatre and examined under anaesthetic with an experienced anaesthetist and a surgeon capable of performing paediatric tracheostomy if required. If the diagnosis is confirmed the team can move straight to intubation, take culture samples and institute antimicrobial therapy. In advanced cases where intubation is impossible, tracheostomy will be life saving, but most cases can be managed medically.

4. C Early tracheostomy

Blunt laryngeal trauma can result in loss of the airway, and prompt intervention might be required. Endotracheal intubation should be avoided as the foreign-body reaction to the tube can result in permanent laryngeal damage. An early tracheostomy is appropriate, with inspection of the larynx and repair of mucosal and cartilage injuries in an attempt to minimise long-term loss of function.

5. D Endoscopic debridement of lesions

Recurrent respiratory papillomatosis is a condition that HPV 6 and 11 cause. Following a biopsy for histological confirmation, the lesions should be excised endoscopically using a microdebrider, cold steel, or laser. This condition is characterised by recurrent growth of papillomas and multiple procedures. The underlying tissues must not be damaged as this condition often improves after puberty and the aim is to maintain the normal function of the larynx as far as possible.

49 Oral/oropharyngeal cancer

Iain J Nixon

Multiple choice questions

→ **Epidemiology**

1. **Which of the following statements are true?**
   A Oral and oropharyngeal cancers account for 2%–4% of all human malignancies.
   B The worldwide incidence of oral/oropharyngeal cancers is falling.
   C Epstiein-Barr virus associated cancers are becoming more prevalent.
   D The incidence in females is greater than that in males.
   E Tobacco and alcohol exert a synergistic carcinogenic effect.

→ **Anatomy**

2. **Which of the following statements are true?**
   A The oral cavity extends from the lower teeth to the soft palate.
   B The oropharynx extends from the oral surface of the soft palate to the level of the hyoid bone.
   C The base of tongue is included in the oropharynx.
   D The hard palate is part of the oral cavity.
   E The retromolar trigone is the most anterior subsite of the oropharynx.

→ **Pathology**

3. **Which of the following statements are true?**
   A Squamous cell carcinoma is the most common cancer of the oral cavity.

B High-risk premalignant lesions include lichen planus and speckled leukoplakia.
C The concept of field change is related to widespread exposure of the upper aero-digestive tract to carcinogens.
D The potential for malignant transformation increases with the age of the patient and the lesion.
E Oral submucous fibrosis is related to chronic cigarette use.

→ **Clinical features**

4. **Which of the following statements are true?**
   A The upper lip is affected by cancer more commonly than the lower lip.
   B A nonhealing ulcer of over 4 weeks duration should be investigated.
   C Neck mass is a common presenting feature of oropharyngeal cancer.
   D Ipsliateral otalgia suggests advanced disease.
   E Trisumus is commonly present in the early stages of oropharyngeal cancer.

→ **Investigations**

5. **Which of the following statements are true?**
   A Early malignancies are generally managed without the need for formal investigations.
   B CT or MRI should be performed to assess the extent of loco-regional disease.

C Bone scans are important to identify sites of involvement of the facial skeleton.

D Fine-needle aspiration cytology should be used to assess neck masses.

E Plain radiology of the mandible and maxilla is now outdated and has no role in preoperative investigation.

→ Treatment

6. Which of the following statements is true?

A Oropharyngeal cancer is more commonly treated with surgery and oral cancer with radiation as primary therapy.

B Previous radiation to the oropharynx is usually a contraindication to further radiotherapy.

C Factors considered in therapy include site, stage, histology and comorbidities.

D Grade of differentiation of squamous cell carcinoma is an important factor in selecting mode of therapy.

E Advanced age is a contraindication to curative therapy.

→ Oral cavity cancers

7. Which of the following statements are true?

A Cancers that require resection of less than one-third of the lip can be excised with a wedge.

B Only 10% of patients with tongue cancer will have nodal metastases at presentation.

C Wound closure following excision of a floor of mouth cancer should approximate the ventral tongue to the labial mucosa.

D Reconstruction is ideal following excision of buccal carcinoma.

E Delayed reconstruction of mandibular defects is preferred to ensure clear margins.

→ Oropharyngeal cancers

8. Which of the following statements are true?

A Surgical access to the base of tongue may require total glossectomy.

B Chemotherapy is combined with radiotherapy for improved results in many cases.

C High rates of occult regional metastases mandate elective treatment of the clinically uninvolved neck.

D Patients treated surgically for multiple neck metastases should undergo selective 'supraomohyoid' neck dissection.

E Swallowing tends to be unaffected by appropriate therapy for oropharyngeal cancer.

→ Outcomes

9. Which of the following statements are true?

A Patients successfully treated for oral/ oropharyngeal cancer do not require follow-up.

B The majority of recurrences occur after 5 years.

C Survival is related to the stage of disease at presentation.

D Cessation of smoking and alcohol should be promoted.

E Extra capsular nodal spread is an important predictor of outcome.

Extended matching questions

1. Staging of oral/oropharyngeal cancer

→ Diagnoses

1 Stage I
2 Stage II
3 Stage III
4 Stage IV

Match the diagnoses with the clinical scenarios that follow:

→ Clinical scenarios

A A 56-year-old man presents with a lateral tongue cancer, which measures 3 cm with no associated nodal or distant disease.
B A 68-year-old presents with a 1-cm cancer of the tonsil with a single ipsilateral enlarged lymph node and no distant disease.
C A 76-year-old man presents with a 2-cm floor-of-mouth cancer, palpable low cervical nodes and evidence of metastases in the lung.
D A 55-year-old lady presents with a 1.5-cm cancer on the hard palate with no evidence of regional or distant disease.

2. Reconstruction following surgical resection

→ Reconstructive approach

1 Advancement of labial mucosa
2 Fibular osseo-cutaneous free flap
3 Pectoralis major rotation flap
4 Primary closure
5 Radial artery forearm free flap

Match the reconstructive approaches with the clinical scenarios that follow:

→ Clinical scenarios

A A 77-year-old man presents with a squamous cell carcinoma invading the posterior mandible who has peripheral vascular disease preventing free flap reconstruction.
B A 52-year-old man presents with a less than one-third lower lip squamous cell carcinoma.
C A 63-year-old presents with a submandibular gland cancer that has invaded the mandible and requires segmental mandibulectomy.
D A 68-year-old woman presents with a 2-cm floor-of-mouth cancer that has invaded the sublingual gland but does not require bony resection.
E A 48-year-old presents with premalignant change affecting the exposed mucosa of the entire lower lip.

Answers to multiple choice questions

Epidemiology

1. A, E

Oropharyngeal and oral cancers account for 2%–4% of human malignancies. The incidence is rising, however, particularly in the developing world. Tobacco and alcohol are recognised carcinogens that have a synergistic effect. HPV-related cancers are also rising, which seems to be associated with the rising incidence seen in the Western world. Males are more commonly affected than females. Interestingly, HPV-related lesions respond more favourably to therapy, although reasons for this are unclear. Indeed, HPV-related oropharyngeal cancers do so well that the traditional staging system seems outdated in this evolving disease.

Anatomy

2. B, C, D

The anatomy of the oral cavity and oropharynx can be confusing. The oral cavity includes all structures from the vermillion border of the lip back to the junction of the soft palate and hard palate. The oropharynx then extends from this level posteriorly. The roof of the oropharynx should be considered during oral respiration, when the soft palate is horizontal at the level of the hard palate. When this is true the oropharynx can be seen to include the base of tongue (region behind the cirumvallate papillae), which leads to the vallecula, which inserts onto the hyoid bone. The lateral walls include the palatine tonsils and lateral pharyngeal wall. Posteriorly, the posterior pharyngeal wall is also included, although rarely involved in cancers. The retromolar trigone is another difficult place to visualise. This area lies posterior to the molar teeth and is the most posterior anatomical site of the oral cavity.

Pathology

3. A, C, D

Although minor salivary gland cancers and lymphomas do occur in the oral and oropharyngeal cavity, the majority of lesions are squamous cell cancers. Most arise denovo, but some will develop from existing premalignant conditions. Although red patches, (erythroplakia), speckled leukoplakia and chronic hyperplastic candidiasis are considered high risk for malignant transformation, lichen planus is not. Increased patient and lesional age are risk factors for malignant transformation, as are further exposure to cigarettes and alcohol. Because the whole upper airway is exposed to carcinogens in smokers and drinkers, it is common for cancers to arise in significantly damaged mucosa. This presents treatment challenges, as the adjacent mucosa might already be dysplastic, which is the concept of field cancerisation or field change. Oral submucous fibrosis is thought to be associated with the use of pan masala areca nut, not cigarettes.

Clinical features

4. B, C, D

The lower lip is far more commonly involved with cancer than the upper lip. Any nonhealing oral ulcer should be investigated further. The mucosa of the oropharynx is folded and might hide early cancers. It is therefore common for such cancers to first present with neck metastases. Otalgia is referred from the cranial nerves (IX and X) and therefore represents advanced disease, which has involved these structures either from the primary site or regional metastases. Trismus is normally due to invasion of the pterygoid muscles. This is a feature of advanced, often surgically unresectable, disease.

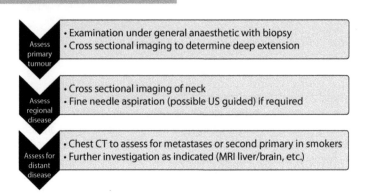

Figure 49.1 Diagnostic algorithm for oropharyngeal cancers.

→ Investigations

5. B, D

All cancers of the upper aerodigestive tract will require investigation. This allows for a pretreatment assessment of the extent of locoregional disease. Cross-sectional imaging with CT or MRI is preferred, and MRI has the benefit of not being affected by dental amalgam artefact. Bone scans tend to overestimate involvement of the facial skeleton and are not in routine use. In contrast, fine-needle aspiration (FNA) is an important investigation and is best performed under ultrasound guidance. One weakness of FNA is the small number of cells obtained, which can make immunohistochemical staining difficult. Core biopsies provide more tissue and can be used to test for HPV status. Although plain radiology (orthopantogram) is a basic investigation it allows an estimation of bony destruction in advanced lesions, which can be useful in the operating room. Although three-dimensional reconstructions of advanced cases are increasingly used, they have not become routine in most centres. A diagnostic algorithm is provided in **Figure 49.1**.

→ Treatment

6. B, C

Primary therapy for oral cancer tends to be surgical and radiation for oropharyngeal cancer. The reasons are complex. Oral cancers are more easily accessed transorally and are partially shielded from radiation by the mandible. In contrast, access to the oropharynx is limited via the transoral route, and these cancers respond well to radiation therapy. Many advanced cancers will be offered combined therapy. Previous radiation is considered a contraindication to further radiotherapy, although in extreme circumstances and unresectable disease, further radiation may be offered. Although grade of differentiation might affect prognosis, it is not usually considered in terms of therapy. Physiological age is more important than chronological age, and some young head and neck cancer patients present with significant comorbidities while older patients might be physiologically more fit. Therefore, age itself is not a contraindication to curative therapy.

Oral cavity cancers

7. A, D

Cancers of the lip should be assessed to consider the extent of resection. Less than one-third can be closed with a wedge, greater than one-third will require rotation or free flaps. Remember that radiation therapy is also very effective for lip cancers. Tongue cancer is the most common oral cancer, and around 30% present with nodal metastases. For this reason, even in clinically negative necks, all but the smallest (<3 mm depth) cancers should be treated with an elective neck dissection. Following excision of a floor-of-mouth or buccal carcinoma, reconstruction is with a vascularised flap. If this is not performed for floor-of-mouth cancers, adhesion between the tongue and lip compromises oral function. Contracture at the site of a buccal cancer resection leads to significant trismus. Cosmetic outcomes are superior with immediate recomstruction of mandibular defects. Ideally they are reconstructed using like for like tissue (e.g.. fibular osseus free flap for mandibular resection).

Oropharyngeal cancers

8. A, B, C

The oropharynx is difficult to access surgically. Particularly for base-of-tongue tumours, wide resections, which might include resection of the tongue (glossectomy), are required to achieve clear surgical margins. This is one of reason why combination chemoradiotherapy has been favoured in recent years. The increasing interest in robotic surgery might provide a surgical solution for accessing this difficult area, and surgical trials are ongoing. The addition of chemotherapy to radiation has been shown to improve outcomes. At least 30% of patients with oropharyngeal cancers have nodal metastases at presentation and therefore even if considered free of disease, the regional lymph nodes should be included in treatment. For those patients with advanced neck disease, surgical treatment should include resection of all lymph nodes in the ipsilateral neck (modified radical or radical neck dissection) rather than selective neck dissection to maximise the chance of controlling neck disease. Even successful treatment of oropharyngeal cancer inevitably results in changes to swallowing and speech functions. The location of the oropharynx means that the structures around are intimately involved in all functions of the pharynx.

9. C, D, E

Patients successfully treated will require regular follow-up to monitor them for recurrent disease and other primary cancers, and to provide support for the side effects of therapy. The majority of disease recurrences happen within 3 years. By 5 years, most patients will be oncologically fit for discharge. Survival is related to the stage of disease at presentation, although for HPV-related cancers, the accuracy of this staging has been questioned. It is increasingly clear that the presence of extra capsular spread of nodal metastases is an important predictor of outcome. Despite this, it has not been formally recognised within the staging system at this point. Alcohol and cigarette use should be ceased in these patients who are at risk of recurrence, second head and neck cancers and other smoking- and alcohol-related diseases. As well as the oncological outcomes, clinicians should be aware that there is a significant pschyco-social element to head and neck cancer. Alteration in speech and swallowing might require adjuncts such as feeding tubes. Patients often need support from many members of the multidisciplinary team involved in managing head and neck cancers for years after the cancer itself has been successfully cured. A standard U.K. follow-up protocol is provided in **Table 49.1**.

Table 49.1 Follow-up protocol for oropharyngeal cancers

Year	Interval Follow-Up*	Support Required
1	1 monthly	Regular support to asses for recurrence and function (pain, nutritional goals, speech and swallowing)
2	2 monthly	
3	3 monthly	Recurrence less likely, medium to long-term side effects of treatment emerging (trismus, strictures, etc.)
	6 monthly	
5	6 monthly	
>5	As required	Ongoing nutritional and psychological support may be required (tubefeeding, chronic pair, etc.)

* Patients should be encouraged to report any symptoms suggestive or recurrence immediately.

Answers to extended matching questions

1. D Stage I
Stage I head and neck cancer must be T1 (<2 cm) N0, M0. This diagnosis can be confirmed for surgical cases where lymph nodes are excised but must be assumed in cases with no evidence of nodal disease who are treated with radiation therapy, as no pathology specimen is obtained.

2. A Stage II
Stage II disease is also limited to the primary site. T2 (2–4 cm), N0, M0 disease. Many of these patients will in fact have occult disease in the neck, but this is only proved if neck dissection is performed. The prefix 'c' refers to clinical staging (cT2N0M0) versus radiological (r) or pathological (p) staging.

3. B Stage III
Neck metastases are considered the strongest prognostic factor in head and neck cancer, halving the chance of survival. A single node increases T1/2 primary cancer to stage III disease. A single node >3 cm in size would be N2a. Multiple nodes on the same side as the primary cancer are called N2b, contralateral nodes are N2c. Any node >6 cm is considered N3. In fact, extra capsular spread is now considered an important prognostic factor but is yet to be formally recognised in the staging systems. Despite this, its presence is used to identify patients who will benefit from postoperative chemotherapy as well as radiation.

4. C Stage IV
Patients with advanced nodal or distant disease are considered stage IVa/b, and those with distant metastases are stage IVc (**Table 49.2**).

Table 49.2 Staging of oropharyngeal cancers

	T1	T2	T3	T4
N0	Stage I	Stage II	Stage III	Stage IVa
N1	Stage III	Stage III	Stage III	Stage IVa
N2	Stage IVa	Stage IVa	Stage IVa	Stage IVa
N3	Stage IVb	Stage IVb	Stage IVb	Stage IVb
		All M1 disease = Stage IVc		

→ Reconstructive approach

1. E Advancement of labial mucosa

In patients who have extensive lower lip changes but who require resection of mucosa only, sufficient mobilisation of the mucosa of the inner lip allows for resurfacing. This provides excellent cosmesis, and the mucosa should be re-approximated along the vermillion border.

2. C Fibular osseo-cutaneous free flap

In patents with adequate peripheral circulation, the fibula provides an excellent reconstructive option following mandibular resection. The flap is reliable and provides sufficient length to reconstruct almost any mandibular defect. In addition, the bone is thick enough to support dental implants once healing has occurred. Skin paddles can be designed to provide oral reconstruction and external reconstruction of skin defects at the same time, if required. Reconstruction with bone prevents the cosmetic deformity seen after soft tissue reconstruction. The projection of the mandible is maintained as is symmetry around the midline. This should be the aim for most mandibular reconstructions.

3. A Pectoralis major rotation flap

Although bony reconstruction for most mandibular defects is ideal, some patients will lack adequate peripheral vasculature to provide free tissue transfer. There are alternatives to the fibula in provision of vascularised bone, including iliac crest, radius and scapula. However, free tissue transfer adds significant anaesthetic time to the procedure and some patients will be deemed unfit for such a long procedure. Posterior mandibular defects suffer less cosmetic deformity if soft tissue reconstruction is used, and in this case a pectorlais major flap is suitable. This flap, previously the workhorse flap in head and neck surgery, is reliable and can be fashioned to provide a large or small tissue volume for reconstruction.

4. B Primary closure

Primary closure is of course the simplest method of reconstruction. IT should be used only when it will not compromise function. Small lip cancers (<1/3) can be closed primarily. Larger tumours will require local flaps. When closing a lip primarily, most attention should be paid to approximation of the vermillion border. This is cosmetically important as the eye is drawn to this region. The lip should be closed in three layers, which are mucosa, muscle and skin. Wounds closed in this manner have an excellent cosmetic and functional outcome, as the orbicularis oris function remains intact.

5. D Radial artery forearm free flap

Following resection of a floor-of-mouth cancer, a few factors should be considered. Assuming that a neck dissection is also performed, there may be continuity between the mouth and neck. If this is so, saliva can drain directly in to the neck and create a salivary fistula. Not only does this compromise healing, but prolonged exposure of the great vessels to the digestive enzymes in saliva can lead to catastrophic bleeding. In addition, functional concerns are important. It is not uncommon that primary closure will be feasible. However, if such an approach tethers the tongue to the lower alveolus this will comprise oral function significantly. Not only will tongue movement be limited, but obliteration of the sulcus on the internal aspect of the mandible prevents denture fitting, which further compromises both cosmesis and function.

In this setting the ideal reconstruction will isolate the mouth and neck, and at the same time provide sufficient tissue to maintain space for a subsequent dental appliance. The radial artery free flap provides thin, pliable and reliable vascularised tissue with which to reconstruct intra-oral defects.

50 Disorders of the salivary glands

Iain J Nixon

Multiple choice questions

→ ### Minor salivary glands

1. **Which of the following statements are true?**

A There are three pairs of minor salivary glands.

B Minor salivary glands contribute 10% of overall saliva flow.

C Most minor salivary gland tumours are benign.

D Presumed benign tumours of the minor salivary glands >1 cm should be managed with excisional biopsy.

E Malignant minor salivary gland tumours are managed with primary surgical resection.

→ ### Sublingual glands

2. **Which of the following statements are true?**

A The sublingual glands occupy the anterior floor of mouth.

B The sublingual glands drain both directly in to the mouth and in to the submandibular duct.

C Tumours of the sublingual glands are rarely malignant.

D The term ranula is applied to mucous retention cysts of the sublingual gland.

E A plunging ranula is the term used to describe a ranula that extends beyond the floor of mouth and in to the neck.

→ ### Submandibular glands (anatomy/surgery)

3. **Which of the following statements are true?**

A The two lobes of the submandibular gland communicate around the posterior belly of the digastric muscle.

B 80% of salivary calculi occur in the submandibular duct.

C Calculi identified posterior to the point where the duct crosses the lingual nerve should be removed via a transoral approach.

D The marginal mandibular nerve is at risk during removal of the gland.

E The lingual nerve is divided during removal of the gland to facilitate dissection of the deep lobe of the gland.

→ ### Submandibular glands (tumours)

4. **Which of the following statements are true?**

A 80% of submandibular gland tumours are benign.

B Submandibular gland masses can be differentiated from lymph nodes by bimanual palpation.

C Facial nerve weakness is a sign suggestive of malignancy.

D Open surgical biopsy is indicated to confirm malignant disease prior to surgery.

E Radiation is the primary modality of treatment for most submandibular gland malignancies.

→ ## The parotid gland (anatomy/surgery)

5. Which of the following statements are true?

A 80% of the parotid gland lies deep to the facial nerve.

B During parotidectomy, the greater auricular nerve should be included in the skin flap to preserve function.

C The facial nerve is identified using landmarks including the tragal pointer and the posterior belly of digastric.

D If a branch of the facial nerve must be sacrificed during dissection, immediate grafting should be performed.

E Frey's syndrome results from inappropriate innervation of sweat glands with parasympathetic fibres within the parotid bed.

→ ## The parotid gland (infection/inflammation)

6. Which of the following statements is true?

A Viral infection of the parotid glands affects both glands symmetrically.

B Dehydrated patients are at risk from bacterial parotitis.

C Recurrent parotitis of childhood tends to result in abscess formation.

D HIV might present with multiple parotid cysts.

E Chronic trauma to the parotid duct may result in obstruction.

→ ## The parotid gland (tumours/ other pathology)

7. Which of the following statements are true?

A The most common tumour of the parotid gland is a pleomorphic adenoma.

B Tumour excision for benign disease involves enucleation of the lesion.

C Malignant tumours should be excised with a cuff of normal tissue including the facial nerve.

D Symmetrical swelling of the parotid glands may be due to excess alcohol intake.

E Sjogrens syndrome is associated with B cell lymphoma.

Extended matching questions

→ ### Diagnoses

1 Bacterial parotitis
2 Minor salivary gland cancer
3 Mucus retention cyst
4 Mumps
5 Parotid gland cancer
6 Pleomorphic adenoma
7 Salivary calculus

Match the diagnoses with the clinical scenarios that follow:

→ ### Clinical scenarios

A A 64-year-old man presents with a unilateral swelling below the left ear lobe. It is 2 cm in size and stable with no skin changes, pain, or facial nerve involvement.

B A 48-year-old presents with a mass at the junction of the hard and soft palate. It is 1.5 cm in size, painless and slowly enlarging.

C A 45-year-old lady presents with unilateral pain under the jaw on mastication.
D A 15-year-old presents with bilateral facial swelling, a raised temperature and CRP but normal white cell blood count.
E A 78-year-old man presents with a rapidly enlarging mass in the right parotid. The skin overlying the mass is erythematous and the facial nerve function is affected.
F A 19-year-old presents with a soft swelling of the lower lip which has increased in size over the past week following minor dental trauma to the area.
G An 89-year-old is admitted from a nursing home with facial swelling and a raised temperature.

Answers to multiple choice questions

1. B, E
There are around 450 minor salivary glands in the upper aerodigestive tract. Although they are present in the nasal cavity, sinuses and larynx, the majority reside in the lip, tongue and palate. Overall, they contribute about 10% of salivary flow. The vast majority of minor salivary gland tumours are malignant. This is in contrast to lesions of the parotid gland. Although small tumours (<1 cm) may be excised to achieve a biopsy, larger lesions should be managed initially with an incisional biopsy. This confirms the diagnosis and guides appropriate therapy. Surgery is the preferred option for benign or malignant lesions, with reconstruction as dictated by the anatomical site and extent of disease.

→ ## Sublingual glands

2. A, B, E
The sublingual glands occupy the anatomical region deep to the mucosa of the floor of mouth. This area, which can be inspected by asking the patient to lift his or her tongue, is bounded by the muscles of the tongue and mandible medially and laterally then by the mylohyoid muscle on its deep aspect and the mucosa on its superficial aspect. The glands drain both into the submandibular duct and directly onto the mucosa. Tumours of the sublingual glands are rare. However, when present, tumours are most commonly malignant (>80%). Although mucous retention cysts do occur, from blocked minor salivary and sublingual glands in this region, the term ranula is reserved to describe an extravasation of saliva. Although this is considered like a cyst, there is no cyst wall. The saliva collects and can be seen through the mucosa of the floor of mouth. If it collects in sufficient volume, the saliva can pass into the neck through the mylohyoid muscle, at which point it is called a plunging ranula. Treatment requires excision of the affected sublingual gland.

→ ## Submandibular glands (anatomy/surgery)

3. B, D
Around 80% of salivary calculi occur in the submandibular duct due to its viscous salvia production and the fact it drains against gravity. For this reason, the anatomy of the gland is important to the general surgeon. There are two lobes that communicate around the posterior edge of the mylohyoid muscle. From the deep lobe runs the duct, which drains into the floor of mouth. Calculi often arises around the region where the duct crosses the lingual nerve. Those anterior to this can be removed transorally; however, those behind the nerve should be approached by removing the gland and identifying the stone within the duct posteriorly to prevent lingual nerve damage. Some units with a special interest might approach even posterior stones transorally, but such an approach requires experience.

Table 50.1 Frequency of benign tumours by salivary gland

Salivary Gland	% of Tumours that are Benign
Parotid	80%
Submandibular	50%
Sublingual	20%
Minor Salivary	10%

During surgery on the gland, the marginal mandibular, lingual and hypoglossal nerve are all at risk and must be preserved. The marginal is preserved by incising straight down onto the gland and reflecting the fascia directly off it, knowing the marginal mandibular nerve will be superficial and therefore protected. The lingual nerve is attached to the gland by the submandibular ganglion, and the anatomy must be delineated prior to division of the ganglion, which allows the lingual nerve to pass up in to the floor of the mouth, out of danger. Some surgeons formally identify the hypoglossal nerve, which lies deep and medial to the gland, to prevent accidental damage.

Submandibular glands (tumours)

4. B, C
The frequency of malignancies within salivary glands is shown in **Table 50.1.** Due to the deep lobe of the gland, which is not present in lymph nodes, bimanual palpation through the mouth facilitates differentiation between these structures. Masses that rapidly increase in size, involve skin changes, facial nerve weakness, or regional lymphadenopathy should all be considered high risk for malignancy. Achieving a diagnostic biopsy in salivary tumours is controversial with many authors recommending no pre-op biopsy. This is because fine-needle aspiration (FNA) biopsy is notoriously inaccurate, particularly in units without a large experience of managing salivary tumours. As therapy for almost all lesions is surgery in the first instance, the impact on treatment approach is minimal whatever the biopsy result. However, most physicians would attempt an FNA, as a positive diagnosis of cancer allows more realistic preoperative counselling and might justify sacrifice of critical structures such as the facial nerve. All authors would agree that open biopsy is never indicated, as it leads to tumour seeding and might compromise the outcomes, whether the lesion is benign or malignant.

The parotid gland (anatomy/surgery)

5. C, E
The parotid gland occupies a space between the mastoid and mandible. It is in this region that the facial nerve leaves the stylomastoid foramen to pass to the muscles of facial expression. The substance of the gland envelops these fibres almost as if poured into the anatomical space. The vast majority (80%) of the gland lies superficial to the nerve, and, crucially, there is rarely if ever a lymph node in the deep lobe. The significance of this is that, unless the deep lobe is involved with tumour, no dissection deep to the nerve is required to remove potentially involved nodes. When raising the skin flap for parotid surgery, the great auricular nerve must be sacrificed. Occasionally the posterior branch might be spared, but patients should be warned that the earlobe will remain numb following surgery. When performing a parotidectomy, the surgeon should be familiar with the landmarks, which allow identification of the facial nerve (**Figure 50.1**). The tragal pointer and posterior belly of digastric are the most commonly used. A plane over the digastric is dissected, as is a plane over the tragal cartilage. Between the two lies the nerve, and it should be dissected

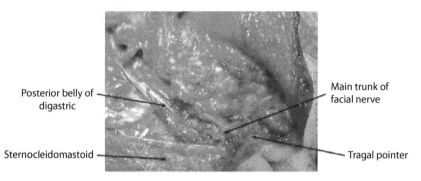

Posterior belly of digastric

Sternocleidomastoid

Main trunk of facial nerve

Tragal pointer

Figure 50.1 Surgical landmarks for the facial nerve.

out by gently and slowly dividing the fibres that attach the parotid gland to the mastoid bone. Often, a small vessel directly overlies the nerve. This can make identification of the nerve challenging, particularly if bleeding is encountered. The surgeon must resist the temptation to use bipolar diathermy indiscriminately at this point, as nerve injury will result. Frey's syndrome occurs as post-ganglionic parasympathetic nerve fibres are transected and regrow to innervate sweat glands in the skin flap. It might be prevented by placing a barrier of muscle or facia between the remaining parotid and skin, although this has not gained universal acceptance.

The parotid gland (infection/inflammation)

6. B, D, E

Mumps is a viral infection of the parotid glands, and although it can present with symmetrical involvement, unilateral atypical viral parotiditis does occur and should be considered when assessing a unilateral painful parotid swelling. Classical patients at risk from bacterial parotid infections include elderly dehydrated patients, and those who have undergone recent surgery. Dehydration promotes viscous saliva and salivary stasis. Ascending infection then results in parotitis. Recurrent parotitis of childhood has a typical history of swelling and pain that responds to antibiotics and rarely results in abscess. It can be seen on sialography with the snowstorm appearance **(Figure 50.2)**. Patients with HIV can present with multiple cysts. These form a 'Swiss cheese' appearance on cross-sectional imaging, and although many will regress when antiretroviral therapy is commenced, some patients might require parotid surgery for cosmesis.

The parotid gland (tumours/other pathology)

7. A, D, E

As stated previously, most parotid gland tumours are benign and the pleomorphic adenoma is the most common benign tumour. Even for benign tumours, enucleation should be avoided. Pleomorphic adenomas have incomplete capsules and so-called pseudopodia (small extensions of disease under the microscope), which lead to high rates of recurrence unless formal excision with a cuff of tissue is undertaken. Almost all tumours of the parotid abut at least one branch of the facial nerve. Even in malignant lesions, however, if the nerve can be dissected off the tumour, no survival advantage has been shown from nerve sacrifice. The majority of such tumours will be treated with postoperative radiation therapy to address microscopic residual disease. Sialosis, or a benign enlargement of the parotid glands, can

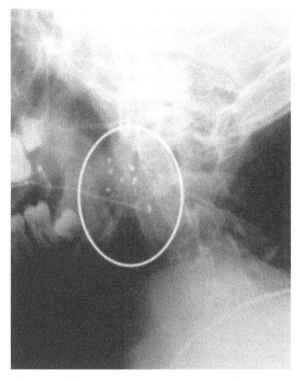

Figure 50.2 Characteristic snowstorm appearance of recurrent parotiditis of childhood.

be associated with malnutrition, drugs, or excess alcohol. Both Sjogrens syndrome and the 'benign lymphoepithelial lesion' of the parotid are associated with lymphoma. Surgery is often required to make a diagnosis in these patients.

Answers to extended matching questions

1. G Bacterial parotitis

Bacterial parotitis is classically seen in dehydrated patients **(Figure 50.3)**. It is not uncommon for elderly patients in care homes to become dehydrated and present in this manner. It can also be seen following surgery. Dehydration promotes salivary stasis and viscous secretions. Ascending infections from the oral cavity can then produce parotitis. Treatment generally consists of rehydration, taking care in patients who might have cardiac compromise and antibiotics. Abscess formation can occur, although this is rare. Ultrasound or cross-sectional imaging will confirm the presence of pus. Incision and drainage might be complicated by facial nerve injury, so in most cases antibiotics are used with milking of secretions from the parotid duct. If the patient's condition requires intervention, a low posterior incision is made and blunt dissection through the parotid tissue with an artery forcep into the abscess cavity may be performed. A dependent drain is then placed for 24–48 hours.

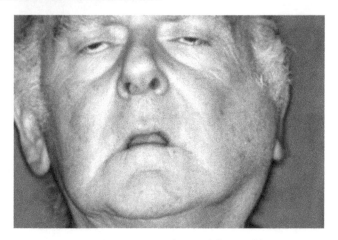

Figure 50.3   Acute bacterial parotitis.

2. B Minor salivary gland cancer

Many of the minor salivary glands are present at the junction of the hard and soft palate (**Figure 50.4**), and when removed surgically it often surprises the surgeon at the depth of the submucosa in this region (**Figure 50.5**). Most tumours of minor salivary glands are malignant, and if <1 cm they can be excised as both a diagnostic and therapeutic procedure. In lesions that are >1 cm however, incisional biopsy is indicated. Investigation of lesions in this area should delineate the locoregional extent of disease, with particular attention to destruction of the bone of the hard palate and presence of regional lymph nodes. Following diagnosis, excision and reconstruction will be required. Attempts should be made to prevent a through-and-through defect allowing communication between the mouth and nose. If this is required given the extent of disease, reconstructive options include rotation palata or temporalis flaps, vascularised free flaps and simple obturation with a dental appliance.

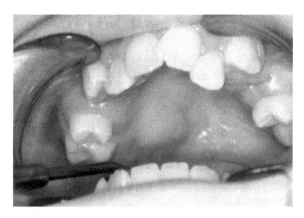

Figure 50.4   Mass at the junction of hard and soft palate.

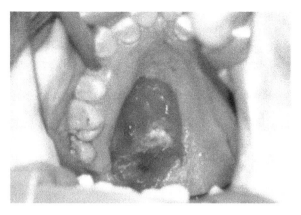

Figure 50.5 Submucosa dissected from perichondrium of the hard palate.

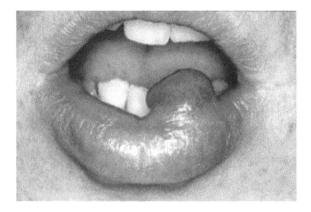

Figure 50.6 Mucus retention cyst.

3. F Mucus retention cyst

Mucus retention cysts are most commonly seen on the lower lip **(Figure 50.6)**. Although aspiration will lead to temporary resolution, excision with the affected minor gland should be undertaken to prevent recurrence. Lesions such as this on the upper lip can be seen but are more suspicious for malignancy.

4. D Mumps

Mumps tends to affect both sides symmetrically. There can also be involvement of the pancreas and testicles, so care must be taken to examine and investigate the patient appropriately. Although less common in the developed world following vaccination programmes, mumps is still seen and even in those considered vaccinated the condition can present. It might also present with unilateral symptoms; therefore, the clinician should be aware of the possibility. Management is expectant, although most clinicians do provide antibiotics to avoid secondary bacterial infection.

5. E Parotid gland cancer

Warning signs here include age, rapid increase in size and facial nerve involvement. Although most parotid gland masses are benign, parotid cancers are not uncommon due to the overall incidence of parotid masses. The first investigation should be a core biopsy or FNA. In addition, cross-sectional imaging will outline the extent of locoregional disease and screen for distant metastases. Primary therapy is surgical, and the clinician should assess the extent of disease for resectability. Particular attention should be paid to the relationship of the mass to the facial nerve. Involvement of the mastoid bone will require a lateral temporal bone resection with resection of the facial nerve to achieve macroscopically clear margins. In addition, adenoid cystic carcinoma has a propensity for perineural invasion, so postoperative therapy that will include radiation should be planned to include the skull base, to try and control microscopic disease extension.

6. A Pleomorphic adenoma

Most parotid masses are benign. FNA may yield a diagnostic sample, although in this case without any other worrying features, surgical resection with a cuff of normal tissue is indicated irrespective of the diagnosis. The majority of masses such as this will be adequately managed with superficial parotidectomy. Many clinicians now order cross-sectional imaging to confirm the position of the mass. The retromandibular vein can be seen on axial contrast-enhanced imaging and marks the junction of the superficial and deep lobes of the parotid. Although approaches are identical between total and superficial parotidectomy, the former puts the facial nerve at higher risk and the patient should be aware of this prior to surgery. Assuming surgery is successful and the mass is excised without rupture of the capsule, recurrence rates are low. In fact if recurrence occurs, it might not present for decades following surgery, so patients should be followed up over a long period. Controversy exists over the management of a ruptured pleomorphic adenoma. The rates of recurrence in this event are thought to be higher, although yet again clinical evidence of recurrence might not present for many years. Some authors advocate postoperative radiation to minimise the risk of recurrence, although side effects, including osteoradionecrosis of the temporal bone, are common. Many authors would consider close follow-up with revision surgery and postoperative radiation reserved only for those patient who do recur.

7. C Salivary calculus

Salivary calculi are most commonly seen in the submandibular duct. This is thought to be because the saliva is more viscous from this gland and that it drains against gravity. Also the duct crosses the lingual nerve, providing a potential area of compression, adding to salivary stasis. Most are radio opaque, and so can be seen without the need for specialist investigation **(Figure 50.7)**. Those stones anterior to the nerve can often be palpated through the mouth. An intraoral incision with a suture placed behind the stone, around the duct to prevent posterior migration, is the classic description. Following removal, the duct should be marsuplialised to prevent stricture on healing. For stones more posterior than this, damage to the lingual nerve is a risk and many authors would advocate submandibulectomy with identification of the stone in the duct from behind and removal. There is growing interest in noninvasive approaches to the salivary

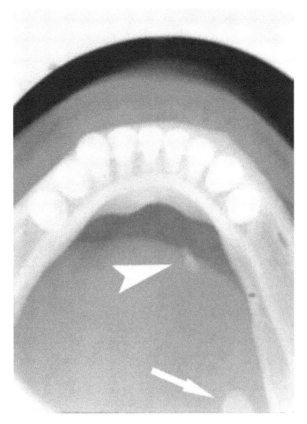

Figure 50.7   Lower occlusal film showing radio-opaque stones in the submandibular ducts (small stone at papilla = arrow head, larger posterior stone = arrow).

ducts. Sialendoscopy and interventional radiology techniques have made previously inaccessible stones targets for procedures that prevent the need for surgical incisions. The equipment and expertise required to perform such procedures, however, has limited its widespread application.

Breast and endocrine glands

51 The thyroid and parathyroid glands

Iain J Nixon, Nandini Rao and Pradip K Datta

Multiple choice questions

→ Surgical anatomy

1. **Which lymph nodes represent the primary echelon of drainage for the thyroid gland?**
A Retropharyngeal nodes.
B Jugulodigastric nodes.
C Central compartment nodes.
D Parapharyngeal nodes.
E Mediastinal nodes.

→ Hyperthyroidism

2. **Which of the following conditions is usually present with hyperthyroidism?**
A Graves' disease.
B Toxic nodule.
C Thyroid malignancy.
D De Quervain's thyroiditis.
E Toxic multinodular goitre.

→ Thyrotoxicosis

3. **What are the manifestations of thyrotoxicosis?**
A Irritability.
B Hair loss.
C Muscle weakness and wasting.
D Hyperkinesias.
E Heart failure.

→ Clinical features of hyperthyroidism

4. **Which of the following are associated with Graves' disease?**
A Pretibial myxoedema.
B Exposure keratitis.
C Optic neuropathy.
D Chemosis.
E Lymphoid hyperplasia.

→ Medical therapy for hyperthyroidism

5. **Which of the following are true regarding medical therapy for thyrotoxicosis?**
A Propranolol and nadolol reduce free T3 (fT3) and free T4 (fT4) levels.
B Antithyroid drugs most often cure thyrotoxicosis due to a toxic nodule.
C Carbimazole can be safely given in pregnancy and lactation.
D Agranulocytosis is an uncommon problem with antithyroid drugs.
E Patients with ophthalmopathy respond best to medical management.

→ Surgery for thyrotoxicosis

6. **Surgery is the preferred option of treatment in which of the following cases of thyrotoxicosis?**
A A diffuse toxic goitre.
B Severe manifestations of Graves' ophthalmopathy.
C Pregnant mothers not adequately controlled with medications.
D Relapse of Graves'.
E Presence of local compressive symptoms.

→ Radioiodine treatment

7. **Which of the following are indications for radioiodine treatment?**
A Relapsed Graves' disease.
B Thyrotoxicosis in young children.
C Multinodular goitre.
D Severe ophthalmopathy.
E Pregnancy and lactation.

→ Neonatal hypothyroidism

8. Which of the following are true in neonatal hypothyroidism?

A Endemic cretinism is due to iodine deficiency.

B Macroglossia is a clinical feature.

C Biochemical screening for hypothyroidism is carried out on all neonates in the United Kingdom.

D Radioactive iodine treatment is safe after the first trimester of pregnancy.

E Women on antithyroid drugs may give birth to a hypothyroid baby.

→ Myxoedema

9. Myxoedema can present as the following:

A Complete heart block.

B Ventricular tachycardia.

C Mania.

D Shortness of breath.

E Sepsis.

→ Biochemical features of hypothyroidism

10. Biochemically hypothyroidism can be associated with the following:

A Hyponatraemia.

B Hyperlipidaemia.

C Thyroid peroxidase (TPO) autoantibodies.

D Raised TSH.

E Low fT3 and fT4.

→ Classification of hypothyroidism

11. Hypothyroidism could be a presenting feature in which of the following conditions?

A Sarcoidosis.

B Pituitary lesions.

C Benzodiazepine treatment.

D Thyroiditis.

E Iodine deficiency.

→ Thyroid cancer

12. Which of the following statements regarding thyroid neoplasms are true?

A Papillary carcinoma is the most common.

B Men and women are equally affected.

C Thyroid cancer is most common after the age of 70 years.

D Medullary carcinoma originates from the C-cells.

E Anaplastic carcinoma is the least common.

→ Thyroglobulin

13. Which of the following statements regarding thyroglobulin are true?

A It is part of normal thyroid function tests.

B It is secreted only by cancerous cells.

C Autoantibodies may interfere with its levels.

D It is a sensitive marker of recurrence of differentiated thyroid cancer.

E Radioiodine treatment affects its concentration.

→ Papillary and follicular cancers

14. Which of the following statements are true?

A Lymph node metastasis is more common in follicular cancer than in papillary cancer.

B In papillary cancer, central lymph node metastases are associated with decreased survival.

C Distant metastasis is more common in the follicular variety.

D Hurthle cell carcinoma is a type of follicular cancer.

E Papillary carcinoma is usually slow-growing.

→ Differentiated thyroid cancers

15. Which of the following statements are true when a preoperative diagnosis of a differentiated thyroid cancer is made?

A Whole-body MRI or CT imaging is essential.

B Lobectomy is recommended for tumours less than 1 cm.

C Elective lateral nodal dissection should be performed.

D Routine central compartment node clearance is not essential for small tumours.

E The absence of a rising thyroglobulin excludes recurrence.

→ Medullary carcinoma of the thyroid

16. Which of the following statements regarding medullary thyroid cancers are true?

A It can present as multiple endocrine neoplasia.
B It is not TSH-dependent.
C It is associated with a poor prognosis.
D Diarrhoea is a common feature.
E High levels of calcitonin and carcinoembryonic antigen (CEA) are typical.

→ Primary hyperparathyroidism

17. Which of the following statements are true?

A Primary hyperparathyroidism is usually sporadic.
B Hypercalcaemia triggers the release of parathyroid hormone (PTH).
C Familial hyperparathyroidism commonly presents as an adenoma.
D Familial hyperparathyroidism is mostly sporadic.
E Hyperparathyroidism can be associated with a pituitary adenoma.

→ Calcium

18. Which of the following suggest a biochemical diagnosis of primary hyperparathyroidism?

A Raised ionised calcium and suppressed PTH levels.
B Raised total calcium and elevated PTH levels.
C Low serum phosphate levels.
D Low urine calcium level.
E Raised ionised calcium and elevated PTH levels.

→ Hypercalcaemia

19. Which of the following are associated with hypercalcaemia?

A Thyrotoxicosis.
B Chronic renal failure (CRF).
C Familial hypocalciuric hypercalcaemia (FHH).
D Sarcoidosis.
E Milk alkali syndrome.

→ Parathyroidectomy

20. Which of the following are operative indications for primary hyperparathyroidism?

A Renal stones.
B Low bone density.
C Renal impairment.
D Serum calcium of 2.75.
E Young age.

→ Primary hyperparathyroidism

21. Regarding operation for primary hyperparathyroidism, which of the following statements are correct?

A Permanent hypoparathyroidism is likely.
B PTH can be measured intraoperatively.
C Recurrent laryngeal nerve damage can occur in about 5%–7% of cases.
D Endoscopic technique is the most favoured operative mode.
E Gamma probes can be used for exploratory purposes.

→ Multiple endocrine neoplasia

22. A 60-year-old retired nurse presents with weight loss, fainting episodes and tiredness. A blood glucose performed is 2.5 mmol/L. An insulinoma is suspected. What are the appropriate tests?

A A short synacthen test.
B Insulin levels.
C C-peptide levels.
D A 24-hour fast.
E All of the above.

→ Imaging and the parathyroid

23. Which of the following statements are true regarding imaging of the parathyroid gland?

A High-frequency ultrasound can identify nearly 75% of enlarged glands.
B Technetium-99m-labelled sestamibi isotope (MIBI) scan identifies around 90% of enlarged glands.
C Single photon emission computed tomography (SPECT) scan can influence surgical approach.

D CT and MRI must be undertaken prior to first-time neck exploration.

E Adenomas weighing less than 500 mg show reduced concordance with imaging.

→ Operative strategies for the parathyroid

24. **Which of the following statements are true regarding operative strategies for the parathyroid?**

A In a conventional approach, a transverse collar incision is made.

B In a targeted approach, a 2–3-cm incision is made over the site of the adenoma.

C In patients with four-gland disease, transcervical thymectomy is not recommended.

D In multiple endocrine neoplasia type 1 (MEN-1), total parathyroidectomy reduces the risk of recurrence.

E Preoperative imaging can identify nearly 10% of patients with mediastinal adenoma.

→ Hypoparathyroidism

25. **Which of the following statements are correct?**

A Serum calcium must be checked within 24 hours of total thyroidectomy.

B Serum calcium levels below 1.9 mmol/L can pose a medical emergency.

C Chvostek's sign is suggestive of hypercalcaemia.

D DiGeorge syndrome is a medical cause of hypoparathyroidism.

E Cardiac arrhythmias can occur during an episode of hypocalcaemia.

→ Management of hypercalcaemia

26. **Which of the following statements are true regarding medical management of primary hyperparathyroidism?**

A Use of diuretics could reduce serum calcium levels by increasing their excretion via the kidneys.

B Cinacalcet is a bisphosphonate used to reduce calcium levels.

C Palmidronate is a bisphosphonate used to reduce calcium levels.

D Intravenous saline is the first line of management in hypercalcaemia.

E Serum calcium over 3.5 mmol/L is a medical emergency.

Extended matching questions

→ Causes of hypercalcaemia and hypocalcaemia

Diagnoses

1 Dehydration
2 FHH
3 Hypoparathyroidism
4 Primary hyperparathyroidism
5 Vitamin D deficiency

Match the diagnoses with the clinical scenarios that follow:

Clinical scenarios

A A 70-year-old man presents with constipation and confusion. His serum calcium is 3.7 mmol/L and his phosphate is 0.5 mmol/L.

B A 40-year-old banker attends a well-man clinic. His serum calcium is 2.9 mmol/L and his phosphate is 0.8 mmol/L. His PTH levels are 9 pmol/L. The urine calcium creatinine ratio is very low.

C An elderly man is recovering from a hernia repair. His bloods are as follows: urea 10.7 mmol/L, creatinine 84 µmol/L and calcium 3.20 mmol/L.

D A young woman underwent a thyroidectomy for a large multinodular goitre. 8 hours after the operation, she developed tingling and numbness around her mouth.

E An elderly woman who is mostly housebound was admitted following a hip fracture. Her serum calcium is 1.8 mmol/L, phosphate is 0.7 mmol/L and serum alkaline phosphatase is 640 IU/L.

Hyperthyroidism

Diagnoses

1 Graves' disease
2 Human chorionic gonadotrophin (HCG) effect
3 Sick euthyroid disease
4 Thyrotoxicosis
5 Toxic nodule

Reference values for thyroid function tests (TFTs) are as follows:

TSH 0.5 – 4 mIU/L
fT3 3.5 – 6.5 pmol/L
fT4 10 – 23 pmol/L

Match the diagnoses with the clinical scenarios that follow:

Clinical scenarios

A An elderly woman presents with sweating and confusion. Her biochemistry is as follows: TSH < 0.1 mIU/L; fT3, 15.8 pmol/L; and fT4, 1.0 pmol/L.

B A 10-week pregnant woman has severe vomiting. Her TFTs are as follows: TSH, 0.02 mIU/L; T3, 5.2 pmol/L; and T4, 11 pmol/L.

C A middle-aged man is in ITU following emergency laparotomy for a bleeding ulcer. His TFTs are as follows: TSH < 0.01 mIU/L; T3, 2.0 pmol/L; T4, 0.5 pml/L.

D A 22-year-old woman with a smooth goitre presents with sweating and weight loss. Her TFTs are as follows: TSH, 0.01 mIU/L; T3, 8.0 pmol/L; and T4, 41 pmol/L.

Hypothyroidism

Diagnoses

1 Amiodarone-induced thyroid disease
2 Autoimmune thyroiditis
3 Heterophil antibodies interference
4 Myxoedema
5 TSH-secreting adenomas (TSHoma)

Match the diagnoses with the clinical scenarios that follow:

Clinical scenarios

A An elderly woman presets to A&E with third-degree heart block. She is overweight and has dry skin and slow reflexes.

B A 44-year-old man underwent chemical cardioversion for atrial fibrillation (AF). His baseline TFTs were normal. He is now hypothyroid.

C A general practitioner (GP) is having difficulty trying to treat a 62-year-old woman for hypothyroidism. Despite thyroxine dosage of 200 µg, her thyroid functions are suggestive of hypothyroidism.

D A young woman with rheumatoid arthritis has discordant TFTs, with TSH, fT3 and fT4 all elevated.

E A 40-year-old woman presents with hypothyroidism and elevated TPO antibodies.

→ Goitre

Diagnoses

1 Follicular carcinoma of the thyroid
2 Graves' disease.
3 Multinodular goitre
4 Toxic nodule

Match the diagnoses with the clinical scenarios that follow:

Clinical scenarios

A A middle-aged woman presents with a long-standing goitre. She is clinically euthyroid.

B A young woman presents with a firm enlarged goitre with bruit. She complains of symptoms suggestive of hyperthyroidism.

C A 60-year-old presents with a firm thyroid nodule that is hot on isotope scanning.

D A 55-year-old presents with thyroid nodule and haemoptysis.

→ Thyroid cancers

Diagnoses

A Anaplastic carcinoma
B Lymphoma
C Medullary Carcinoma
D Papillary Carcinoma

Match the diagnoses with the clinical scenarios that follow:

Clinical scenarios

A An 82-year-old woman presents with a thyroid nodule, weight loss, backache and hypercalcaemia.

B An elderly woman with previous history of Hashimoto's thyroiditis presents with an irregular, hard nodule in her right thyroid lobe.

C A 12-year-old boy presents with a nodule and regional lymph node enlargement.

D A 28-year-old has a parathyroid adenoma and elevated levels of calcitonin.

→ Hyper- and hypoparathyroidism

Diagnoses

1 Hypopararthyroidism
2 Primary hypoparathyroidism
3 Secondary hyperparathyroidism
4 Tertiary hyperparathyroidism
5 Tetany

Clinical features

A A 35-year-old man complains of vague abdominal pains associated with bone pains and periodical nausea. He was on dialysis since the age of 22 for 10 years, after which he received a renal transplant which has been successful so far. On examination he has a fistula in his forearm and a transverse lower abdominal scar.

B A 46-year-old woman has been readmitted to the surgical unit complaining of numbness around her mouth with paraesthesia and numbness in her fingers. She has had a few episodes of muscle spasms in her forearms. One week ago she underwent total thyroidectomy with bilateral lymph node dissection for papillary thyroid carcinoma.

C A 58-year-old man complains of a general feeling of ill health for several months for which he did not bother to seek medical advice. Recently, however, he has developed abdominal pain radiating to the back. Three years ago he had a proved attack of right ureteric colic for which no further treatment was necessary after the stone passed spontaneously. His GP performed routine blood tests, which were as follows:

Hb	13.2 g/dL	Na	140 mmol/L
MCV	86 fl	K	4.8 mmol/L
MCH	30 pg	Cl	102 mmol/L
MCHC 35 g/dL		HCO$_3$	26 mmol/L
		calcium	2.9 mmol/L
		Phos	0.5 mmol/L

D A 52-year-old woman complains of pain in the bones of her hands and feet, pruritis and muscle weakness resulting in reduced mobility. This has become worse recently. She has suffered from chronic renal failure for which she has been on haemodialysis for 5 years.

E A 55-year-old man with a long history of duodenal ulcer presents with intermittent projectile vomiting for 4 weeks. The vomitus contains stale food and is nonbilious. He is dehydrated, with a visible gastric peristalsis and succussion splash. His blood results are the following:

Hb	16 g/dL
WCC	9 x 10^9/L
Na	130 mmol/L
K	2.8 mmol/L
Cl	92 mmol/L
Urea	14 mmol/L
Cr	155 µmol/L
pH	7.5
PCO$_2$	6.8 kPa
PO$_2$	10.2 kPa
HCO$_3$	34 mmol/L

Answers to multiple choice questions

→ Surgical anatomy

1. C

The thyroid gland has a rich lymphatic supply and drains primarily to the central compartment or level VI nodes. These can be further subdivided in to prelaryngeal (Delphian nodes), pretracheal and paratracheal regions. Although most lesions of the thyroid drain to these regions, occasionally drainage from the upper poles can be to the parapharyngeal region. Papillary thyroid cancer (the most common malignancy of the thyroid) metastasises often and early, so many nodes in central and lateral compartments of the neck may be involved, although this is not always obvious on clinical examination or even imaging. Interestingly, even though micrometastases are present in up to 40% of patients considered free of disease, micrometastases rarely progress to cause clinical recurrence and therefore elective neck dissection is not routinely advocated.

→ Hyperthyroidism

2. A, B, D, E

Graves' disease is a common autoimmune condition that usually occurs in young women and is associated with eye signs. Abnormal TSH receptor antibodies produce a disproportionate and prolonged effect. It can be associated with other autoimmune conditions such as Addison's disease, type 1 diabetes, pernicious anaemia and coeliac disease. Toxic nodular goitre is often seen in middle age or in the elderly and is rarely associated with eye signs. A solitary toxic nodule is often autonomous and its hypertrophy or hyperplasia is not associated with TSH receptor antibodies.

Thyroid cancer very rarely presents as hyperthyroidism. Thyroid inflammation, especially postpartum, can cause hyperthyroidism.

→ Thyrotoxicosis

3. A, B, C, D, E

Thyrotoxicosis is characterised by the clinical, physiological and biochemical changes that result when tissue is exposed to excess thyroid hormone. It can present with symptoms of hyperactivity, insomnia and heat intolerance, weight loss with increased appetite, palpitations and fatigue. The signs often are fine tremor, warm moist skin, proptosis palmar erythema, onycholysis, hair loss, high output heart failure and, rarely, periodic paralysis, which is associated with hypokalaemia.

→ Clinical features of hyperthyroidism

4. A, B, C, D, E

The exophthalmos in thyroid eye disease is due to retrobulbar infiltration of tissue with fluid and round cells. Oedema of the eyelids and conjunctival injection might be worsened by compression of ophthalmic veins. Urgent action (orbital decompression) is necessary in the case of corneal ulceration, congestive ophthalmopathy, or optic neuropathy. Treatment with steroids and orbital radiotherapy is sometimes necessary. Thyroid dermopathy is caused by deposition of hyaluronidase in the dermis and cutis.

→ Medical therapy for hyperthyroidism

5. D

Carbimazole (first drug of choice) and propylthiouracil (given during pregnancy and lactation) are the common antithyroid drugs used; 30%–40% of patients remain euthyroid 10 years after discontinuation of therapy. However, rarely, relapses are corrected with medication.

Large goitres, younger patients and very elevated fT3 and fT4 rarely benefit from medical management. A toxic nodule is autonomous in nature and will relapse if medications are stopped. Agranulocytosis occurs in only 0.1%–0.5% of patients on antithyroid drugs. Beta-blockers reduce the adrenergic effects of thyroxine in peripheral tissue.

→ Surgery for thyrotoxicosis

6. A, B, C, D, E

Cure can be offered by surgery, reducing the mass of overactive tissue. However, there is a risk of permanent hypothyroidism in total thyroidectomy and recurrence of toxicity in subtotal resections. Recurrence can also occur in 5% of cases if less than a total thyroidectomy has been performed. Parathyroid insufficiency occurs in <5% of cases undergoing surgery. The following are also indications for surgery: presence of suspicious thyroid nodule by FNAC, pregnant women inadequately controlled on medications and large thyroid glands with relatively low radioiodine uptake.

→ Radioiodine treatment

7. A, C

Radioiodine treatment requires the administration of enough radioiodine to achieve normal thyroid status. Hypothyroidism occurs in 15%–20% at 2 years. It is contraindicated in young children and pregnant and lactating mothers. It is the definitive choice of treatment in cases of relapsed Graves' disease and in multinodular goitre and adenomas.

→ Neonatal hypothyroidism

8. A, B, C, E

Cretinism is a consequence of inadequate thyroid hormone production during the foetal and early neonatal periods. Endemic cretinism is due to dietary deficiency, whereas sporadic cases are due to inborn error of thyroid metabolism or complete or partial agenesis of the gland. Immediate diagnosis and treatment are essential to prevent long-term physical and mental developmental delay. In hyperthyroid pregnant women, drugs such as propylthiouracil are preferred as they limit ability to induce hypothyroidism in the foetus.

→ Myxoedema

9. A, B, C, D, E

Myxoedema is associated with accentuated signs and symptoms of hypothyroidism. There is often a malar flush, yellow tinge to the skin and altered mental state. It can present as bradycardia and hypothermia with its associated tachy- and bradyarrhythmias. Heart failure and infections are associated with increased mortality.

→ Biochemical features of hypothyroidism

10. A, B, C, D, E

Biochemically, hypothyroidism is characterised by low free t3 and free t4 hormones. As a compensatory attempt, the pituitary secretes TSH, which is elevated. It can present as hyponatraemia and raised total cholesterol and LDL cholesterol.

→ Classification of hypothyroidism

11. A, B, D, E

Hypothyroidism can be classified as the following: goitrous (iodine deficiency, Hashimoto's thyroiditis, or drugs such as lithium, amiodarone, iodides and aminosalicylic acid); nongoitrous (atrophic thyroiditis, post-radiation); pituitary-related (panhypopituitarism); neoplastic; infiltrative (sarcoidosis); or infective (rare).

→ Thyroid cancer

12. A, D, E

Depending on the cells of origin, thyroid cancers can be classified as originating from:

- Follicular cells (papillary/follicular/Hurthle cell/anaplastic carcinomas)
- Lymphocytes – lymphoma
- C-cells – medullary carcinoma.
- Mesenchymal cells (sarcoma which is very rare)

The relative incidence of primary malignant tumour of the thyroid cancer is as follows: papillary cancer, 80%; follicular or Hurthle cell carcinoma, 10%; the remainder are medullary cancers and other malignancies including lymphoma. The annual incidence of thyroid cancer is increasing rapidly. This is thought to be due to rising use of imaging rather than a true increase in incidence of disease. The female:male sex ratio of differentiated thyroid cancer is 3:1. It is most common in adults ages 40–50. Anaplastic carcinoma presents in older patients and might be due to de-differentiation of prior differentiated thyroid cancer. Medullary carcinoma may present at any age, with familial cases (around 25% overall) sometimes presenting in childhood and being prevented with prophylactic thyroidectomy.

→ Thyroglobulin

13. C, D, E

Thyroglobulin is secreted by normal thyroid tissue and differentiated thyroid cancer cells. It can be a sensitive marker of recurrence of differentiated thyroid cancer. The aim of therapy for high-risk differentiated thyroid cancer is to render the patient without detectable thyroglobulin. To achieve this, total thyroidectomy and appropriate neck dissection should be performed. Postoperative radioactive iodine therapy will then be used to destroy microscopic deposits of normal and malignant thyroid tissue. Thyroglobulin can then be used as an effective tumour marker, particularly in the absence of autoantibodies, which can interfere. For lower-risk patients, lobectomy alone will be appropriate. In this setting thyroglobulin never becomes undetectable, but trends can be followed to indicate possible recurrence.

→ Papillary and follicular cancers

14. C, D, E

Compared with most cancers, the prognosis in differentiated thyroid cancers is excellent. Papillary cancers are encapsulated and slow-growing but do spread to regional nodes often and early. They are confined to the neck in >95% of cases. Despite the rates of metastasis, this does not predict survival. Indeed, early studies suggested that regional metastases might actually be protective. Experience, however, has shown that this was due to the fact that young patients tend to present with neck nodes, and age is the strongest predictor of all. Central neck metastases do not predict survival. Lateral neck metastases, however, particularly in older patients, are more predictive. Follicular cancer and the associated Hurthle cell carcinoma arise from thyroid epithelium. They more commonly spread via the haematogenous route than papillary cancers.

→ Differentiated thyroid cancers

15. B, D

This is a controversial subject. When a preoperative diagnosis has been made, the patient should have ultrasound screening of the neck at least. If there is widespread nodal metastases, cross-sectional imaging is encouraged to visualise the extent of disease and in particular the mediastinum, which is poorly seen on ultrasound. Small, low-risk tumours (<1 cm) are well treated by lobectomy alone. Most international guidelines recommend total thyroidectomy if tumours are >1 cm or have any risk factors such as nodal metastases. Although papillary cancers routinely metastasise to the central and lateral neck, if these metastases are occult, both the central and lateral neck can be observed safely. Some authors recommend elective central neck dissection for larger or more aggressive tumours; however, few support elective lateral neck dissection due to the high rates of morbidity. Although a rising thyroglobulin indicates disease recurrence, if a tumour de-differentiates, it will stop producing thyroglobulin, so an absence of a rise does not exclude recurrent disease.

Medullary carcinoma of the thyroid

16. A, B, D, E
Medullary carcinoma refers to tumours of the parafollicular C cells and as such is not TSH-dependent. Surgery is the only primary therapy, as the tumour cells do not concentrate iodine. Instead of thyroglobulin, it is characterised by high levels of serum calcitonin and CEA. Diarrhoea is present in 30% of cases and might be due to 5-hydroxytryptamine produced by tumour cells. This is a particular problem in end-stage disease. Like many endocrine neoplasms, the progression of disease may be slow. It can occur with phaechromocytoma and hyperparathyroidism in a syndrome called multiple endocrine neoplasia type 2A (MEN 2A).

Primary hyperparathyroidism

17. A, E
The prevalence of primary hyperparathyroidism increases with advancing age. Most cases are sporadic. Nearly 85% of these patients have an adenoma; 13% have hyperplasia of the glands; and a very small proportion have multiple adenomas or cancer.

Familial hyperparathyroidism is genetically determined and associated with MEN-1 (primary hyperparathyroidism, pituitary adenoma and pancreatic tumours such as insulinoma, gastrinoma and VIPoma) and MEN 2 (primary hyperparathyroidism, medullary carcinoma of thyroid and phaeochromocytoma). The familial variety can also exist as isolated hyperparathyroidism and as hyperplasia.

Calcium

18. B, C, D, E
Hypercalcaemia normally suppresses the release of PTH by the parathyroid gland. Calcium circulates in the plasma mostly bound to albumin; however, it is the ionised or free calcium that is biologically active. Measurement of ionised calcium is tedious and albumin-adjusted (corrected) calcium is just as good. Hyperparathyroidism is associated with raised serum calcium, low serum phosphate and hypercalciuria.

Hypercalcaemia

19. A, B, C, D, E
Chronic renal failure is associated with vitamin D deficiency and hypocalcaemia initially; these result in stimulation of the parathyroid gland and release of PTH, causing secondary hyperparathyroidism. However, long-standing stimulation of the parathyroid results in autonomous secretion of PTH by the gland, causing tertiary hyperparathyroidism. Granulomatous conditions such as tuberculosis and sarcoidosis cause hypercalcaemia.

Parathyroidectomy

20. A, B, C, E
Surgery is the only curative option for this condition. Medical therapy such as calcium receptor agonists and bisphosphonate therapy are helpful along with eradication of drugs that induce hypercalcaemia (diuretics, lithium). Surgery is indicated in the presence

of hypercalcaemia with serum calcium over 2.9 mmol/L (especially in the presence of symptoms), presence of falling bone density, or presence of osteoporosis and renal stone disease or renal impairment.

Primary hyperparathyroidism

21. A, B, E

Preoperative discussion for a parathyroidectomy must include the possibility of recurrent laryngeal nerve injury (1%), postoperative haemorrhage (1%) and recurrent and permanent hypoparathyroidism. PTH has a very short half-life and will disappear within a few minutes of excision of the gland. High levels, despite excision, suggest residual gland. PTH levels are measured in an operative setting to guide the surgeon if the gland has been completely removed. A conventional thyroidectomy incision is most frequently used. A gamma probe can be used to guide exploration following preoperative injection of MIBI.

Multiple endocrine neoplasia

22. B, C, D

An insulinoma is a tumour that originates from the pancreas; it is biochemically confirmed by demonstrating hyperinsulinaemia despite hypoglycaemia with elevated levels of proinsulin and C-peptide. It is often very difficult to diagnose, as imaging with MRI may not always pick up these small lesions (<4 mm). A supervised 24 h fast may be necessary. Insulinoma can be a part of MEN associated with hyperparathyroidism and pituitary adenoma (type 1) and medullary carcinoma (type 2). Assessment of bone profile, PTH levels, and genetic testing are other tests required.

Imaging and the parathyroid

23. A, C, E

High-frequency ultrasound is noninvasive and can identify 75% of enlarged glands. However, despite good resolution it has poor penetrance and cannot visualise the mediastinum. Technetium-99m-labelled sestamibi isotope scans can identify 75% of glands and the area scanned must include the mediastinum to detect ectopic glands. SPECT scan gives a three-dimensional approach and can influence surgical approach.

Operative strategies for the parathyroid

24. A, B, D

Confident preoperative localisation permits a 2–3-cm incision located over the site of the adenoma. This is placed to permit extension to a formal bilateral exploration incision if the imaging is suboptimal. In a conventional approach, the patient is positioned in reverse Trendelenburg and a transverse incision is made, the subplatysmal plane is developed superiorly and inferiorly and the deep cervical fascia incised. In four-gland disease, a transcervical thymectomy is considered to reduce the risk of recurrence or recurrent primary hyperparathyroidism. Preoperative imaging identifies around 1% of patients with a mediastinal adenoma.

Hypoparathyroidism

25. A, B, D, E

Signs and symptoms of hypocalcaemia are related to the duration and level of hypocalcaemia. It could range from mild circumoral and digital numbness to tetany with carpopedal spasm, neuromuscular excitability, cardiac arrhythmias and seizures. Serum calcium below 1.90 must be treated as an emergency and 10-mL or 10% calcium gluconate must be given IVI slowly;

10% magnesium infusion is also considered. In milder cases, 1 g of oral calcium can be given three or four times daily.

→ Management of hypercalcaemia

26. C, D, E
Intravenous saline is first-line therapy to correct dehydration. Medical management of primary hyperparathyroidism involves a low-calcium diet and withdrawal of drugs that aggravate hypercalcaemia, such as diuretics and lithium. Cinacalcet is a calcium receptor agonist and reduces calcium levels. Bisphosphonates such as palmidronate are also useful.

Answers to extended matching questions

→ Causes of hypercalcaemia and hypocalcaemia

1. C Dehydration
Dehydration is a very common cause for mild hypercalcaemia.

2. B Familial hypocalciuric hypocalcaemia
Familial hypocalciuric hypocalcaemia is another differential for primary hyperparathyroidism. It causes the same biochemical features as primary hyperparathyroidism apart from low urinary calcium excretion. Most patients are asymptomatic and the problem is in the calcium-sensing receptors in the parathyroid gland.

3. D Hypoparathyroidism
Serum calcium levels can come down when the parathyroid glands are inadvertently removed. Levels must always be checked within 24 hours of any thyroid surgery.

4. A Primary hyperparathyroidism
Primary hyperparathyroidism is associated with raised serum calcium and low phosphate levels. The PTH levels are not suppressed despite the hypercalcaemia.

5. E Vitamin D deficiency
Vitamin D deficiency is common in housebound and institutionalised individuals. It causes hypocalcaemia and hypophosphataemia in severe cases. Alkaline phosphatase is elevated in osteomalacia. However, recent fracture could also raise the ALP levels.

→ Hyperthyroidism

1. D Graves' disease
Graves' disease is an autoimmune condition characterised by a smooth goitre, strong family history and female preponderance.

2. B Human chorionic gonadotrophin (HCG) effect
Pregnancy can be associated with hyperthyroidism. Beta-HCG increases exponentially in early pregnancy. This causes suppression of TSH. The thyroid-binding globulin levels are altered as well.

3. C Sick euthyroid disease
Thyroid functions are not helpful in the immediate period after an acute illness or stress. Sick euthyroid disease causes suppression of TSH and free thyroid hormones.

4. A Thyrotoxicosis
Thyrotoxicosis can present with all features of thyroid excess. Due to rapid conversion of T4 to T3, T4 levels are often low.

→ Hypothyroidism

1. B Amiodarone-induced thyroid disease
Amiodarone is a popular antiarrhythmic. It contains a very high iodine load, however, and can cause both overactivation and understimulation of the thyroid gland.

2. E Autoimmune thyroiditis
Thyroid peroxidase antibodies (TPO) are associated with autoimmune hypothyroidism.

3. D Heterophil antibodies interference
Autoantibodies, especially found in rheumatoid arthritis, can interfere in the fT4 levels and cause discordant TFTs. They can be corrected by performing tests on another analyser or the use of heterophil-blocking antibodies.

4. A Myxoedema
Myxoedema can present with heart block, hypothermia and sometimes coma.

5. C TSH-secreting adenomas (TSHoma)
TSHoma is a rare tumour from the anterior pituitary secreting TSH. Thyroid hormone resistance is another cause of elevated TSH levels, despite adequate thyroxine replacement.

→ Goitre

1. D Follicular carcinoma of the thyroid
Follicular carcinoma of the thyroid is the second most common after papillary carcinoma. It arises later in life and is prone to bloodborne metastasis. Secondaries to the lung are the most common cause of death.

2. B Graves' disease
Graves' disease is an autoimmune disease due to the presence of TSH receptor antibodies. Exophthalmos, diffuse goitre with a bruit with clinical and biochemical hyperthyroidism, is characteristic.

3. A Multinodular goitre
Multinodular goitre is due to relative iodine deficiency. It is long-standing. FNAC should be undertaken if there is a doubt about the diagnosis.

4. C Toxic nodule
Solitary toxic nodule could represent a single active nodule in a multimodal goitre, thyroid adenoma (scan shows normal or decreased uptake), or toxic adenoma (increased uptake with hyperthyroid features).

→ Thyroid cancers

1. A Anaplastic carcinoma
Anaplastic carcinoma tends to occur in the elderly and is poorly differentiated and one of the most aggressive tumours in humans.

2. B Lymphoma
Lymphoma can arise in a gland affected by Hashimoto's thyroiditis.

3. D Medullary carcinoma
Medullary carcinoma of the thyroid can form part of the MEN syndrome. It occurs in young adults and carries a good prognosis. These carcinomas secrete calcitonin from the parafollicular cells.

4. C Papillary carcinoma
Papillary thyroid cancers are the most common thyroid cancer in children and adults. They are well differentiated and commonly associated with metastasis to the regional lymph nodes.

Hyper- and hypoparathyroidism

1. B Hypoparathyroidism

This patient's early symptoms of tetany are from hypocalcaemia caused by hypoparathyroidism from inadvertent damage to the parathyroid glands. This may be due to injury, removal, or ischaemia during major neck surgery. The level of calcium at which symptoms of tetany develop can vary and is unpredictable.

This is a medical emergency, particularly if the level is less than 1.9 mmol/IL An intravenous drip of 10% calcium gluconate might be necessary. This is supplemented by oral calcium and Vitamin D; magnesium supplements may also be required. If the hypocalcaemic symptoms are minimal with the serum level in the region of 2.0 mmol/L, oral calcium supplements of 1 g in divided doses is given. Less than 1% of patients undergoing such surgery will have such a complication permanently.

The normal serum calcium is 2.2 to 2.6 mmol/L. Of the total calcium in the body, 50% is free ionised; of the rest 40% is bound to plasma proteins, whilst the remainder is bound with anions – citrate, phosphate and sulphate.

When an abnormal serum calcium level is obtained from the laboratory, it is important to estimate the corrected serum calcium level, particularly in the presence of hypoalbuminaemia where the corrected serum calcium will be higher.

The regulation of calcium homeostasis is the result of an interplay between parathormone (PTH) secreted by the parathyroids, the kidneys, the absorption of Vitamin D and calcitonin secreted by the parafollicular 'C' cells of the thyroid. This is explained in **Figure 51.1**. When there is a drop in serum calcium, there is increased secretion of PTH acting in the form of a feedback mechanism as shown in **Figure 51.2**. PTH acts in concert with 1,25- dihydroxycholecalciferol (1,25-DHCC, 1,25 vitamin D) and calcitonin on kidney and gut to maintain a constant blood-ionised calcium, which is necessary for nerve and muscle excitability and blood coagulation. PTH has a greater role in the regulation of serum calcium than calcitonin.

The control of serum calcium by PTH is explained in **Figure 51.3**. The role of calcitonin is to cause a reduction in serum calcium and is explained in **Figure 51.4**. Serum calcium regulation is also linked to plasma phosphate (PO) levels. The normal PO level is 0.8 to 1.4 mmol/L; PTH

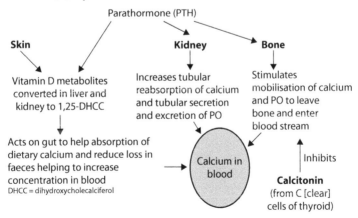

Figure 51.1   Role of parathormone in calcium metabolism.

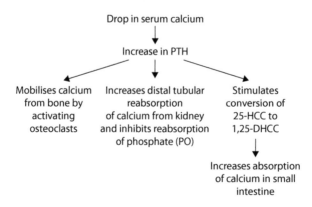

Figure 51.2 Feedback mechanism between PTH and drop in serum calcium.

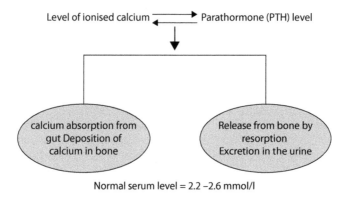

Normal serum level = 2.2 –2.6 mmol/l

Figure 51.3 Control of serum calcium by parathormone.

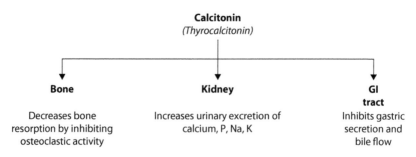

Figure 51.4 Role of calcitonin in calcium metabolism.

increases the excretion of PO while increasing renal tubular reabsorption of calcium. Variations in plasma PO levels affect serum calcium. In renal failure, there is increase in plasma PO that stimulates the parathyroids causing secondary hyperparathyroidism.

2. C Primary hyperparathyroidism.

Primary hyperparathyroidism, a condition resulting from an excessive secretion of PTH, is caused by a solitary parathyroid adenoma in 85% of patients; in 13%–14%, the cause might be multiglandular hyperplasia, whilst the remainder might be due to a carcinoma or multiple adenomas. The most common presentation of primary hyperparathyroidism from an adenoma is when it is discovered in an 'asymptomatic' patient who undergoes a routine biochemical screening. When hypercalcaemia is found routinely and the cause is an adenoma and it is removed, patients admit to a huge sense of well being. In the past they had ascribed their insidious symptoms to ageing. Thus, strictly speaking, in retrospect the patient was not 'asymptomatic' but had symptoms that could not be pinpointed. Women are more often affected. It is said that 1% of the adult population is found to have hypercalcaemia on routine biochemical screening.

The condition may be familial when it is a part of multiple endocrine neoplasia (MEN) syndrome. When symptomatic, the clinical features reflect hypercalcaemia and hypophosphataemia: bone pain with x-ray changes in the hands (osteitis fibrosa cystica), skull (pepper-pot skull) and abdominal pain from peptic ulcer, recurrent pancreatitis and constipation. In almost one-third of patients there might be psychiatric symptoms. Renal disease in the form of nephrocalcinosis **(Figure 51.5)** and recurrent ureteric colic may be a presentation when a raised serum calcium alerts one to the diagnosis. These protean manifestations **(Figure 51.6)** have been traditionally summarised as 'stones, bones, psychic moans and abdominal groans', although such a florid presentation is rarely seen. Rarely, patients might present as a metabolic emergency due to acute hyperparathyroid hypercalcaemic crisis. The patient's corrected serum calcium should be carried out. For this the serum albumin is done (see previous section). The next step is to do the serum PTH. Elevated

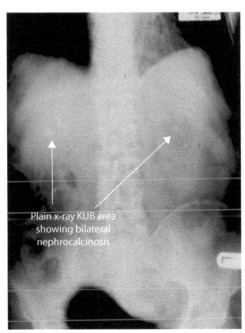

Figure 51.5 Plain x-ray KUB (kidney, ureter, bladder) area showing bilateral nephrocalcinosis.

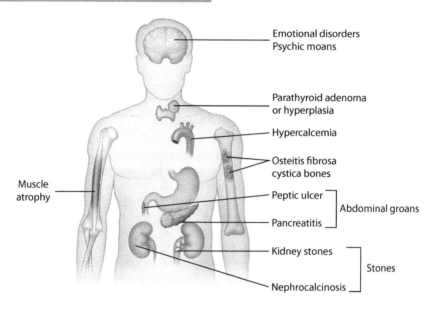

Figure 51.6 Clinical features of primary hyperparathyroidism.

levels of PTH with hypercalcaemia and hypophosphataemia and increased excretion of calcium in the urine confirms a diagnosis of primary hyperparathyroidism.

The next step is to localise the site of the adenoma. This is done by technetium-99 m labelled sestamibi scan and ultrasound to include the mediastinum to exclude an adenoma in an ectopic gland. In primary hyperparathyroidism, systematic bilateral neck exploration is done in cases of parathyroid hyperplasia where removal of three-and-a half glands is carried out with the remaining gland being marked with a metal clip or nonabsorbable suture or transplanted into the forearm. However, targeted parathyriodectomy through a small unilateral incision for an adenoma is the procedure of choice in the vast majority as solitary adenoma is the most common cause of primary hyperparathyroidism.

3. D Secondary hyperparathyroidism
The main cause for secondary hyperparathyroidism is chronic renal failure (CRF), which is the cause in this patient. The other causes are chronic hypocalcaemia from vitamin D deficiency and malabsorption. The following can occur as a result of CRF:

- Vitamin D is not converted into 1,25 Dihydroxycholecalciferol, which in turn inhibits absorption of calcium in the gut.
- Reduced intestinal calcium absorption results in low-serum calcium and increased-serum PO due to failure of the kidney to excrete PO.
- Hyperphosphtaemia and hypocalcaemia is present causing increased PTH secretion, thus producing secondary hyperparathyroidism.

Such patients present with bone pain, muscle weakness and ectopic calcification in muscles of limbs or chest wall.

This patient's serum calcium will be low or at the lower limit of normal. The management is medical initially with phosphate restriction and calcium and vitamin D supplementation. Hyperparathyroidism is usually due to multiple gland disease, which requires total parathyroidectomy. The causes of hypercalcaemia are shown in **Figure 51.7**.

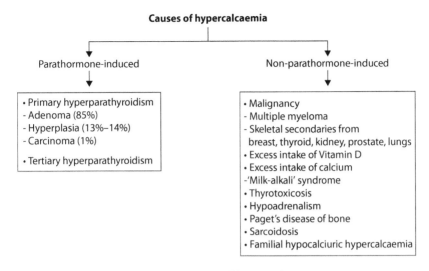

Figure 51.7   Causes of hypercalcaemia.

4. A Tertiary hyperparathyroidism

Tertiary hyperparathyroidism occurs after long-standing secondary hyperparathyroidism, which in turn has resulted from prolonged chronic renal failure. Even after the renal failure has been successfully treated with a transplant, after a long period of parathyroid hyperplasia of all four glands, one of them becomes autonomous and turns into a dominant adenoma.The patient is investigated on the same lines as in primary hyperparathyroidism. These patients have hypercalcaemia and a dominant adenoma is found in the midst of hyperplastic glands. The treatment is total or subtotal parathyroidectomy, depending upon the scan findings. If subtotal parathyroidectomy is carried out, about 50 mg of one gland is autotransplanted into the forearm

The summary of hyperparathyroidism is shown in **Figure 51.8**.

5. E Tetany from gastric outlet obstruction.

A long-standing healed duodenal ulcer produces cicatrisation with scarring and complete stenosis of the duodenum wrongly called 'pyloric stenosis' – a misnomer because it is

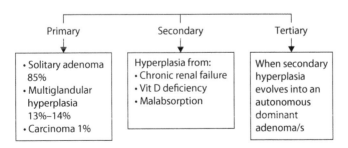

Figure 51.8   Summary of types of hyperparathyroidism.

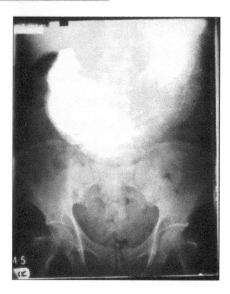

Figure 51.9 Barium meal showing gastric outlet obstruction from cicatrizing duodenal ulcer.

actually duodenal stenosis. A barium meal **(Figure 51.9)** would show smooth cut-off at pyloroduodenal junction where there is total obstruction with massive gastric dilatation with a large amount of food residue.

Prolonged vomiting causes loss of H^+, K^+ and Cl^- with increase in HCO_3^- resulting in hypcholraemic, hypokalaemic metabolic alkalosis. Fluid loss causes extreme dehydration seen clinically as sunken eyes, dry tongue and loss of skin turgor. The patient has carpo-pedal spasm because of tetany. Tetany is liable to occur in any form of alkalosis, in this case metabolic. This is because loss of H^+ (normally bound to albumin) releases a place that is taken up by free ionised Ca^{++}, which is now bound to albumin thus reducing ionised Ca^{++}, resulting in tetany.

The patient should be resuscitated by intravenous normal saline with added potassium chloride, indwelling catheter and CVP line; a large-bore stomach tube is inserted to wash out the stomach to empty semisolid stale food. Confirmation of the diagnosis is made by OGD. During OGD an attempt might be made to do balloon dilatation of the stenosis as a form of treatment that may only be temporary. The definitive surgical procedure is gastrojejunostomy – posterior, retro-colic, iso-peristaltic, short loop. Some surgeons might consider adding a truncal vagotomy to prevent a future anastomotic ulcer.

52 The adrenal glands and other abdominal endocrine disorders

Nandini Rao

Multiple choice questions

Multiple endocrine neoplasia (MEN) (epidemiology and genetics)

1. **Which of the following statements are true?**
   A MEN1 is characterised by tumours in the pituitary, pancreas and parathyroids.
   B Medullary thyroid carcinoma (MTC) plays a key role in MEN2 subtypes.
   C The mode of inheritance is autosomal dominant in both MEN1 and 2.
   D The penetrance of the mutation is low.
   E Screening of family members of the affected individual is essential.

MEN1 Clinical presentation

2. **The following statements are true except:**
   A Nephrolithiasis is a common clinical presentation.
   B Pancreatic endocrine tumours (PET) are a common cause of death.
   C Insulinomas are the most common pancreatic tumours in MEN1.
   D All pituitary tumours must be surgically resected.
   E Adrenocortical carcinomas frequently develop.

Surgical treatment in MEN1

3. **Which of the following statements are true?**
   A Selective resection of the parathyroid is a preferred treatment option.

B MEN1 gastrinomas and insulinomas must be operated on.
C All nonfunctional adrenal tumours can be left alone.
D All nonfunctional PETs can be left alone.
E Most procedures related to the pituitary can be performed through the trans-spenoidal approach.

MEN2

4. **Which of the following statements are true?**
   A MTC is a late manifestation of MEN2a.
   B Primary hyperparathyroidism (pHPT) is an early manifestation of MEN2.
   C Diagnostic work up for MEN2 must include scintigraphy.
   D Mutation carriers of MEN2 must be offered a thyroidectomy.
   E Unilateral or bilateral sub-total resection of a phaeochromocytoma in MEN2 is appropriate.

Adrenal incidentalomas

5. **Which of the following statements are true?**
   A A diagnostic work up is unnecessary if it is <6 cm.
   B Most incidentalomas are nonfunctioning.
   C A 1-mg overnight dexamehasosne suppression test is helpful in diagnosis.
   D An adrenal biopsy is always indicated.
   E Adrenal metastasis is more likely in patients with a history of cancer elsewhere.

→ **Adrenal glands anatomy and hormones**

6. The following statements are true except:

A The weight of a normal adrenal gland is 15 g.

B Adrenals are retroperitoneal organs.

C The right adrenal vein drains into the right renal vein.

D Dehydroepiandrosterone is produced in the zona glomerulosa.

E Aldosterone is produced in the zona reticularis.

Extended matching questions

→ Adrenals

Diagnoses

1 Addison's disease
2 Congenital adrenal hyperplasia
3 Cushing's syndrome
4 Cushing's syndrome due to ectopic ACTH production
5 Pheochromocytoma

Match the diagnoses with the clinical scenarios that follow:

A A 68-year-old alcoholic and smoker presents with weakness, weight loss, hyper-pigmentation and cough. His blood pressure (BP) is 170/90 mmHg and is cachectic. Blood glucose is 7.0 mmol/L, Na is 135 mmol/L and is K 2.5 mmol/L. Morning cortisol and midnight cortisol are 719 nmol/L and 675 nmol/L, respectively.

B A 50-year-old woman sees her general practitioner (GP) with symptoms of palpitations, abdominal pain, sweating and panic attacks. Her BP is fluctuant and ranges between 140/80 and 180/98 mmHg; thyroid function tests (TFT) are normal.

C A middle-aged woman is concerned about hirsuitism and weight gain. She is found to have abdominal striae, BP is 160/90 mmHg and BMI is 30. Her blood glucose is 11.6 mmol/L, Na is 140 mmol/L and K is 3.5 mmol/L. She shows elevated urinary cortisol excretion, which fails to suppress after dexamethasone.

D A 19-year-old slim-built diabetic woman presents to A&E with an episode of collapse. Her tests are as follows: Na 129 mmol/L, K 5.6 mmol/L and blood glucose 11.2 mmol/L.

E An ill male infant presents with vomiting and diarrhoea. Na is 130 mmol/L, K is 5.0 mmol/L, blood glucose is 7.0 mmol/L and cortisol is 50 nmol/L.

→ Hypoglycaemia

Diagnoses

1 Diabetes Mellitus
2 Disorder of carbohydrate metabolism
3 Hypoglycaemia secondary to oral hypoglycaemic agents
4 Insulinoma
5 Insulin overdose

Match the diagnoses with the clinical scenarios that follow:

A A middle-aged-man with a BMI of 29 presents to the GP feeling dizzy especially after large meals. He has noticed nocturia and blurred vision. His fasting blood glucose on two occasions is 7.3 and 7.8 mmol/L.

B A 42-year-old diabetic on insulin and a sulponylurea feels dizzy and unsteady. He sustained a fit 2 weeks ago. Blood glucose at the time was 2.2 mmol/L. Plasma insulin levels and proinsulin levels are elevated.

C An 80-year-old diabetic man on insulin and metformin presents with shakiness, sweating and anxiety. He has features of dementia and is awaiting placement at a nursing home. Blood glucose is 2.5 mmol/L. Insulin levels are within normal limits in blood and proinsulin is undetectable.

D A 48-year-old man finds that he becomes dizzy, anxious and confused in the mornings. These symptoms are relieved after eating. He has felt these symptoms after exercise. He also has abdominal pain and diarrhoea.

E A 7-month-old infant is admitted with a seizure and noted to have a blood glucose of 2.1 mmol/L. The child also has hepatomegaly and lactic acidosis.

Endocrine disorders

Diagnoses

1 Carcinoid syndrome
2 Conn's syndrome
3 Hyperthyroidism
4 Metastatic liver disease
5 Phaeochromocytoma

Match the diagnoses with the clinical scenarios that follow:

A A 46-year-old woman presents with intermittent explosive diarrhoea and colicky abdominal pain for 3 months. It is associated with wheeze and flushing. On examination, she is slightly jaundiced and her liver is enlarged, hard and nodular. She has a midline scar for a right hemicolectomy carried out 8 years ago.

B A young woman complains of intermittent diarrhoea, weight loss and anxiety. On examination she is slightly jaundiced, has marked pedal oedema, tremor and a smooth goitre.

C A middle-aged man presents with constipation and diarrhoea, weight loss and poor appetite. He has lost nearly 8 kg over the past 3 months. On examination he is pale and jaundiced and shows an enlarged, hard, nodular liver. A mass is felt in the left iliac fossa.

D An elderly woman with hypertension, anxiety and depression was found to have an adrenal mass when being screened for an abdominal aortic aneurysm. Her 9 am cortisol was 565 nmo/L, 24-hour urine cortisol was normal and 24-hour urine catecholamines were elevated.

E A young man is found to have poorly controlled hypertension despite being on three types of antihypertensive drugs. He was started on a diuretic but felt very unwell. His blood results are the following: Na 145 mmol/L, K 2.5 mmol/L, Cl 101 mmol/L and HCO₃ 20 mmol/L.

Answers to multiple choice questions

→ ## Multiple endocrine neoplasia (MEN) (epidemiology and genetics)

1. A, B, C, E

MEN1 is associated with a triad of anterior pituitary tumours (prolactinoma or nonfunctional tumours), primary hyperparathyroidism (pHPT) and pancreaticoduodenal tumours (PET). MEN2 have the following three subtypes: familial medullary carcinoma, MEN2a (MTC, pHPT and phaeochromocytoma) and MEN2b (features of MEN2a and neuromas and a marfanoid habitus). They are all inherited in an autosomal dominant manner, and genetic counselling with screening of family members is helpful.

The prevalence of the syndrome is 0.04–0.2 cases per 1000 population per year, but the penetrance of the mutation is high with almost 100% of carriers developing the syndrome. In particular MEN2 shows a good genotype-phenotype correlation.

→ ## MEN1 (Clinical presentation)

2. C, D, E

Pituitary tumours are found in 30%–60% of MEN1 sufferers. They are most often microprolactinomas or nonfunctional tumours and are medically treated. The adrenals can be involved in 40%–50% of patients, but most tumours are nonfunctioning ones.

In total, 90%–100% of persons affected with MEN1 develop pHPT characterised by multiglandular hyperplasia. Renal stone disease is a common presentation. Measurement of serum parathyroid hormone (PTH) levels and Ca, PO4 in both serum and urine confirms pHPT. Pancreatic endocrine tumours (PET) occur in 50%–60% of MEN1 patients. They are mostly multiple, recur after surgery and are a cause of syndrome associated death. Gastrinomas are the most common functional PET followed by insulinomas.

→ ## Surgical treatment in MEN1

3. B, E

MEN1 gastrinomas and insulinomas must be removed to prevent liver metastasis and control hormone excess. For gastrinomas located in the gastrinoma triangle **(Figure 52.1)**,

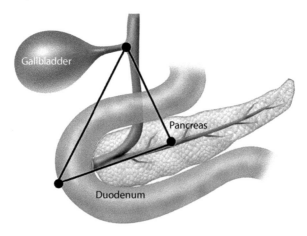

Figure 52.1 Gastrinoma triangle.

partial pancreaticoduodenectomy is recommended. MEN1 insulinomas require distal pancreatectomy with enucleation of the tumours. Anterior pituitary tumours that fail medical therapy or symptomatic nonfunctional tumours must be considered for trans-spenoidal surgery.

As multiglandular disease is present in all cases, total parathyroidectomy, cervical thymectomy or 3 ½-gland resection leaving behind half of one gland of parathyroid tissue is the preferred procedure. Non functional PETs >1 cm and nonfunctional adrenal tumours > 4cm in size must be operated upon.

MEN2

4. C, D, E

Diagnostic work up for a phaeochromocytoma includes measurement of urinary catecholamines, abdominal CT or MRI, iodine 131-MIBG scintigraphy. The operative approach is laparotomy or laparoscopic. A subtotal resection which retains the healthy part of the gland is preferred and prevents long-term dependence on glucocorticoids or mineralocorticoid. The likelihood of developing MTC is 100% for most mutations and hence operative therapy is offered to patients detected by genetic screening. Depending on the mutation detected, risk groups have been defined to determine the appropriate age for thyroidectomy.

MTC is almost always the first manifestation of the syndrome. MTC occurs early and is most aggressive in MEN2b with lymph node metastasis present in early stages. pHPT is present in 20%–30% of patients with MEN2a. Most patients are asymptomatic with it.

Adrenal incidentalomas

5. B, C, E

Nonfunctioning incidentalomas account for 78%. Functioning adenomas are the following: Cushing's adenoma (17%), adrenocortical carcinoma (4%) and phaeochromocytoma (4%), and the remaining are rarer causes such as metastasis, cysts and Conn's adenomas.

All adrenal masses require a complete history, physical examination and biochemical tests for hormone excess (elevated midnight cortisol, elevated 24-hour urinary cortisol or catecholamine, failure of cortisol to suppress after an overnight dexamethasone suppression test, increased aldosterone-rennin in primary hyperaldosteronism) and additional imaging to exclude a functioning or malignant adrenal tumour.

Any nonfunctioning adenoma >4 cm, functional tumours and smaller tumours that are growing must be resected. Nonfunctional tumours <4 cm should be followed up regularly with hormonal and imaging tests.

CT and MRI must precede FNAC only after a phaeochromocytoma has been excluded biochemically.

Adrenal glands anatomy and hormones

6. A, C, D, E

A normal adrenal gland weighs just 4 g and is situated near the upper poles of the kidneys in the retroperitoneum within Gerota's capsule. The right gland is located between the right lobe of the liver and diaphragm, behind the IVC. The left gland is close to the upper pole of the left kidney and renal pedicle. The adrenals are very vascular organs. The arterial supply shows considerable variation, but it receives blood from the aorta and diaphragmatic and renal arteries. A large adrenal vein drains on the right side into the IVC and on the left side into the renal vein. It is hence difficult to access the left adrenal vein in procedures such as adrenal venous sampling.

It has two functional parts, which are the cortex and medulla. Catecholamines (adrenaline, noradrenaline, dopamine and metanephrines) are secreted by the adrenal medulla. Cells of the zona glomerulosa of the adrenal cortex secrete aldosterone (regulates sodium homeostasis). Cells of the zona fasciculata and zona reticularis synthesize cortisol and adrenal androgens such as dehydroepiandrosteron.

Answers to extended matching questions

→ Adrenals

1. D Addison's disease

Addison's disease is associated with other autoimmune condition such as type 1 DM, vitiligo, etc. Tuberculosis remains a leading cause of primary adrenal failure globally. Hypotension, hyponatraemia, hyperkalaemia and hypoglycaemia are commonly observed. The diagnosis is confirmed by high 9 am ACTH levels (reduced cortisol production causes a negative feedback and rise in ACTH drive by the pituitary) and inability of serum cortisol to elevate following a short synacthen test.

2. E Congenital adrenal hyperplasia

Congenital adrenal hyperplasia is a group of autosomal recessive disorders of steroid synthesis, resulting in decreased cortisol secretion. The age and type of clinical presentation varies widely from neonatal emergencies to young adults presenting with features of androgen excess. Associated mineralocorticoid deficiency is associated with hypotension and sodium wasting.

3. C Cushing's syndrome

Cushing's syndrome is characterised clinically **(Figure 52.2a** and **b)** by weight gain (abdominal obesity), hirsuitism, easy bruising, thin skin, stria, proximal myopathy, glucose

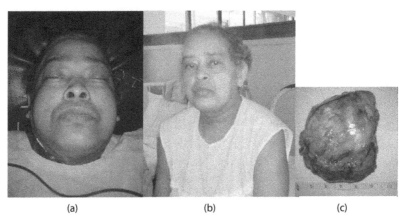

(a)   (b)   (c)

Figure 52.2 (a) Cushing's syndrome. (b) Cushing's syndrome – postoperative. (c) Adrenal tumour: Cushing's syndrome – same patient as (a) and (b). (Courtesy of Dr. Nissanka Jayawardhana, MB BS, MS, FRCSEd, Consultant General Surgeon, District General Hospital, Kegalle, Sri Lanka.)

intolerance and hypertension. It is due to exogenous steroid usage or related to in vivo production of cortisol. Cortisol excess is diagnosed by the following:

- Elevated morning and midnight plasma cortisol levels, possibly with loss of diurnal rhythm.
- Dexamethasone fails to suppress 24-hour urinary cortisol excretion.
- Serum ACTH levels discriminate ACTH-dependent from ACTH-independent disease treatment is open **(Figure 52.2c)** or laparoscopic excision.

4. A Cushing's syndrome due to ectopic ACTH production

ACTH-dependent cortisol excess might be due to a pituitary disease (associated with a corticotrophin microadenoma) when it is Cushing's disease or related to ectopic ACTH secretion by a variety of tumours (most often small cell carcinoma of the bronchus) Malignancy associated Cushing's presents with pigmentation, weight loss and severe hypokalaemic alkalosis.

5. B Phaeochromocytoma

Phaeochromocytomas are mostly adrenal in origin (90%). It is often referred to as a '10% tumour' because 10% occur in children, 10% are inherited, 10% are malignant, 10% are extra-adrenal and 10% are bilateral. They present with features of hypertension – headaches, palpitations and episodes of anxiety. A patient presenting with the triad of headaches, palpitations and sweating should arouse the suspicion of a phaeochromocytoma. Excessive metanephrine and normetanephrine in a 24-hour urine specimen is almost diagnostic.

The tumour classically shows a 'Swiss cheese' configuration. The next step is localisation. A ^{123}I-MIBG (metaiodobenzylguanidine) single-photon emission computed tomography (SPECT) will identify about 90% of primary tumours and is essential for the detection of multiple extra-adrenal tumours and metastases. PET scanning using FDG PET or DOPA PET is yet more sensitive in detecting metastatic foci.

Management requires good teamwork between the endocrinologist, anaesthetist and surgeon. Preoperative preparation by α- blockers is essential, with immediate postoperative care being in the ICU. Laparoscopic adrenalectomy is now the routine. However, if the tumour is >8 cm or malignancy is suspected, open operation should be carried out.

Hypoglycaemia

1. A Diabetes mellitus

Reactive or prandial hypoglycaemia occurs in diabetes mellitus, alimentary hypoglycaemia and alcohol induced. Symptoms typically occur 2 to 5 hours after a meal and are predominantly of adrenergic origin (anxiety, restlessness, sweating and palpitation). Neuroglycopenic symptoms (dizziness, confusion, paraesthesia, weakness, seizures and coma) rarely occur.

2. E Disorder of carbohydrate metabolism

Glycogen storage disorders are a group of inherited metabolic disorders associated with fasting hypoglycaemia. It occurs due to the deficiency of enzymes required to break down and use glycogen. The liver and other organs become enlarged with accumulated glycogen. It presents in infancy with fasting hypoglycaemia. Infants and children require constant feeding (approximately once every 2 hours) to prevent hypoglycaemia.

3. B Hypoglycaemia secondary to oral hypoglycaemic agents

Hypoglycaemia might be associated with increased or inappropriate plasma insulin levels in conditions such as insulinoma, sepsis, drugs such as quinine and pentamidine, overdosage or administration of insulin, or a sulphonylurea (which increase proinsulin release). A urine drug screen can confirm the excess of sulphonylurea within the body.

4. D Insulinoma

Pancreatic endocrine tumours (PET) account for 5% of all detected pancreatic tumours. They can be benign or malignant, functional or nonfunctional. Insulinomas are the most common PET and represent 70%–80% of all PET's. Insulin-producing tumours cause Whipple's triad, i.e., symptoms of hypoglycaemia after fasting or exercise, plasma glucose <2.8 mmol/L and relief of symptoms on administration of glucose. Being aware of the condition is the secret in suspecting the diagnosis. High secretion of insulin, proinsulin and C-peptide in serial measurements is diagnostic in almost 80%. Once suspected, endoscopic ultrasound (EUS) helps in localisation supplemented by intraoperative ultrasound. Treatment is excision or enucleation.

5. C Insulin overdose

All confirmed hypoglycaemic events must be evaluated in relation to food (fasting or prandial) and presence of detectable insulin or not at the time of hypoglycaemia. Those associated with suppressed insulin levels include hypopituitarism, adrenal insufficiency, chronic renal impairment, liver disease, malnutrition, exercise-induced and drugs such as salicylates and beta blockers.

Endocrine disorders

1. A Carcinoid syndrome

Carcinoid tumours are neuroendocrine tumours mostly found in the small bowel. The tumours produce serotonin and cause carcinoid syndrome in patients with large liver metastasis or tumour invading the inferior vena cava. The cause of this syndrome is excessive secretion of 5-hydroxytryptamine (5-HT, serotonin). Diagnosis is made by history, examination and assessment of 24-hour urine for 5-hydroxy-indoleacetic acid (HIAA). Somatostatin-receptor scintigraphy will show tumour deposits in organs, provided they are large enough to have a high burden.

The clinical manifestations are protean in nature. They are the following:

Vasomotor: Flushing in face and neck and sun-exposed areas
Gastrointestinal: Mild to explosive diarrhoea, abdominal pain, bloating and tenesmus
Cardiopulmonary: Hypotension during flushing attacks, right-sided heart failure, pulmonary and tricuspid stenosis, bronchospasm
Nutritional: Weight loss, features of pellagra: Dementia and skin lesions from niacin deficiency

Diagnosis is confirmed by CT scan, which shows multiple liver secondaries. The ideal palliation is hepatic artery chemoembolisation.

2. E Conn's syndrome

Primary hyperaldosteronism (PHA), or Conn's syndrome, is defined by hypertension, as a result of hyper secretion of aldosterone by the adrenal cortex. Among hypertensives, the incidence of PHA is around 2%. The most frequent cause of PHA with hypokalaemia is a unilateral adrenocortical adenoma. Biochemical diagnosis involves assessment of potassium (low) and aldosterone to rennin ratio (elevated). Once the biochemical diagnosis is confirmed, MRI or CT should be performed to distinguish unilateral from bilateral disease.

Selective adrenal vein catheterisation can help to decide on nonsurgical treatment with spironolactone and anti-hypertensives or surgical treatment with unilateral laparoscopic adrenalectomy in the presence of unilateral disease or subtotal resection in case of a single Conn's adenoma.

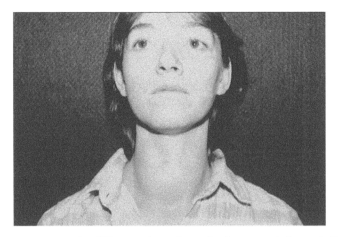

Figure 52.3 Smooth, diffuse goitre of medically treated Graves' disease.

3. B Hyperthyroidism

Graves' disease is an autoimmune condition characterised by hyperthyroidism, pretibial myxoedema and a smooth goitre. Symptoms related to hyperthyroidism include anxiety, sweatiness, diarrhoea and unintended weight loss. Thyroid function tests (TFTs) show a suppressed TSH and elevated fT3 and fT4. The patient will have cardiovascular and neurological features of thyrotoxicosis, with a smooth diffuse goitre **(Figure 52.3)**.

The patient is treated by the physician with anti-thyroid drugs over a period of time and closely monitored. In due course a discussion is had with the patient regarding the ideal long-term management among drug therapy, radioactive iodine and surgery. After full-informed consent, the choice is made by the patient with help and advice from the physician and surgeon. If the patient chooses surgery, nowadays the choice is between near-total thyroidectomy and total thyroidectomy whilst a minority of surgeons still may perform subtotal thyroidectomy.

4. C Metastatic liver disease

A middle-aged person with significant weight loss, cachexia and presence of a palpable mass and liver involvement is strongly suggestive of metastatic bowel cancer. A detailed history and examination is followed by confirming the diagnosis, staging the disease and then instituting definitive treatment after discussion in a multidisciplinary meeting.

The diagnosis is confirmed by colonoscopy and biopsy; staging is done by CECT of abdomen and liver US and CXR. Depending upon the staging, the patient would undergo neoadjuvant chemotherapy +/– radiotherapy followed by the appropriate surgery to the bowel.

5. D Phaeochromocytoma

The prevalence of adrenal masses increases with advancing age. Incidentalomas are detected in 1% of patients undergoing imaging. A phaeochromocytoma must be excluded (24-hour urinary catecholamines and metanephrines) and the patient managed appropriately (please see previous section).

53 *The breast*

Selvi Radhakrishna and P Raghu Ram

Multiple choice questions

→ Benign breast disease

1. Which of these following statements are true?

A Nipple retraction always indicates an underlying malignancy.

B *Staphylococcus aureus* is the most common cause for lactational mastitis.

C Fibroadenomas should always be offered excision, as they are associated with a high risk of malignancy.

D The histology of phyllodes tumour may be benign, intermediate or malignant.

E Blood-stained nipple discharge is usually due to a breast carcinoma.

→ Carcinoma of the breast

2. Which one of the following statements are false?

A Hormone replacement therapy (HRT) increases the risk of breast cancer.

B Inflammatory breast cancer is caused by infection in the breast.

C Medullary carcinoma in the breast is associated with a poor prognosis.

D Van Nuy's scoring system is used to decide further management after local excision in patients with ductal carcinoma in situ (DCIS).

E Oestrogen receptor negative tumours are treated with tamoxifen or aromatase inhibitors.

3. Which one of the following statements are true?

A Paget's disease of the breast is usually associated with an underlying invasive carcinoma.

B The survival outcome following breast-conserving treatment and mastectomy are equal.

C Positive resected margins are a significant predictor of recurrence after breast-conserving surgery.

D Sentinel lymph node biopsy should not be offered in clinically node-negative axilla.

E The pectoralis minor and major muscles are removed in Patey's mastectomy.

4. Which of the following statements are false?

A Adjuvant chemotherapy is not given to post-menopausal women with ER-positive breast cancer.

B Tamoxifen reduces the risk of contralateral breast cancer.

C Cyclophosphamide chemotherapy is as effective as anthracycline- and taxane-based chemotherapy.

D Neoadjuvant chemotherapy improves breast conservation rates in women with slightly larger primary tumour.

5. Which if the following statements are true?

A Lymphoedema in the arm after treatment usually indicates a recurrence.

B Radiotherapy after implant reconstruction of the breast gives poor cosmetic results.

C Chemotherapy is safe in second and third trimester in women with pregnancy-associated breast cancer.

D Male breast cancer carries a poor prognosis when compared with female breast cancer.

Extended matching questions

Choose and match the correct diagnosis or investigations with each of
the case scenarios that follow:

1. ANDI (Aberration of normal development and involution)
2. BRCA 1 and 2 tests
3. Breast abscess
4. Breast cyst
5. Core needle biopsy
6. Duct ectasia
7. Fibroadenoma
8. Galactocele
9. Gynaecomastia
10. Male breast cancer
11. MRI scan of the breasts
12. Phyllodes tumour
13. Vacuum-assisted biopsy

A. A 26-year-old breast-feeding mother presents as an emergency with pain, swelling in the right breast and fever for 2 days.

B. A 58-year-old woman underwent a screening mammogram and was recalled for further assessment. She was found to have fine linear branching micro-calcifications.

C. A 49-year-old woman woke up to find a lump in the right breast with pain. She is very anxious.

D. A 35-year-old woman presents with breast pain and lumpiness in both breasts. It is particularly worse before her periods.

E. A 32-year-old woman attends the breast clinic with a strong family history of breast cancer. Two of her sisters, her mother and her maternal aunt's daughter had breast cancer at an early age. She wants to know her risk of getting breast cancer.

F. A 42-year-old woman presented with a painless mass in the right breast, which has been rapidly increasing in size. On examination she has a large mass in the right breast with skin stretched and shiny over it.

G. A 48-year-old woman feels a hard lump that is painless and gradually increasing in size over the past 4 months. Her mammogram shows a spiculated mass in the right breast.

H. A 26-year-old young woman presents with a painless mass in the left breast. She stopped breastfeeding 1 month ago, following which she noticed this lump.

I. A 14-year-old boy presents with enlarging breasts which are embarrassing him.

J. A 45-year-old woman has been diagnosed with a lobular carcinoma in the right breast.

K. A 52-year-old woman presented with a greenish black nipple discharge on both sides.

L. A 28-year-old woman presents with a discrete lump in the breast. The lump is painless and moves freely within the breast.

M. A 49-year-old man presents with a painless mass just under the nipple and areola on the right side of 3 months duration.

Answers to multiple choice questions

→ Benign breast disease

1. B, D

Nipple retraction might be noticed during puberty when the breasts develop and the etiology is unknown. This might cause difficulty in breastfeeding due to retained secretions.

Recent retraction of nipple, particularly in older women, might be of considerable pathological significance. A slit-like retraction might be caused by duct ectasia and chronic periductal mastitis, whereas a circumferential nipple retraction is likely to be due to a malignancy.

Staphylococcus aureus is the most common cause of lactational infections. Fifty percent of infants harbour staphylococci in the nasopharynx. A cracked nipple might initiate the mastitis and blocked lactiferous ducts with stagnant milk will allow organisms to multiply, leading to breast abscess.

Early recognition and treatment with antibiotics, such as flucloxacillin or comoxiclav, can prevent an abscess formation. Once abscess is formed, then pus should be aspirated under ultrasound guidance. Some patients will require a mini incision and drainage. MRSA (methicillin-resistant *Staphylococcus aureus*) infections can sometimes occur, particularly if the infection is hospital-acquired.

Fibrodenomas are not associated with a high risk of malignancy. They are offered excision if they are large or have a suspicious cytology or when a patient desires to have them removed.

Phyllodes tumours are usually single, unilateral, painless palpable breast masses. On clinical examination the phyllodes tumours feel firm, well-circumscribed like fibroadenoma and might be slightly larger when first detected. It is impossible to differentiate smaller phyllodes tumour from fibroadenoma clinically. Features that alert a clinician to a phyllodes tumour include the following:

1. Older age of the patient
2. Larger tumour size
3. History of rapid growth

Phyllodes tumor is classified as benign, intermediate and malignant. The degree of stromal cellular atypia, mitotic activity per 10 high-power field, presence or absence of stromal overgrowth (defined as single 40 times field of pure stroma devoid of epithelium), infiltrative or expansile margins are the criteria used to subclassify phyllodes as benign, borderline, or malignant.

Blood-stained nipple discharge might be caused by duct ectasia, a duct papilloma, or carcinoma. When due to a duct papilloma or a carcinoma, it is often solitary and spontaneous. Cytology of nipple discharge might not yield any useful information.

Mammogram is rarely useful to evaluate nipple discharge, but sometimes might show an underlying mass or calcifications. A high-resolution ultrasound scan might show a dilated duct with intraductal solid component. Ductogram and ductoscopy can be done to visualise the ductal system.

→ Breast cancer

2. B, C, E

Long-term use of combined preparation of HRT does significantly increase the risk of developing breast cancer. The million women study has shown that the current use of HRT is associated with an increased risk of incidence of fatal breast cancer. The effect is substantially greater for oestrogen and progesterone combination than for other types of HRT. There has been a decrease in the incidence of breast cancer in the 50s to 60s cohort of women due to a decrease in the use of HRT in the United States and United Kingdom.

Inflammatory breast cancer is not related to infection. It is a rare, aggressive type of breast cancer, presenting with swelling, redness, warmth and pain in the breast with oedema. It mimics a cellulitis or abscess, but the findings are due to blocked subdermal lymphatics with tumour cells. The presence of cancer cells in the subdermal lymphatics confirms the diagnosis of inflammatory breast cancer. They used to be rapidly fatal, but with recent advances in systemic therapy, the prognosis has improved considerably.

Medullary carcinomas are rare breast cancers that have characteristic histopathological findings that show solid sheets of large cells with lymphoplasmacytic infiltration. They are often oestrogen receptor (ER) and progesterone receptor (PR) negative. Medullary cancers, despite having an aggressive histological picture and being triple negative, often have a better prognosis than infiltrating duct carcinoma not of an otherwise specified type.

Ductal carcinoma in situ of the breast represents a broad spectrum of disease with a range of treatment options. The van Nuy's prognostic index is a tool that quantifies measurable prognostic factors like the tumour size, grade, margin width, necrosis and age.

Scores 4,5, 6 – Excision alone
Scores 7, 8, 9 – Radiotherapy after excision
Scores 10, 11, 12 – Mastectomy should be considered

Women with ER-negative breast cancers should not be offered hormone manipulation. Oestrogen receptor expression is the main indicator of potential response to endocrine therapy. Approximately 70% of breast cancers are ER positive and therefore hormone dependent. Premenopausal ER patients are treated with tamoxifen, which competes with oestrogen to block the oestrogen receptor selectively. The blockade prevents further downstream signaling for the tumour cells to divide and multiply. Postmenopausal ER-positive women are treated with tamoxifen or, more recently, aromatase inhibitors. Drugs like letrozole, anastrozole, or exemestane inhibit the aromatase enzyme, thereby preventing the peripheral conversion of androstenadione to oestradiol.

3. A, B, C
Paget's disease of the nipple is an eczema-like condition of the nipple and areola and usually is associated with an underlying invasive carcinoma. A punch biopsy of the nipple areola should be done if there is any doubt. Microscopically, Paget's disease is characterised by the presence of large ovoid cells with abundant clear pale-staining cytoplasm in the epidermis.

Evidence from several randomized controlled trials has shown that long-term survival outcome is equal between breast-conservation surgery along with radiotherapy and mastectomy (**Table 53.1**). Breast-conservation therapy should be followed up with radiation. The local recurrence rates are high when radiotherapy is omitted following breast-conservation surgery.

Younger age, positive resection margins, high-grade tumours, presence of extensive ductal carcinoma-in-situ (DCIS) and presence of lymphovascular invasion are all important

Table 53.1 Options in local treatment to breast in cancer

Score	1	2	3
Size	≤15	16–40	>41
Margin width	>10 mm	1–9 mm	<1 mm
Grade	Low/Intermediate without necrosis	Low/Intermediate with necrosis	High grade with or without necrosis
Age	>60	40–60	<40

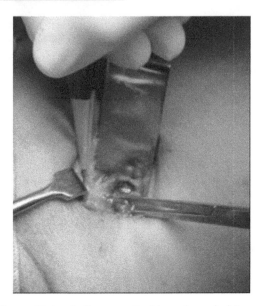

Figure 53.1   Axillary sentinel lymph node biopsy.

determinants of risk of local recurrence. If resected margins are involved, re-excision should be done. If the new re-excised margins are also involved, then mastectomy should be considered. Radiotherapy does not compensate for involved margins to prevent local recurrence.

Sentinel lymph nodes in the axilla are the first echelon of lymph nodes draining the breast. Subareolar injection of patent blue dye and radioactive tracer, locates the sentinel lymph node during surgery. The sentinel nodes are removed and evaluated for the presence of metastases from the primary tumour **(Figure 53.1)**. If metastasis is not found, then axillary dissection is not required, thereby reducing the risk of lymphoedema.

Pectoralis major muscle is preserved and the minor is removed in Patey's mastectomy. A modification of Patey's mastectomy, where the pectoralis minor muscle is just retracted to provide access to the level 2 and 3 axillary lymph nodes is more widely practiced now.

4. A, C, D
Adjuvant chemotherapy is increasingly being offered to high-risk post-menopausal women. Prognostic indices such as the Nottingham prognostic index and more recently computer-aided programs such as Adjuvant! Online or UK Predict have been used to counsel patients for risk and benefits of adjuvant systemic therapy. Gene signatures are increasingly used to tailor systemic therapy based on the recurrence scores.

Tamoxifen has been used widely in the hormonal management of breast cancer for more than four decades. Along with its intended benefit to reduce recurrence rate and death from breast cancer, it also significantly reduces the risk of contralateral breast cancer.

The results of various studies comparing CMF versus anthracycline-containing regimens suggest a modest advantage for anthracycline regimens. Inclusion of taxanes further improve the disease-free survival and overall survival. Hence, CMF is no longer considered adequate for adjuvant therapy.

Neoadjuvant chemotherapy was initially used to downsize locally advanced tumours to facilitate surgery. It was then used in operable breast cancer to decrease the tumour size to facilitate breast conservation. However, neoadjuvant chemotherapy has no additional advantage over disease-free survival or overall survival when compared with standard adjuvant therapy.

5. B, C, D

Lymphoedema of the arm is a troublesome complication of breast cancer treatment that can occur anytime from months to years after treatment. The incidence of lymphoedema is significantly higher when axillary dissection is combined with axillary radiation. It is less seen now as axillary dissection and radiotherapy to the axilla are rarely combined.

Besides, sentinel lymph node biopsy has been widely adopted as the standard of care in clinically node-negative axilla.

Radiotherapy after implant-based reconstructions can lead to fibrosis and capsular contracture surrounding the implant, resulting in unacceptable results. Implant-based reconstruction after the chest wall has been treated with radiotherapy is also associated with several problems. Delayed or poor wound healing can occur due the effects of radiotherapy. Autologous reconstructions are a better option if radiotherapy to the chest wall is anticipated.

Chemotherapy should be avoided in the first trimester, but it appears to be safe in the second and third trimester. Therefore, chemotherapy might be administered as neoadjuvant or adjuvant therapy in the second or third trimester.

Stage for stage, the treatment and prognosis of male breast cancer is similar to female breast cancer. Male breast cancer accounts for <1% of all breast cancers. Mastectomy is more often required as the breast size in proportion to the lump is usually small.

Answers to extended matching questions

1. D ANDI

There is sound clinical evidence that many benign breast conditions, especially cyclical pain, nodularity and cysts are likely to have their pathogenesis in hormonal events during reproductive life. ANDI is a term used to describe most benign breast diseases. It is based on the fact that most benign breast disorders are relatively minor aberrations of the normal processes of development, cyclical hormonal response and involution. Patients may give a history of cyclical mastalgia and nodularity. Persistent dominant nodules that are palpable clinically might require imaging evaluation and histopathological correlation.

2. E BRCA1 and 2 tests

Women who are thought to be gene carriers may be offered BRCA 1 and BRCA 2 tests. *BRCA 1* gene is located in the long arm of chromosome 17 and *BRCA2* in the short arm of chromosome 13. Genetic counseling should be offered before testing. Those who test positive have a 50%–80% risk of developing breast cancer and 15%–45% risk of developing ovarian cancer in their lifetime.

3. A Breast abscess

Lactation-associated infections are the most common infections in the breast. It occurs normally within 6 to 8 weeks following delivery. Patients often present with pain, swelling and redness along with fever and chills. There might be a tender, palpable lump with stretched, discolored, shiny skin. The abscess starts to point, and with skin necrosis the pus is discharged. *Staphylococcus aureus* is the most common organism.

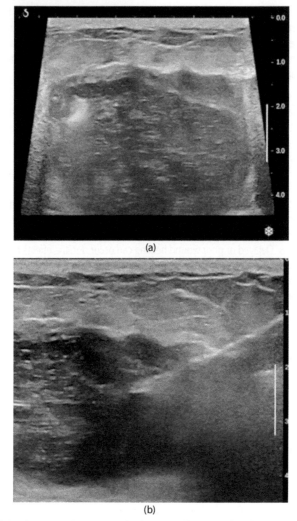

(a)

(b)

Figure 53.2 (a) Ultrasound image of a breast abscess. (b) Shows aspiration under ultrasound guidance.

On ultrasound, abscess cavity appears as an ill-defined hypoechoic collection that can sometimes be multi-loculated. The wall of the abscess cavity is often thick, irregular and echogenic with increased vascular flow. Acoustic enhancement is present due to fluid content (**Figure 53.2a** and **b**).

The majority of lactation-associated breast abscesses can be drained by ultrasound-guided aspiration, and this is the preferred method of treatment. Flucloxacillin or augmentin are usually the antibiotics of choice. In patients with penicillin sensitivity, erythromycin or clarithromycin can be given.

4. C Breast cyst
Symptomatic cysts present with a palpable breast mass or masses that might develop suddenly and be associated with pain and tenderness. Clinically detected breast mass cannot be characterised as a cyst on the basis of physical findings alone.

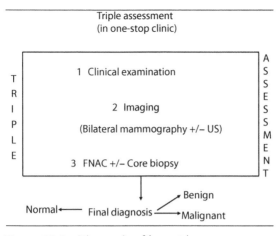

Figure 53.3   Diagnosis of breast lump.

Any breast mass in a woman above 40 years of age should be investigated with a mammogram and breast ultrasound after a clinical breast examination (triple assessment) (**Figure 53.3**). Cysts develop as a result differential of involution of breast acinar tissue and ductules. They might be small or large, single, or multiple. Large tension cyst might typically present with a painful lump in the breast and cause great anxiety to the patient. Mammogram may show single or multiple masses, and breast ultrasound clearly distinguishes cyst from a solid mass (**Figures 53.4a, b** and **c**). Guided aspiration provides instant relief. Cytology of the cyst aspirate is not done routinely.

5. G Core needle biopsy
Spiculated lesion on a mammogram (**Figures 53.5a, b** and **c**) is very suspicious of a malignancy. She requires a core needle biopsy of the lesion. Core needle biopsy allows a definitive diagnosis, with the possibility of differentiation between in situ and invasive disease (**Figure 53.6**). It is also possible to obtain estrogen and progesterone receptors and HER2 receptor status for treatment planning. It is particularly important to do a core biopsy before neoadjuvant chemotherapy. Although fine-needle aspiration (FNAC) is quick, easy and much more cost effective to do, it is associated with high false-negative results and inconclusive smears.

6. K Duct ectasia
Bilateral greenish black discharge in a premenopausal woman is likely to be due to duct ectasia. Duct ectasia is usually due to progressive involution of ducts. With increasing age, the myoepithelial layer of the major ducts loses its elasticity and contractility resulting in progressive duct dilatation and thickening of its walls. The stagnant secretions within the blocked duct gets thicker and inspissated. Most women with duct ectasia are asymptomatic, and it is often an incidental finding on ultrasound. Some describe a feeling of intense surge resembling the milk surge with breastfeeding. Some women present with multiple episodes of greenish-brown to black nipple discharge. There might also be associated nipple retraction because of shortening of ducts due to repeated inflammation. The retraction is slit-like (letterbox nipple) in contrast to retraction due to malignancy, where the entire nipple gets pulled in.

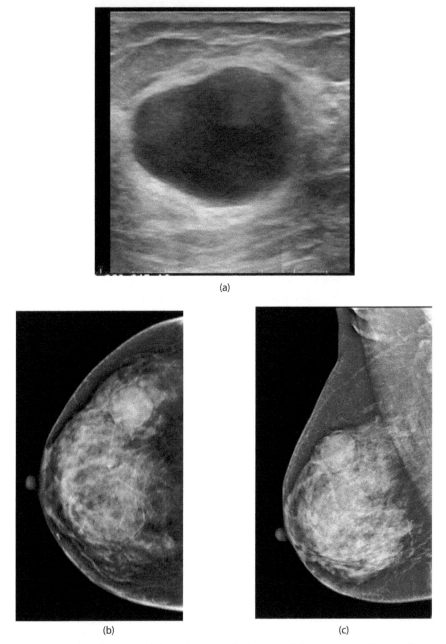

(a)

(b)   (c)

Figure 53.4   (a) Ultrasound showing anechoic cyst, thin imperceptible wall, posterior acoustic enhancement. (b and c) CC and MLO view of mammogram showing rounded dense opacity with partial halo and partly obscured margins.

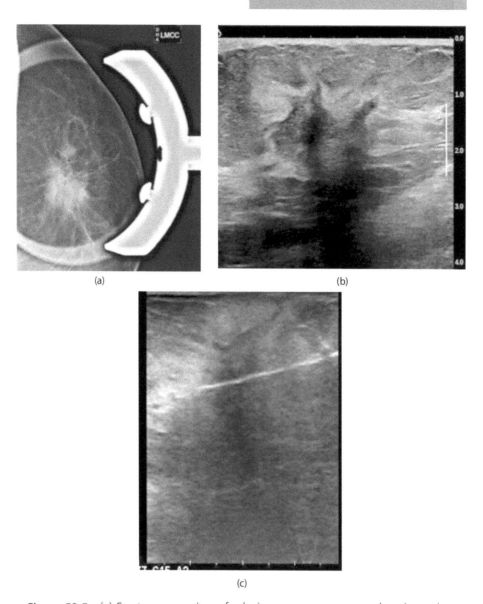

(a) (b)

(c)

Figure 53.5 (a) Spot compression of a lesion on mammogram showing spiculated lesion. (b) Ultrasound appearance of a spiculated irregular hypoechoic lesion. (c) Ultrasound guided core needle biopsy of the suspicious lesion.

7. L Fibroadenoma

Fibroadenomas are firm, rubbery, elliptical, or gently lobulated in shape. They are freely mobile and often described as a 'breast mouse.' They are encapsulated by a thin rim of compressed breast tissue. Histologically they are of two types—intracanalicular and pericanalicular. Pericanalicular fibroadenomas have stromal tissue surrounding the ducts and intracanalicular fibroadenomas have the ducts compressed into slits by the stroma **(Figure 53.7)**.

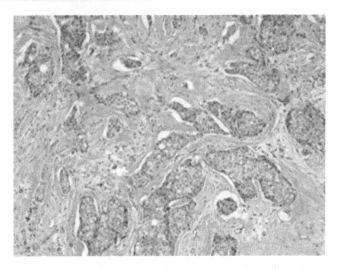

Figure 53.6   Core biopsy histology: Invasive ductal carcinoma.

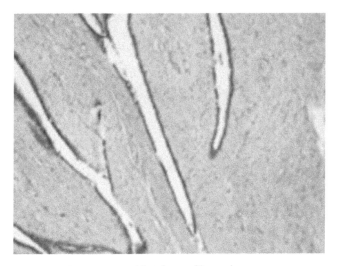

Figure 53.7   Histology: fibroadenoma.

Breast ultrasound is a very useful tool in very young women with dense breasts in whom mammogram is very difficult to interpret. Ultrasound reliably distinguishes a solid from a cystic mass and is very useful in characterising masses. Well-delineated, transversely oriented, hypoechoic mass with edge shadows is likely to be a benign fibroadenoma **(Figure 53.8)**.

8. H Galactocoele

A painless lump that occurs following cessation of lactation is likely to be a galactocele. Patients typically present with a painless breast lump occurring over weeks to months. It is essentially a milk-retention cyst. Ultrasound appearances show a cyst, sometimes with fat fluid levels **(Figure 53.9)**. Aspiration yields milky fluid. It might become thick and inspissated if it has been present for a long duration. Galactoceles usually resolve with aspiration. Secondary infection may result in a breast abscess.

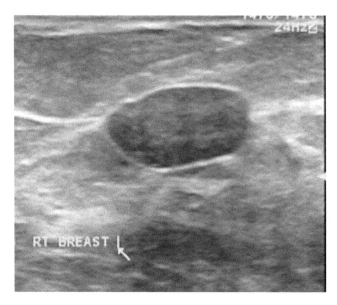

Figure 53.8   Ultrasound image of an ovoid hypoechoic, well-delineated lesion with a capsule, suggestive of a fibroadenoma.

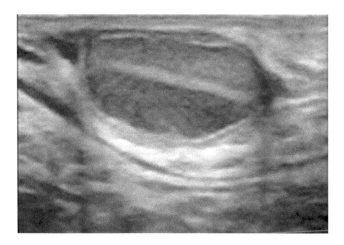

Figure 53.9   Ultrasound image showing a cystic lesion with fat fluid levels suggestive of a galactocele.

9. I Gynaecomastia

Gynaecomastia is a common benign condition that mainly affects teenage boys and older men, although it can affect men at any age. The causes are listed in **Figure 53.10**. The presentation varies from minor enlargement of breast tissue just behind the nipple to enlargement of the entire breast. Diagnosis is based on clinical breast examination and ultrasound of the breast or breasts. Most often, reassurance is all that is necessary. For some, removing the cause of gynaecomastia, such as changing medication and reducing alcohol intake, will reduce extra breast tissue. Occasionally, gynaecomastia might be treated by

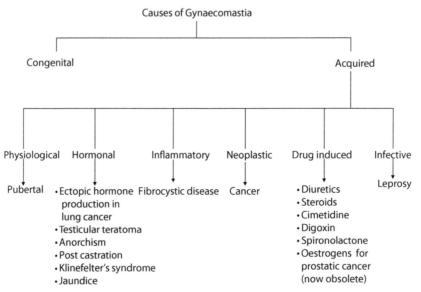

Causes of Gynaecomastia

Congenital   Acquired

Physiological   Hormonal   Inflammatory   Neoplastic   Drug induced   Infective

Pubertal
- Ectopic hormone   Fibrocystic disease   Cancer
  production in
  lung cancer
- Testicular teratoma
- Anorchism
- Post castration
- Klinefelter's syndrome
- Jaundice

Leprosy

- Diuretics
- Steroids
- Cimetidine
- Digoxin
- Spironolactone
- Oestrogens for
  prostatic cancer
  (now obsolete)

Figure 53.10 Causes of gynaecomastia.

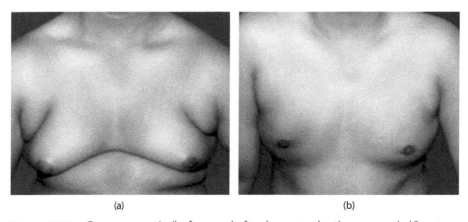

(a)   (b)

Figure 53.11 Gynaecomastia (before and after breast reduction surgery). (Courtesy of N. Hemanth Kumar, Consultant Plastic Surgeon, KIMS, Hyderabad, India.)

short-term hormonal therapy such as tamoxifen. Surgery is recommended if gynaecomastia has not improved with conservative measures and if it is affecting quality of life. The aim of surgery is to restore a normal- looking chest **(Figure 53.11)**.

10. M Male breast cancer

About 1% of breast cancers occur in men. Men with Klinefelter's syndrome are at a high risk of developing male breast cancer. BRCA2 mutations in men are also associated with a higher risk of breast cancer. Typically a patient presents with a lump in the breast. The assessment and treatment for male breast cancer is the same as in female breast cancers. The prognosis for male breast cancer is similar to that of female breast cancer **(Figures 53.12a,b and c)**.

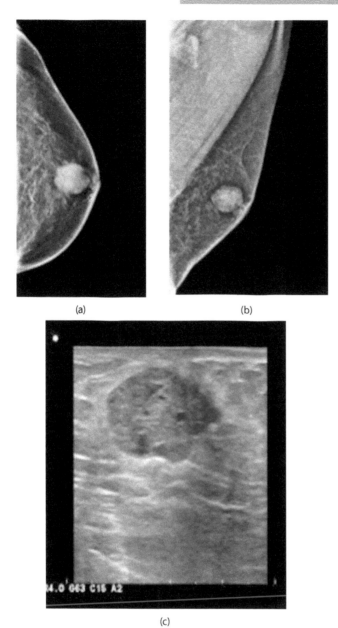

(a) (b)

(c)

Figure 53.12 (a and b) CC and MLO view of a male breast showing a rounded dense mass in the retro-areolar region. (c) Ultrasound image showing a hypoechoic lesion with micro-lobulations and an echogenic halo.

11. J MRI scan of breasts

Lobular cancer accounts for about 10% of all invasive cancers and is often multicentric and bilateral. MRI is useful to assess multicentricity and also will evaluate the contralateral breast to rule our bilateral breast cancers **(Figure 53.13)**. Histologically the duct lobular units are distended by tumour cells, which exhibit round nuclei and small nucleoli. The cancer cells form solid clusters that pack and distend lobular acini **(Figure 53.14)**.

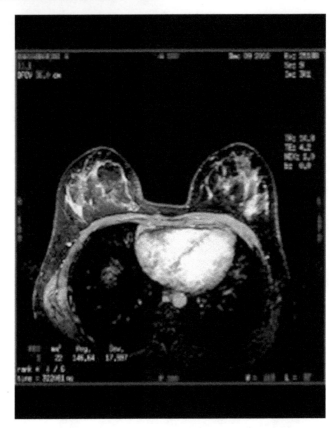

Figure 53.13   MRI of breasts demonstrating bilateral lobular cancers in a 32-year-old woman (premarked and marked images demonstrating bilateral lobular breast cancer).

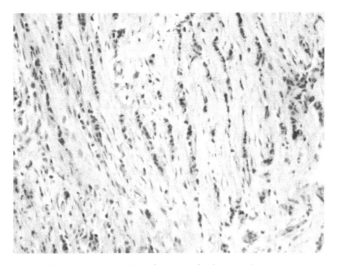

Figure 53.14   Histology: Lobular carcinoma.

12. F Phyllodes tumour

Phyllodes should certainly be considered as a possibility in older woman presenting with a rapidly enlarging breast mass. The rapidity of growth by itself does not indicate malignant potential. Because of the rapidity of growth, the mass may produce visible bulging when it expands quickly, with shiny and stretched skin with dilated veins over the mass as it pushes against the skin. The skin may ulcerate secondary to ischemia due to pressure on the overlying skin.

On a mammogram most phyllodes tumours appear as circumscribed lobulated, high-density masses **(Figure 53.15a)**. On breast ultrasound **(Figure 53.15b)** they are seen as large, well-circumscribed, ovoid heterogeneous hypoechoic lesion with cystic cleft-like space. Phyllodes can be benign, intermediate, or malignant. Wide excision with good margins will be required. For more aggressive and very large lesions, mastectomy is recommended.

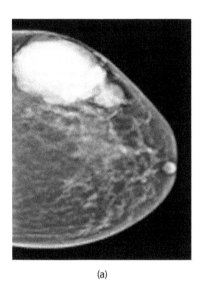

(a)

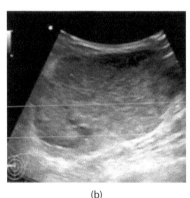

(b)

Figure 53.15 (a) CC view of mammogram showing a dense lobulated large mass. (b) Ultrasound image of the same lesion showing a large hypoechoic mass with cleft-like spaces suggestive of a phyllodes.

13. B   Vacuum-assisted biopsy (Figures 53.16a,b and c).
Large core biopsy with a large core technique allows more extensive sampling of nonpalpable pleomorphic or fine linear branching calcifications, as these may represent ductal carcinoma in situ. Sampling error decreases and diagnostic accuracy improves with large biopsies with vacuum systems.

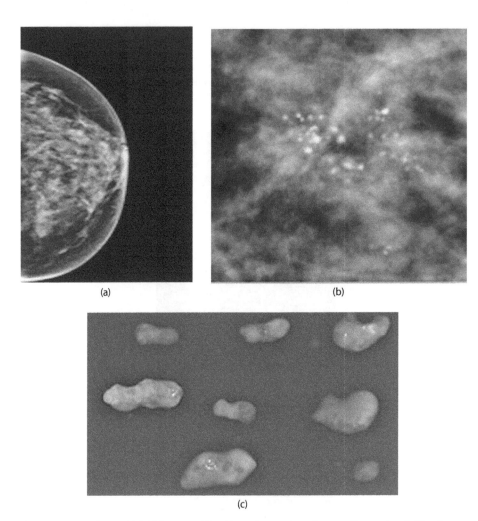

(a)   (b)

(c)

Figure 53.16   (a and b) CC, magnification views showing malignant calcifications. (c) Specimen x-ray of the cores obtained after vacuum-assisted biopsy showing calcifications.

54 Cardiac surgery

Dumbor L Ngaage

Multiple choice questions

→ ## Cardiopulmonary bypass

1. All of the following statements are true except:

A Cardiopulmonary bypass can be used in any procedure where the function of the heart and lungs need to be replaced temporarily.

B The cardiopulmonary bypass circuit consists of a venous reservoir, oxygenator, heat exchanger, filter and roller pump.

C Patients require full-dose heparin with the use of cardiopulmonary bypass.

D Cardiopulmonary bypass is used exclusively for cardiac surgery procedures.

E Cardiopulmonary bypass can cause serious systemic complications.

2. Which of the following is NOT a potential complication of cardiopulmonary bypass?

A Pulmonary embolism.

B Intestinal ischaemia or infarction.

C Post-cardiotomy syndrome.

D Neurological dysfunction.

E Bleeding disorders.

→ ## Ischaemic heart disease

3. Which of these is not a risk factor for ischaemic heart disease?

A Obesity.

B Female gender.

C Advancing age.

D Reduced physical activity.

E Smoking.

→ ## Coronary artery bypass surgery

4. Which of the following statements are true?

A Coronary artery bypass surgery affords symptomatic and prognostic benefit for subsets of patients with ischaemic heart disease.

B Coronary artery bypass grafting can be performed with cardiopulmonary bypass, or off-pump, and by minimally invasive approach (MIDCAB).

C Selective coronary angiography is the 'gold standard' investigation and demonstrates coronary stenosis and coronary characteristics helpful in planning surgery.

D An estimate of the operative mortality can be calculated using risk-scoring systems.

E The left internal mammary (or thoracic) artery does not confer any advantage compared to long saphenous vein grafts.

→ ## Valvular heart disease

5. Which of these statements are true?

A Biological valves are obtained from animals (xenograft or heterograft), dead humans (allograft or homograft) and the patient (autograft).

B Mechanical valves are more durable than biological valves.

C Lifelong anticoagulation is required for all prosthetic valves.

D Age is the only determinant of the choice of prosthetic valve.

E Biological valves are not at risk of prosthetic valve endocarditis.

6. **All of the following statements are true except:**

A Mitral stenosis causes left atrial enlargement, pulmonary hypertension, atrial fibrillation and haemoptysis.

B Severe symptoms, as assessed by the New York Heart Association (NYHA) functional classification, are the indication for surgery in mitral valve disease (regurgitation and stenosis).

C Acute and chronic mitral regurgitation have similar pathophysiology and clinical presentation.

D Mitral valve repair is preferable to mitral valve replacement but more technically demanding.

E Percutaneous mitral valve repair (MitraClip) can be used to treat subsets of high-risk patients with mitral valve regurgitation.

7. **Which of the following statements are false?**

A Aortic stenosis is associated with a risk of sudden death related to the severity of stenosis.

B Aortic stenosis and aortic regurgitation present with similar clinical features, which makes it difficult to distinguishing between both on clinical grounds alone.

C Rheumatic heart disease can cause aortic stenosis and aortic regurgitation.

D Aortic valve repair is not a common practice like mitral valve repair.

E Aortic stenosis can be managed by transcatheter aortic valve implantation (TAVI) is select patient groups.

→ Congenital heart disease

8. **All of the following statements are true except:**

A Cyanotic heart diseases are often more complex compared with acyanotic diseases, and result from a right-to-left shunt or a pulmonary circulation that runs in parallel with systemic circulation, or abnormal connection of blood vessels to the heart.

B Acyanotic heart diseases are more common than cyanotic heart diseases and usually cause heart failure in infancy.

C The coexistence of ventricular septal defect, overriding aorta, pulmonary stenosis and right ventricular hypertrophy is referred to as Fallot's tetralogy.

D Four types of atrial septal defects are perimembranous, muscular, atrioventricular and subarterial.

E In septal defects (atrial and ventricular) a left-to-right shunt causes an increase in pulmonary blood flow and pulmonary vascular resistance. Progressive changes occur if the defects are not closed, leading to Eisenmenger's syndrome.

9. **Which of these are not acyanotic heart diseases?**

A Patent ductus arteriosus.
B Total anomalous pulmonary venous drainage.
C Transposition of the great vessels.
D Patent foramen ovale.
E Coarctation of the aorta.

→ The thoracic aorta and pericardial disease

10. **Which one of these statements is false?**

A Common causes of thoracic aortic aneurysm are atherosclerosis and connective tissue disorders.

B Indication for surgery in thoracic aneurysm depends on the part of the thoracic aorta involved.

C Paraplegia, renal failure and ventricular dysfunction are some complications of descending aneurysm repair.

D Stanford types A and B aortic dissection require emergency repair.

E Pericardial effusion causes an increase in intrapericardial pressure and compression of the atria when this pressure exceeds the atrial pressure. This decreases venous return, cardiac output and blood pressure (cardiac tamponade).

Extended matching questions

→ Cardiac disease and management

1 Computed tomography (CT) scan of the chest
2 Echocardiography
3 Emergency resternotomy
4 Ischaemic heart disease
5 Mitral regurgitation

Choose and match the most appropriate diagnosis or management for the clinical scenarios that follow:

→ Clinical scenarios

A A patient is informed during consent for a procedure for a cardiac disease that, in addition to a procedure-related mortality of about 2%, there is a risk of neurological dysfunction of less than 2%, cardiac arrhythmia up to 30% and significant bleeding up to 5%. What condition is this procedure for?

B A patient who had undergone cardiac surgery through a median sternotomy suffers an asystolic cardiac arrest on the fourth postoperative day. Basic life support is commenced promptly, and initial measures fail to resolve the arrest. Suspecting cardiac tamponade, the next appropriate step should be to perform the following test(s) or intervention?

C A patient with chronic stable angina presents with new-onset dyspnoea on mild exertion, bilateral basal crepitations and a new loud apical pansystolic murmur. Chest radiograph shows cardiomegaly and pulmonary congestion, but electrocardiography does not show evidence of recent myocardial infarction. What is the likely diagnosis?

D Clinical examination of a Marfan's syndrome patient with aneurysmal dilatation of the ascending aorta reveals wide pulse pressure, water-hammer pulse and a mid-diastolic murmur. What procedure is appropriate at this stage in the management of this patient?

E On routine chest radiography, a 78-year-old male is suspected of having an aneurysm of the descending thoracic aorta. What is the appropriate investigation?

Answers to multiple choice questions

→ Cardiopulmonary bypass

1. D
Cardiopulmonary bypass provides cardiac and respiratory support when the function of the heart and lungs needs to be temporarily interrupted. Advances in cardiopulmonary bypass have resulted in miniaturised circuits with possible advantages of reduced systemic inflammatory response, and the related complications. Cardiac surgery remains its principal domain, but it can be used in the management of patients outside cardiac surgery. For example, it facilitates the resection of renal and hepatic tumours invading the inferior vena cava, highly vascular tumours, extensive arteriovenous malformations and rewarming of patients with severe hypothermia.

2. A
Complications can occur at the commencement, during and end of cardiopulmonary bypass. Exposure of blood to the non-physiological surfaces of the cardiopulmonary bypass circuit evokes a systemic inflammatory response that can lead to multi-organ dysfunction. Whereas

systemic embolic complications due to air and microemboli can occur with cardiopulmonary bypass, pulmonary embolism is not usually related to cardiopulmonary bypass. In fact, fully heparinising the patient should have a protective effect against pulmonary embolism in the early postoperative period. However, patients at risk for pulmonary embolism tend to develop this complication from about the seventh postoperative day especially if they are not commenced on deep vein thrombosis prophylaxis and mobilised early.

→ Ischaemic heart disease

3. B
Male gender is a risk factor for ischaemic heart disease. However, studies have shown that female gender is associated with a worse outcome after surgical revascularisation.

→ Coronary artery bypass surgery

4. A, B, C, D
Survival benefit of surgery over angioplasty and stenting has been demonstrated in patients with the following:

- >50% stenosis of the left main stem
- >70% stenosis of the proximal left anterior descending artery
- >70% stenosis of all three major coronary arteries (right coronary, left anterior descending and circumflex)
- Coronary artery stenosis with poor left ventricular function

Recent studies have also shown similar outcomes for diabetic patients and patients with severe calcific coronary artery disease (high SYNTHAX score).

Coronary artery bypass grafting is performed using cardiopulmonary bypass (on-pump) and without cardiopulmonary bypass (off-pump). The prospect of eliminating the systemic inflammatory response syndrome associated with cardiopulmonary pass led to an upsurge in the use of off-pump more than a decade ago, but this practice has introduced a different set of concerns related to poor long-term graft patency. Recent data have shown that while early operative outcomes were similar, a higher re-intervention rate was observed with off-pump. Nevertheless, off-pump seems to have good outcomes in subsets of patients with renal failure and neurological dysfunction. Minimally invasive coronary artery bypass (MIDCAB) is used for single vessel (left anterior descending artery) bypass and has been shown recently to have better outcome than stenting.

Selective coronary angiography demonstrates coronary anatomy and enables the visualisation of coronary artery size, evaluation of the site, extent and complexity of stenosis and assessment of the distal coronary to help plan surgery. It also allows an estimation of left ventricular function. Rare lesions that can affect outcome of surgery, such as coronary artery aneurysm and fistula, are also revealed. Selective coronary angiography provides comprehensive information, not possible with other imaging techniques, that is useful in developing a strategy for surgery. There is a growing role for CT angiography, which is noninvasive and better demonstrates the degree of calcification of proximal parts of the coronary arteries. Its role in current practice is largely supplementary to coronary angiography.

Risk-scoring systems, like the EuroSCORE (European system for cardiac operative risk evaluation) and STS (The Society of Thoracic Surgeons) risk score, allocate scores to each risk factor in a patient that are added up to calculate the predicted operative mortality. These risk calculators are available online and used routinely to provide an estimate of the operative mortality for patients' informed consent.

Venous and arterial grafts are the major conduits used for coronary artery bypass surgery. The long saphenous vein is the most common vein conduit used and the left internal mammary artery is the most common arterial conduit, and the graft of choice for the left anterior descending artery. Venous grafts are susceptible to atherosclerosis, resulting in a 10-year patency rate of 50%–60% for the long saphenous vein. By comparison, arterial grafts are better protected against atherosclerosis. The left internal mammary artery has a 10-year patency rate of 90%. There is a growing trend to use the right internal mammary artery as emerging evidence supports its longer-term patency compared with vein grafts. The concept of total arterial revascularisation (the use of only arterial conduits) where appropriate, is promising and continues to be investigated.

Valvular heart disease

5. A, B

Biological valves are made or obtained from animal or human tissue. While valves obtained from humans (homograft and autograft) are harvested and implanted without major alteration of the configuration, valves made from animal tissue (heterograft) are constructed to resemble human valves and are mounted on a frame (stented) or frameless (stentless). Among biological valves, heterografts are most commonly used; specifically, stented heterografts are the most frequently implanted. Biological valves are non-thrombogenic, so do not require lifelong anticoagulation.

Biological valves, unlike mechanical valves, are subject to degenerative changes, which lead to structural failure, and hence their durability is limited. Younger patients are probably more vulnerable. The need to replace a prosthetic valve also arises if there is a paravalvular leak causing haemodynamic instability or haemolytic anaemia, thrombosis of the valve, thromboembolism related to the valve and infection of the valve (prosthetic valve endocarditis). Homografts and autografts (entirely human tissues) are less susceptible to thrombosis or thromboembolism and infection. Mechanical valves and the other biological valves have low risks of paravalvular leak, infection and thrombosis or thromboembolism.

The choice of the valve type to implant in a patient is influenced by age and other factors, including clinical considerations (like co-existing medical conditions such as bleeding disorders), patient lifestyle (heavy alcohol use) and patient choice.

6. B, C

Surgery is performed in mitral valve disease to relieve symptoms and improve survival (prognostic). Severe symptoms, however, are not the only indication for surgery. For mitral regurgitation, progressive left ventricular dilatation or dysfunction and severe onset of regurgitation are the other indications. With increasing numbers of mitral regurgitation being repaired rather than replaced, and the low mortality risk of repair in the early phase of the disease, there is a trend to advocate surgery even in asymptomatic patients with morphological changes (increase in cardiac dimensions) and functional changes (impaired left ventricular function) with or without new onset atrial fibrillation. For mitral stenosis, the other indications are the severity of stenosis (moderate and severe stenosis with valve area of ≤ 1.5 cm^2) and systemic emboli.

The onset of mitral regurgitation has implications for changes in cardiac morphology and function, and consequently the strategy for surgical correction. In mitral regurgitation, retrograde ejection leads to an increase in left ventricular volume load. The amount of retrograde ejection increases slowly in chronic mitral regurgitation, allowing adaptive changes like progressive left ventricular dilatation and hypertrophy, and left atrial dilatation, to develop without substantial pressure increase. As a result the pulmonary circulation is protected from developing a sudden increase in pressure. Acute mitral regurgitation does not allow time for these compensatory changes. High-volume retrograde flow into a small left atrium causes a sudden surge in left atrial pressure and a back-pressure increase affecting the pulmonary venous circulation, leading to pulmonary congestion and oedema. Chronic mitral regurgitation, however, ultimately causes congestive cardiac failure when the compensatory mechanisms are overwhelmed.

Acute mitral regurgitation presents with sudden onset and rapidly progressive dyspnoea with clinical and radiological evidence of pulmonary oedema. Chronic mitral regurgitation is usually asymptomatic until pulmonary congestion and left ventricular failure develop. Then symptoms like fatigue, dyspnoea on exertion, orthopnoea and atrial fibrillation (due to left atrial enlargement) occur, and left ventricular enlargement becomes apparent radiologically. A loud apical pansystolic murmur is audible in both acute and chronic mitral regurgitation.

7. B
Aortic stenosis and chronic aortic regurgitation are usually asymptomatic until cardiac decompensation occurs. Compensatory mechanisms include ventricular hypertrophy (increase in wall thickness) to overcome the left ventricular outflow obstruction of aortic stenosis and left ventricular dilatation to accommodate the increased left ventricular volume load due to aortic regurgitation. With cardiac decompensation, and acute aortic regurgitation, patients develop exertional dyspnoea and angina. Syncope is also common with aortic stenosis.

Marked differences exist with clinical findings. A harsh systolic ejection murmur, heard loudest in the aortic area and radiating to the carotids, is typical of aortic stenosis.

The distinctive features of aortic regurgitation are due largely to a wide pulse pressure and include the following:

- Collapsing pulse (water-hammer pulse)
- Visible capillary pulsation in the nail bed (Quincke's sign)
- Pulsatile head bobbing (de Musset's sign)
- Visible pulsation of neck arteries (Corrigan's sign)
- 'Pistol shot' sound on auscultation of the femoral artery (Traube's sign)
- Uvular pulsation (Müller's sign).

In aortic regurgitation also, the apex beat is often visible and displaced laterally. The characteristic murmur of aortic regurgitation is high-pitched, mid-diastolic and best heard at the left sternal border. The electrocardiographic and radiological appearances are not usually distinctive.

→ Congenital heart disease

8. D
Three main types of atrial septal defect (defect in the septum between the right and left atria) described are the following: ostium secundum, ostium primum and sinus venosus.

The defects listed in D (perimembranous, muscular, atrioventricular and subarterial) are the four types of ventricular septal defects. In atrial and ventricular septal defects, a left-to-right shunt occurs and in the long term can cause Eisenmenger's syndrome from high-volume pulmonary blood flow, high pulmonary pressure and reversal of shunt.

9. B, C
In total anomalous pulmonary venous drainage, pulmonary venous return is into the systemic venous circulation usually through a communication with the inferior vena cava, superior vena cava, coronary sinus, or right atrium, instead of left atrium. The typical presentation is cyanosis after the first week of life. If there is a co-existent atrial septal defect, cyanosis is minimal even with high pulmonary flow.

The aorta arises from the right ventricle and the pulmonary artery from the left ventricle in transposition of the great vessels. This arrangement allows the pulmonary and systemic circulation to run in parallel rather than in series. As oxygenated blood is confined to the pulmonary circulation and deoxygenated blood to the systemic circulation, this condition is not compatible with life. Associated defects like foramen ovale and ventricular septal defect provide channels for mixing of blood. Transposition of the great vessels is the most common congenital heart disease, causing cyanosis in the newborn period, and, in general, the second-most common cyanotic congenital heart disease after tetralogy of Fallot.

⇨ The thoracic aorta and pericardial disease

10. D

Aortic dissection originating (defect or intimal flap) in the ascending aorta is type A, and one that originates in the descending aorta (beyond the origin of the left subclavian artery) is type B, according to the Stanford classification. Type A requires emergency surgical intervention, but type B is best managed conservatively initially. The indications for surgery in type B aortic dissection include the following:

* Worsening chest pain indicating imminent rupture
* Progressive expansion of lesion on serial chest imaging (radiograph or CT scan)
* Malperfuson syndrome resulting in organ dysfunction, such as renal failure, or limb and neurological complications

Recent advances in the management of aortic disease include the transluminal placement of stents across the site of aortic aneurysm and localised dissection of the descending aorta in select patients. Thoracic endovascular repair (TEVAR) is less invasive and is performed percutaneously.

Answers to extended matching questions

⇨ Cardiac disease and management

1. E Computed Tomography (CT) scan of the chest

The diagnosis of thoracic aneurysm can be confirmed by CT of the chest. The site, size and presence of thrombi can be assessed. As descending thoracic aneurysm is often managed conservatively, CT is useful for serial assessment of the aneurysm to determine when surgery is indicated, due to acute enlargement or progressive increase in size to more than 6 cm.

2. D Echocardiography

Marfan's syndrome is associated with cystic medial necrosis of the vessel wall, causing weakness and dilatation of the vessel. The aortic root and ascending aorta are commonly affected. Aortic regurgitation due to aortic root dilatation is common. The presence of clinical features of aortic regurgitation in the setting of ascending aortic aneurysm warrants further investigation. Echocardiography assesses the severity of regurgitation, diameter of the aortic root, aortic valve morphology and left ventricular dimensions and function. The information provided by echocardiography is vital in deciding the optimal type of surgical repair.

3. B Emergency resternotomy

Emergency resternotomy contributes to the high survival rate reported for cardiac arrests following cardiac surgery. Early re-sternotomy is strongly recommended if a stable cardiac output is not achieved within 5 minutes of the onset of the cardiac arrest. Internal cardiac massage should be performed at a rate of 100 beats per minute, with an aim to achieve systolic arterial pressure of at least 60 mmHg. Emergency resternotomy should be considered until 10 days postoperatively. In some situations, it might be necessary to institute cardiopulmonary bypass.

4. A Ischaemic heart disease

Surgical revascularisation for ischaemic heart disease is achieved by coronary artery bypass grafting, one of the most investigated surgical procedures with well and consistently documented complications. An estimate of the operative mortality can be calculated using risk-stratification systems like the EuroSCORE or STS score. Surgery for mitral valve disease is associated with a higher operative risk, approximately 5%–6%, and greater risk for neurological complications.

5. C Mitral regurgitation

Even with stable symptoms due to adequate medical therapy, ischaemic heart disease can still cause morphological complications and remains a common cause of mitral regurgitation (ischaemic mitral regurgitation) as a result of its local or global effects. Regional myocardial ischaemia and myocardial infarction cause papillary muscle dysfunction or rupture. Global myocardial ischaemia causes left ventricular dysfunction and dilatation, which pull the mitral leaflets apart so that functional mitral regurgitation occurs in the presence of grossly normal mitral valve leaflets.

55 The thorax

Dumbor L Ngaage

Multiple choice questions

→ ## Introduction

1. All of the following statements are true except:

A The lungs are derivatives of the primitive foregut.

B Lymphatic drainage of the lungs to numbered lymph node stations is important in lung cancer staging.

C Bronchial arteries arise directly from the thoracic aorta to provide systemic blood supply to the trachea and bronchi.

D Anatomical differences between the right and left main bronchi favour the inhalation of foreign bodies into the right.

E The left lung has more lobes and segments than the right lung.

2. Which of the following statements is false?

A Pulmonary function tests assess the functional capacity and severity of pulmonary disease, and help to predict response to treatment.

B The peak expiratory flow rate is reliable and reproducible but is effort-dependent.

C Forced expiratory volume in 1 second (FEV1) might be normal in people with poor gas exchange.

D The gas transfer factor is a test of the integrity of the lung's alveolar-capillary surface area for gas exchange and not affected by haemoglobin level.

E Spirometry readings improve with bronchodilators for obstructive lung diseases, but no change is observed for restrictive lung diseases.

→ ## Pleural space disease

3. Which one of these is not an indication for surgical intervention in pneumothorax?

A Bilateral spontaneous pneumothoraces.

B First ipsilateral spontaneous pneumothorax in a young, tall male.

C First contralateral spontaneous pneumothorax.

D Pneumothorax in professionals at risk like divers and pilots.

E Persistent air leak following drain insertion or failure of the lung to re-expand.

4. Which of the following statements are true?

A Tension pneumothorax can cause haemodynamic compromise.

B Pleural effusions due to cardiac failure, renal failure, hepatic disease, inflammatory disease and malignancy have different protein content.

C Infection of the pleural space (empyema) results from iatrogenic and noniatrogenic causes.

D Chest drains are no longer critical to the management of chest disease.

E Video-assisted thoracoscopic surgery (VATS) plays a major role in the management of pleural space diseases.

→ ## Presentation of lung disease

5. All of the following are false except:

A Repeated haemoptysis is always due to malignant lung tumour.

B Chest computed tomography (CT) scan is the most important investigation for repeated haemoptysis.

C Repeated haemoptysis should be investigated with chest x-ray and bronchoscopy.

D Patients with repeated haemoptysis should only have regular full blood count and be kept under close observation.

E Traumatic haemoptysis usually resolves spontaneously, so no investigation is necessary.

→ Malignant lung tumours

6. Which one of these statements is false?

A Lifetime burden of cigarette smoking, quantified as 'pack-years', is the major risk factor for bronchial carcinoma.

B Compared with non-small cell cancer, small-cell lung cancer, formerly known as oat cell cancer, is less common, metastasises early and is less amenable to surgery.

C Finger clubbing and hypertrophic pulmonary osteoarthropathy are clinical features of advanced lung cancer and do not resolve after resection of primary lung cancer.

D The appropriate treatment strategy is dependent on tumour type, tumour stage and the general fitness and lung function of the patient.

E Haemorrhagic pleural effusion is a poor prognostic sign for primary lung cancer.

7. Which one of these statements is true?

A Chest radiograph yields useful information about primary lung cancer.

B CT is only useful for guiding fine-needle aspiration (FNAC).

C Positron emission tomography (PET) has high specificity for bronchial carcinoma.

D Sputum cytology has a high sensitivity.

E Invasive procedures such as endobronchial ultrasound, endoscopic ultrasound, mediastinoscopy, mediastinotomy and thoracoscopy are not staging procedures.

8. All of the following statements are true except:

A Perihilar lymph node sampling or en bloc dissection is not necessary in patients undergoing surgery with a curative intent.

B Video-assisted thoracoscopic surgery prevents rib-spreading and might reduce postoperative pain and length of hospital stay.

C Surgery for early-stage non-small cell lung cancer (T1-3, N0-1) should be with curative intent.

D The choice of lung resection for lung cancer is influenced by the fitness of the patient.

E Posterolateral thoracotomy is the standard route into the thoracic cavity.

Extended matching questions

→ Procedures

1 Bronchoscopy
2 Chest drain insertion
3 CT scan of the chest
4 Pulmonary function tests
5 Thoracotomy
6 VATS

Match the procedures with the clinical scenarios that follow:

→ Clinical scenarios

A A middle-aged patient presents with spontaneous repeated haemoptysis, and clinical examination reveals no abnormal findings. Her chest radiograph is normal. What is the next procedure of choice?

B After reading the information booklet about his proposed procedure, an anxious patient being consented for a procedure is worried about the post-procedural complications of pain and possible rib fractures. What procedure is planned for this patient?

C Following a right pneumonectomy, the postoperative recovery of a patient is complicated by bronchopleural fistula, which presents with pyrexia, expectoration of large amounts of purulent sputum and a high fluid level on chest radiograph. In addition to positioning the patient to lie on the operated side, what procedure is urgently required?

D A mediastinal mass is found incidentally on the chest radiograph of a 65-year-old nonsmoker who is otherwise healthy, with no significant past medical history. Which procedure would you recommend to this patient at this time?

E A 75-year-old man who suffers from emphysema is referred for surgical resection of a left upper-lobe lung cancer. Which procedure is required to assess his fitness for lung resection?

F An 69-year-old retired builder with suspected pleural mesothelioma and an indeterminate histological diagnosis from a CT-scan-guided biopsy is referred with recurrent right pleural effusion for surgical management. What is the most appropriate procedure?

Answers to multiple choice questions

→ Introduction

1. E
The left lung is divided into an upper lobe and lower lobe by the oblique fissure. There are five segments in the upper lobe and four in the lower lobe. Each segment is an anatomically defined unit with named bronchi, pulmonary artery branch and pulmonary vein tributary.

The right lung, on the other hand, has three lobes. An oblique fissure separates the upper and lower lobes. The upper lobe is further separated from a middle lobe by a horizontal fissure. The right lung also has the same number of segmental divisions distributed as follows: three in the upper, two in the middle and four in the lower lobe.

2. D
The gas transfer factor, also called 'diffusion capacity' (DLCO) is a measure of the overall ability of the lungs to transfer gases from the alveoli to blood. It is a test of the integrity of the alveolar-capillary surface area of the lungs for gas exchange and is affected by the patient's haemoglobin level. The test involves the inhalation of a test gas that contains a small amount of carbon monoxide. The uptake of carbon monoxide into blood is affected by the haemoglobin concentration. Low haemoglobin concentration as is seen in anaemia will reduce the uptake (transfer) of carbon monoxide, while high haemoglobin levels as occur in polycythaemia vera will increase the transfer factor.

→ Pleural space disease

3. B
The first episode of an ipsilateral spontaneous pneumothorax is not an indication for surgical intervention. Current management recommendation is the insertion of small-bore Seldinger-type chest drains, ideally under ultrasound guidance.

Only about one-third of these patients have a recurrence. However, patients who have a second episode of spontaneous pneumothorax should have a surgical intervention, as one-half will have a recurrence.

4. A, B, C, E
In tension pneumothorax, positive pressure builds up in the hemithorax as air accumulates through a breach in the visceral pleura, which acts like a valve allowing a unidirectional flow of

air out of the lung. The high intrapleural pressure results in compression of the ipsilateral lung, flattening of the hemidiaphragm, mediastinal distortion and shift and impairment of venous return to the heart and hence a reduction of cardiac output.

Pleural effusion results from interference with either the mechanisms of pleural fluid production by capillaries of parietal pleura or absorption by the capillaries of the visceral pleura. Depending on the protein concentration, pleural effusions are classified as transudates (less than 30 g/L) or exudates (30 g/L or more).

In cardiac failure, the pulmonary capillary pressure is elevated, leading to increased production of pleural effusion with low protein content.

Renal and hepatic failures are associated with low plasma protein and intravascular oncotic pressure. The pleural effusion that results from reduced pleural fluid absorption is low in protein content. Inflammatory diseases increase pleural capillary permeability to cause the accumulation of fluid and protein. Malignancy obstructs the lymphatic system and causes a protein-rich pleural effusion.

The pleural cavity is sterile but the bronchial tree is not. A breech of the sterile barrier between the pleura and bronchial system on one hand (endogenous), and between the pleura and external environment (exogenous) on the other, increases the risk of empyema (infection within the pleural space). Iatrogenic introduction of bacteria into the pleural space can occur during aspiration of effusions, insertion of chest drains, thoracoscopy and thoracotomy. Traumatic haemothorax provides a favourable culture medium for infection. Endogenous spread can occur from pneumonia, bronchiectasis, tuberculosis, fungal infections and lung abscess.

Video-assisted thoracoscopic surgery (VAT) is a less invasive method for investigating and treating thoracic pathologies, including pleural diseases such as pneumothorax, pleural effusion and empyema. VAT plays a major role in the management of thoracic diseases.

Intercostal chest drains are fundamental to the management of chest disease. The insertion of chest drains can be lifesaving, and they are used as sole therapeutic interventions or adjunctive to other thoracic procedures.

→ Presentation of lung disease

5. C

Patients presenting with repeated haemoptysis should be investigated with a chest radiography and bronchoscopy, at the minimum. A detailed history is crucial to elucidate associated symptoms and signs of the underlying cause, which could be lung carcinoma, nonmalignant lung tumour or lung infections, or, indeed, disease conditions not affecting the lungs like mitral stenosis.

The findings of chest radiography and bronchoscopy will determine the need for and timing of a computed tomography scan of the chest.

→ Primary lung cancer

6. C

Finger clubbing and hypertrophic pulmonary osteoarthropathy are clinical findings seen in some patients with primary lung cancer. The direct association with lung cancer is demonstrated by regression of these muscular and skeletal abnormalities when the cancer is resected.

7. A

Most lung cancer lesions or their secondary effects are detected on chest radiograph. Pleural effusion, distal lung collapse or consolidation due to bronchial obstruction and raised hemidiaphragm due to invasion of phrenic nerve are some secondary effects of lung cancer seen on chest radiograph.

CT is central to further characterisation of primary lung cancer with regard to site, tumour size (T stage), proximity to chest wall and mediastinal structures and mediastinal lymph node status (N stage). It also facilitates percutaneous biopsy for peripheral lesions.

Positron emission tomography shows high uptake of fluorodeoxyglucose (FDG) by lesions with high metabolism, so in addition to cancer, infections and other inflammatory lesions show avid uptake of FDG. Therefore, it does not have a high specificity for lung cancer.

Sputum cytology has a high false-negative rate because it relies on the probability of obtaining a sample with exfoliated tumour cells, which can be low for peripheral lung cancers.

Endobronchial ultrasound (EBUS), endoscopic ultrasound (EUS) mediastinoscopy, mediastinotomy and thoracoscopy are techniques for obtaining mediastinal lymph node biopsies, and are useful in assessing the extent of tumour spread (staging) and sometimes for establishing histological diagnosis.

8. A
The principle of surgery with curative intent for lung cancer is to excise all the cancer tissue in the lung and the lymph nodes, while conserving as much unaffected lung tissue as possible. Surgical excision of lung cancer can be achieved by anatomical resections such as segmentectomy, lobectomy, bilobectomy and pneumonectomy, and nonanatomical resection such as wedge resection. This should be combined with removal of mediastinal lymph nodes that are involved. This is accomplished by either excision of enlarged lymph nodes (sampling) or en bloc dissection of the mediastinal lymph nodes (systematic dissection).

Answers to extended matching questions

1. A Bronchoscopy
Haemoptysis is commonly caused by bronchopulmonary trauma, infection, or neoplastic (benign and malignant) lesions of pulmonary system. The underlying pathologies are usually in direct or indirect communication with the bronchial tree. Bronchoscopy affords the ability to visualise the lesion, the potential to obtain biopsies or treat, or the insight to plan further treatment. The flexible bronchoscope can be advanced into segmental bronchi and is useful for obtaining sputum and tissue biopsies. As the calibre is small and suction limited, flexible bronchoscopes might not have optimal diagnostic and therapeutic yield soon after an episode of haemoptysis because blood clots obscure visualisation. Rigid bronchoscopy overcomes these setbacks but requires general anaesthesia.

2. C Chest drain insertion
Morphological changes such as mediastinal shift, elevation of the hemidiaphragm and crowding of the ribs occur after pneumonectomy to contract the pneumonectomy space, which fills with tissue fluid. Dehiscence of the bronchial stump occurs in bronchopleural fistula to establish communication between colonised bronchial tree and sterile pneumonectomy space. Invariably, the pneumonectomy space and contained fluid get infected due to the bronchopleural fistula. Signs of systemic infection (pyrexia) with clinical (expectorating purulent sputum) and radiological (high fluid level) evidences of infected collection in the chest warrant immediate chest drain insertion, to control the source of sepsis. Further management of bronchopleural fistula is undertaken in specialised centres.

3. D Computed tomographic (CT) scan of the chest
A mediastinal mass on chest radiograph deserves further investigation with CT scan of the chest to define the site, size, nature and attachments of the mass and surrounding structures,

and, where possible, to obtain a guided percutaneous biopsy for histological diagnosis. On the basis of the location in the mediastinum, the possible cause of the mass can be suspected. Common mediastinal masses in different parts of the mediastinum are the following:

- Superior mediastinum – lymphoma, thyroid and parathyroid
- Anterior mediastinum – thymoma, lymphoma and germ cell tumour
- Middle mediastinum – cystic lesions, lymphoma and mesenchymal tumours
- Posterior mediastinum – neurogenic tumours, cystic lesions and mesenchymal tumours.

4. E Pulmonary function tests

To determine the fitness of patients for lung resection, and the extent of resection they can tolerate, pulmonary function tests are necessary. Peak expiratory flow rate, forced expiratory volume in 1 second (FEV_1), forced vital capacity (FVC), diffusion capacity (DLCO) and arterial blood gases provide useful information. Patients with borderline fitness based on pulmonary function test can be subjected to cardiopulmonary exercise testing or shuttle walk testing.

5. B Thoracotomy

Thoracotomy involves muscle cutting, rib-spreading and parietal pleura breeching. Sometimes rib fractures occur, and the intercostal nerves are bruised during rib-spreading. In the early postoperative period, therefore, thoracotomy pain can be severe and difficult to control. The functional consequence of post-thoracotomy pain leads to other complications such as impairment of mobilisation and normal breathing and gas exchange. The strategies commonly used to manage early post-thoracotomy pain include oral analgesia with paracetamol, and intravenous opiates used as patient-controlled analgesia (PCA) or local anaesthesia delivered via catheters into the paravertebral or extrapleural space.

6. F Video-assisted thoracoscopic surgery (VATS)

VATS enables complete drainage of the pleural effusion and sampling the effusion for cytological assessment, direct visualisation of the pleural cavity and making a clinical judgement, guided multiple pleural biopsies for histological analyses and talc pleurodesis. The role of VATS in managing pleural disease is well established and clearly of advantage because of its less-invasive nature and faster postoperative recovery compared to thoracotomy.

Vascular

56 Arterial disorders

Pradip K Datta

Multiple choice questions

→ Arterial stenosis and occlusion

1. The following statements are true except:

A Pain of intermittent claudication (IC) comes on after taking the first step.

B Rest pain occurs at night.

C Clinical presentation reflects the site of obstruction.

D Severity of symptoms depends upon the size of the vessel and if the onset is acute or chronic.

E The most common cause is atheroma.

→ Investigations for arterial occlusive disease

2. Which of the following statements is not true?

A Concomitant diseases must be excluded in all patients.

B Doppler ultrasound should be the initial vascular investigation.

C Duplex scanning is ideal to visualise the aorto-iliac segment.

D A treadmill accurately assesses the claudication distance.

E Angiography, the roadmap, should be done in all patients.

→ Management of arterial stenosis or occlusion

3. Which of the following statements are true?

A Intervention (surgical or radiological) should be considered at the first consultation before the obstruction gets worse.

B Conservative management must be the first line of treatment in all cases.

C Drugs can be used in selected patients.

D Percutaneous transluminal angioplasty (PTA) should be the first interventional procedure to be tried.

E Operations for vascular reconstruction is carried out in severe disease where PTA has failed.

→ Other sites of atheromatous occlusive disease

4. The following statements are true except:

A Transient ischaemic attacks (TIAs) are a symptom of internal carotid stenosis.

B Subclavian steal syndrome is the result of vertebrobasilar insufficiency.

C Thoracic inlet syndrome can cause vascular insufficiency of the upper limb.

D Renovascular hypertension is always due to atherosclerotic stenosis.

E Ischaemic colitis is due to occlusion of the superior mesenteric artery.

→ Gangrene

5. Which of the following statements are true?

A Wet gangrene occurs when there is infection.

B Neuropathy is an important factor in diabetic gangrene.

C Frostbite is gangrene caused by cold injury to the vessel wall.

D Bedsore is a type of gangrene.

E Amputation of the affected limb should be done in all cases at the earliest to prevent the spread of life-threatening sepsis.

→ Acute arterial occlusion

6. Which of the following statements are not true?

A Acute thrombosis is the most common cause of acute arterial occlusion.

B When acute thrombosis is diagnosed, thrombolysis should always be the first line of treatment.

C When an embolus is the cause of arterial occlusion, a left ventricular mural thrombus is the usual source.

D Embolectomy should be the treatment for an arterial embolus.

E Compartment syndrome is a complication that might occur after embolectomy.

→ Amputation

7. Which of the following statements are true?

A Amputation sometimes might have to be carried out in the absence of gangrene.

B Distal amputations are possible in diabetic gangrene.

C Below-knee (BK) amputation gives the best chance of walking again, with a prosthesis.

D Presence of a femoral pulse guarantees healing of a BK amputation.

E Long posterior flap technique is the more common method of BK amputation.

→ Aneurysms

8. The following statements are true except:

A 95% of abdominal aortic aneurysms (AAA) are infra-renal.

B When an AAA presents as an emergency, it is due to intraperitoneal rupture.

C An AAA of more than 5.5 cm in diameter should be operated upon.

D A thrombosed popliteal artery aneurysm can be confused for an abscess.

E Berry aneurysms occur along the trunks of the vessels that form the Circle of Willis.

→ Arteritis and vasospastic conditions

9. Which of the following statements are true?

A Thromboangiitis obliterans mainly affects the large vessels of the limbs.

B Arteritis occurs in association with rheumatoid arthritis, systemic lupus erythematosus (SLE) and polyarteritis nodosa.

C Cystic myxomatous degeneration presents with claudication.

D Raynaud's disease and Raynaud's syndrome are different.

E Sympathectomy is an effective surgical treatment in Raynaud's disease.

Extended matching questions

→ Diagnoses

1 Abdominal aortic aneurysm (AAA)
2 Abdominal compartment syndrome (ACS)
3 Acute femoro-popliteal embolus
4 Acute femoro-popliteal thrombosis
5 Aortoiliac occlusion
6 Arteriovenous fistula
7 Diabetic gangrene
8 Femoro-popliteal occlusion
9 Internal carotid artery (ICA) stenosis
10 Limb compartment syndrome
11 Popliteal artery aneurysm
12 Raynaud's disease

13 Ruptured AAA
14 Subclavian steal syndrome
15 Thoracic inlet (outlet) syndrome
16 Thromboangiitis obliterans (TAO)

Match the diagnoses with the clinical scenarios that follow:

➡ Clinical scenarios

A A 70-year-old man has been brought as an emergency complaining of sudden onset of severe left-sided abdominal pain radiating to the back. He has a systolic blood pressure of 90 mmHg, pulse rate of 120 per minute and is cold and clammy with a tender distended abdomen and a pulsatile mass.

B A 52-year-old man complains of a weak grip in his left hand with tingling and numbness along the inner side of his arm and palm. When using his arm he has pain, and his palm has a dusky discoloration of the fingertips. His left radial pulse is weaker than the right.

C A 73-year-old woman complains of attacks of sudden blindness in her right eye that last for a few minutes. At the same time, she has episodic weakness of her upper limb. A systolic bruit can be heard over the bifurcation of her carotid artery.

D A 68-year-old man, who is a heavy smoker, complains of pain in his right thigh and buttocks on walking about 400 metres. Once he stops, the pain disappears and returns when he walks a similar distance again.

E A 60-year-old woman, who is a heavy smoker and works as a domestic, gets syncopal attacks when she is working scrubbing floors using her right upper limb vigorously. This makes her quite uneasy and at times she feels faint.

F A 68-year-old woman complains of sudden onset of severe pain in her right thigh, calf and leg of 6 hours duration. She has lost sensations from the mid-thigh distally, cannot move her foot or knee, her skin feels very cold and she looks pale. There are no pulses. She had a myocardial infarction 6 weeks ago.

G A 32-year-old woman complains of episodes of pain in the fingers of both her hands when it is cold. The fingers go white, swollen and dusky when she is unable to make any fine movements. After some time, this subsides when the fingers become red.

H A 28-year-old man, who is a heavy smoker, complains of pain in his right lower limb on walking. He has developed a tender cord-like structure along his long saphenous vein with some tenderness and a generally swollen leg.

I A 74-year-old man complains of epigastric discomfort and throbbing backache for 4 months. On examination he has a mass in his epigastrium extending on to umbilical region, which shows expansile pulsation.

J A 64-year-old man, who is a postman, complains of intermittent claudication in his calf for 8 months. He has a claudication distance of 200 metres and is a type 2 diabetic.

K A 70-year-old man, who is a long-term heavy smoker, complains of onset of severe pain in his left calf and thigh of 2 days duration. Prior to this he had suffered from intermittent claudication, with a claudication distance of 50 metres. He is unable to walk now.

L A 45-year-old woman complains of a lump on the left side of her forehead for many years. This has gradually become larger and gives her a continuous headache. On examination the lump has a to-and-fro thrill and a machinery murmur.

M A 55-year-old woman who has been an insulin-dependent diabetic for 35 years has developed necrotic skin patches in her right forefoot following a fall from a bicycle. In spite of good immediate and ongoing treatment from her doctor's surgery, she has developed necrotic skin patches in her distal foot.

N A 66-year-old man presented with a tender lump over his right popliteal fossa and severe pain in his leg for 48 hours. The lump was there a couple of years, but only over the last couple of days it has become extremely tender, the leg has become cold and he is unable to walk.

O A 70-year-old man underwent emergency operation for a leaking AAA. While in the ITU, after 2 days, he became oliguric and has abdominal distension and cardio-respiratory compromise. His CVP is 10 cm of water. He is still on the ventilator.

P A 65-year-old woman with atrial fibrillation underwent a successful lower limb embolectomy under local anaesthetic. A couple of days later she developed in the same limb severe throbbing pain over a period of 4 hours; the limb looked pink.

Answers to multiple choice questions

1. A
The pain of IC does not come on after taking the first step. It comes on after walking a certain distance and is relieved by stopping. This fact clinically differentiates it from arthritic pain, which comes on after taking the first step and is not relieved by rest. The pain-free distance that a patient can walk is called the claudication distance. Rest pain typically occurs at night and is felt in the distal foot. The pain is relieved by keeping the foot dependent and hanging it by the bedside or sleeping in a chair. The site of arterial obstruction can be diagnosed clinically. In aortoiliac disease, the patient complains of thigh and buttock claudication whilst calf claudication indicates superficial femoral artery obstruction.

The severity of symptoms depends upon the size of the original vessel and duration of onset. In acute onset the presentation would be sudden and severe, whereas in chronic disease the presentation will be gradual because there would have been time for collaterals to develop. The clinical presentation will also be influenced by the organ affected and size of the artery occluded: transient ischaemic attack or stroke in internal carotid artery stenosis, angina or myocardial infarction (MI) in the case of coronary artery, hypertension in renal artery stenosis and IC in lower limb vessel obstruction. The most common cause is atheromatous obstruction the pathophysiology of which is explained in **Figure 56.1**.

2. C, E
Duplex scanning is a major noninvasive technique that uses B-mode ultrasound to obtain an image of the vessels. The aorto-iliac segment is not ideally suited to this investigation, as obesity obscures the image; CT angiography is best for this segment. Duplex scanning is best to visualise the carotid. Angiography should not be done in all patients. It is done only when the decision has been made on clinical grounds to intervene, either radiologically or surgically.

In all patients with arterial occlusive disease, intercurrent illnesses must be excluded. Haematological and biochemical investigations are done to exclude anaemia, diabetes, renal impairment and polycythaemia or thrombocythaemia. An ECG and CXR will exclude cardiopulmonary problems, which are not uncommon in this age group. A cardiac echo and pulmonary function tests would be necessary in more severe disease for anaesthetic assessment, particularly when major arterial surgery is contemplated.

The ideal initial vascular investigation is a Doppler ultrasound, which would help to calculate the ankle-brachial pressure index (ABPI) that gives an objective assessment of the degree of ischaemia. The claudication distance is best measured by the treadmill in the vascular laboratory.

3. C, D, E
Drug treatment is required for concomitant diseases such as diabetes and hypertension. Treatment of the latter with β-blockers may worsen the claudication. Raised blood lipids are treated with statins, which also have a stabilising effect on atherosclerotic plaques; aspirin

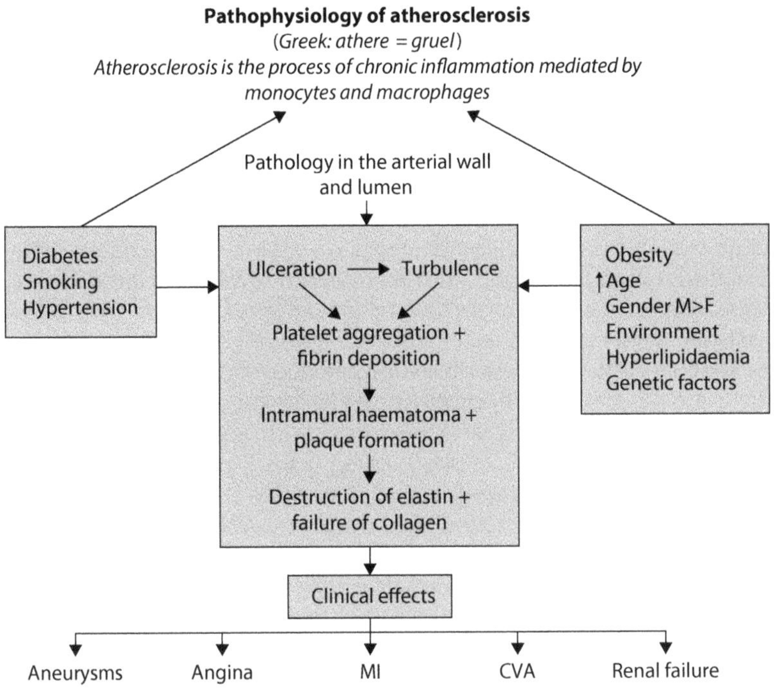

Pathophysiology of atherosclerosis
(Greek: athere = gruel)
Atherosclerosis is the process of chronic inflammation mediated by
monocytes and macrophages

Figure 56.1   Pathophysiology of atherosclerosis.

(75 mg) as an anti-platelet agent or clopidogrel as an alternative is useful. Vasodilators provide no benefit.

Intervention is necessary when the symptoms of the patient are threatening the limb (critical ischaemia), livelihood and lifestyle. The first port of call should be the interventional radiologist for PTA. In the iliacs, the procedure is followed by insertion of a stent. Vascular reconstruction by open surgery is performed when PTA is not possible due to extensive disease or has failed. Depending upon the site of obstruction the procedures are aortofemoral or aorto-bi-femoral bypass, femoro-popliteal, or femoro-distal bypass. In patients with severe comorbid disease who have aortoiliac obstruction, extra-anatomic bypass graft in the form of axillo-femoral or femoro-femoral should be considered as a limb-salvage procedure.

4. D, E

Renovascular hypertension from renal artery stenosis is not always due to atherosclerotic stenosis. It can be due to fibromuscular hyperplasia. In the latter all other vessels would be normal, while the narrowing would be smooth and confined to the main trunk of the artery without involvement of the origin; when atherosclerosis is the cause the neighbouring vessels would be involved, including the origin from the aorta. Ischaemic colitis occurs due to atherosclerosis of the inferior mesenteric artery, causing post-prandial pain and rectal bleeding.

Transient ischaemic attacks (TIAs) are the classical presentation of internal carotid artery (ICA) stenosis. In addition, patients may present with amaurosis fugax, sudden episodic blindness and reversible intermittent neurological deficit, and a systolic bruit in the neck. Subclavian steal syndrome occurs when there is atherosclerotic obstruction of the first part of the subclavian artery. Such patients, when they use the upper limb vigorously, suffer syncopal attacks because the subclavian artery responds to increasing demand by stealing blood from the vertebral artery causing cerebral ischaemia. Thoracic inlet syndrome may cause compression of the subclavian artery from a cervical rib or fibrous band. This might result in a stenosis with post-stenotic dilatation and atherosclerosis; small emboli from a thrombus get dislodged causing distal ischaemia of the hand.

5. A, B, C, D

Wet gangrene typically occurs when infection has supervened upon a part of the limb where there is tissue necrosis from vascular occlusion. This results in putrefaction. Clinically crepitus is felt denoting infection from gas-forming organisms, a situation typical of diabetic gangrene. Neuropathy is a major pathological change that contributes to diabetic gangrene. This is due to sensory loss as a result of which the patient is unaware of minor injuries, which therefore go unnoticed. Motor neuropathy causes neuropathic joints with loss of reflexes. Callosities form, which are a portal of entry of infection that spreads quickly along subfascial planes.

Frostbite is gangrene caused by exposure to very low temperatures. It is seen in mountain climbers, the elderly and vagrants, the latter when exposed to unexpected cold spells. Cold injury damages the blood vessels, resulting in leakage of fluid and swelling with severe pain. There is blistering followed by gangrene and clear demarcation of devitalised tissue. Bedsores are a form of localised gangrene caused by pressure commonly seen in the elderly, debilitated and immunocompromised. The typical sites are ischial tuberosity, greater trochanter, sacrum and heel. The underlying pathology consists of the following: prolonged weight bearing → mechanical shear forces on soft tissues over bony prominences → increase in pressure across small vessels → reduced tissue perfusion → ischaemic necrosis → ulceration.

Amputation should not be carried out at the earliest. Attempts must be made to salvage as much tissue as possible by considering revascularisation by surgery or interventional radiology. These procedures, with a period of conservative management, might help in performing a more distal amputation.

6. A, B

The most common cause of sudden arterial occlusion is an arterial embolus, not thrombosis. Moreover, the presentation of acute thrombosis is not as acute and dramatic as that of an embolus. If acute thrombosis is diagnosed, thrombolytic therapy is not the first line of treatment in all patients. Many vascular surgeons would perform revascularisation procedures straightaway so as not lose valuable time in trying thrombolysis. The latter may not be successful at all or be only partially successful.

An embolus, the most common cause of sudden arterial occlusion, usually originates from a mural thrombus in the left ventricle following a myocardial infarction (**Figure 56.2**). Embolectomy should be the treatment of choice carried out under general or local anaesthetic, depending upon the clinical condition of the patient who would just be recovering from a MI. Whilst an arterial thrombus is the most common cause of an embolus, there are several causes (**Figure 56.3**). Following an embolectomy, revascularisation injury in the form of compartment syndrome is a real worry. The surgeon should be on the lookout for such a complication, the treatment for which is fasciotomy.

7. A, B, C, E

Amputation might have to be performed in the absence of gangrene, in the presence of severe rest pain in critical limb ischaemia where vascular reconstruction is not possible. It is also necessary when there are joint contractures following paralysis where the limb is a liability and in irreparable traumatic damage. In these situations, the limb is referred to as a 'dead loss' limb. Distal amputations such as ray amputations and transmetatarsal and midtarsal amputations are possible in the diabetic because the ischaemia is due to microangiopathy as evidenced by a warm distal foot.

Pathophysiology of arterial embolus

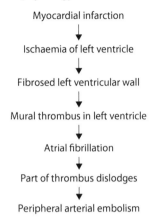

Figure 56.2   Pathophysiology of arterial embolus.

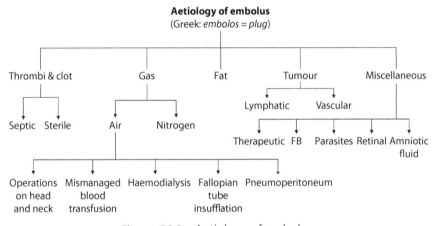

Figure 56.3   Aetiology of embolus.

The amputee has the best chance of walking with a prosthesis after a BK amputation. The presence of the knee joint gives good proprioception, enabling early and better mobilisation. BK amputation is performed by two techniques – a long posterior flap and a skew flap. The former is more commonly performed because it is simpler.

Almost one-quarter of BK amputations will need conversion to an above-knee (AK) amputation because of failed healing. Presence of a femoral pulse does not guarantee healing of a BK amputation. Several tests such as Doppler pressures, oximetry, isotope clearance, arteriography, thermography and plethysmography have been used to predict the success of healing of a BK amputation. However, the simplest indicator of success of primary healing continues to be clinical judgement with the amount of bleeding at the incision site.

8. B, E

Emergency presentation of rupture or leak of AAA is retroperitoneal in the vast majority. This is because the anterior part of the aneurysm is occupied by clot and so leak occurs into the retroperitoneal space as a haematoma. Only a small minority rupture intraperitoneally; they usually do not survive. Berry aneurysms that occur along the Circle of Willis are always at the bifurcation of the vessels and not along the trunk. This is because the bifurcation is the weakest part, as the tunica media is absent at the site.

The cause of AAA is atheromatous disease and 95% are infra-renal. A patient with an AAA that is 5.5 cm or more in diameter is advised to undergo an operation even if it is asymptomatic because the patient has a greater risk of rupture. A popliteal artery aneurysm can often result in thrombosis. The patient then presents with distal ischaemia and a painful red tender swelling mimicking a popliteal abscess.

9. B, C, D
In connective tissue disorders such as rheumatoid arthritis, SLE and polyarteritis nodosa, arteritis is a common feature. Although the domain of the physician, the surgeon is involved when amputation of digits is necessary for distal gangrene. Cystic myxomatous degeneration mainly affects the popliteal artery where there is accumulation of jelly-like material causing narrowing of the vessel presenting with claudication. Duplex scan is the investigation of choice. The treatment is excision of the myxomatous material.

Raynaud's disease and the syndrome by the same name are different. Raynaud's disease usually affects the hands of young women where the small arteries of the digits are constricted, causing the fingers to turn white. Typically the condition is episodic, with each attack consisting of blanching of the digits, dusky cyanosis, red engorgement and pain. Raynaud's syndrome (or phenomenon) is the term applied when there is an established cause. It is an arterial manifestation of collagen diseases such as SLE and rheumatoid arthritis and might occur after prolonged use of vibrating tools. This might also be part of CREST syndrome – Calcinosis, Raynaud's syndrome (sometimes called Raynaud's phenomenon), oEsophageal motility disorder, Scleroderma and Telengiectasis. The clinical features mimic Raynaud's disease but are much more intense.

Thromboangiitis obliterans (TAO) or Buerger's disease affects the small and medium-sized arteries of the limbs causing occlusion; thrombophlebitis of the superficial and deep veins is also present. It is a disease of male smokers under the age of 30. There are inflammatory changes in the walls of the arteries and veins, resulting in thrombosis. Sympathectomy has no role in the surgical treatment of Raynaud's disease.

Answers to extended matching questions

1. I Abdominal aortic aneurysm
The various methods of presentation are shown in **Figure 56.4**. Once a clinical diagnosis is made, the first investigation is an ultrasound **(Figure 56.5)** to assess the size. If the aneurysm is 5.5 cm or more in diameter or is symptomatic, operation is carried out. A plain abdominal x-ray, taken for an unrelated cause, might show up an AAA **(Figure 56.6)**. Further preoperative investigations are carried out, the details of which are in **Table 56.1**.

The patient is treated by an open operation **(Figure 56.7)** or endovascular repair (EVAR), the choice depending upon the deliberations of the vascular surgeon and vascular radiologist.

2. O Abdominal compartment syndrome (ACS)
Raised intra-abdominal pressure (IAP) can occur in various conditions, one of them being ruptured AAA. High IAP leads to reduced blood flow and global ischaemia causing multi-organ failure – renal impairment, decreased cardiac output from reduced preload and increased afterload, increased ventilation pressures because of diaphragmatic splinting resulting in decreased lung compliance, and reduction in visceral perfusion.

Presentation of abdominal aortic aneurysm

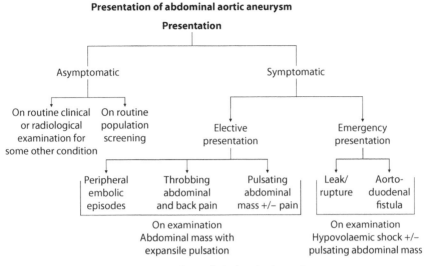

Figure 56.4   Presentation of abdominal aortic aneurysm.

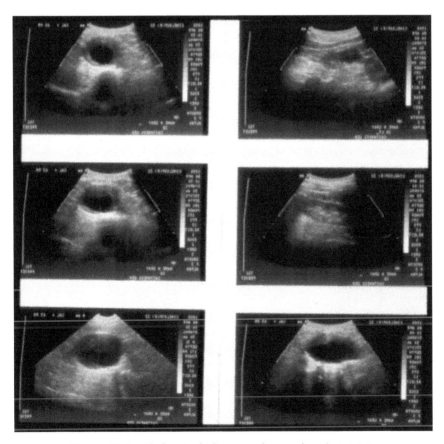

Figure 56.5   Abdominal ultrasound scan showing AAA.

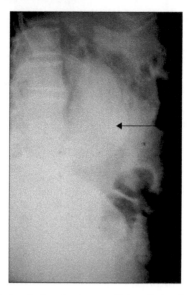

Figure 56.6 Plain abdominal x-ray (lateral view) showing AAA.

Table 56.1 Investigations for abdominal aortic aneurysm

In asymptomatic patients, if US scan shows the size to be <5.5 cm, patient is observed. In symptomatic patients or those with size of 5.5 cm or more operation is advised. The following investigations are done if surgery is considered.
Routine: Haematology, biochemistry, CXR, ECG
       Pulmonary function tests, Echocardiography
Specific: Ultrasound, CT   When endovascular repair
       Contrast enhanced spiral CT   (EVAR)
       MR angiography   is considered

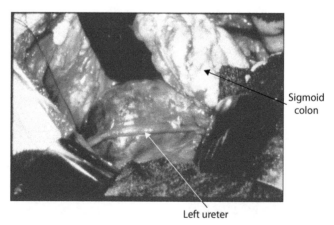

Sigmoid colon

Left ureter

Figure 56.7 Open operation for elective AAA.

Table 56.2 Differences between arterial embolus and acute thrombosis in acute limb ischaemia

Symptoms	Embolus	Thrombosis
Pain	Sudden and severe	Not as sudden and severe
Duration	In hours	In days (2 to 3 days)
Past history	Recent MI	Long term IC
Cardiac signs	AF	Chronic ischaemia
6 'P's	Very obvious	Not as obvious
Treatment	Embolectomy + anticoagulation	Bypass surgery May be preceded by attempt at thrombolysis

Ideally this should be prevented by laparostomy – leaving the incision open and covering the abdominal contents with a mesh or a plastic saline-soaked bag (Bogota bag); once the tension has subsided, the abdomen is closed at a later date. If it has occurred, the abdominal incision is re-opened and the wound is left open as described above. The condition has a high mortality and if the patient survives, incisional hernia is almost inevitable.

3. F Acute femoro-popliteal embolus
This patient, with a recent past history of MI, has a typical femoro-popliteal embolus – pain, pallor, pulselessness, paraesthesia, paralysis and perishing cold (six 'S's). The six classical features might not always be present. This is a clinical diagnosis. In case of doubt a Doppler ultrasound might be carried out, and if it cannot be distinguished from acute thrombosis an angiogram is done. **Table 56.2** shows the differences between an embolus and thrombosis.

The patient is given analgesia and 5000 units of intravenous heparin. An embolectomy is carried out under local or general anaesthesia. Following the operation the patient is heparinised for 3 to 4 days, after which she is stabilised on warfarin, which should be continued for 6 months. The patient should be closely observed for the development of compartment syndrome (see the following).

4. K Acute femoro-popliteal thrombosis
This patient is given analgesia and has to undergo an urgent angiogram to see the extent and exact site of thrombosis. Depending upon the local protocol and policy of the vascular and radiology units, the patient should undergo thrombolysis or a bypass procedure. If it is decided to give thrombolysis a chance initially, the angiogram catheter is left in place, through which tissue plasminogen (TPA) is infused. Repeat angiograms are done at regular intervals during the next 24 hours to see the outcome, and the patient remains under very close observation.

Depending upon the success of thrombolysis (complete, partial, or none), the patient might not require any surgery or have to undergo an angioplasty or bypass. This requires very close teamwork between the vascular surgeon and interventional radiologist. Following a successful outcome one should be on the lookout for compartment syndrome.

5. D Aortoiliac occlusion
This patient who has a claudication distance of almost one-quarter of a mile should first be managed by conservative measures – lose weight with dietary advice, give up smoking, and undertake regular exercises and walking within the limits of his disability. He should be started on statins, aspirin, or clopidogrel (if aspirin intolerant). The patient is kept under follow up.

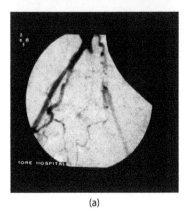 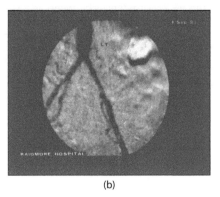

(a) (b)

Figure 56.8 Digital subtraction angiography (DSA) showing left iliac occlusion (a) and after angioplasty (b). (Courtesy of Dr David Nicol, Former Consultant Radiologist, Raigmore Hospital, Inverness, Scotland.)

If his symptoms are threatening his livelihood or severely affecting his lifestyle, then intervention is discussed. An angiogram **(Figure 56.8a** and **b)** is carried out with a view to angioplasty and stenting or aorto-femoral bypass, depending upon the findings.

6. L Arteriovenous fistula (A-V fistula)

These are found in the head, neck and extremities **(Figure 56.9)**. This patient has one in the head called cirsoid aneurysm, which is a localised A-V fistula of congenital origin. It exhibits a to-and-fro thrill and a machinery murmur on auscultation. When they occur in the lower limbs, they produce local gigantism and in the long term might result in high-output cardiac failure.

The true extent of the malformation is seen by magnetic resonance angiography. Treatment is by therapeutic embolisation or occlusion of the feeding vessel with excision of the mass. This procedure for head-and-neck lesions can be dangerous, as it may cause

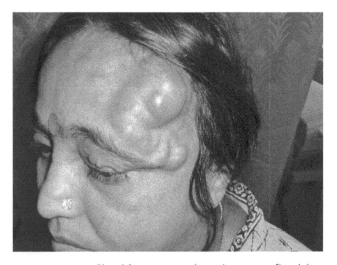

Figure 56.9 Cirsoid aneurysm (arteriovenous fistula).

a stroke. Therefore, such a procedure should be carried out only by a very experienced radiologist after careful consideration of the symptoms.

7. M Diabetic gangrene

This patient has diabetic gangrene. This is an outcome of the pathological triad of ischaemia, neuropathy and sepsis. Ischaemia is secondary to small vessel atherosclerosis (microangiopathy); peripheral sensory neuropathy leads to trophic ulcers and the immunosuppression of hyperglycaemia predisposes to infection. Motor neuropathy with loss of reflexes might result in neuropathic joints.

Management consists of making sure that the diabetes is under good control. The infection is treated by drainage procedures and local amputations under appropriate antibiotic cover. An angiogram is carried out to map the blood supply to determine the possibility of revascularisation, which might render the limb salvageable or allow more distal amputations.

8. J Femoro-popliteal occlusion

This patient has symptoms of femoro-popliteal occlusion with a short claudication distance. It is possible that his IC is affecting his job. If the condition progresses his livelihood may be under threat. Active conservative management must be advised – good control of his diabetes, total abstinence from smoking and weight-loss regimen. If his symptoms persist in spite of a good period of nonsurgical management, then revascularisation should be advised. An angiogram is carried out and depending upon the findings, the appropriate procedure performed.

In localised obstruction (stenosis) **(Figure 56.10a** and **b)** PTA is carried out. In a long obstruction (occlusion) of the superficial femoral artery a femoro-popliteal bypass is done using the patient's own long saphenous vein. This can be used in situ or reversed, a choice that depends on the individual surgeon. If the angiogram shows the obstruction to be in the posterior tibial artery, then a femoro-distal bypass should be the procedure.

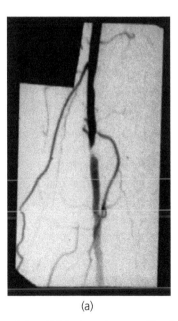 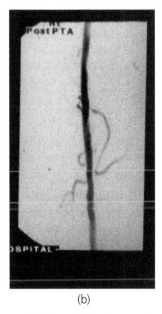

(a)   (b)

Figure 56.10   DSA showing popliteal stenosis (a) and (b) after angioplasty. (Courtesy of Dr David Nicol, Former Consultant Radiologist, Raigmore Hospital, Inverness, Scotland.)

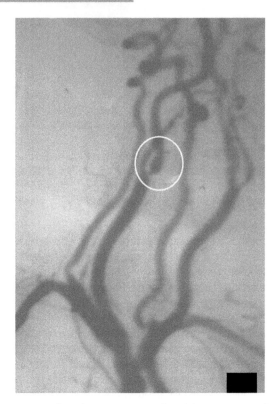

Figure 56.11   DSA showing ICA stenosis with post-stenotic dilatation.

9. C Internal carotid artery (ICA) stenosis

This patient has ICA stenosis causing her symptoms of transient ischaemic attacks (TIA) such as amaurosis fugax and minor strokes. This is caused by platelet emboli into the cerebral circulation; the emboli arise from the atheromatous segment of the ICA where there might be a post-stenotic dilatation **(Figure 56.11)**. These symptoms are a warning sign of an impending stroke and hence the patient should be treated urgently.

A duplex scan is carried out, followed by ICA endarterectomy. Instead of an open operation, PTA with stenting can also be considered, the choice of the procedure depending upon the policy of the vascular and radiology unit. In patients who have an asymptomatic stenosis picked up by a carotid bruit, intervention is advised when the stenosis is more than 70%.

10. P Limb compartment syndrome

This patient has developed compartment syndrome, which is a form of revascularisation injury. Following limb revascularisation procedures, some vascular units routinely measure compartment pressures (normal: up to 8 mmHg). A rising pressure is an indication for urgent fasciotomy where long incisions are made in the calf as the posterior compartment is the tightest. Later, skin grafting might be required.

The typical clinical features are severe pain out of proportion to the injury or operation, inability to discern two-point discrimination, extreme pain on passive movement of the muscles, and swollen tense compartment. Pressure studies can be unreliable, and fasciotomy must be performed on clinical grounds. However, in the unconscious patent pressure studies must be carried out. This condition also occurs following orthopaedic operations, burns, and crush injuries.

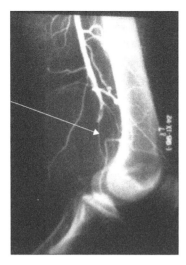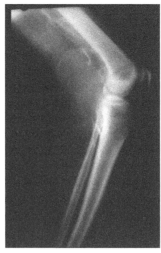

Figure 56.12   Angiogram showing thrombosed popliteal aneurysm (Courtesy of Calcutta Medical Research Institute, Kolkata, India.)

11. N Popliteal artery aneurysm

This patient has a popliteal artery aneurysm which accounts for 70% of all peripheral aneurysms. The history is typical of thrombosis in the aneurysm (**Figure 56.12**), a recognised complication. An angiogram is done to see the 'run off' followed by femoro-distal bypass using the patient's reversed long saphenous vein. Surgery can be unsuccessful because the distal vessels are thrombosed; 50% of such limbs are not salvageable. An asymptomatic aneurysm should be repaired if the diameter is 2.5 cm or more to prevent complications such as distal emboli or thrombosis.

12. G Raynaud's disease

This patient has intermittent digital vasospasm where no underlying cause can be found. The three typical phases are digital blanching from arterial spasm; swollen, blue and painful fingers from stagnant anoxia from local cyanosis; red and tingling of the digits due to recovery and reactive hyperaemia from vasodilatation. All three phases are not always present. In extreme cases there might be constant pain with ulceration and skin necrosis. Although the cause is unknown, it is thought that abnormality in the α-receptors of the vascular smooth muscle produces problems with smooth muscle contraction and elasticity of the arterial wall.

Certain investigations are done routinely, including full blood count, urea and electrolytes, ESR, CRP, cryoglobulins, antinuclear factor, rheumatoid antibodies, anti-mitochondrial antibodies, antithyroid antibodies and x-ray of the thoracic inlet. The management is conservative and consists of avoidance of cold, tobacco abstinence and use of heated gloves. Cervical sympathectomy, used in the past, sometimes has dramatic but short-lived effect. As the procedure can be done by minimal access surgery (transthoracic endoscopic), it is sometimes still used albeit after full-informed consent.

13. A Ruptured AAA

This is a typical emergency presentation of AAA. In 80% of these patients the presentation is a posterior leak as the aneurysm anteriorly is occupied by clot. This gives the patient a chance to get to the hospital and perhaps survive. In 20%, it is a true rupture into the peritoneal cavity when the patient dies before getting to the hospital. The combined mortality (community and hospital) of these patients is around 80%–90%. Hence, the benefit of screening for AAA in certain parts of the NHS.

This patient should be immediately resuscitated with two wide-bore intravenous cannulas for volume expansion with crystalloids, although the blood pressure should not be raised above 90–100 mmHg. Permissive hypotension should be the policy as it would be counterproductive to raise the blood pressure any higher. An indwelling urinary catheter is introduced and the patient taken to theatre for immediate operation.

With the triad of severe abdominal and back pain, hypovolaemic shock and pulsatile abdominal mass, precious time should not be lost by doing investigations. In the rare instance when the diagnosis is uncertain, a CT scan or a bedside US is carried out. CT scan is necessary if EVAR is being contemplated. The treatment is an emergency operation, which, in the vast majority, is an open procedure.

14. E Subclavian steal syndrome

This woman has subclavian steal syndrome. There is obstruction of the first part of the subclavian artery from atheroma proximal to the origin of the vertebral artery. Vigorous exercise of the upper limb demands extra blood supply. In this patient, as there is narrowing of the subclavian artery, the extra demand for more blood is met by the subclavian artery stealing blood from the vertebral artery. Thus there is vertebro-basilar insufficiency leading to cerebral ischaemia, giving features of syncope. Confirmation is by digital subtraction angiography and treatment is PTA.

15. B Thoracic inlet (outlet) syndrome

This condition is caused by compression of the subclavian artery and the lowest cord of the brachial plexus (C8 and T1) by one of several anatomical abnormalities: cervical rib, prominent transverse process of the C7 vertebra, fibrous band extending from the C7 transverse process to the first rib, and a sharp edge of the scalene muscles. The clinical features can be of vascular, neurological and local factors **(Figure 56.13)**.

The vascular symptoms are from compression of the subclavian artery, causing it to narrow with post-stenotic dilatation and intraluminal thrombus. Small emboli are released from the thrombus, causing digital ischaemia with pain and in extreme cases skin necrosis of the digits. The neurological symptoms are from compression of the lower cord of brachial plexus with neurological deficiency in the distribution of the ulnar nerve. The local symptoms are pain and discomfort in the supraclavicular area from a bony lump, which is the abnormal rib. Rarely, the subclavian vein may be obstructed with swelling of the arm and subclavian vein thrombosis.

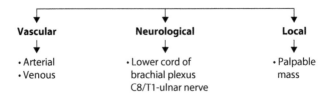

Vascular	Neurological	Local
• Arterial	• Lower cord of	• Palpable
• Venous	brachial plexus	mass
	C8/T1-ulnar nerve	

Figure 56.13 Clinical features of thoracic inlet (outlet) syndrome.

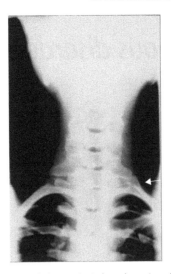

Figure 56.14 X-ray of thoracic inlet showing left cervical rib.

An x-ray of the thoracic inlet is useful in the presence of a rib **(Figure 56.14)**. A Doppler ultrasound might help to elucidate the actual abnormality in the subclavian artery. The treatment is to remove the cause surgically.

The differential diagnosis of thoracic inlet syndrome is cervical spondylosis, syringomyelia, progressive muscular atrophy and Pancoast's tumour (bronchogenic carcinoma of the lung apex).

16. H Thromboangiitis obliterans (TAO) (Buerger's disease)

This young man has typical TAO, which is an occlusive inflammatory disease of the small- and medium-sized arteries of the extremities. The additional features are thrombophlebitis of the superficial and deep veins and Raynaud's syndrome (see above). Usually all the features of the triad are not present. Involvement of the endothelium with neutrophil infiltrates leads to thrombosis and obliteration of the lumen. These histological changes might extend to the neighbouring veins and nerves.

Total abstinence from smoking is mandatory; this will arrest although not reverse the disease. Sympathectomy relieves the rest pain because there is an element of vasospasm in the diseased vessels; the procedure might also help to heal distal patches of skin necrosis and nailbed infection.

57 Venous disorders

Pradip K Datta

Multiple choice questions

→ **Anatomy of venous system of the limbs**

1. **Which of the following statements are true?**

A The saphenofemoral junction is situated 2.5–3 cm below and lateral to the pubic tubercle.

B The long saphenous vein (LSV) is accompanied by the saphenous nerve in front of and above the medial malleolus.

C The short saphenous vein (SSV) lies behind the lateral malleolus with the sural nerve.

D The basilic and cephalic veins unite to form the axillary vein.

E Perforating veins (perforators) joining the superficial and deep veins of the calf have valves.

→ **Venous pathophysiology**

2. **The following statements are true except:**

A The capillaries have a pressure of 32 mmHg at the arterial end and 12 mmHg at the venular end.

B The venous pressure in a foot vein when stationary is 100 mmHg.

C Patent deep veins, perforators and superficial veins, all with competent valves, are necessary to keep the venous pressure down to normal.

D Perforator incompetence is a potent cause of venous hypertension.

E In post-thrombotic syndrome the drop in ambulatory venous pressure is big.

→ **Varicose veins (VVs)**

3. **Which of the following statements are true?**

A The CEAP classification for chronic venous disorders is widely used.

B Tourniquet tests should be done in all patients prior to surgery.

C Continuous wave handheld Doppler is very accurate in assessment.

D Duplex ultrasound scanning is the mainstay of varicose vein imaging.

E Varicography as an investigation might sometimes be necessary.

→ **Management**

4. **Which of the following statements is false?**

A Thigh length compression hosiery is more effective than knee length.

B In ultrasound-guided foam sclerotherapy in a single session the maximum volume should be no more than 20 mLs.

C Endovenous laser ablation (EVLA) is not suitable in severely tortuous veins.

D Endovenous interventions may result in thromboembolic and phlebitic complications.

E After traditional varicose vein surgery the complication rate is up to 20%.

→ **Venous thrombosis**

5. **Which of the following statements are true?**

A The three factors in venous thrombosis are endothelial damage, stasis and thrombophilia

B Deficiencies of antithrombin, activated protein C and protein S predispose to venous thrombosis.

C Homan's sign is specific and clinically confirmatory of deep vein thrombosis (DVT).

D A duplex compression ultrasound scan of the deep veins is confirmatory.

E Radionucleotide imaging should be used in preference to CT pulmonary angiography (CTPA) for pulmonary embolism.

6. Which of the following statements is not true?

A Unfractionated heparin and warfarin are normally used in the prophylaxis of DVT.

B All patients undergoing surgery should be considered for DVT prophylaxis.

C Pharmacological methods are more effective than mechanical methods in the prophylaxis of DVT.

D On confirmation of DVT, the patient should be treated with heparin and warfarin.

E Patients at high risk of pulmonary embolism (PE) should have an inferior vena caval filter inserted.

Leg ulceration

7. Which of the following statements are true?

A Venous disease is the cause in 60% to 70% of all ulcers in the lower leg.

B Venous hypertension is a cause.

C In a minority an arterial cause might also be present.

D Squamous carcinoma can occur in a venous ulcer.

E Look for a nonvenous cause if the ulcer is not on the gaiter area.

Extended matching questions

Diagnoses

1 Axillary vein thrombosis
2 Deep vein thrombosis (DVT)
3 Klippel–Trenaunay syndrome
4 Superficial thrombophlebitis
5 Varicose veins
6 Venous malformation
7 Venous ulcer

Match the diagnoses with the clinical scenarios that follow:

Clinical scenarios

A A 33-year-old woman complains of aching and heaviness of her left lower limb, which is much worse at the end of the day after working as a shop assistant. On examination she has large varicosities along the medial side of her entire left lower limb.

B A 14-year-old boy complains of an unsightly lump occupying most of his lower lip. This has been there almost all his life, is painless and feels soft and compressible.

C A 74-year-old man complains of a tender cord-like structure along the medial side of his entire right lower limb of two months duration. He was investigated for abdominal and back pain and weight loss. US and CT scans of the abdomen showed a solid mass in the body of the pancreas.

D A 65-year-old man who underwent an anterior resection for rectal cancer complains of pain in his left calf on the first postoperative day. On examination he has low-grade pyrexia and the calf looks swollen with shiny skin and is tender.

E A 72-year-old woman complains of an ulcer on the medial side of her left leg over 5 months. This started as a small ulcer and has gradually become larger. Many years ago she suffered from recurrent swollen legs following the birth of her three children, who are now in their forties.

F   A 38-year-old man complains of marked swelling of his entire right upper limb of 24 hours duration. He woke up with it, having worked very hard as a bricklayer the day before. On examination there is marked uniform swelling of his right upper limb, extending from the supraclavicular region.

G   A 28-year-old man complains of extensive varicose veins on the outer side of his entire left lower limb, where he has had a prominent big vein over the whole leg. Since he was a teenager, his left lower limb has felt larger than the right and has a large capillary naevus.

Answers to multiple choice questions

1. A, B, C, E

The saphenofemoral junction is situated 2.5–3 cm below and lateral to the pubic tubercle. This anatomical landmark is important when making an incision to perform groin dissection for varicose vein surgery. The LSV starts at the medial part of the dorsal venous arch of the foot and is accompanied by the saphenous nerve in front of and above the medial malleolus. This anatomical fact is important when performing a venous cut-down for open intravenous access and not to strip a varicose vein down to the ankle.

The SSV originates on the lateral aspect of the dorsal venous arch and lies behind the lateral malleolus with the sural nerve. It ascends along the lateral edge of the Achilles tendon in the subcutaneous fat covered by skin and superficial fascia. In its ascent, it passes between the two heads of the gastrocnemius to terminate in the popliteal vein above the knee joint. In the calf and thigh, there are several perforating veins with valves that join the superficial to the deep venous system.

In the upper limb, the axillary vein is not formed by the union of the basilic and cephalic veins. The basilic vein drains the medial side of the forearm and hand, piercing the deep fascia at the elbow where it joins the venous tributaries of the brachial artery to form the axillary vein. The cephalic vein ascends along the lateral aspect of the forearm and arm and empties into the axillary vein after piercing the deltopectoral fascia in the deltopectoral groove.

2. E

In post-thrombotic syndrome there is venous hypertension and therefore the drop in ambulatory venous pressure is small. At the same time, the recovery period is short. In primary varicose veins the drop in pressure is the same as in a normal leg, but the recovery time is shorter than in the normal leg. At rest, the venous pressure in the foot is 100 mmHg. The blood passing through the arterioles into the capillaries has a pressure of 32 mmHg at the arteriolar end and 12 mmHg at the venular end. In a healthy limb, this pressure difference of 20 mmHg is maintained at a constant level to maintain a stable fluid balance without causing oedema or venous hypertension (**Figures 57.1a** and **b**).

Patent superficial veins, perforator veins and deep veins with their competent valves account for reduction in the venous pressure at rest and during walking. However, when there is pathology in the veins or incompetence of the valves, there will be venous hypertension with all the accompanying clinical problems of post-thrombotic syndrome.

3. A, D, E

The CEAP classification for chronic venous disorders is used widely and acts as a form of a good scoring system to decide on the management. It is an acronym for **C**linical, **E**tiology, **A**natomy, **P**athophysiology. The clinical class of the acronym has eight subsets, whilst the other

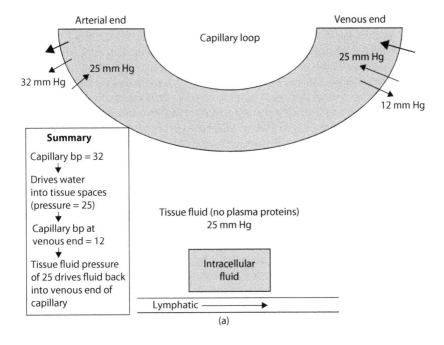

Arterial end

Venous end

Capillary loop

25 mm Hg

25 mm Hg

32 mm Hg

12 mm Hg

Summary

Capillary bp = 32
↓
Drives water
into tissue spaces
(pressure = 25)
↓
Capillary bp at
venous end = 12
↓
Tissue fluid pressure
of 25 drives fluid back
into venous end of
capillary

Tissue fluid (no plasma proteins)
25 mm Hg

Intracellular
fluid

Lymphatic ⟶

(a)

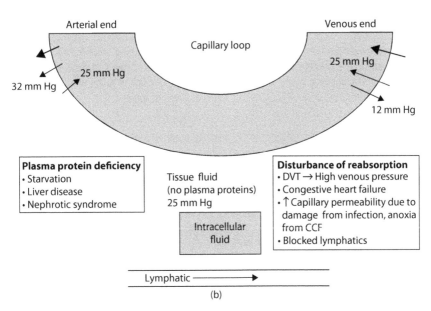

Arterial end

Venous end

Capillary loop

25 mm Hg

25 mm Hg

32 mm Hg

12 mm Hg

Plasma protein deficiency
• Starvation
• Liver disease
• Nephrotic syndrome

Tissue fluid
(no plasma proteins)
25 mm Hg

Intracellular
fluid

Disturbance of reabsorption
• DVT → High venous pressure
• Congestive heart failure
• ↑ Capillary permeability due to
  damage from infection, anoxia
  from CCF
• Blocked lymphatics

Lymphatic ⟶

(b)

Figure 57.1 (a and b) Pathophysiology of the venous system.

three classes have four each. Each clinical class is further subdivided into 'S' for symptomatic and 'A' for asymptomatic. For the details, the reader is asked to refer to a textbook.

Duplex ultrasound imaging is the 'gold standard' for varicose vein imaging in recurrent varicose veins and particularly when intervention is planned. It will determine which saphenous junctions are incompetent and the site, extent of reflux, number, location and diameter of the incompetent perforators, competence of deep veins and whether there is any thrombosis. Varicography is an invasive investigation, occasionally performed in recurrent varicose veins with complex anatomy.

The tourniquet tests have been given up except as a teaching tool very occasionally. Continuous wave handheld Doppler combined with clinical evaluation will miss almost one-third of perforators and information on affected veins. It is to be used only as a substitute when duplex scan is not available.

4. A, B
The principle of using compression hosiery is that graduated external pressure improves deep venous return. There is no evidence that thigh length hosiery is more effective than knee length; hence keen-length stockings are more often prescribed, resulting in greater patient compliance. Compression hosiery is classed according to the pressure exerted and does improve symptoms. In ultrasound-guided foam sclerotherapy, sodium tetradecyl sulphate is used. In a single session the maximum permitted amount of foam is 10–12 mLs.

EVLA, although suitable for the vast majority of patients, is not suitable for patients who have excessively tortuous varicosities; it is unsuitable also for those with thrombophlebitis and needle phobia. The other endovenous modality of treatment is radiofrequency ablation (RFA). This is a form of minimally invasive endovascular therapy that uses bipolar catheter to generate thermal energy to ablate the vein. These procedures might result in complications such as thrombophlebitis in about 5% and embolism in about 1%.

Following open surgery of saphenofemoral ligation and long saphenous stripping or saphenopopliteal junction ligation and short saphenous vein stripping, complications occur in up to one in five patients, with wound infection being the most common. Following long saphenous vein stripping, injury to the saphenous nerve occurs in up to 7% whereas sural nerve neuropraxia occurs in 4% after short saphenous vein stripping.

5. A, B, D
The three factors, first described by the German pathologist Rudolf Virchow – changes in the vessel wall in the form of endothelial damage, stasis and coagulability of the blood – contribute to the development of venous thrombosis. While there are multiple factors leading up to the formation of DVT, there are many predisposing causes, chief among which are major operation, musculo-skeletal injury, pregnancy, immobility, obesity and oral contraceptive pill. Deficiencies of antithrombin, activated protein C and protein S are predisposing factors in the young. Confirmation of the diagnosis on clinical suspicion is by duplex ultrasound examination of the deep veins, which should be located and compressed. Filling defects in the flow and lack of compressibility confirm thrombosis.

Clinically Homan's sign (resistance of the calf muscle to forcible dorsiflexion) is nonspecific and should not be elicited for fear of dislodging the thrombus producing a pulmonary embolism (PE). Other clinical features should be sought – pain, swelling and tenderness of calf, shiny skin, pyrexia. Radionucleotide imaging as a first-line investigation has largely been replaced by CT pulmonary angiography, which would show filling defects in the pulmonary arteries; moreover, the procedure can be used therapeutically for thrombolysis.

6. A, B
Unfractionated heparin and warfarin are rarely used in the prophylaxis of DVT. Patients in need of prophylaxis are started on low-molecular-weight heparin subcutaneously once per

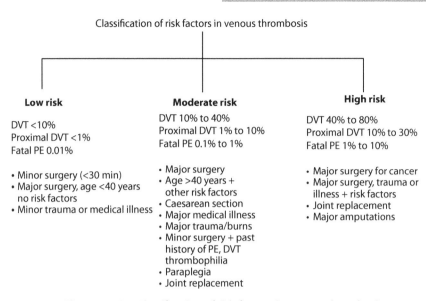

Figure 57.2 Classification of risk factors in venous thrombosis.

day. All patients undergoing surgery do not need DVT prophylaxis. Patients undergoing surgery are categorised as low risk, moderate risk and high risk (**Figure 57.2**), the low-risk patient being exempted from prophylaxis.

Moderate- and high-risk patients are given prophylaxis in the form of pharmacological and mechanical methods, the latter consisting of graduated elastic compression stockings and external pneumatic calf compression. Used by itself, pharmacological methods are more effective than mechanical methods although the downside is the slight increased risk of bleeding. Established DVT is treated initially by heparin followed by warfarin, the latter continued as a maintenance dose monitored by regular blood tests. Thrombolytic therapy might be considered in iliac vein thrombosis when diagnosed early. Patients who are at high risk for developing PE should have an inferior venal caval filter inserted.

7. A, B, C, D, E

Venous disease is the cause for up to 70% of all leg ulcers particularly when they occur in the lower leg. Nonvenous causes are ischaemia, rheumatoid arthritis, inflammatory bowel disease, trauma, diabetic neuropathy, neoplasm and infections (in developing countries). Venous hypertension that occurs as a result of long-term DVT is the underlying cause, which is compounded by incompetent valves and perforators. The hypertension leads to leakage of fibrin and red cells, the former causing the formation of a pericapillary fibrin cuff while the latter causes haemosiderin deposition and pigmentation. This results in anoxia, lipodermatosclerosis and ulceration (**Figure 57.3**).

In about one-fifth of the patients, ischaemia may be a contributory factor. Pedal pulses might not be palpable because of the indurated skin; therefore, ankle-brachial pressure index should be assessed by Doppler studies. In long-standing nonhealing ulcers, squamous cell carcinoma (Marjolin's ulcer) should be excluded by biopsy especially when the edge looks raised and everted. Typically venous ulcer occurs in the gaiter area. Therefore if the ulcer is seen on the foot or high up in the calf the diagnosis of a venous ulcer must be reconsidered.

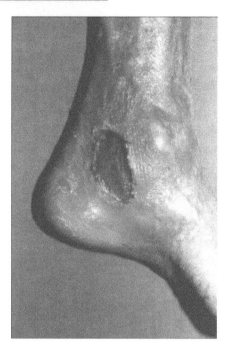

Figure 57.3 Venous ulcer.

Answers to extended matching questions

1. F Axillary vein thrombosis

This patient has axillary vein thrombosis, which is typically seen in a young muscular man after heavy use of the arm. This should be confirmed by a Duplex ultrasound scan. At the same time, an x-ray of the thoracic inlet is done to exclude a cervical rib that might have precipitated the thrombosis by compression of the vein.

The condition is of short duration. Hence, an attempt should be made to cannulate the vein and treat by thrombolysis using tissue plasminogen activator. After treatment, further imaging must be done to see the outcome. If a cervical rib is confirmed, causing thoracic inlet syndrome, then it is removed in due course.

2. D Deep vein thrombosis (DVT)

This patient has deep vein thrombosis. A D-dimer measurement is carried out, followed by Wells score. If the score is more than 4, DVT is diagnosed. However, a duplex compression ultrasound examination should be performed. This would show up the filling defects in flow and lack of compressibility, which indicates the presence of thrombosis.

Treatment should be commenced immediately on low-molecular-weight heparin and anticoagulated with warfarin according to the local protocol. Usually it is 10 mg, 10 mg and 5 mg, on three consecutive days monitored by daily prothrombin time. The dose is adjusted such that the reading of INR (international normalised ratio) is about 3. The patient is maintained on warfarin for at least 6 months.

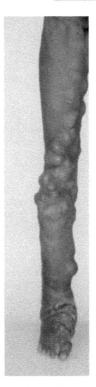

Figure 57.4 Haemangioma of right leg: Klippel–Trenaunay syndrome. (Courtesy of Professor Ahmad Fahal, MD, FRCS, FRCP, Professor of Surgery, Khartoum, Sudan).

3. G Klippel–Trenaunay (K-T) syndrome (Figure 57.4)

This syndrome is a rare mesodermal abnormality often associated with lymphatic and other congenital abnormalities where there is venous and lymphatic hypoplasia and aplasia. It consists of cutaneous naevus, varicose veins and bone and soft tissue deformity. These patients have an increased incidence of DVT and PE.

Treatment is mainly conservative, with elastic support stockings. Superficial veins are removed if symptoms are not relieved by stockings after making sure the deep veins are normal. Laser ablation of the naevus might be considered. Excessive limb growth might have to be controlled by epiphyseal stapling or heel raise of the opposite limb.

4. C Superficial thrombophlebitis

This patient suffers from superficial thrombophlebitis. In spite of its name, inflammation is rare. Common causes are trauma, intravenous infusion of hyperosmolar solutions or drugs and visceral malignancy (as in this patient). In patients with visceral malignancy different veins might be affected at different times; hence the term thrombophlebitis migrans. Coagulation disorders such as polycythaemia, thrombocytosis and sickle cell disease might predispose to this condition.

Full blood count, coagulation screen and a duplex scan are carried out. Treatment is with nonsteroidal anti-inflammatory drugs, and the condition usually resolves spontaneously. Some authorities advocate saphenofemoral ligation if ultrasound shows the thrombus to have extended to the saphenofemoral junction.

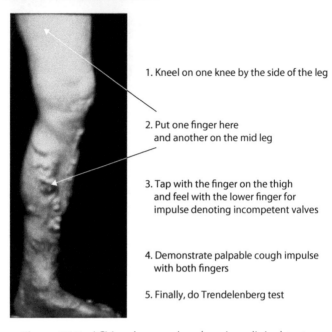

1. Kneel on one knee by the side of the leg

2. Put one finger here
   and another on the mid leg

3. Tap with the finger on the thigh
   and feel with the lower finger for
   impulse denoting incompetent valves

4. Demonstrate palpable cough impulse
   with both fingers

5. Finally, do Trendelenberg test

Figure 57.5   LSV varicose veins showing clinical tests.

5. A Varicose veins (VV)

This patient with symptomatic VVs would be classified in CEAP as C3S. In a surgical examination such a patient would be a common clinical case. The clinical signs to be demonstrated are the cough impulse, percussion or tap sign and Trendelenburg test without using the tourniquet **(Figure 57.5)**. Sometimes at the groin a saphena varix may be seen **(Figure 57.6)**.

Young patients with primary symptomatic VVs would require treatment. A duplex ultrasound imaging is carried out to map the exact sites of valvular incompetence; extent of reflux; number, location and diameter of incompetent perforators; and state of the deep venous system. Having confirmed the extent of the patient's pathology, the choices are given to the patient include conservative management by the use of compression hosiery, ultrasound-guided foam sclerotherapy, endovenous laser or radiofrequency ablation and surgery involving saphenofemoral ligation and stripping of LSV.

When intervention is carried out, the short-to-medium-term results are similar between endovenous and open surgery. However, in the immediate postoperative period, endovenous methods are superior in that recovery is quicker with earlier return to work and normal activities.

6. B Venous malformation

A venous malformation is almost always congenital in origin. It is soft, compressible and painless **(Figures 57.7a and b)**. The main problem is cosmetic and embarrassment and bullying in children. The malformation consists of veins, lymphatics, arterioles, muscles and skin; rarely it might involve the bone.

The extent can be delineated by contrast CT or MRI. Treatment is unsatisfactory. Excision is not curative. Embolisation and sclerotherapy can be tried but might be dangerous if the malformation is near the central nervous system.

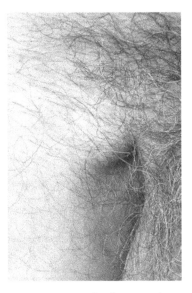

Figure 57.6 Saphena varix.

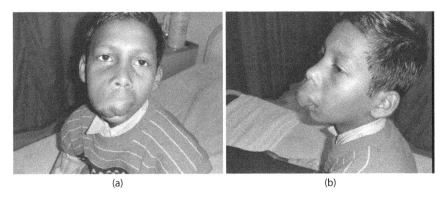

(a)   (b)

Figure 57.7 (a and b) Venous malformation.

7. E Venous ulcer

In the majority of patients a venous ulcer is the long-term complication of DVT causing venous hypertension **(Figure 57.8)**. Ischaemia as a contributory factor must always be excluded by doing arterial Doppler measurements because pedal pulses, even when present, might not be felt in the presence of pericapillary fibrin cuff and lipodermatosclerosis, which are normally predisposing factors in a venous ulcer. In an ulcer of long duration, biopsy from the edge should be taken to exclude malignant transformation. Diabetes must be excluded.

Investigations to be carried out are full blood count, blood glucose, ESR, C-reactive protein, rheumatoid factor, sickle cell test if appropriate and duplex scan. Once a diagnosis of venous ulcer has been made, most often by a process of exclusion, ideally these patients are

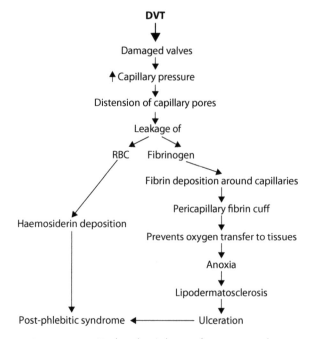

Figure 57.8 Pathophysiology of a venous ulcer.

managed in a specialised ulcer clinic as this is a long-term undertaking. Patients are treated by a compression bandaging regimen, of which there are three types. In suitable patients excision and mesh grafting have shown healing in 50% at 5 years. Preventing recurrence can be a challenge. Patients who have saphenous and perforator reflux should be offered an operation to cure this problem only after confirming that the deep veins are patent.

58 Lymphatic disorders

Pradip K Datta

Multiple choice questions

→ Anatomy and physiology of the lymphatic system

1. Which of the following statements are true?

A Lymphatic trunks are lined by endothelial cells.

B Lymph from the lower limbs and abdomen drain through the cisterna chyli into the thoracic duct.

C The lymphatic system comprises of lymphatic channels, lymphoid organs and circulating elements.

D The major part of lymph flow is from superficial to deep.

E Pressures of up to 30 to 50 mmHg have been recorded in normal lymph trunks.

→ Lymphangitis

2. Which of the following statements is not true?

A The commonest organisms causing acute lymphangitis are *Pseudomonas* and *Bacteroides*.

B Erythematous streak is a typical early sign.

C It might result in septicaemia.

D It might go on to produce lymphoedema.

E Underlying systemic disease may be a cause.

→ Lymphoedema

3. Which of the following statements are true?

A Lymphoedema can be primary or secondary.

B Lymphoedema typically involves the foot.

C Malignancy can develop in long-standing lymphoedema.

D Primary lymphoedema is from an inherited abnormality.

E Lymphoedema developing late in life (after 50 years) usually is from an underlying malignancy.

→ Secondary lymphoedema

4. The following statements are true except:

A The causes can be traumatic, infective, neoplastic and inflammatory.

B The most common cause worldwide is filariasis.

C Lymphoedema can co-exist with chronic venous insufficiency.

D Lymphangiography as an investigation should be performed in all patients.

E Limb volume measurement is very helpful in the diagnosis.

→ Management of lymphoedema

5. Which of the following statements are true?

A All patients must be thoroughly investigated by imaging techniques available.

B Management aims to relieve pain, reduce swelling and prevent complications.

C Amoxycillin is the treatment of choice in acute inflammatory episode.

D Reduction of swelling is achieved by decongestive lymphoedema therapy (DLT).

E Surgery is indicated in a small minority of patients.

6. **Which of the following statements are not true?**

A Vigorous anaerobic and isometric exercises have a beneficial effect.

B Diuretics have a beneficial effect in pure lymphoedema.

C Liposuction has some benefit in lymphoedema with non-pitting oedema.

D Limb reduction procedures are indicated when the condition interferes with mobility and livelihood.

E Lymphatic bypass procedures are disappointing.

Extended matching questions

→ Diagnoses

1 Acute lymphangitis
2 Filariasis
3 Primary lymphoedema
4 Secondary lymphoedema

Match the diagnoses with the clinical scenarios that follow:

→ Clinical scenarios

A A 58-year-old man complains of swelling of his right lower limb of 2 months duration. The swelling started in the region of his groin and spread distally. The limb feels very heavy and uncomfortable. On systemic questioning, he admits to having passed painless blood clots in his urine during this period.

B A 48-year-old man complains of swelling of his entire lower limb for many years during which time he worked as a farmer in the African continent. He has presented because he developed pain, redness and some discharge from the skin of the affected swollen leg.

C A 27-year-old woman presented with pain, swelling and redness in her right upper limb after working in her garden. She thinks she might have sustained an injury that she did not notice. On examination she has pyrexia, with a swollen right forearm and arm with red streaks up to her axilla where a tender lump can be felt.

D A 30-year-old woman complains of swelling of her right leg for many years ever since her puberty. Recently, she has noticed some swelling in the other leg too. The limb feels heavy and uncomfortable, and she wishes to have some relief of her symptoms. Her 33-year-old sister also has a similar problem but not as bad.

Answers to multiple choice questions

1. A, B, C, E

The structure of lymph trunks are similar to that of veins. They are lined by a layer of endothelial cells on a basement membrane overlying smooth muscle cells innervated by the autonomic nervous system. Lymph from the lower limbs and abdomen drains into the cisterna chyli, which is a sac-like structure under the right crus of the diaphragm in front of the first and second lumbar vertebrae. The upper end continues as the thoracic duct, which enters the point of confluence of the left internal jugular and subclavian veins. Lymph from the head and right arm drains through a separate right lymphatic trunk (might sometimes be two or three) into the commencement of the right brachiocephalic vein.

The lymphatic system consists of the lymphatic channels, the lymphoid organs which comprise the lymph nodes, spleen, Peyer's patches, thymus, and tonsils and circulating cells (lymphocytes and mononuclear immune cells). The mechanism of lymph transport is governed by Starling's forces. The distribution of fluid and protein between the vascular system and the interstitial fluid depends on the hydrostatic pressure and oncotic pressure (Starling's forces) **(see Figures 56.1a and b)**. In normal lymph trunks pressures of up to 30 to 50 mmHg have been recorded. About 90% of lymph is transported against venous flow from the deep to the superficial in epifascial lymph trunks.

2. A

Streptococcus pyogenes and *Staphylococcus aureus* are the most common organisms that cause acute lymphangitis. A typical early sign is a red streak along the line of the lymphatic channel. This might extend along the limb up to the regional lymph nodes, which might show tender lymphadenopathy with a swollen limb. If the condition is not promptly treated it might progress on to bacteraemia and septicaemia.

In the long term, because of damage to the lymphatic channels, lymphoedema might result. Those with lymphoedema are prone to recurrent acute inflammatory episodes. The condition should be promptly treated with intravenous antibiotics and the part (usually a limb) rested and elevated. If the patient does not improve within 48 hours in spite of prompt and appropriate antibiotics, an underlying abscess should be suspected. Otherwise, it might be denote an undiagnosed malignancy or immunodeficiency.

3. A, B, C, D, E

Lymphoedema can be broadly classified as primary where a cause cannot be found or secondary where there is an underlying cause. Primary lymphoedema is from an inherited abnormality of the lymphatic system referred to as 'congenital lymphatic dysplasia'. These may be familial (hereditary), such as Milroy's disease, or part of an inherited syndrome. The following types are described: lymphoedema congenita where the onset is within 2 years of birth and more common in males and usually bilateral; lymphoedema praecox where the onset can be anytime up to 35 years and is more common in females and more often unilateral; lymphoedema tarda develops after 35 years and is associated with obesity. In general, characteristically lymphoedema affects the foot and extends proximally usually stopping at the knee.

When the condition has been going on for 20 years or more, lymphangiosarcoma can develop. Ulceration, nonhealing bruises and raised satellite lesions should arouse the suspicion of malignant transformation. The condition is also known to occur in oedema following mastectomy when it is called Stewart-Weber syndrome. Biopsy confirms the diagnosis and amputation is the only treatment.

When the condition develops in any patient over the age of 50 years, an underlying pelvic malignancy should be suspected and appropriately investigated. Carcinoma of the urinary bladder, uterus, or rectum causing obstruction to the lymphatics causes lymphoedema, which typically starts proximally.

4. D, E

Although regarded as 'gold standard' to show structural abnormalities, lymphangiography has become obsolete. As a procedure it can be technically difficult, unpleasant for the patient and cause injury to the lymphatics. Limb volume measurement is not helpful in the diagnosis. It is a useful tool, not often used, to find out the severity of the disease, guide management and assess response to treatment.

Causes of secondary lymphoedema are best classified as the following: traumatic as following radiotherapy or lymph node dissection; infective as in filariasis; neoplastic as in infiltrative pelvic malignancy; and inflammatory as in rheumatoid arthritis and sarcoidosis. Worldwide, the most common cause is filariasis due to infection from the parasite Wuchereria bancrofti. It is particularly prevalent in Africa, India and South America.

Lymphoedema and chronic venous insufficiency often co-exist in the same patient, as both conditions are common. Superficial venous thrombophlebitis and DVT can both lead to lymphatic obstruction and secondary lymphoedema. Duplex ultrasound scan will help confirm venous disease. If there is superficial venous reflux, varicose vein surgery should not be undertaken as superficial venous reflux rarely causes limb swelling; surgery on the veins would make the patient worse.

5. B, C, D, E
The three principles of management are relief of pain, reduction of swelling and prevention of complications, particularly relating to skin. The overall management has to be a multidisciplinary approach. If a cause is obvious, such as post-mastectomy lymphoedema, that needs to be addressed. Opioid or non-opioid analgesics, steroids, tricyclic antidepressants, nerve blocks and physiotherapy should all be considered. In the prevention of complications, skin care is of the utmost importance. Acute inflammatory episodes are due to infection from group A β-haemolytic streptococci or staphylococci, for which amoxycillin is the treatment of choice.

There are several approaches for reduction of swelling. The term used for this is deconges-tive lymphoedema therapy (DLT). Under the umbrella of DLT is manual lymphatic drainage (MLD) and multi-layer lymphoedema bandaging (MLLB). This is administered in the following two phases: the first phase is a therapist-led short intensive period followed by the second phase of maintenance self-care regimen professionally supervised at regular intervals. The details of these regimes are beyond the scope of this book. Surgery is indicated in a very small minority.

Investigations, such as any imaging, are hardly necessary unless secondary lymphoedema from a malignancy is strongly suspected. In the vast majority, it is possible to diagnose and manage lymphoedema in a holistic manner by good history and examination. Routine blood tests are all that is necessary.

6. A, B
Vigorous anaerobic and isometric exercises will tend to exacerbate lymphoedema. Patients should be advised to avoid prolonged static activities. Slow rhythmic isotonic movements as in swimming will increase venous and lymphatic return and are beneficial. Diuretics are of no value in pure lymphoedema. They will be harmful because of electrolyte disturbances.

Surgery is of the following three types: liposuction, reduction procedures and bypass pro-cedures. Liposuction, used in chronic lymphoedema, is reserved for patients with non-pitting oedema. Following a procedure, the success can be maintained by using compression hosiery for at least 1 year. There are several limb-reduction procedures, a sure indication of the unsatisfactory outcome of this group of procedures, which are indicated when the condition is interfering with mobility and livelihood. Cosmesis is not an indication, as all the procedures leave the patient with severe scarring. Bypass procedures, such as lyphaticovenular anasto-mosis by supermicrosurgical techniques, have disappointing results. The results are better when carried out in the upper limb for the complication of axillary clearance or radiotherapy.

Answers to extended matching questions

1. C Acute lymphangitis
This young woman has acute lymphangitis from trauma sustained while gardening. It has spread to the axillary lymph nodes causing lymphadenitis. This must to be managed promptly

to prevent the condition from progressing to bacteraemia or septicaemia. The patient should be given analgesia and blood sent for culture and full blood count, which will show polymorphonuclear leucocytosis. Blood cultures are often negative because the signs are the result of the release of toxins into the circulation that stimulate a cytokine-mediated systemic inflammatory response. The most likely organisms are *Staphylococcus aureus*, β-haemolytic streptococci, or clostridia.

She should be started on the 'best guess' antibiotics intravenously. Benzylpenicillin and flucloxacillin should be the drugs of choice. The arm should be elevated to reduce swelling and rested to reduce lymph drainage. If the patient does not improve within 48 hours, the antibiotic regime should be reconsidered.

2. B Filariasis

This patient has filariasis **(see Chapter 6)**, the most common cause worldwide of lymphoedema. It is caused by the parasite *Wucheria bancrofti*, which is carried by the mosquito. Immature parasites (microfilariae) are inoculated by the mosquito. Having entered the bloodstream, the parasite travels along the lymphatics to reside in the lymph nodes. Here, due to direct damage and immune response from the host, fibrosis and obstruction to the lymphatic system causes the clinical presentation. Adult parasites lodge in the proximal lymphatics resulting in massive oedema in the long term, the clinical picture being termed elephantiasis **(Figure 58.1)**.

As with all parasitic infestations, eosinophilia is present. Treatment is with diethylcarbamazine, which will kill the parasites but not reverse the pathological changes. These patients are prone to recurrent attacks of infection (as in this patient), which need to be promptly treated.

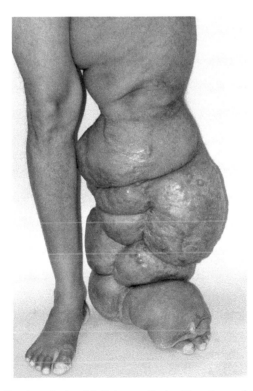

Figure 58.1 Elephantiasis of left lower limb. (Courtesy of Professor Ahmad Fahal, MD, FRCS, FRCP, Professor of Surgery, University of Khartoum, Sudan.)

3. D Primary lymphoedema

This patient has primary lymphoedema, the cause of which is an inherited abnormality of the lymphatic system referred to as 'congenital lymphatic dysplasia'. The history is suggestive of Milroy's disease. The condition is estimated to occur in 1 in 6000 births and is inherited in an autosomal dominant manner. The disease causes brawny lymphoedema of both legs, which develops from birth or childhood. Lymphangiography shows aplasia or hypoplasia.

Depending upon the age of onset, the following three types are recognised: lymphoedema congenita (onset at or within 2 years of birth) commoner in males and usually bilateral; lymphoedema praecox (onset from 2 to 35 years) more common in women and usually unilateral; and lymphoedema tarda (onset after 35 years) often associated with obesity.

This patient requires detailed history and examination. After full discussion in a multi-disciplinary team meeting, the indication for a lymphangiogram is discussed. The patient is appraised of the entire gamut of choices of treatment and managed appropriately after full-informed consent.

4. A Secondary lymphoedema

Any patient who presents with lymphoedema after the age of 50 (as this patient) has secondary lymphoedema. This should arouse the strong suspicion of a pelvic malignancy blocking off the lymphatics. Typically in these patients, the swelling starts proximally in the thigh and spreads distally. With a history of haematuria, this patient has a urinary bladder cancer. He should be referred urgently to the urologist. An urgent cystoscopy and examination under anaesthesia, biopsy and CT scan for staging is carried out, followed by discussion in a multidisciplinary team meeting. The presentation indicates advanced disease, which is appropriately treated according to the staging.

Abdominal

59 History and examination of the abdomen

Pradip K Datta

Multiple choice questions

→ **Gathering information**

1. **Which of the following statements are true?**

A Observing the patient prior to taking a history is important.
B It is best to ask leading questions right from the start.
C History of presenting complaint should give an idea of the system involved.
D Relevant past history is essential.
E System review and family history is to be done followed by summary given to the patient.

→ **Clinical presentation of abdominal problems**

2. **The following statements are true except:**

A Abdominal pain might be a symptom from non-surgical conditions.
B Altered bowel habit usually indicates obstructive and inflammatory pathology.
C A hernia causing abdominal symptoms will always be obvious.
D An inebriated person with abdominal pain should be diagnosed as alcoholic gastritis.
E Abdominal pain related to food habits and associated with other symptoms usually denote pathology in the biliary tract or stomach and duodenum.

→ **Pathophysiological basis of common abdominal symptoms and signs**

3. **Which of the following statements is not true?**

A Abdominal wall and parietal peritoneum are supplied by the somatic nervous system.
B Abdominal organs and the visceral peritoneum are innervated by the autonomic nervous system.
C Pain arising from pathology in the midgut is localised to the epigastrium.
D Colicky abdominal pain indicates underlying obstructive pathology.
E Pain away from the site of abdominal pathology denotes referred pain.

→ **Examination of the abdomen**

4. **Which of the following statements are true?**

A Abdominal examination must always be preceded by general examination.
B Abdominal discoloration at specific sites denotes underlying serious pathology.
C Free movement of abdominal wall on respiration excludes peritonitis.
D Rebound tenderness is best tested by gentle percussion.
E An intra-abdominal lump becomes prominent when the patient tenses the abdomen or lifts the head from the bed.

Extended matching questions

→ Diagnoses

1 Abdominal aortic aneurysm
2 Acute pancreatitis
3 Biliary colic
4 Carcinoma of caecum
5 Distal small bowel obstruction
6 Incisional hernia
7 Perforated duodenal ulcer
8 Secondary metastases in liver

Match the above diagnosis with the clinical scenarios below. Please note that no details of the above conditions will be discussed in this chapter. Details of the conditions are discussed in the appropriate chapters. Here the EMQs are used as a diagnostic clinical exercise.

→ Clinical scenarios

A A 58-year-old man complains of a lump in his abdomen deep to an incision for 2 years. This started 3 months after he had an emergency operation for intestinal obstruction when he underwent a right hemicolectomy. The lump is increasing in size and becomes prominent when he coughs and sits up.

B A 72-year-old man complains of throbbing backache and a feeling of his heartbeat in his 'stomach'. On examination a pulsatile mass can be seen in his epigastrium, which looks full.

C A 35-year-old woman complains of severe colicky abdominal pain of 6 hours duration. It is in the epigastrium and right upper quadrant and radiates to the back. The pain comes and goes, and in between the attacks she is left with a dull ache in the right subcostal region.

D A 74-year-old woman complains of generalised abdominal pain and distension for 36 hours. This started with greenish vomiting, which has now been replaced with brownish faeculent material. She is dehydrated with a distended abdomen and a small tender lump in her right groin of which she is unaware.

E A 62-year-old woman complains of undue shortness of breath while going about her daily activities. On examination she looks very pale with an irregular non-tender lump in her right iliac fossa.

F A 45-year-old man, who admits to being a chronic alcoholic, complains of severe pain in his epigastrium radiating to the back of 8 hours duration. He is sweaty, with a pulse rate of 122 beats per minute, blood pressure (BP) of 110/80 mmHg and with a tense, tender abdomen with rigidity.

G A 70-year-old woman presents with jaundice and vague abdominal pain of 6 weeks duration. On examination she is jaundiced with a long midline scar and an enlarged hard nodular liver. The midline scar is from a left hemicolectomy for carcinoma of the splenic flexure.

H A 55-year-old man complains of sudden onset of very severe pain in his epigastrium, radiating to the back, of 6 hours duration. On examination his BP is 130/90 mmHg, pulse rate is 90 beats per minute, the abdominal wall does not move with respiration and he has thoracic respiration. Over the past hour he has been having pain in his right shoulder tip. In the past he has suffered from 'indigestion' for a long time.

Answers to multiple choice questions

1. A, C, D, E

A major amount of information can be gleaned by observing the patient even before the first question is asked. Initial observations obtained by direct eye contact are important. Looking at the patient while he or she is giving the history will help the clinician to realise whether the patient is any pain. Patients who do not make eye contact might be shy or are not giving the correct history. General appearance of the patient, gait, position in bed, facial expression and tone of speech, provide preliminary information.

The patient's presenting complaint gives an idea of the system involved. For example, upper abdominal pain related to food might be connected with pathology in the stomach or gallbladder; altered bowel habit would indicate something wrong with the small and large bowel. Taking past history is very important, particularly if the patient has had an operation before. This might have bearing on the present problem – a recurrence if the operation was for cancer or adhesive obstruction. Toward the end it is essential to do a system review to exclude comorbid disease. Then, summarising the history given by the patient is useful to help the patient recollect anything in the history that he or she might have forgotten.

Right at the start, it is not a good idea to ask leading questions. This gives the impression to the patient that the surgeon is impatient and interested in only a 'box-ticking exercise'. The best way to start a clinical interview is to say at the outset 'Tell me in your own words how it all started' and then look intensely interested with eye contact. The patient realises that the surgeon is a 'listening doctor' and will open up with very useful information. In an emergency, however, if the patient is in severe pain, the clinician might have to resort to leading questions, because the patient might be in far too much pain to volunteer a good history.

2. C, D

A hernia causing abdominal symptoms will not always be clinically obvious. This is particularly true when an elderly obese lady presents with features of distal small bowel obstruction from an obstructed femoral hernia, which can easily be missed unless the groins are examined meticulously. When an inebriated patient presents as an emergency with abdominal pain, the diagnosis of alcoholic gastritis should never be made automatically. Although the history might be straightforward in view of his mental status, thorough examination and investigations must be carried out to exclude acute pancreatitis, perforated duodenal ulcer, or acute exacerbation of the same.

Abdominal pain can well be a clinical manifestation of medical conditions such as right lower lobe pneumonia, angina, porphyria and diabetic ketoacidosis. A history of altered bowel habit with abdominal symptoms indicates an inflammatory (inflammatory bowel disease), infective (parasitic or tuberculosis depending upon the geographical area), or obstructive (large bowel carcinoma) pathology. Upper abdominal pain points to hepatobiliary, pancreatic, or upper gastrointestinal pathology. Painless weight loss associated with anorexia might point to a gastric carcinoma.

3. C

Pain that arises from pathology in the midgut such as small bowel, appendix and right colon is localised in the periumbilical region. Pain in the epigastrium denotes pathology in the foregut such as the stomach and duodenum. The abdominal wall and parietal peritoneum are supplied by somatic nerves, while the autonomic nervous system innervates the abdominal organs and visceral peritoneum. That is the reason for the migration of pain from the periumbilical area in appendicular colic to the right iliac fossa where the pain settles as an ache when the parietal peritoneum is affected.

Pain of autonomic origin is deep and poorly localised. When the pain is transmitted to the appropriate somatic distribution (from T1 to L2), the pain is localised to the surface of the abdominal wall. Such an example is seen in Murphy's sign. Here the pain of acute cholecystitis from the inflamed gallbladder, as it comes into contact with the parietal peritoneum on taking a deep breath, is felt in the right upper quadrant and scapular region in the back.

Colicky abdominal pain is a classical symptom of obstruction of a hollow tube such as the intestines, ureter and common bile duct. In small bowel, because the origin of pain is from pathology in a midgut structure, the colic is central abdominal. The pain comes on as the peristaltic wave tries to overcome the obstruction. Disappearance of the peristaltic wave coincides with the relief of colicky pain that is replaced by a dull ache.

Pain might often be felt at a site well away from the pathology. A perforated hollow viscus such as a duodenal ulcer will cause collection of fluid and air underneath the right dome of diaphragm. This irritates the visceral surface of the diaphragm, which is supplied by the phrenic nerve (principally C4). Hence pain is felt in the right shoulder tip, which has the same segmental nerve supply. This phenomenon is called referred pain.

4. A, B, C, D

General examination of the patient is absolutely essential before abdominal examination, both in the emergency and elective situation. In the emergency, looking at the patient gives the following very important information: apprehensive patient lying motionless is in pain, sweaty patient (in normal room temperature) is in shock, thoracic respiration and immobility of the abdomen denotes peritonitis. In the elective situation the clinician should be aware of the following: weight loss which is apparent if a patient has loose-fitting clothes with holes in the belt having gone up a couple of notches; anaemia when the patient looks pale; and jaundice when there is yellowish discoloration of the skin and conjunctiva. The three features of weight loss, anaemia and jaundice might turn out to be a manifestation of the same condition – disseminated malignancy.

Discoloration of the abdominal wall, particularly in an emergency, is very significant – Cullen's and Grey–Turner's signs indicate intra-abdominal bleeding from acute haemorrhagic pancreatitis, leaking abdominal aortic aneurysm, ruptured ectopic pregnancy, or ruptured liver or spleen. Cullen's sign is haemorrhagic discoloration around the umbilicus while Grey–Turner's sign is the same in the right flank **(Figure 59.1)**. One must be aware that in an elective patient hyperpigmentation of the skin may indicate adrenal insufficiency – Addison's disease.

In an emergency, a good clinician would ask the patient to take deep breaths in and out before feeling the abdomen. Lack of movement of the abdominal wall on breathing will show that the patient has thoracic respirations, a clear sign of peritonitis; this means that abdominal palpation should be done with the utmost gentleness. To follow on, when it comes to testing for rebound tenderness, a sign of peritonitis, gentle percussion shows finesse on the part of

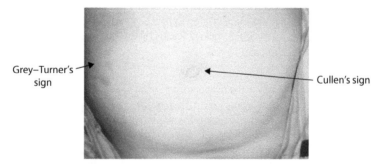

Figure 59.1   Abdominal wall showing Cullen's and Grey–Turner's signs. In this patient, they were from acute haemorrhagic pancreatitis.

the clinician. Even before this, asking the patient to cough would indicate peritonitis when the patient winces or experiences severe pain.

Examination of a child with acute abdominal pain (for ease of reading, the male gender is used generically in this paragraph):

Examining a child with an acute abdomen can be quite a challenge for a clinician not trained in paediatrics. The following technique can be quite useful. After detailed observation of the child, ask the child to put his hand over the sore area. The clinician should then place his hand over the child's hand and continue the palpation using the child's hand with his own. To look for rebound tenderness, coughing is the best way to start. A child with peritonism will not cough. Also to look for rebound, ask the child to press his abdomen and then suddenly 'let go'. In peritonitis he will wince with pain. The aim should be to elicit rebound tenderness without even feeling the abdomen, or, at the most, very gentle percussion.

In the elective patient with an obvious abdominal lump, when the patient tenses the abdomen by the Valsalva manoeuvre or raising the head off the bed, an intra-abdominal lump will become less prominent or disappear depending upon the size. If it becomes prominent, it means that the lump is in the abdominal wall or is a hernia. Palpation of the nine quadrants of the abdomen is carried out in a systematic manner.

Answers to extended matching questions

1. B Abdominal aortic aneurysm (AAA)
This man complains of throbbing backache with a pulsatile sensation in his abdomen. He has a pulsatile abdominal epigastric mass. The backache is from the AAA eroding into the lumbar vertebral bodies. Typically an AAA is best seen when observed from the side by the clinician squatting by the bedside so as to keep the eyes at the same level as the anterior abdominal wall. The suspicion is confirmed by demonstrating an expansile pulsatile mass on palpation (**see Chapter 56**).

2. F Acute pancreatitis
The history of alcohol abuse in this patient with acute abdominal pain should arouse the suspicion of acute pancreatitis. He has the clinical features of an acute abdominal emergency with features of shock. A working diagnosis of acute pancreatitis should be made unless otherwise proved and investigations carried out accordingly (**see Chapter 68**).

3. C Biliary colic
This young woman has all the characteristics of biliary colic. As opposed to acute cholecystitis, she does not have features of infection such as fever and generally feeling unwell with a positive Murphy's sign. Here the pathology is mainly obstructive, whereas in acute cholecystitis it is obstructive and infective. In biliary colic the patient feels relatively well in between attacks (**see Chapter 67**).

4. E Carcinoma of caecum
Clinical features of chronic anaemia, such as undue tiredness or shortness of breath on routine daily activities is typical of anaemia, the classical elective presentation of a right-sided colonic carcinoma such as the one arising from the caecum. This is confirmed on clinical examination by the presence of a mass in the right iliac fossa (**Figure 59.2a** and **b**) (**see Chapter 69**).

5. D Distal small bowel obstruction
This elderly woman has distal small bowel obstruction with clinical features of abdominal distension, vomiting and abdominal pain. Faeculent vomiting is classical of distal small bowel

obstruction. This would be associated with signs of dehydration such as sunken eyes, dry tongue and loss of skin turgor. The finding of a tender lump in her right groin indicates an incarcerated femoral hernia as the cause of intestinal obstruction (**see Chapter 60**).

6. A Incisional hernia

This patient has an incisional hernia. Typically the lump becomes prominent when the intra-abdominal pressure is raised. The lump is deep to an abdominal scar and has a cough impulse. Lumps that arise from the abdominal wall musculature also become prominent on raising the intra-abdominal pressure (**see Chapter 60**).

7. H Perforated duodenal ulcer

This patient has the typical presentation of a perforated hollow viscus. With features of peritonitis as seen from a rigid abdomen and thoracic respiration, he complains of pain in his right shoulder tip, which is from irritation of the diaphragm. History of long-standing indigestion points to a duodenal ulcer perforation (**see Chapter 63**).

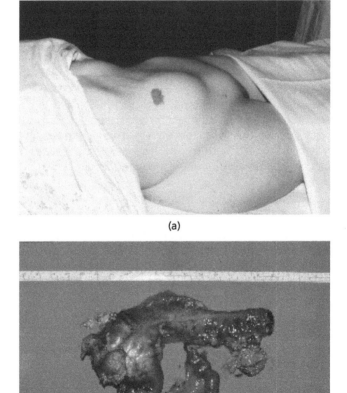

(a)

(b)

Figure 59.2 (a) Lump in the right iliac fossa from carcinoma of the caecum. (b) Specimen of right hemicolectomy of patient in (a).

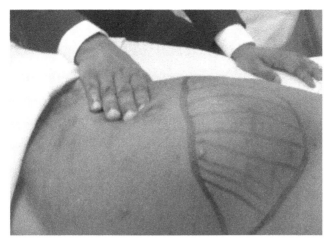

Figure 59.3 Malignant hepatomegaly demonstrating how to palpate an enlarged liver.

8. G Secondary metastasis in liver

This patient who has jaundice and an enlarged hard liver has the hallmarks of pathology in the liver **(Figure 59.3)**. The fact that she has had a left hemicolectomy for a left colonic carcinoma points to secondary liver metastasis causing her jaundice and hepatomegaly **(see Chapter 65)**.

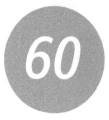

60 Abdominal wall, hernia and umbilicus

Stephen J Nixon

Multiple choice questions

→ ## Inguinal and femoral hernia

1. Which of the following statements are true?

A Inguinal hernia is more common in men than in women.

B Femoral hernia is more common than inguinal hernia in women.

C Femoral hernia is felt below and medial to the pubic tubercle.

D The risk of bowel strangulation is greatest in femoral hernia, less in indirect inguinal hernia and least in direct inguinal hernia.

E A 'sliding' inguinal hernia can pass either medial or lateral to the inferior epigastric vessels.

→ ## Surgery for inguinal hernia

2. Which of the following statements are true?

A Open repair of inguinal hernia should always involve placement of a mesh.

B The Lichtenstein Open Repair has the lowest recurrence rate of any type of repair.

C Laparoscopic repair has been shown to have less postoperative pain, less chronic pain, accelerated postoperative recovery and fewer wound complications.

D Approximately 5% of cases of inguinal hernia will be bilateral and 10% will be on patients with recurrent inguinal hernia after previous surgery.

E Chronic postoperative pain occurs in more than 20% of cases after surgery.

→ ## Mesh for hernia repair

3. Which of the following are true?

A Mesh should not be used in the presence of infection.

B Mesh is mainly used to induce fibrosis, thus making a strong repair.

C Polypropylene mesh is hydrophobic and monofilament.

D Simple polypropylene is ideal for intra-peritoneal use.

E Synthetic, nonabsorbable meshes can contract in size by up to 50% over time.

→ ## Surgery for femoral hernia

4. Which of the following are true?

A There is no place for laparoscopic surgery in femoral hernia.

B Skin discolouration over the hernia suggests possible strangulation.

C There is a decreased risk of femoral hernia after open inguinal hernia repair.

D A high, abdominal, McEvedy approach is best in patients presenting with a strangulating femoral hernia.

E The femoral nerve is at risk due to its proximity to the neck of a femoral hernia.

→ ## Incisional hernia and its repair

5. Which of the following are not true?

A Most incisional hernias will occur within 2 years of the surgery.

B Jenkins Rule states that in closing an abdominal incision the length of suture used should be four times the length of the incision. However, this has been disproved.

C Transverse abdominal incisions are less likely to herniate than vertical incisions.

D Non-absorbable meshes placed at initial surgery will reduce the risk of subsequent incisional herniation.

E Open mesh repair of incisional hernia has a higher wound infection rate but lower recurrence rate when compared with laparoscopic mesh repair.

Extended matching questions

→ ## 1. Diagnoses of abdominal wall hernias

1 Direct inguinal hernia
2 Divarication of recti
3 Epigastric hernia
4 Femoral hernia
5 Incisional hernia
6 Indirect inguinal hernia
7 Paraumbilical hernia
8 Port-site hernia
9 Spigelian hernia
10 Umbilical hernia

Match the diagnoses with one of the scenarios that follows:

A A 6-month-old infant has a history of lump over the belly-button that increases in size when the baby cries.

B A 26-year-old presents with a lump over his left groin. Examination reveals cough impulse and a reducible hernia extending into the scrotum. Pressure over the internal ring controls the hernia.

C A 60-year-old obese woman has a painful lump just above her umbilicus. Examination confirms a round smooth tender mass with no cough impulse.

D A 78-year-old woman has a suspected enlarged left groin lymph node. Examination reveals a 2-cm hard, tender and irreducible lump below and lateral to the pubic tubercle with no cough impulse.

E A 40-year-old woman describes a gradually increasing lump in the lower, right abdomen. She has had three caesarean sections. There is a Pfannenstiel scar with a reducible mass at its lateral end.

F A 76-year-old man has a 2-year history of small swellings in both groins, causing no real discomfort. Examination confirms reducible hernias, which are not controlled by pressure over the deep inguinal ring.

G A 50-year-old man presents with a lump below but well lateral to the umbilicus. You suspect an inguinal hernia but the mass seems to be slightly too high and too lateral for this diagnosis.

H A 22-year-old fit male presents with tender, firm, 2-cm nodule in the midline just below the xiphisternum. There is no cough impulse. The patient believes that the lump increases in size on exercise.

I A 62-year-old labourer is referred with an abdominal hernia. When lying down, no mass is visible but on raising his head from the bed, a broadly based swelling appears between the xiphisternum and umblilicus.

J A 45-year-old woman has a 3-cm firm mass at the umbilicus. She had a laparoscopic cholecystectomy 2 years ago.

→ ## 2. Treatment of abdominal wall hernias

1 Wait and watch
2 Laparoscopic inguinal hernia repair (TEP or TAPP)
3 Open Lichtenstein repair
4 Open or laparoscopic mesh repair
5 Non-surgical
6 Open suture or plug repair
7 Open suture or mesh repair

Choose and match the most appropriate operation with each of the conditions that follow:

A Uncomplicated primary unilateral inguinal hernia
B Recurrent inguinal hernia – post-open repair
C Infantile umbilical hernia
D Recurrent inguinal hernia – post-laparoscopic repair
E Divarication of recti
F Complex incisional hernia in patient known to have extensive adhesions
G Small paraumbilical hernia

→ ## 3. Named operations and techniques in hernia surgery

1 Desarda operation
2 Lichtenstein operation
3 Mayo repair
4 Ramirez technique
5 Shouldice operation
6 Stoppa operation

Match the operation to the description that follows:

A Suture repair of inguinal hernia with double breasting of posterior wall of inguinal canal.
B Open pre-peritoneal mesh repair for complex inguinal hernia.
C Suture repair of paraumbilical hernia with double breasting of anterior sheath.
D Suture repair of inguinal hernia employing external oblique aponeurosis.
E Open mesh repair of inguinal hernia.
F Muscle release to aid abdominal wall closure in large incisional hernia.

Answers to multiple choice questions

1. A, D

Inguinal hernia is more common in men than in women due to the expansion of the deep inguinal ring to allow the testis and accompanying structures to pass. Other factors might be increased abdominal pressures due to prostatic symptoms, higher incidence of smoking and chest conditions. More than 50% of femoral hernia cases present as an emergency with high risk of strangulation, as the neck of the femoral canal is small and rigid. All cases of femoral hernia should be operated on as soon as possible. Inguinal hernia is less likely to present as an emergency. Indirect inguinal hernias often contain bowel, which may extend into the scrotum and become adherent to the sac. This may lead to bowel obstruction and strangulation. Direct inguinal hernias rarely present as an emergency with bowel involvement.

Femoral hernia is more common in women than in men, but inguinal hernia is still common in women than femoral hernia. A femoral hernia is palpated below and lateral to the pubic tubercle. They are often non-reducible and misdiagnosed as an inguinal lymph gland or missed altogether if the groin is not examined, particular in elderly female patients presenting with symptoms of abdominal pain. A 'sliding' inguinal hernia is always of the indirect, lateral type passing through the deep inguinal ring. In a sliding hernia extra-peritoneal tissue initially passes through the deep inguinal ring pulling bowel with it, often the caecum on the right side, and sigmoid colon on the left.

2. C, D, E

Many trials compare laparoscopic and open repair for inguinal hernia and confirm that laparoscopic surgery accelerates postoperative recovery and reduces postoperative and chronic pain. There is a reduction in wound haematoma, seroma and wound infection. However, laparoscopic surgery is technically demanding and might take longer to perform. One in 20 patients present to the surgeon with bilateral herniae, but more detailed tests find that 20% of patients will have an occult contralateral hernia. One in three patients who undergo unilateral surgery will require repair of the opposite side in later life. 10% of patients undergoing surgery will have had a previous operation on the same side. Laparoscopic surgery is particularly beneficial in both recurrent and bilateral cases. Chronic postoperative pain is the most common complication of all forms of inguinal hernia surgery and occurs in more than 20% of cases but is more severe after open surgery compared with laparoscopic.

Most surgeons use mesh routinely for inguinal hernia, the most popular operations being the open Lichtenstein repair and laparoscopic TEP repair. There are open suture repair techniques including the Shouldice repair, Moloney Darn and Desarda operation, which have reported excellent results, comparable to Lichtenstein repair. These operations do not use a mesh. Early studies of the Lichtenstein repair suggested that recurrence rates were less than with suture repairs, but more recent studies have shown comparable recurrence rates. Also trials of Lichtenstein repair versus laparoscopic repair have generally shown equal recurrence rates.

3. C, E

Polypropylene is hydrophobic and monofilament, enhancing its antimicrobial properties. Polyethylene is hydrophilic and multifilament, which enhances its tissue incorporation. Synthetic meshes 'shrink' up to 50% due to fibrous infiltration and later contraction of the collagen. Lighter-weight meshes with large pore sizes are less susceptible to shrinkage. It is important to use large meshes with sufficient overlap so that shrinkage will not re-expose the hernia defect and cause recurrence.

Absorbable meshes can be used in the presence of infection. More recent reports have shown that large pore, non-absorbable meshes are more resistant to infection and can also be used. They have been used prophylactically to reduce the incidence of para-stomal hernia in the presence of faecal peritonitis. Synthetic meshes are stronger than the human abdominal wall, and fibrosis is not required to add further to strength. Too much fibrosis leads to chronic pain and excessive shrinkage. Minimal fibrosis holds the mesh in position and is all that is required. Polypropylene causes adhesions if placed within the peritoneal cavity. It should not be used in the peritoneal cavity unless coated with a 'non-stick' layer.

4. B, D

A reddish discolouration or bruising suggests that hernia contents are strangulating, leading to surrounding infection or seepage of blood-stained fluid into the tissue. Discolouration of the skin over any hernia is a warning sign and urgency of surgical management is indicated. When choosing between a low, inguinal, or high approach in femoral hernia the risk of bowel resection should be considered. In emergency cases, the risk of bowel infarction requiring resection is high and therefore a high approach, allowing easy access to the peritoneal cavity, is best.

Laparoscopic approaches have been used in elective femoral hernia repair and the finding of an occult femoral hernia during inguinal hernia surgery is not unusual. The mesh is placed to cover the deep inguinal ring, Hasselbach's triangle and femoral canal, thus protecting against indirect inguinal, direct inguinal and femoral hernia. Studies have shown an increased risk of femoral hernia after open inguinal hernia repair, possibly due to widening of the femoral canal. In some cases, it might be that there was an error of diagnosis and an inguinal hernia repair was done when the patient actually had a femoral hernia. The femoral vein runs immediately lateral to the femoral canal and is at risk during surgery. The femoral artery is more lateral and the nerve more lateral still. They are unlikely to be damaged.

5. A, B

Long-term follow-up studies have shown that whilst there is a increased rate of herniation in the first 18 months after surgery, the rate of failure then remains constant at least for the next 10 years and that this rate of late failure is similar for suture and mesh repair. Jenkins rule does state that the suture length should be four times the length of the abdominal wound and has been proved by more recent publications. It should be obeyed to reduce the risk of incisional hernia.

Transverse incisions are less likely to result in incisional hernia than vertical incisions, but the difference is relatively small. Studies have shown that, in high-risk patients, e.g., bariatric surgery, the use of prophylactic meshes will reduce the rate of incisional hernia. Mesh placed around a bowel stoma also reduces the risk of para-stomal herniation. In comparative studies, open repair of incisional hernia is associated with a higher risk of infection but lower risk of recurrence compared with laparoscopic repair. Risk of complications should be discussed with the patient prior to surgery.

Answers to extended matching questions

→ ## 1. Diagnoses of abdominal wall hernias

1. F Direct inguinal hernia

In elderly men it is not uncommon to see bilateral groin bulges lying medial to the deep inguinal ring. These are early direct hernias. If truly asymptomatic, a wait and watch policy might be adopted (sometimes called watchful waiting) but surgery should be recommended if symptoms develop or the masses are clearly increasing in size.

2. I Divarication of recti

To the patient, a divarification is like a hernia but in fact the linea alba has simply stretched to allow the bulging. They do not contain bowel and therefore cannot strangulate. The results of surgery are poor and therefore operation is not recommended. There may be an accompanying epigastric or paraumbilical hernia which might require surgery.

3. H Epigastric hernia

Epigastric hernias are often irreducible and have no cough impulse. On examination they feel like a lipoma, as they normally only contain extraperitoneal fat. There is no risk of bowel strangulation but an operation is advised to treat the pain.

4. D Femoral hernia

It is easy to miss a small groin lump or for it to be misdiagnosed as a lymph node. Early exploration should be recommended. A low approach may be used in this case and local anaesthesia might be used in the unfit patient.

5. E Incisional hernia

An incisional hernia is the most likely diagnosis in this case, indeed any hernia close to a surgical incision is likely to be an incisional hernia.

6. B Indirect inguinal hernia

At this age, an early operation would be required as the hernia is likely to affect his work. There is also higher risk of complications in an indirect inguinal hernia, suggested by control with pressure at the deep inguinal ring.

7. C Paraumbilical hernia

Paraumbilical hernia is common in adults. Small painless hernias might not require surgery, but the pain in this case and irreducibility suggest complications are likely and thus surgical invention is required.

8. J Port-site hernia

Port-site hernias occur in approximately 1% of cases after laparoscopic surgery, almost always at the site of 10-mm ports (or larger) and 75% at the umbilicus. They are treated like para-umbilical hernias.

9. G Spigelian hernia

This is the most common site of a Spigelian hernia, most of which occur at the level of the arcuate line but in fact can occur at any site along the Spigelian line, which is the junction of muscle and aponeurosis of the transverses abdominis muscle. The hernia is described as interstitial because it expands in a plane between the three muscles. An ultrasound or CT scan is helpful in diagnosis. Operation is advised.

10. A Umbilical hernia

Most infantile umbilical hernias resolve spontaneously and no surgical treatment is indicated under the age of 2 years unless complications occur.

2. Treatment of abdominal wall hernias

1. C Wait and watch

Infantile umbilical hernias will most often resolve and therefore surgery is delayed until beyond 2 years unless complications occur.

2. B Laparoscopic inguinal hernia repair (TEP or TAPP)

When an inguinal hernia recurs after open surgery, a laparoscopic repair should be recommended as the surgery is minimally affected by postoperative scarring. Laparoscopic repair is also recommended in bilateral hernias.

3. D Open Lichtenstein repair

Recurrent inguinal hernia after laparoscopic repair is best re-repaired using an open mesh technique, the most common being a Lichtenstein operation. It is extremely difficult to re-enter the extraperitoneal space laparoscopically due to the mesh causing dense fibrosis.

4. A Open or laparoscopic mesh repair

Current guidelines suggest that both open and laparoscopic mesh repairs can be recommended for primary inguinal hernia depending on the experience of the surgeon.

5. E Non-surgical

It is better not to operate for simple divarification of the rectus as results are poor and complications of the divarification are unlikely.

6. G Open suture or plug repair
Small paraumbilical hernias may be repaired by suturing or the use of a small plug or mesh. Laparoscopic repair is possible but expensive.

7. F Open suture or mesh repair
When a patient is known to have extensive adhesions, a laparoscopic approach is unlikely to be successful with a high risk of bowel injury. Open surgery is preferred by using suture or mesh.

3. Named operations and techniques in surgery

1. D Desarda operation
The Desarda technique for inguinal hernia isolates a strip of external oblique aponeurosis, which is still attached both medially and laterally and sutures this down between the inguinal ligament and conjoint tendon, thus reinforcing the posterior wall of the inguinal canal.

2. E Lichtenstein operation
The Lichtenstein open mesh repair remains the most common technique for repair of inguinal hernia because of its relative simplicity and low recurrence rates. It can be performed under local anaesthesia.

3. C Mayo repair
The Mayo repair is used in paraumbilical hernia, making a transverse incision in the anterior rectus sheath and then closing the defect in two layers. This operation is being replaced by the use of non-absorbable mesh.

4. F Ramirez technique
The Ramirez muscle separation technique is used in large incisional hernias where the surgeon has difficulty in closing the abdomen. Lateral-releasing incisions allow the separation of the three muscle layers so that muscle mass can be moved medially to close a central defect.

5. A Shouldice operation
The Shouldice repair for inguinal hernia is a modified Bassini operation where the posterior wall of the inguinal canal is opened from the deep inguinal ring to the pubic tubercle then closed in two overlapping layers.

6. B Stoppa operation
The Stoppa operation is an open preperitoneal operation placing a large mesh over the posterior aspect of the inguino/femoral canal area, useful in complex, recurrent inguinal hernia.

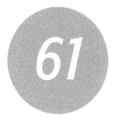

61 The peritoneum, omentum, mesentery and retroperitoneal space

Pradip K Datta

Multiple choice questions

→ ## Anatomy and physiology

1. Which of the following statements are true?

A The surface area of the peritoneum is nearly equal to that of the skin.
B The parietal peritoneum is poorly innervated.
C The peritoneum has the capacity to absorb large volumes of fluid.
D The peritoneum has the ability to produce fibrinolytic activity.
E When injured, the peritoneum produces an inflammatory exudate.

→ ## Peritonitis – microbiology

2. The following organisms are a gastrointestinal (GI) source of peritonitis except:

A *Escherichia coli.*
B Streptococci.
C *Chlamydia.*
D *Bacteroides.*
E *Clostridium.*

→ ## Peritonitis – local and diffuse

3. Which of the following statements are true?

A Peritonitis gets localised because of anatomical factors.
B The greater omentum plays an important role in localising infection.
C Diagnostic peritoneal lavage (DPL) has a vital role in diagnosis.
D CT scan is useful for both diagnostic and therapeutic purposes.
E Operation is not necessary in all patients with peritonitis.

→ ## Peritonitis – management

4. Which of the following statements is not true?

A All patients should be thoroughly resuscitated.
B A paracolic abscess on CT scan must have open surgery.
C Septic shock might follow.
D Nutritional support must be instituted in certain patients.
E Young children do not have the natural barrier against the spread of peritonitis.

→ ## Special forms of peritonitis

5. The following statements are true except:

A Bile peritonitis is usually a feature following operation.
B A leucocytosis of >30,000 with 90% polymorphs is suggestive of pneumococcal peritonitis.
C Tuberculous ascites may be loculated.
D Tuberculosis (TB) spreads from the ileocaecal region.
E Diagnostic smear will be positive in the vast majority of cases of tuberculosis.

Intraperitoneal abscess

6. Which of the following statements are correct?

A The pelvis is the commonest site of intraperitoneal abscess.

B Pus can also collect in four other intraperitoneal sites.

C The usual cause is postoperative.

D Pain may be a feature well away from the site of pathology.

E Open operation and drainage is the treatment of choice.

Ascites

7. Which of the following statements are not true?

A Imbalance between plasma and peritoneal colloid osmotic and hydrostatic pressure causes ascites.

B Shifting dullness is a classical sign in all cases of ascites.

C The protein content determines if the ascitic fluid is a transudate or an exudate.

D A peritoneovenous shunt should be considered in all cases of ascites.

E Chylous ascites is most commonly caused by malignancy.

Tumours of the peritoneum

8. Which of the following statements are true?

A Secondary tumours are more common.

B Carcinomatosis peritonei is usually a terminal event.

C Pseudomyxoma peritonei arises from a primary tumour from the appendix.

D Repeated 'debulking surgery' in pseudomyxoma peritonei gives relief.

E Peritoneal loose bodies are malignant in origin.

Adhesions

9. The following statements are true except:

A Ischaemic tissue inhibits fibrinolysis encouraging formation of adhesions.

B Laparoscopic surgery reduces adhesion related complications.

C Adhesions are responsible for two-thirds of small bowel obstructions.

D Prevention of adhesions can be actively achieved.

E Intestinal obstruction from sclerosing encapsulating peritonitis should be treated by surgery.

The omentum and mesentery

10. Which of the following statements are true?

A Torsion of the omentum always presents as an emergency.

B Mesenteric injury occurs as a seatbelt syndrome.

C Acute nonspecific ileocaecal mesenteric adenitis can be confused with acute appendicitis.

D A mesenteric cyst clinically presents as a fixed periumbilical mass.

E Chylolymphatic cyst is the commonest type of mesenteric cyst.

The retroperitoneal space

11. Which of the following statements is not true?

A Idiopathic retroperitoneal fibrosis can present as chronic renal failure.

B An AAA can cause retroperitoneal fibrosis.

C Retroperitoneal fibrosis is always a benign condition.

D Retroperitoneal abscess may be a manifestation of vertebral tuberculosis.

E Retroperitoneal lipoma is often a sarcoma.

Extended matching questions

Diagnoses

1 Idiopathic retroperitoneal fibrosis

2 Mesenteric cyst

3 Retroperitoneal liposarcoma

4 Right subhepatic abscess
5 Small bowel obstruction from adhesions
6 Tuberculous ascites

Match the diagnoses with the clinical scenarios that follow:

A A 62-year-old man presents with generalised colicky abdominal pain with bilious vomiting for 48 hours. His symptoms have been intermittent. He has a distended abdomen with generalised tenderness without any rigidity or rebound tenderness. Following an operation for left hemicolectomy 3 years ago through a long midline incision, he has had several such episodes some of them requiring admission.

B A 58-year-old man complains of malaise, bilateral backache, nausea and occasional vomiting for 2 months. Clinically there is nothing to find except for bilateral hydroceles of which the patient was not aware. His general practitioner performed routine blood tests, which are as follows: Hb 10 g/dL, ESR 88, CRP 292, urea 22 mmol/L, creatinine 256 mmol/L, K 6.1 mmol/L, Na 135 mmol/L, Cl 98 mmol/L and HCO_3 18 mmol/L.

C A 45-year-old woman complains of an abdominal lump that she noticed in the bath 6 weeks ago. She has some generalised discomfort in her abdomen. On examination she looks well, with a smooth fluctuant periumbilical mass freely mobile in a diagonal plane from the right subcostal to the left iliac fossa.

D A 50-year-old man underwent a laparoscopic closure of a perforated duodenal ulcer. His postoperative period during the first 4 to 5 days was uneventful. Thereafter he complained of hiccoughs with pain in the right subcostal area and right shoulder tip. He had swinging pyrexia, was toxic, tachypnoeic and tender in the right upper quadrant with oedema of the overlying skin.

E A 38-year-old woman, who arrived from the Indian subcontinent 1 year ago, complains of general malaise, cough and low-grade evening temperature for 6 months. She has lost some weight and abdominal examination shows central abdominal distension with a feeling of an encysted periumbilical mass.

F A 47-year-old woman complains of generally feeling unwell with weight loss for 6 months. She complains of some discomfort over her entire left side of the abdomen associated with constipation. On examination she has a marked fullness in her left lumbar region and loin.

Answers to multiple choice questions

1. A, C, D, E

As the largest cavity in the body, the peritoneum has a surface area of 2 square metres in the adult – almost equal to that of the skin. It is composed of flattened polyhedral cells and consists of two parts, a visceral peritoneum enveloping the organs and a parietal part lining the surfaces of the abdominal cavity. The peritoneum has the capacity to absorb large amounts of fluid, a particular function that is utilised therapeutically for peritoneal dialysis in renal failure. In intra-abdominal pathology, fibrinolytic activity is a function of the peritoneum. When injured the peritoneum produces an inflammatory exudate, hence the fluid exudation in peritonitis.

The parietal peritoneum is richly innervated, as a result of which pain originating from the parietal peritoneum is severe and well localised. In contrast, the visceral peritoneum is poorly innervated as the nerves travel along the blood vessels; this results in poor localisation when pain originates from the organs.

2. C

In women, ascending infection via the Fallopian tubes due to colonisation with *Chlamydia* resulting in pelvic inflammatory disease (PID) is the most common non-gastrointestinal cause of peritonitis – gonococcus being another. These organisms might also cause the infection to ascend to the liver, causing perihepatitis by involving the Glisson's capsule producing 'violin string' adhesions giving rise to Fitz-Hugh–Curtis syndrome, a diagnosis that can be confused with acute cholecystitis.

Organisms from the GI tract usually are in the form of two or more strains, the common flora being *E. coli*, Streptococci, *Bacteroides* and *Clostridia*. The bacterial colonisation is low in the small bowel and much higher distally; this is exacerbated when there is pathology such as obstruction and inflammation. The same is true of the biliary and pancreatic systems. Endotoxins and exotoxins released from the bacteria exert their effect by the release of tumour necrosis factor (TNF) from the host leucocytes. In serious cases they may result in endotoxic shock.

3. A, B, D, E

A knowledge of the anatomy of the peritoneal cavity helps in understanding the sites and methods of localisation of peritonitis. The general peritoneal cavity is divided into a greater sac and lesser sac, the two communicating through the foramen of Winslow. The greater sac is subdivided into the subdiaphragmatic (subphrenic) spaces, pelvis and general peritoneal cavity. The lesser sac, also called the omental bursa, is the space behind the stomach. There are seven subdiaphragmatic spaces, four intraperitoneal and three extraperitoneal. The general peritoneal cavity is divided by the transverse colon and mesocolon into supra- and infra-colic compartments. These anatomic divisions have a bearing on the localisation of intraperitoneal infection.

The greater omentum plays a major role in localising peritonitis. It envelops the inflamed organ to localise the infection such as a perforated sigmoid diverticulum. This function as a barrier to the spread of infection prompted Rutherford Morison to give it the metaphorical name of 'abdominal policeman'. When intraperitoneal infection is suspected, a contrast-enhanced CT scan is the ideal imaging of choice. It will show the site of the collection of pus such as a paracolic abscess and the cause such as perforated diverticulitis. The procedure can be used to drain the pus and leave a catheter. Operation is not necessary in many patients, because image-guided drainage (US or CT) by the interventional radiologist is often successful.

Diagnostic peritoneal lavage (DPL), an invasive method not without its complications, is now obsolete with the availability of alternative diagnostic methods such as high-quality US and CT.

4. B

A paracolic abscess diagnosed on CT scan hardly ever will require open surgery. This should be drained by CT guidance and a catheter left in place. The catheter can also be used to irrigate the abscess cavity. Once the patient has recovered, detailed investigations are carried out and the pathology dealt with definitively.

All patients should be thoroughly resuscitated by correction of fluid, electrolyte and acid-base disturbance; an indwelling urinary catheter and a nasogastric tube are inserted and the patient started on the appropriate broad-spectrum antibiotic to cover aerobic and anaerobic organisms. Good analgesia is essential; an epidural might be considered. If the patient is not promptly and effectively managed, septic shock might follow. Assessing the patient early will give an idea as to the need for nutritional support, which will help toward quicker recovery.

For example, if the patient has had a laparotomy for diffuse peritonitis removal of the cause is carried out with thorough peritoneal lavage with several litres of warm normal saline. This should be followed by a feeding jejunostomy for long-term nutrition. Young children do not have a well-developed omentum. Therefore, they do not have the natural protection to localise peritonitis; the surgeon should therefore consider early surgery.

5. E
Diagnostic smears for acid-fast bacilli are positive in less than 3% of patients. Cultures take 4 to 8 weeks without any guarantee of a positive result. Laparoscopy with peritoneal biopsy and macroscopic intraperitoneal findings confirms the diagnosis. Caseating peritoneal nodules are common. Ascites is present in all patients with TB; this can be a generalised form or be loculated. The disease originates from the ileocaecal region, spreading via the mesenteric lymph nodes or directly from the bloodstream usually from the miliary form of the disease. Peritoneal involvement occurs in the vast majority.

The diagnosis of bile peritonitis is usually made at laparotomy unless the patient had an operation on the biliary tract in the recent past. If the patient has not had an operation, the most common cause is perforated cholecystitis. Postoperative causes are the following: postcholecystectomy with cystic duct blow-out or CBD injury, leak following biliary-enteric bypass, or duodenal stump leak after Polya gastrectomy. Bile peritonitis might also result from liver injury.

6. A, B, C, D
The pelvis is the most common site for an intraperitoneal abscess. This is because it is the most dependent site, and postoperatively the patient usually sits up. Also one of the most common causes is after an operation for pelvic appendicitis and tubo-ovarian infections causing pelvic inflammatory disease. Besides, the other intraperitoneal sites of abscesses are four in number, two on either side – right subphrenic, right subhepatic and left subphrenic and left subhepatic (**Table 61.1**). The causes in the vast majority are postoperative (**Tables 61.2 and 61.3**).

While the clinical presentation might be insidious, the patient develops swinging pyrexia, looks toxic and typically complains of pain in his right shoulder tip when the right subphrenic or subhepatic spaces are involved. This is because pus collection under the right dome of the diaphragm causes irritation of the diaphragmatic peritoneum and pain travels along the sensory fibres of the phrenic nerve. This classically produces referred pain to the right shoulder tip in the distribution of C4.

The management of an intraperitoneal abscess is to localise the site of abscess by imaging such as US or CT scan, followed by image-guided drainage. Open operation is almost obsolete, the interventional radiologist having taken over the task.

Table 61.1 Involvement of the subphrenic spaces on both sides

- Involvement of right spaces is more common than left.
- Left subphrenic space is bounded by the splenorenal, gastrosplenic and phrenicocolic ligaments which produce a partial barrier to the left paracolic gutter.
- Hence collections occur less often in the left subphrenic space.
- Collections in left subphrenic space are after surgery on the stomach, spleen and tail of pancreas.
- Collection in the left subhepatic space (lesser sac) is usually a pseudo-cyst of the pancreas.

Table 61.2 Causes of subphrenic abscesses – right side

Right subphrenic abscess	Right subhepatic abscess
• Perforated gall bladder	• Retrocaecal appendicitis
• Perforated duodenal ulcer	• Perforated gall bladder
• Perforated retrocaecal appendicitis	• Leak after right hemicolectomy
	• Perforated duodenal ulcer

Table 61.3 Causes of subphrenic abscesses – left side

Left subphrenic abscess	Left subhepatic abscess
After operations on the:	• Commonest cause of collection is a pseudo-cyst of pancreas which is a sterile collection after acute pancreatitis
• Stomach	
• Pancreas	• Infected pseudo-cyst of pancreas
• Spleen	• Perforated gastric ulcer which gets walled off
• Splenic flexure of colon	

7. B, D

In a patient with normal body habitus, for ascites to be clinically diagnosed there must be more than 1.5 litres of intraperitoneal fluid. Shifting dullness and fluid thrill are the clinical signs of ascites. However, shifting dullness cannot be elicited when there is a huge amount of fluid as there would be no free space in the peritoneal cavity for the fluid to be shifted. As a means of treating ascites by intervention, a peritoneovenous shunt is considered only rarely in selected cases.

Ascites is the accumulation of excess fluid in the peritoneal cavity. It occurs when there is a disturbance between the plasma and peritoneal colloid and hydrostatic pressures. This can be due to several causes, including cardiac, hepatic, renal and local. When the amount of protein in the ascitic fluid is >25 g/L it is called an exudate, while it is called a transudate when the protein content is <25 g/L. Capillary hydrostatic pressure is increased when there is a generalised water retention, as in heart failure, liver cirrhosis, portal vein thrombosis, or hepatic vein obstruction (Budd-Chiari syndrome); plasma colloid osmotic pressure is lowered in starvation, intestinal malabsorption, abnormal protein loss, or defective protein synthesis as in the cirrhotic.

Chylous ascites most commonly is the result of malignant obstruction of the thoracic duct usually a lymphoma; other causes are filariasis, TB and nephrotic syndrome. The fluid looks milky from excess of chylomicrons (triglycerides).

8. A, B, C, D

Secondary tumours of the peritoneum are much more common and referred to as carcinomatosis peritonei (peritoneal metastases) and usually a terminal event. The primary can be from any intra-abdominal organ and also breast and bronchus. The malignancy takes the form of discrete nodules, plaques of varying sizes, or diffuse adhesive lesions giving a 'frozen pelvis'. There is blood-stained or straw-coloured ascites. The condition can be mistaken for tuberculous peritonitis.

Pseudomyxoma peritonei, a rare condition and more common in women, arises from a primary tumour of the appendix that implants on to the ovaries. It fills the abdomen with yellow jelly-like mucinous material that might be encysted in the form of mucinous cystic tumours. Adenocarcinoma of the appendix resembles ovarian mucinous adenocarcinoma, and hence it is thought that most ovarian mucinous tumours are seeded from the appendix.

The diagnosis is suspected on ultrasound and CT scan. Good palliation is obtained by repeated debulking laparotomies when carried out in specialist units.

Peritoneal loose bodies are benign small lumps found loose in the peritoneal cavity incidentally at laparotomy. It is the outcome of an appendix epiploica that has undergone torsion and become detached following necrosis.

9. D, E

Major research has been ongoing for many years for the prevention of adhesions. Many drugs have been tried without much success. Various barrier methods have been used in trials. Although there has been reduction in adhesion formation, the findings do not translate to reduction in adhesion-related clinical problems. The outcomes of several trials have shown that the use of barrier products has reduced the incidence, extent and severity of adhesions, but this was not reflected in the clinical outcome in reducing the incidence or surgical intervention for intestinal obstruction. Sclerosing encapsulating peritonitis, which is the result of long-term peritoneal dialysis, is a form of severe adhesions that produces bowel obstruction. In this situation, surgery should be avoided.

Adhesions form in the absence of fibrinolysis. Ischaemic tissue inhibits fibrinolysis, as it does not have the ability to break down fibrin; hence all attempts must be made to prevent ischaemia. Two-thirds of cases of small intestinal obstruction are caused by adhesions. Reducing the production of ischaemic tissue by good surgical technique is the hallmark in the prevention of adhesions. Further, the advent of laparoscopic surgery has resulted in reduction of readmissions for problems related to adhesions.

10. A, B, C, E

Torsion of the omentum is a diagnosis made at an emergency operation carried out for a mistaken diagnosis of acute appendicitis. Usually the sufferer is a middle-aged obese man who presents as an emergency with pain and tenderness in the right iliac fossa. At operation there is a gangrenous mass, which is a black piece of twisted omentum. This is ligated and excised. The normal appendix is usually removed at the same time to prevent confusion in diagnosis in the future, as the patient would have a gridiron incision.

Injury to the mesentery is the aftermath of blunt abdominal injury occurring as a result of the seat belt crushing against the anterior abdominal wall from deceleration injury from a road-traffic accident. This causes a tear in the mesentery with haemorrhage and bowel ischaemia, which will require resection and end-to-end anastomosis. The presentation might be delayed.

Acute nonspecific ileocaecal mesenteric adenitis is a classical differential diagnosis of acute appendicitis especially in children. It is suspected when there is shifting tenderness that is poorly localised and there are symptoms of upper-respiratory infection with cervical, axillary and groin lymphadenopathy. In situations where the diagnosis remains uncertain and acute appendicitis cannot be ruled out, an emergency appendicectomy has to be carried out.

Mesenteric cysts can be chylolymphatic (commonest type), enterogenous, dermoid and urogenital remnant; the diagnosis might be confused with congenital hydronephrosis. The typical presentation is a painless mobile lump that has a classical physical sign of moving diagonally up and down at right angles to the attachment of the mesentery (Tillaux's sign). Confirmation is by ultrasound.

11. C

Retroperitoneal fibrosis is not always a benign condition. It can be the result of a lymphoma or secondary lymph nodal deposits from a testicular tumour or other malignancies. In the majority a cause of the fibrosis cannot be found and hence is called idiopathic retroperitoneal fibrosis. The condition can cause involvement of both ureters, causing them to be pulled medially and lying in front of the vertebral bodies. This results in insidious chronic renal failure. AAA can cause retroperitoneal fibrosis. This happens when it is an inflammatory aneurysm, which involves the left ureter causing hydronephrosis and hydroureter. Such an aneurysm is very adherent to the neighbouring structures particularly the duodenum. It is suspected when the patient has a high ESR and CRP.

A retroperitoneal abscess is a psoas abscess that tracks along the psoas sheath down into the femoral triangle to the lesser trochanter. Clinically a fluctuant mass is palpable in the iliac fossa and the femoral triangle that exhibits cross fluctuation. In developing countries it is still commonly seen, as the cause is vertebral tuberculosis resulting in a cold abscess. The retroperitoneal space-occupying lesion is a lipoma, which is often a liposarcoma. Women are more often affected, complaining of vague abdominal pain; the swelling can be very big and the diagnosis made by ultrasound and CT scan.

Answers to extended matching questions

1. B Idiopathic retroperitoneal fibrosis
A rare condition, retroperitoneal fibrosis results in the formation of greyish-white plaques in the retroperitoneum that spreads laterally to envelop adjacent organs such as the ureters, vessels and aorta. The causes may be benign resembling other fibromatoses such as Dupuytren's contracture and Peyronie's disease, inflammatory type of AAA and certain drugs. The malignant causes are lymphoma and secondary lymph nodal deposits. Histologically there may be active inflammation with high cellularity and collagen bundles; there may be mature fibrosis with calcification.

Patients with the idiopathic benign disease present with chronic renal failure. Diagnosis is confirmed by ultrasound and contrast CT showing bilateral hydronephrosis and hydroureters, the latter being pulled medially by the fibrotic process.

The patient may require treatment for the renal failure such as dialysis. The urologist should take the patient over to perform the operation of ureterolysis with the ureters being wrapped around by omentum to prevent recurrence.

2. C Mesenteric cyst
These occur more often in the small bowel mesentery. Their origin can be chylolymphatic (most common), enterogenous, urogenital remnant and dermoid. They are relatively asymptomatic and found as an abdominal lump. Diagnosis is by ultrasound and CT scan.

Treatment is resection. In about a third of patients undergoing removal of the cyst, the bowel attached to the cyst will also require resection and end-to-end anastomosis.

3. F Retroperitoneal liposarcoma
These are rare tumours, the other histological types being leiomysarcoma and malignant fibrous histiocytoma. Patients usually present late because of the capacious retroperitoneal space, which allows the tumour to grow very large before its presence is felt by nonspecific symptoms. Diagnosis is by CT scan and MRI and confirmation is by image-guided biopsy.

A multidisciplinary team approach gives the best results. At operation three-quarters of resections will entail removal of at least one of the adjacent organs (parts of bowel and kidney). Survival rates even after complete resection are in the region of 35% to 50%.

4. D Right subphrenic abscess
A subphrenic abscess is to be suspected when a patient, particularly after an intra-abdominal operation for a potentially septic condition, does not make a smooth recovery. The classical adage is 'Pus somewhere, pus nowhere, pus under the diaphragm'. After an initial uneventful

few days postoperatively, the patient typically fails to progress, has swinging pyrexia and is toxic. The most common site being the right side, the patient has right upper abdominal pain, with features of right basal pneumonia due to sympathetic right pleural effusion. The patient has polymorphonuclear leucocytosis; confirmation of the diagnosis is by US and CT scan.

The subdiaphragmatic spaces are named in **Figure 61.1**. The anatomic arrangement of the spaces are diagrammatically shown in **Figure 61.2** and **Figure 61.3**. Involvement of the spaces

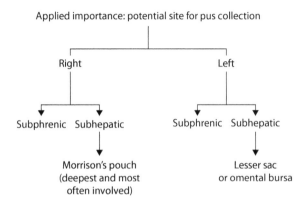

Figure 61.1 Names of subdiaphragmatic spaces.

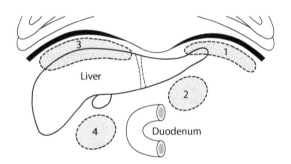

Figure 61.2 Subdiaphragmatic spaces – saggital section.

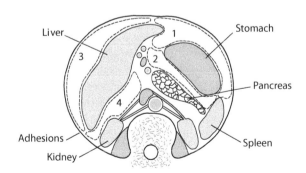

Figure 61.3 Intraperitoneal abscess on transverse section: (1) left subphrenic space (2) left subhepatic space or lesser sac (3) right subphrenic space (4) right subhepatic space or Morison's pouch.

on the right side is more common than on the left. This is explained in **Table 61.1**. The various postoperative causes on the right and left sides are enumerated in **Tables 61.2** and **61.3**.

After the diagnosis is made, having being confirmed by US or CT scan, the abscess is drained under image guidance by the interventional radiologist and a catheter is left in the abscess cavity. As the patient is toxic, after blood cultures have been sent, intravenous broad-spectrum antibiotics are started. Sometimes the aspiration might have to be repeated if there are several loculi.

In rare instances an open operation may have to be performed. For a right anterior subphrenic abscess a right subcostal incision is made and the abscess drained extraperitoneally. For a posterior abscess, an oblique right loin incision is made and the 12th rib is excised subperiosteally followed by a transverse incision on the abscess cavity taking care not to enter the pleural cavity. Drains are left after open drainage.

5. A Small bowel obstruction from adhesions

Small intestinal obstruction is the most common adhesion-related complication, being responsible for almost two-thirds of the causes of intestinal obstruction. Pelvic adhesions are responsible for the majority of causes of secondary infertility. Adhesions as a cause of chronic abdominal and pelvic pain remains unproved; division of adhesions reducing chronic abdominal pain has yet to be convincingly shown in trials. Nevertheless, significant research continues into prevention of postoperative adhesions.

This patient needs to be resuscitated with analgesia, intravenous fluids, nasogastric suction and an indwelling urinary catheter. A supine plain abdominal x-ray will show dilated loops of small bowel in the form of valvulae conniventes (jejunal dilatation) and featureless ileum (ileal dilatation). This patient will be hypokalaemic, which needs to be corrected. As long as the patient has no signs of strangulation (compromise of blood supply), conservative management should be given a fair trial.

Laparotomy is avoided as long as possible as most of these patients do settle down. Moreover, laparotomy for release of adhesions would result in further future adhesions. Faeculent vomiting or aspirate is a sinister finding. This or clinical features of tachycardia, rebound tenderness and toxicity (signs of strangulation) are an indication for laparotomy.

6. E Tuberculous ascites

This condition has an insidious onset with general malaise, vague abdominal symptoms, occasional nausea and vomiting, sometimes alternating constipation and diarrhoea, weight loss, evening pyrexia, night sweats and abdominal distension. Abdominal examination gives a 'doughy' feel from the matted greater omentum studded with tubercles. Localised encysted ascitic collections might give the false impression of an abdominal mass.

A strong Mantoux test suggests the diagnosis, which is strongly supported with a raised ESR and CRP. Chest x-ray (for pulmonary TB) and abdominal US and CT scan are necessary, the latter to confirm ascites. Laparoscopy is the ideal diagnostic avenue and will reveal typical tubercles on the bowel serosa, multiple strictures, a high subhepatic caecum and enlarged lymph nodes. Biopsies are taken from the omentum and lymph nodes for confirmation.

The patient should be managed by the physician with full chemotherapy with involvement of the public health authorities. Surgeons are involved only in case of intestinal obstruction.

62 *The oesophagus*

Pradip K Datta

Multiple choice questions

→ ## Anatomy

1. Which of the following statements are true?

A The oesophagus is 30 cm long.
B The oesophagus has five natural constrictions.
C The gastro-oesophageal junction is 40 cm from the incisors.
D The oesophagus is lined by stratified squamous epithelium.
E The oesophageal opening in the diaphragm is at the level of T10 vertebra.

2. The following statements are true except:

A The lower oesophageal sphincter (LOS) is an area of high pressure.
B The normal length of the LOS is 3 to 4 cm.
C The three phases of swallowing, oral, pharyngeal and oesophageal, are involuntary.
D Pharyngeal diverticulum occurs because of the incoordination of the pharyngeal phase of deglutition.
E The pressure in the LOS is 10–25 mmHg.

→ ## Oesophageal symptoms

3. Which of the following statements are false?

A Dysphagia (difficulty in swallowing) is a cardinal symptom of oesophageal carcinoma.
B Dysphagia associated with cough is a symptom of impending tracheo-oesophageal fistula.
C Dysphagia in the oral and pharyngeal phases of swallowing indicates a neurological rather than a mechanical problem.
D Odynophagia (painful swallowing) is always of cardiac origin.
E Regurgitation and reflux are the same and caused by dysphagia.

4. The following statements are true except:

A Anginal pain can be confused with heartburn.
B Heartburn with weight loss is a 'red flag' symptom.
C Barium swallow is the ideal investigation in a patient with heartburn.
D Dysphagia to liquids more than solids is typical of achalasia of cardia.
E Oesophagogastroduodenoscopy (OGD) is the first line investigation in suspected spontaneous rupture of oesophagus.

→ ## Oesophageal investigations

5. Which of the following statements are true?

A A barium meal should be the first line of investigation in a patient presenting with heartburn.
B 24-hour pH monitoring is the most accurate method to assess gastro-oesophageal reflux disease (GORD).
C Laparoscopy should be undertaken prior to oesophagectomy.
D Manometry is essential in the diagnosis of motility disorders.
E Raman spectroscopy detects early molecular changes in Barrett's mucosal neoplasia.

→ ## Treatment of oesophageal conditions

6. Which of the following statements are false?

A Injection of botulinum toxin is a modality of treatment in achalasia.

B The operation for resection of carcinoma of middle one-third of oesophagus is Heller's procedure.

C Endoscopic mucosal resection is a surgical option in very early mucosal neoplasia in Barrett's oesophagus.

D All patients with oesophageal perforation should be treated with surgical repair.

E The ideal surgical treatment for a Zenker's diverticulum is excision through an incision on the left side of the neck followed by cricopharyngeal myotomy.

Extended matching questions

→ Diagnoses

1 Achalasia of cardia
2 Carcinoma of oesophagus
3 Diffuse oesophageal spasm
4 Gastro-oesophageal reflux disease (GORD)
5 Pharyngeal diverticulum
6 Rolling hiatus hernia

Match the diagnoses with the clinical scenarios that follow:

→ Clinical scenarios

A A 68-year-old woman complains of recurrent cough that is worse at night when she is woken up from her sleep. She is embarrassed by halitosis. Her general practitioner (GP) has treated her for chest infection several times with antibiotics. Examination shows some signs of basal penumonitis.

B A 48-year-old man complains of intermittent dysphagia for almost 1 year. He has some postprandial discomfort, which is relieved by belching and occasional regurgitation of food. This is associated with retrosternal pain and pressure sensation. An ECG is normal. Chest x-ray shows a gas bubble behind the heart.

C A 42-year-old man complains of dysphagia with retrosternal chest pain. This has been intermittent. On one occasion the pain was very severe with pain radiating along the arms. He was admitted as an emergency to the medical ward where his ECG and cardiac enzymes were normal.

D A 72-year-old man, a long-standing smoker, complains of progressive dysphagia with food sticking behind his mid-sternum for 3 months. The problem started with solids, but now he has difficulty with liquids. He has lost 14 kg of weight during this time. On examination the weight loss is obvious from his loose, ill-fitting clothes.

E A 35-year-old man complains of dysphagia of almost 2 years duration. Occasionally he has regurgitation of foul-smelling stale food and frothy sputum. He has been treated for chest infection a few times by his GP. He has lost some weight and looks slightly malnourished.

F A 42-year-old woman complains of retrosternal burning pain, which she refers to as heartburn, epigastric discomfort and repeated regurgitation. Her symptoms are worse after fatty and spicy foods and by stooping. She has also experienced painful swallowing when she felt an acidic taste in her throat. On examination she is obese with signs of chest infection.

Answers to multiple choice questions

→ Anatomy

1. C, D, E

The gastro-oesophageal junction is normally 40 cm from the incisors. The oesophagus is lined by non-keratinised stratified squamous epithelium. Should there be columnar epithelium, it is regarded as abnormal and occurs as a result of gastro-oesophageal reflux disease (GORD). The oesophageal opening is at the level of the tenth thoracic vertebra behind the left seventh costal cartilage, the surface marking being 2.5 cm to the left of the midline.

The oesophagus is 25 cm long. It has three natural constrictions. The first at the cricopharyngeal junction which 15 cm from the incisors, the second at 25 cm from the incisors where it is crossed by the aortic arch and left main bronchus (although the latter is slightly lower) and finally the cardio-oesophageal junction, which is at 40 cm. The surgical importance is that foreign bodies are prone to arrest at these sites.

2. C

The three phases of swallowing are not all involuntary. The oral phase where the food is shifted from the mouth into the oropharynx is voluntary. Thereafter the pharyngeal and oesophageal phases are involuntary. The food bolus is propelled along the oesophagus through the LOS.

Incoordination in swallowing in the pharyngeal phase where the cricopharyngeus muscle does not relax, causes a high pressure within the pharynx; this is the basis of a pharyngeal (Zenker's) diverticulum. The LOS, about 3 to 4 cm long, is an area of high pressure, the pressure being in the region of 10–25 mmHg. This helps to prevent gastro-oesophageal reflux.

Oesophageal symptoms

3. D, E

Odynophagia is painful swallowing. It is not always of cardiac origin although a cardiac cause must be excluded. It is a symptom of oesophageal motility disorders, particularly diffuse oesophageal spasm. Regurgitation and reflux are not the same and do not always result from dysphagia; patients might have difficulty distinguishing the two. Regurgitation, often the effect of a mechanical obstruction such as carcinoma, is the return of swallowed food contents that do not travel down. Reflux is the involuntary return of stomach contents such as acid into the oesophagus or pharynx.

Dysphagia (difficulty in swallowing) is the first symptom of an oesophageal carcinoma. When associated with cough it is of much more sinister significance as it indicates an impending tracheo-oesophageal fistula. Dysphagia in the initial stages of swallowing (oral and pharyngeal) usually has a neurological cause.

4. C, E

Barium swallow is not the ideal investigation in a patient with heartburn. The ideal investigation is oesophagogastroduodenoscopy (OGD). This enables the endoscopist to assess the type of reflux, quantity of reflux, state of the mucosa and site of the gastro-oesophageal junction, and to take biopsies. This investigation should not be carried out in suspected oesophageal rupture where the investigation should be a chest x-ray followed by contrast CT scan.

Anginal pain can easily be confused with heartburn so much so patients with angina often complain of 'indigestion'. Heartburn with weight loss might indicate the onset of a peptic stricture or malignancy in a Barrett's oesophagus and hence a 'red flag' symptom. Patients with achalasia often complain of dysphagia to liquids more than solids.

Oesophageal investigations

5. B, C, D, E

GORD is best assessed by 24-hour pH monitoring. It is particularly useful in patients who are unresponsive to medical treatment and without significant oesophagitis on OGD. This might be combined with pH-impedence recording. In oesophageal carcinoma, when preliminary investigations suggest that a resection is possible, laparoscopy as a staging procedure is undertaken to exclude small peritoneal secondaries. Motility disorders always warrant manometry for confirmation. In high-grade dysplasia bordering on very early malignancy, a diagnosis can be achieved by Raman spectroscopy, which can detect early mucosal changes.

Barium meal is not a good investigation for patients presenting with heartburn (see previously). It is an obsolete investigation for this symptom.

→ Treatment of oesophageal conditions

6. B, D, E
The operation for resection for carcinoma of middle one-third of oesophagus is called an Ivor-Lewis procedure. Heller's operation is done for achalasia of the cardia. All patients with oesophageal perforation do not require surgical repair. A contrast-enhanced CT scan will show the extent of the perforation. This should help to decide whether the patient needs an operation. Besides how early the patient is seen is another factor to be taken into consideration prior to surgery. A fair number of these patients will not require surgery. Zenker's diverticulum is ideally treated by minimal access surgery by endoscopic-stapling diverticulotomy and not open surgery.

Botulinum toxin injection into the LOS is a treatment modality used particularly in the elderly with comorbidities. This acts by interfering with the cholinergic neural activity; the procedure might have to be repeated.

Answers to extended matching questions

1. E Achalasia of cardia
Patients with achalasia of cardia (cardiospasm) complain of long-standing dysphagia, particularly for liquids while solids tend to go down better. This is associated with repeated chest infections from regurgitation of food into the tracheo-bronchial tree; halitosis is often present. On examination the only physical findings are evidence of weight loss and chest infection.

A barium swallow is the investigation of choice to be followed by OGD. The contrast study shows a massively dilated oesophagus with food residue and smooth narrowing of the lower end, typically described as a 'bird beak' appearance **(Figure 62.1)**. On OGD, the endoscopist has a feeling of 'entering a cave' with a large amount of stale food **(Figure 62.2)**. The gastro-oesophageal opening is eccentric in position. Biopsies are taken, the entire procedure being carried out with extra caution because of the risk of perforation.

Depending upon the severity of the condition, at initial OGD, balloon dilatation may be tried. In the elderly, injection of botulinum toxin (see previously) is worthwhile although the procedure might have to be repeated. The definitive surgical procedure is Heller's cardiomyotomy where a longitudinal incision is made on the muscle of the lower oesophagus and cardia. Intraoperative OGD is carried out to ensure the efficacy of the myotomy. Because of the complication of gastro-oesophageal reflux, most surgeons add some form of anti-reflux procedure. The operation is carried out laparoscopically, the open transthoracic or transabdominal approaches now being almost obsolete.

2. D Carcinoma of oesophagus
Patients, normally heavy smokers, complain of increasing dysphagia of short duration with chest symptoms and weight loss. A barium swallow shows an irregular stricture with typical shouldering **(Figure 62.3)**. OGD confirms the diagnosis **(Figure 62.4)**. Prior to taking biopsy, endoluminal ultrasound (EUS) is carried out which gives an accurate idea of the local extent and mediastinal lymph nodal metastasis. Biopsy would show a squamous carcinoma. CT scan is done to assess loco-regional staging. If after these investigations, resection is regarded as a possibility, laparoscopy with laparoscopic ultrasound (US) is carried out.

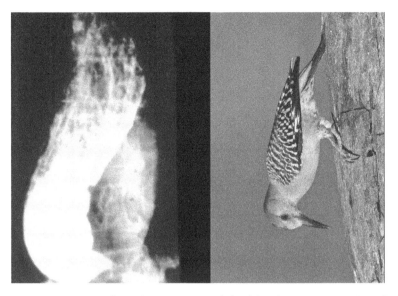

Figure 62.1   Barium swallow showing typical 'bird beak' appearance in achalasia with a large amount of food residue inside the oesophagus.

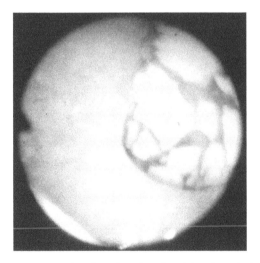

Figure 62.2   OGD showing food residue in achalasia.

If resection is considered, possible only in a minority, the procedure is Ivor-Lewis operation. In this the first stage is a midline laparotomy to mobilise the stomach and lower oesophagus, preserving the right gastric and gastro-epiploic vessels and performing a pyloroplasty. After closing the abdomen, a right posterolateral thoracotomy is carried out to mobilise and resect the oesophagus with part of the fundus. Gastro-oesophageal anastomosis is carried out just below the aortic arch.

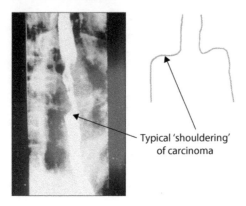

Typical 'shouldering'
of carcinoma

Figure 62.3 Barium swallow showing irregular stricture with shouldering typical of carcinoma.

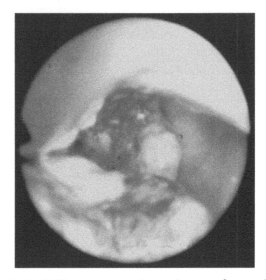

Figure 62.4 OGD appearance in carcinoma of oesophagus.

Sometimes it might be possible to give the patient adjuvant chemotherapy or radiotherapy to downstage the tumour and then proceed to the operation.

The vast majority of patients are seen too late to be suitable for surgical resection. Radiotherapy and chemotherapy with the insertion of a self-expanding metallic stent are the methods of palliation. This might be supplemented by laser ablation, a procedure that might have to be repeated.

3. C Diffuse oesophageal spasm

The usual sufferer is a middle-aged patient who complains of intense odynophagia of short duration. After excluding cardiac causes of the pain, the diagnosis might be confirmed by a barium swallow when the appearance is likened to a 'corkscrew' **(Figure 62.5)**. OGD might show the increased peristalsis **(Figure 62.6)**. Manometric pressures might be as high as 400–500 mmHg, the abnormal contractions being more common in the lower two-thirds. When pressures are persistently more than 180 mmHg in the presence of chest pain, the condition is referred to as nutcracker oesophagus.

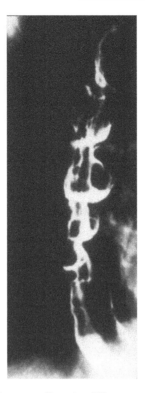

Figure 62.5 Barium swallow in diffuse oesophageal spasm showing a 'corkscrew' oesophagus.

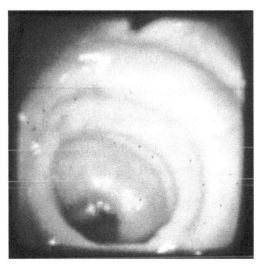

Figure 62.6 OGD appearance in diffuse oesophageal spasm showing hyperperistalsis.

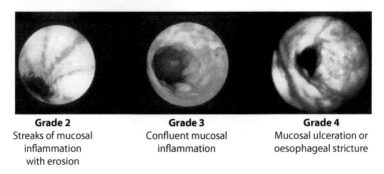

Grade 2	Grade 3	Grade 4
Streaks of mucosal inflammation with erosion	Confluent mucosal inflammation	Mucosal ulceration or oesophageal stricture

Figure 62.7   OGD appearance in oesophagitis in GORD.

Once a cardiac cause has been excluded, reassurance helps. Calcium channel blockers, vasodilators and endoscopic dilatation have only temporary benefit. If symptoms are bad enough to cause malnutrition, surgery in the form of long myotomy up to the aortic arch might be tried. However, this procedure is more effective in alleviating dysphagia than chest pain. Therefore, it is better not carried out if chest pain happens to be the predominant symptom.

4. F Gastro-oesophageal reflux disease
The usual triad is heartburn, epigastric pain radiating to the back and regurgitation, the latter resulting in chest infections. OGD should be the initial investigation. This will show if there is shortening of the oesophagus indicating a sliding hiatus hernia, the type and content of reflux, competence of the LOS and degree of oesophagitis, which is graded **(Figure 62.7)**. Biopsies are taken to assess the inflammation, exclude *H. pylori* and look for dysplasia.

It is essential to exclude Barrett's oesophagus where the squamo-columnar junction is seen proximally. Biopsy might show metaplasia into specialised columnar epithelium, which has a propensity for adenocarcinoma. Presence of intestinal metaplasia is a sinister finding. Therefore these patients must be kept under strict endoscopic surveillance to detect increasing degree of dysplasia. During OGD, Raman spectroscopy can be carried out to detect very early carcinoma in situ, which may be suitable for endoscopic mucosal resection (EMR).

The vast majority of patients are treated by the following conservative measures: lifestyle changes, medical treatment with proton pump inhibitors (PPI), *H. pylori* eradication and H2-receptor antagonist. When medical treatment is unsuccessful, the anti-reflux procedure of fundoplication is carried out by the laparoscopic route. In this operation an adequate length of intra-abdominal oesophagus (5 cm) is created and the mobilised gastric fundus is placed behind the intra-abdominal oesophagus and sutured to itself partially or completely. The diaphragmatic hiatus is narrowed behind the oesophagus.

5. A Pharyngeal (Zenker's) diverticulum
This is pulsion diverticulum that occurs through the two parts of the inferior constrictor muscle, the thyropharyngeus and circopharyngeus. It occurs because the cricopharyngeus muscle fails to relax during the pharyngeal phase of deglutition. When it reaches a significant size it presents with repeated attacks of chest infection due to spillage of food contents into the tracheobronchial tree. Rarely a large diverticulum might be felt as a soft lump on the left

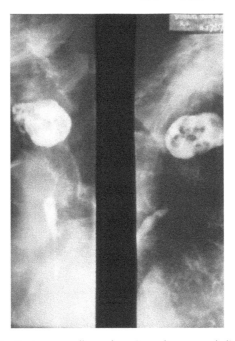

Figure 62.8   Barium swallow showing pharyngeal diverticulum.

side of the neck. The diagnosis is made on barium swallow when a pouch is seen in the lower neck and upper chest **(Figure 62.8)**.

A small asymptomatic diverticulum found incidentally is left alone. When it produces symptoms it should be excised. This is best carried out by the head and neck surgeon by minimal access surgery. The open procedure of excision through an incision on the left side of the neck has now been superseded by Dholman's endoscopic stapling diverticulotomy and cricopharyngeal myotomy. Prior to excision, the pouch is emptied and inspected to make sure that there is no suspicion of a squamous carcinoma (a rare complication) in which case open excision should be carried out.

6. B Rolling hiatus hernia

Also called paraoesophageal hernia, this is rare. Most of the rolling hernias are mixed where the cardio-oesophageal junction is displaced into the chest along with the greater curve of the stomach. As the stomach rolls up into the chest, it rotates, forming a volvulus, a potentially dangerous problem. Colon and small bowel might be in the hernial sac. Dysphagia and chest pain relieved by belching is a typical symptom. Rarely the hernia might present as an emergency with strangulation, gangrene and perforation.

A chest x-ray might show a gas bubble and fluid level behind the heart. A barium meal **(Figure 62.9)** is the method to diagnose the condition, as OGD may be confusing. If a patient

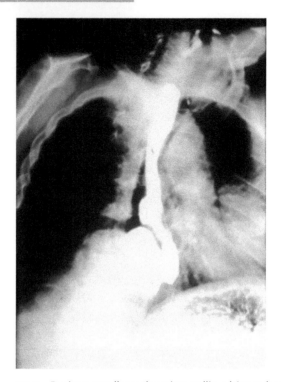

Figure 62.9   Barium swallow showing rolling hiatus hernia.

presents as an emergency and is not in extremis, nasogastric decompression of the stomach followed by elective surgery is carried out. The operation consists of reduction of the hernia, excision of the sac and narrowing the diaphragmatic crus followed by fundoplication, the latter being an effective method to retain the stomach in the abdomen and at the same time preventing gastro-oesophageal reflux.

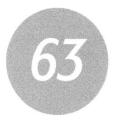

Stomach and duodenum

BV Praveen and Pradip K Datta

Multiple choice questions

→ ## Gross anatomy of the stomach and duodenum

1. Which of the following statements are true regarding blood supply?

A The stomach has an arterial supply on both lesser and greater curves.

B The right gastric artery arises from the common hepatic artery.

C The gastroduodenal artery passes behind the second part of duodenum.

D The short gastric arteries are branches of the left gastric artery.

E The right gastroepiploic artery runs along the greater curvature of the stomach.

2. Which of the following statements are true regarding the nerve supply?

A The intrinsic nerves exist principally in two plexuses, the myenteric plexus of Auerbach and the submucosal plexus of Meissner.

B There are fewer ganglia in the sub-mucosal plexus of the antrum of the stomach.

C The extrinsic supply is mainly derived from the vagus nerves.

D The vagal fibres are only efferent.

E The sympathetic fibres are derived from the thoracic ganglia.

→ ## Microscopic anatomy of the stomach and duodenum

3. The following statements are true except:

A The parietal cells are in the body of the stomach.

B The chief cells produce pepsinogen.

C The endocrine cells are in the antrum and produce gastrin.

D The endocrine cells in the duodenum produce secretin and cholecystokinin.

E Histologically the chief cells are found at the mucosal surface.

→ ## Physiology of the stomach and duodenum

4. Which of the following statements are true regarding gastric acid secretion?

A Hydrogen ions are produced in the parietal cells by the proton pump.

B The most important factor acting on the chief cell is histamine.

C Vagus nerve is responsible for the gastric phase of acid secretion.

D Secretin stimulates acid secretion.

E Somatostatin inhibits acid secretion.

5. Which of the following are functions of the stomach?

A Reservoir for ingested food.

B Mechanically breaks down ingested food.

C Starts the process of digestion.

D Produces mucus.

E Proximal stomach exhibits peristaltic activity.

→ ## Investigations of the stomach and duodenum

6. Which of the following statements are true?

A Flexible endoscopy is the primary investigation of choice.

B Endoscopic ultrasound is useful in determining the 'T' status of tumours.

C CT scan is useful in the staging of gastric cancer.

D PET/CT scan can help avoid radical surgery in approximately 10% of patients with gastric cancer.

E Laparoscopy is helpful in evaluating posterior extension of tumours.

→ Type A and B gastritis

7. The following statements are true except:

A Type A gastritis is an autoimmune condition.

B Type A gastritis produces hypochlorhydria and achlorhydria.

C Type B gastritis is associated with *Helicobacter pylori.*

D Type B gastritis most often affects the body and fundus of the stomach.

E Both type A and B gastritis predispose to gastric cancer.

→ Erosive gastritis

8. Which of the following statements are true?

A It is caused by increased production of acid.

B It is associated with the inhibition of COX-1 receptor enzyme.

C The production of cytoprotective prostaglandins is reduced in this condition.

D Long-term use of selective COX-2 inhibitors may cause cardio-vascular side effects.

E The beneficial anti-inflammatory effects of NSAIDS are mediated via COX-2 receptors.

→ Menetrier's disease

9. The following statements are true except:

A Menetrier's disease is characterised by gross hypertrophy of the gastric mucosal folds.

B Hyperchlorhydria is an associated finding of Menetrier's disease.

C Menetrier's disease is caused by the reduced expression of transforming growth factor alpha (TGF-α).

D Menetrier's disease might present with hypoproteinaemia and anaemia.

E The treatment for Menetrier's disease is gastrectomy.

→ Stress gastritis

10. Which of the following statements are true?

A Usually it occurs in patients who are in the intensive care unit (ICU).

B It is due to avascularity of the gastric mucosa.

C The usual presentation is perforation of an ulcer.

D Prevention is the keystone in management.

E *H. pylori* has no role in its aetiology.

Extended matching questions

→ Diagnoses

The following conditions are discussed. You are expected to match the diagnosis with the clinical features.

1 Benign gastric ulcer
2 Carcinoma of stomach
3 Gastric lymphoma
4 Gastric outlet obstruction
5 Gastritis
6 Leiomyoma of stomach
7 Perforated duodenal ulcer
8 Periampullary carcinoma

Match the previously listed diagnoses with the clinical scenarios of the various conditions that follow.

Clinical features

A   A 48-year-old man, a heavy smoker, has been admitted with sudden onset of very severe pain in the epigastrium radiating to the back and right shoulder tip of 3 hours duration. His pulse is 88 beats per minute and his blood pressure (BP) is 120/70 mmHg; his abdomen has board-like rigidity and does not move with respiration, which is mainly thoracic.

B   A 55-year old man complains of epigastric pain for 6 months, the pain not related to food. His appetite has been poor and he has lost 10 kg of weight during this period. There was nothing to find in his abdomen except for evidence of weight loss. An OGD showed diffuse mucosal thickening of the entire pylorus with some ulceration. Histology showed lymphoid hyerplasia with lymphoid cells expanding the lamina propria.

C   An 80-year-old woman presents with severe itching and her relatives noticed that she was becoming yellow over the last couple of months. Recently she has had vomiting, the vomitus not being bile stained. On examination she has lost a considerable amount of weight and has scratch marks all over her body and a smooth globular mass in the right upper quadrant of her abdomen.

D   A 69-year-old man presents with acute haematemesis. He has been well until his presentation, except that recently he has had a feeling of early satiety after small amounts of food. An urgent OGD showed a large submucosal mass with an ulcerated area, which was the site of bleeding.

E   A 52-year-old woman complains of epigastric pain on and off for 3 years for which she took medicines from across the counter. Almost 6 months ago she underwent a repeat OGD and biopsy that showed *H. pylori* infection in a gastric ulcer for which she was treated. She was well after that, but recently the pain has returned. Her haemoglobin is 11.9. Repeat OGD shows a 2-cm diameter punched- out ulcer on the lesser curve with overhanging edges.

F   A 65-year-old man complains of anorexia and weight loss for 3 months. He has intermittent vomiting associated with malaise. On examination he looks anaemic and has a firm mobile mass in the epigastrium and right hypochondrium.

G   A 35-year-old man, a bus driver, complains of epigastric pain radiating to the back on and off for several months. He has some backache, for which he took some NSAIDs, and occasionally consumes alcohol. Following a bout of drinking, he vomited and the vomitus was streaked with blood.

H   A 60-year-old man complains of incessant vomiting for 2 weeks. The vomitus contains stale food ingested a few days ago. There is no abdominal pain, although many years ago he suffered from prolonged 'indigestion' for which he took antacids from across the counter on and off for years. On examination he has sunken eyes, dry tongue and loss of skin turgor, and his epigastrium looks full. While being examined he had an attack of carpo-pedal spasm.

Answers to multiple choice questions

1. A, B, E

The stomach has a very rich blood supply with vascular arcades along the greater and lesser curves. The left gastric artery is a short stout vessel arising from the coeliac axis and anastomoses with the right gastric artery, a branch of the common hepatic artery, along the lesser curvature. The branches of the left gastric artery also pass toward the cardia. The gastroduodenal artery, which is a branch of the hepatic artery, passes behind the first part of the duodenum; a penetrating duodenal ulcer will erode into the gastroduodenal artery, causing torrential haemorrhage. Here it divides into the superior pancreaticoduodenal artery and the right gastroepiploic artery.

The superior pancreaticoduodenal artery anastomoses within the C-loop of the duodenum with the inferior pancreaticoduodenal artery, which arises from the superior mesenteric artery (anastomosis between the arteries of the foregut and the midgut). The right gastroepiploic artery runs along the greater curvature of the stomach anastomosing with the left gastroepiploic artery, a branch of the splenic artery. The short gastric arteries (vasa brevia) are branches of the splenic artery and supply the fundus of the stomach. The right gastric and the right gastroepiploic arteries form the vascular pedicle, which feeds the stomach tube that is formed during the abdominal procedure of an Ivor-Lewis oesophagectomy for cancer.

2. A, C
The stomach and duodenum possess both intrinsic and extrinsic nerve supplies. The intrinsic nerves are contributed by two plexuses – the myenteric plexus of Auerbach and submucosal plexus of Meissner. The extrinsic supply is derived from the 10th cranial nerve, vagus nerve, the larger of which is the right which lies on the posterior surface of the oesophagus and the left plastered on the anterior surface.

In the antrum, the ganglia of the myenteric plexus are well developed; they are fewer in the fundal area. Vagal fibres are both afferent (sensory) and efferent (motor). The efferent fibres are involved in the receptive relaxation of the stomach, stimulation of gastric motility and secretory function. It was to abolish the secretory function that was utilised in the procedure of vagotomy for the surgical treatment of duodenal ulcer in days gone by. The sympathetic supply is derived mainly from the coeliac ganglia.

Microscopic anatomy of the stomach and duodenum
3. E
In a gastric gland, histologically, the parietal and chief cells are found in the gastric crypts. The basophilic chief cells are in the deepest layer. The mucus-secreting cells are at the mucosal surface, and the eosinophilic parietal cells lie superficially in the glands. The parietal cells are in the body of the stomach (acid-secreting portion). They produce the hydrogen ions actively secreted by the proton pump to form hydrochloric acid.

The chief cells lie proximally in the gastric crypts to produce pepsinogen I and pepsinogen II, the former produced only in the stomach. Pepsinogen is activated in the stomach to produce pepsin. The stomach has endocrine cells. In the antrum there are G cells that produce gastrin. All over the body of the stomach there are enterochromaffin-like cells, which produce histamine, the driving factor in gastric acid secretion. There are also somatostatin-producing D cells throughout the stomach, the hormone somatostatin having a negative regulatory role. The duodenal endocrine cells produce secretin and cholecystokinin, the latter regulating the contraction of the gall bladder.

Physiology of the stomach and duodenum
4. A, B, E
Hydrogen ions are produced in the parietal cell by the proton pump. Although numerous factors can act on the parietal cell, the most important of these is histamine, which acts via the H2-receptor. Enterochromaffin-like (ECL) cell produces histamine in response to a number of stimuli that include the vagus nerve and gastrin. Gastrin is released by the G cells in response to the presence of food in the stomach.

There are three phases of gastric secretion. The cephalic phase is mediated by vagal activity, secondary to sensory arousal. The gastric phase is a response to food within the stomach, which is mediated principally by gastrin and not influenced by the vagus. In the intestinal phase, the presence of chyme in the duodenum and small bowel inhibits gastric emptying, and the acidification of the duodenum leads to the production of secretin, which inhibits gastric acid secretion. Somatostatin is released by D cells in response to a number of factors including acidification. This peptide acts on the G cell, ECL cell and parietal cell itself to inhibit the production of acid.

5. A, B, C, D

The stomach acts as a reservoir for ingested food that is mechanically broken down with the actions of acid and pepsin, thus converting into chyme and starting the process of digestion. The acid chyme on entering the duodenum is neutralised by the alkaline environment caused by the bicarbonate from the pancreas and duodenum. Mucus is produced by the mucus-producing cells of the stomach and the pyloric glands. This produces a viscid layer of mucopolysaccharides, which is an important physiological barrier preventing the gastric mucosa from mechanical damage and the effects of acid and pepsin; bicarbonate ions in the mucus also help as a buffer.

Following a meal proximal stomach exhibits relaxation, thus acting as a reservoir. Most of the gastric peristaltic activity is found in the distal stomach, which is referred to as the 'antral mill'. The antral contraction against the closed pyloric sphincter helps in the milling activity of the stomach.

Investigations of the stomach and duodenum

6. A, B, C, D

Flexible endoscopy (oesophagogastroduodenoscopy, OGD) is the best first-line investigation in suspected upper gastrointestinal (stomach and duodenum) pathology. It is generally a safe investigation; however, those undertaking these procedures should be adequately trained and resuscitation facilities always available. The dose of the sedation should be decided upon according to the age and comorbidities of the patient, being increased in small amounts under careful monitoring. Complications might occur from the sedation such as bradycardia, cardiac arrest, respiratory arrest and allergic reactions whilst perforation is a complication of the procedure.

Endoscopic ultrasound is the most sensitive technique in the evaluation of the 'T' stage of gastric cancer, this being assessed with 90% accuracy. Identification of enlarged lymph nodes is possible with 80% accuracy. As a staging process in gastric cancer, axial multislice imaging on CT scan is useful in detecting gastric wall thickening as in linitis plastica **(Figure 63.1)**. Positron emission tomography (PET) is a form of functional imaging that depends on the uptake of a tracer by metabolically active tumour tissue. When combined with CT (CT/PET), one obtains functional and anatomical information and demonstrates occult metastases

Gross diffuse thickening of entire stomach wall

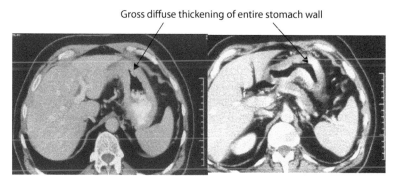

Figure 63.1   CT scan of stomach showing gross thickening of stomach wall and contracted stomach – typical of linitis plastica.

thus preventing unnecessary major surgical resection; it is estimated that in 10% of gastro-oesophageal cancers CT/PET would help to avoid a futile major resection.

Laparoscopy, much as it is a very useful staging procedure, does not help in delineating posterior extension of the tumour. It is useful in detecting peritoneal secondaries and when combined with US detects lymph nodal and hepatic metastases.

Type A and B gastritis

7. D

Type B gastritis mainly affects the antrum; hence these patients are mostly affected by peptic ulcer. Sometimes there is pangastritis. Type B gastritis is associated with *Helicobacter pylori* infection and hence is the cause of peptic ulcer disease. Type A gastritis is an autoimmune disease caused by antibodies against the parietal cell. This causes atrophy of the parietal cell mass resulting in hypochlorhydria going on to achlorhydria. As parietal cells also produce intrinsic factor, this is also depleted causing malabsorption of vitamin B12, which, if not treated, will cause pernicious anaemia, the precursor of gastric cancer.

Type B gastritis, which can produce pangastritis, results in intestinal metaplasia; when this is associated with dysplasia, there is a high chance of the development of cancer. Therefore, cancer stomach might be the outcome of type A and type B gastritis although the mechanism is different in the two types. Under the circumstances, regular OGD surveillance is appropriate for patients with both types of gastritis.

Erosive gastritis

8. B, C, D, E

Erosive gastritis is caused by agents such as NSAIDs and alcohol, which disturb the gastric mucosal barrier. The NSAID-induced gastric lesion is associated with inhibition of the cyclo-oxygenase type 1 (COX-1) receptor enzyme, thus reducing the production of gastric cytoprotective prostaglandins. The beneficial anti-inflammatory activities of NSAIDs are mediated by COX-2, and the use of specific COX-2 inhibitors reduces the incidence of these side effects. However, cardiovascular complications can occur if this is used in the long term.

Menetrier's disease

9. B, C

Hypochlorhydria is the typical feature. The disease is a result of the overexpression of the transforming growth factor alpha (TGF-α). It presents with hypoproteinaemia and anaemia. On OGD there is gross hypertrophy of the gastric mucosal folds. The condition is premalignant and hence gastrectomy is recommended.

Stress gastritis

10. A, B, D, E

This typically occurs in seriously ill patients who are being treated in the intensive care unit or recovering from major surgery, trauma, illness, or burns. Much as the stomach is an extremely vascular organ, it is most sensitive to ischaemia as a result of hypovolaemia as shown by gastrointestinal tonometry. This measures intramucosal pH and PCO_2 as an indicator of mucosal ischaemia and hence ICU mortality and morbidity. Ischaemia causes breakdown in the gastric mucosal barrier, resulting in gastritis going on to ulceration. *H. pylori* has no role in the aetiology. The classical presentation is sudden, severe haemorrhage.

It is much easier to prevent than treat this condition. Hence the routine use of prophylaxis in these patients with H_2-antagonists and barrier agents such as sucralfate given orally or by the nasogastric route. Effective prevention has reduced the incidence.

Answers to extended matching questions

1. E Benign gastric ulcer

Chronic gastric ulcer, more common in the developing world and in the lower socioeconomic groups, presents with abdominal pain coming on within a few minutes of eating. *H. pylori* and long-term use of NSAIDs are the causative factors. Ulcers on the lesser curvature are associated with chronic gastritis, whilst those on the greater curve are the result of ingestion of NSAIDs. OGD and biopsy is essential to exclude carcinoma.

The complications are perforation, bleeding and gastric outlet obstruction. Rarely a benign gastric ulcer turns malignant; probably less than 1% of gastric cancers originate in a benign gastric ulcer. When perforation occurs anteriorly into the peritoneal cavity, the patient presents with features of generalised peritonitis. Sometimes the perforation might occur posteriorly into the lesser sac. In such a case, the peritonitis is contained with a resultant perigastric abscess. Perforation requires resuscitation followed by operation – biopsy and closure of the perforation.

Bleeding might occur slowly when the patient presents with anaemia and faecal occult blood (FOB) is positive. Acute haematemesis and melaena is the emergency presentation of a bleed. This happens when the ulcer penetrates into the anastomosis between the left and right gastric arteries along the lesser curve or when the ulcer is in the middle of the body on the posterior wall and penetrates into the splenic artery causing torrential haemorrhage and hypovolaemic shock. The management of acute upper gastrointestinal haemorrhage is summarised in **Figures 63.2** and **63.3**. A chronic prepyloric gastric ulcer might cicatrise, resulting in pyloric stenosis causing gastric outlet obstruction. This will produce vomiting resulting in acid-base disturbances (for details see the following in 4H).

The treatment in general is medical consisting of modification of lifestyle, eradication of *H. pylori* and proton pump inhibitors. If in the rare instance healing does not occur or relapse occurs, partial gastrectomy should be done **(Figure 63.4)**. The same procedure might rarely have to be carried out when severe haemorrhage cannot be controlled by minimal access surgical means **(Figure 63.5)**.

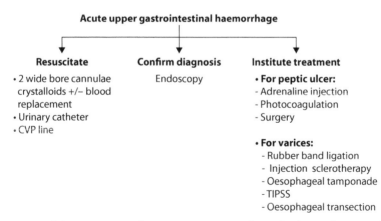

Figure 63.2   Management of acute upper gastrointestinal tract haemorrhage.

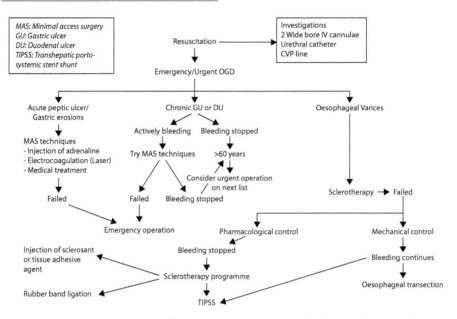

Figure 63.3 Management of acute upper gastrointestinal tract haemorrhage.

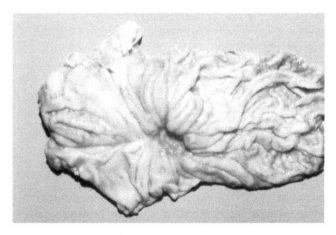

Figure 63.4 Partial gastrectomy in benign gastric ulcer.

2. F Carcinoma of stomach

Traditionally gastric cancer has been described as presenting with the three A's – anaemia, asthenia and anorexia. It is said that any male over the age of 45 years who complains of anorexia for no known reason of more than 4 weeks duration should undergo an OGD to exclude cancer. This is to prevent late diagnosis as usually by the time diagnosis is made, the disease is advanced and hence has a poor outlook.

Patients complain of early satiety, bloating, abdominal distension, vomiting from gastric outlet obstruction and malaise from iron deficiency anaemia. A palpable mass usually denotes a late stage of the disease. The proximal stomach is the most

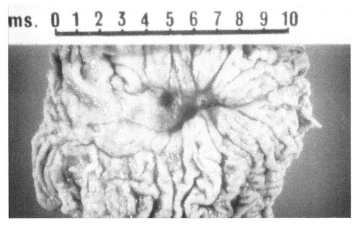

Figure 63.5 Partial gastrectomy for bleeding benign gastric ulcer.

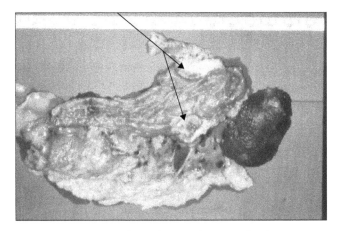

Figure 63.6 Ulcerative carcinoma of pylorus.

common site of gastric cancer in the West. As many adenocarcinomas arise in the lower oesophagus, it is estimated that 60% of cancers in this region occur in the oesophagogastric junction.

Once suspected, the diagnosis is confirmed by OGD and biopsy. Histologically, the following two broad types are recognised: intestinal gastric cancer and diffuse gastric cancer. In the former it takes the form of an ulcerative **(Figure 63.6)** or polypoid lesion, which carries a better prognosis than the diffuse variety that infiltrates into the entire stomach wall often called a linitis plastica **(Figure 63.7)**, which has a dismal prognosis. Thereafter, accurate staging is carried out by CT scan, CT/PET and US. If curative resection is on the cards, then laparoscopy +/- US is the final staging procedure before discussion in MDT prior to surgery.

Gastric cancer spreads directly, by lymphatics, bloodstream and by the transcoelomic route. The staging is by the TNM staging of UICC. Distant spread usually does not occur in the absence of lymphatic secondaries. After staging, if curative operation is envisaged,

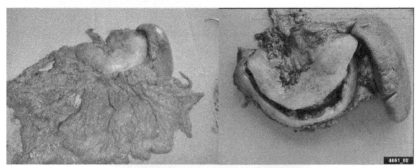

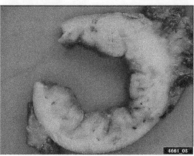

Figure 63.7 Linitis plastic (same patient as in Figure 63.1). (Courtesy of Mr Appou Tajimarane, Consultant Surgeon and Dr James McPhie, Consultant Pathologist, Raigmore Hospital, Inverness.)

neoadjuvant chemotherapy is given prior to surgery. Surgery can be in the form of total or subtotal radical gastrectomy depending upon the exact site of the cancer. The most common type of operation is D2 type of gastrectomy, which involves clearing lymph nodes at the major arterial trunks. For growths that cannot be cured, if resectable, palliative partial gastrectomy should be considered. Further details of operation for gastric cancer are beyond the scope of this book.

3. B Gastric lymphoma

Gastric lymphoma can occur as a separate entity or might be a part of generalised lymphoma. The stomach is the most common site, accounting for 20% of extranodal non-Hodgkin's lymphomas. The tumour arises from *M*ucosa-*A*ssociated *L*ymphoid *T*issue, hence the acronym MALToma. These are low-grade β-cell tumours that arise in untreated *H. pylori* gastritis with lymphoid hyperplasia. These tumours account for 5% of all gastric malignancies. Involvement of lymph nodes is late.

On OGD the findings are very similar to those in linitis plastica – small, contracted, non-distensible stomach with diffuse mucosal thickening and loss of detail within the gastric mucosa, which is infiltrated by the lymphomatous process over a large area. Biopsy confirms the diagnosis.

The management initially requires thorough staging to make sure that the tumour is a primary gastric lymphoma and not a part of a generalised lymphomatous process. This is done by full haematological investigations, CT scan of the chest and abdomen and bone marrow biopsy.

The treatment in localised disease is gastrectomy. The use of postoperative chemotherapy is contentious; some oncologists believe that the condition can be treated by chemotherapy alone. In very early cases when *H. pylori* is isolated, eradication of the organism has been known to cause regression of the tumour.

4. H Gastric outlet obstruction (GOO)

Gastric outlet obstruction in the adult is from long-standing duodenal ulcer or a carcinoma of the pylorus. A rare condition called adult hypertrophic pyloric stenosis also causes GOO. It might occur in a 4-week old infant, usually a male, from congenital hypertrophic pyloric stenosis.

The history in this patient indicates the cause to be a long-standing healed duodenal ulcer, which has produced cicatrisation with scarring and complete stenosis of the duodenum. Clinical presentation is prolonged vomiting with loss of H^+, K^+ and Cl^- with increase in HCO_3^- resulting in hypcholraemic, hypokalaemic metabolic alkalosis. Fluid loss causes extreme dehydration seen clinically as sunken eyes, dry tongue and loss of skin turgor. As a result of dehydration the patient will also have haemoconcentration causing high haemoglobin. Clinically abdominal examination might show visible gastric peristalsis and succussion splash. In extreme cases of alkalosis, the patient might develop tetany because of reduction in ionised Ca^{++}.

The management consists of resuscitation, confirmation of the diagnosis and definitive treatment. Resuscitation should consist of haematological and biochemical blood investigations, intravenous normal saline with added potassium chloride, indwelling catheter and CVP line; a large bore stomach tube is inserted to wash out the stomach to empty semi-solid stale food material – several wash-outs might be necessary. The diagnosis is confirmed by OGD; during OGD an attempt might be made at balloon dilatation of the stenosis as a form of treatment, which might only have a temporary effect. The definitive operation is gastrojejunostomy – posterior, retro-colic, iso-peristaltic, short loop. Some surgeons might consider adding a truncal vagotomy to prevent a future anastomotic ulcer. When the GOO is from a pyloric cancer, the management should be on the lines described previously as for cancer of stomach.

5. G Gastritis

For summary, please see **Figure 63.8**. **Type A autoimmune gastritis** is an atrophic gastritis related to pernicious anaemia. It is diffuse, occurs in the body and fundus and might develop dysplasia followed by carcinoma. Regular endoscopic screening is advocated. **Type B gastritis** results from *H. pylori* infection usually involving the antrum. This causes intestinal metaplasia going on to produce pangastritis, which might result in cancer. Eradication of *H. pylori* infection is essential. **Reflux gastritis** occurs after gastric surgery where there is a gastro-jejunal anastomosis; this results from bile reflux. Symptomatic treatment is the mainstay; very rarely in intractable cases revisional surgery in the form of a Roux-en-Y procedure is undertaken. It might rarely occur without previous gastric surgery. **Erosive gastritis** is caused by alcohol and NSAIDs, which disturb the gastric mucosal barrier causing

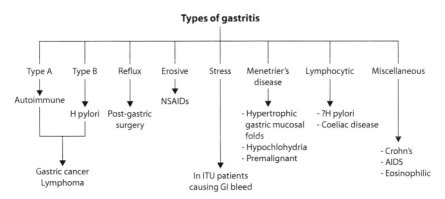

Figure 63.8   Types of gastritis.

minimal inflammation. Prevention by excluding the causative agent is the treatment. **Stress gastritis** occurs in patients in the intensive care unit (ICU); they tend to develop ischaemia of the gastric mucosa causing ulceration, which presents as acute haematemesis. This is best prevented by putting all patients in the ICU on routine prophylactic H_2 receptor antagonist. **Menetrier's disease** is a precancerous condition (see previously). **Lymphocytic gastritis**, might be associated with coeliac disease. The gastric mucosa is infiltrated by T cells and may have *H. pylori* infection, which, if present, is eradicated. It is rare. **Miscellaneous types of gastritis** are **granulomatous** due to Crohn's disease, **AIDS-related** due to infection with Cryptosporidium and **eosinophilic,** which might be due to food allergies. Treatment is directed toward the cause.

6. D Leiomyoma of stomach

This is a form of gastrointestinal stromal tumour (GIST). The stomach harbours 50% of such tumours, which are of mesenchymal origin. The cut surface of the tumour is whorled, consisting of spindle-shaped cells embedded in a collagenous stroma. The presence of this tumour is detected when the patient has haematemesis due to ulceration of the tumour through the mucosa. Therefore most often diagnosis is made on OGD. Rarely if a barium meal is carried out, the appearance is very typical – smooth filling defect within the body of the stomach with a speck of barium stuck in the middle where the tumour has ulcerated through **(Figure 63.9)**.

Once the diagnosis is established on OGD, the patient is operated upon urgently on the next operating list, although an emergency procedure might be necessary if the patient re-bleeds while waiting. At operation local resection is the treatment of choice. Depending upon the exact site of the tumour in the stomach, a partial gastrectomy may be necessary.

7. A Perforated duodenal ulcer

These patients present as an emergency with sudden onset of severe upper abdominal pain radiating to the back and rest of the upper abdomen. Soon the patient might complain of pain in the right shoulder tip – pain referred from diaphragmatic irritation. The patient

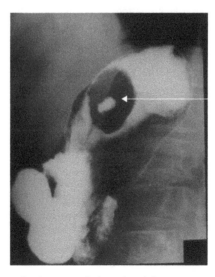

Figure 63.9 Barium meal showing leiomyoma of stomach.

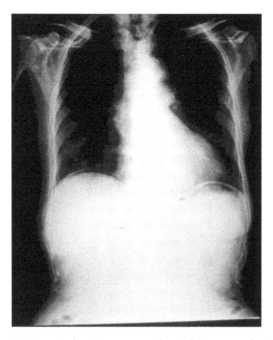

Figure 63.10   CXR erect showing gas under right dome of diaphragm from perforated duodenal ulcer.

likes to lie still with an abdominal wall that does not move with respiration which is mainly thoracic. Abdominal palpation reveals typical 'board-like' rigidity with obliteration of the liver dullness due to subdiaphragmatic air. Confirmation is by CXR showing gas under the right dome of the diaphragm **(Figure 63.10)**, which might not always be present. Should there be any doubt about the diagnosis when there is no gas under the right dome of the diaphragm, a diagnostic laparoscopy is performed. If perforation is confirmed, it is closed laparoscopically if the expertise is available. If not, the procedure described below is carried out.

As a surgical emergency, the patient needs to be resuscitated immediately followed by his definitive treatment. Resuscitation should be in the form of analgesia of 100 mg of pethidine, intravenous access with crystalloids, naso-gastric suction and intravenous antibiotics. After anaesthetic assessment, the patient is taken to theatre.

The abdomen is opened through an upper midline incision. On entering the peritoneal cavity, the sound of free gas is heard. In perforated duodenal ulcer there will be free turbid, odourless, greenish fluid from the right upper quadrant. A perforation will be seen on the anterior wall of the first part of the duodenum. The free fluid is sucked clear. The perforation is isolated; at least three vicryl sutures (depending upon the size) are inserted through the perforation, which is now closed. The sutures are left long with haemostats at the ends. A patch of omentum is then put in between the sutures, covering the closure. The same sutures are now used to tie over the omentum. Thorough peritoneal lavage with warm normal saline is performed. The abdomen is closed.

8. C Periampullary carcinoma

Adenocarcinoma of the duodenum, although rare, arises in the periampullary region. The other conditions that give rise to a similar clinical picture are carcinoma of head of pancreas and carcinoma of lower end of common bile duct (CBD), although the latter does not produce gastric outlet obstruction. However, there is a subtle difference in the presentation of periampullary cancer where the jaundice is not progressive but waxes and wanes. This is because the periampullary carcinoma outgrows its blood supply; as a result the growth obstructing the ampulla sloughs off allowing bile to drain causing the jaundice to lessen. At the same time the size of the distended gall bladder gets smaller only for the whole process to repeat itself as the growth enlarges again. In the presence of jaundice if there is a distended gall bladder, the underlying pathology is a malignancy and not gall stones because the latter would result in a thick and contracted gall bladder (Courvoisier's law).

The initial management is to confirm the diagnosis and stage the disease. Confirmation is done by OGD and biopsy. Staging is next carried out by CT scan and chest x-ray. Should these staging procedures give an indication that a radical resection is possible, a laparoscopy (+/- ultrasound) is then done to exclude any peritoneal secondaries. If the patient is deemed suitable for curative resection by a MDT, then radical resection is carried out. At the time of presentation 70% are deemed to be resectable. A Whipple's pancreatoduodenectomy is the procedure carried out, following which the 5-year survival rate is 20%.

When the condition is unresectable, itching, which is very distressing for the patient, requires palliation. Insertion of a stent into the CBD alleviates itching whilst a stent in the pyloro-duodenal junction would achieve the same for gastric outlet obstruction. If for any reason a stent cannot be inserted into the CBD (such as previous gastric surgery or a duodenal diverticulum), an open procedure has to be done. This would consist of cholecystojejunostomy, jejuno-jenostomy (sometimes not done) and an anterior gastrojejunostomy (triple anastomosis).

64 *Bariatric surgery*

Pawanindra Lal

1. **Which of the following defines morbid obesity?**
   A BMI greater than 32 Kg/m²
   B BMI greater than 35 Kg/m² with cormorbidity
   C BMI greater than 40 Kg/m²
   D BMI greater than 45 Kg/m²
   E BMI greater than 50 Kg/m²

2. **Which of the following constitute the selection criteria for performing bariatric surgery as per international norms?**
   A Minimum of 5 years obesity.
   B Failure of conservative treatment.
   C No alcoholism or major untreated psychiatric illness.
   D Avoid if likely to get pregnant within 1 year.
   E Acceptable operative risk on preoperative assessment.

3. **Preoperative nutritional screening of morbidly obese patients includes which of the following?**
   A Vitamins A, D and E, parathyroid hormone.
   B Glucocorticoids and mineralocorticoids.
   C Magnesium, calcium and phosphate.
   D Ferritin, vitamin B12, folate and coagulation screen.
   E Zinc, selenium, copper and C-reactive protein.

4. **Roux-en-Y gastric bypass is which type of bariatric procedure?**
   A Restrictive
   B Malabsorptive
   C Combined restrictive and malabsorptive
   D Type of bowel transposition
   E Uses band prosthesis

5. **Which of the following are specific complications of bariatric procedures?**
   A Internal herniation in gastric bypass and bilio-pancreatic diversion (BPD).
   B Staple line or anastomotic leak in gastric bypass, sleeve gastrectomy and BPD.
   C Pouch dilatation in gastric band, gastric bypass and sleeve gastrectomy.
   D Erosion in BPD and sleeve gastrectomy.
   E Band slippage in gastric banding.

→ Surgical procedures

1 Bilio-pancreatic diversion (BPD)
2 Gastric banding
3 Ileal transposition
4 Roux-en-Y gastric bypass
5 Sleeve gastrectomy

Choose and match the correct surgical procedures with each of the scenarios that follow:

A A 50-year-old man weighing 105 kg and with a height of 180 cm presents with a history of progressive and poorly controlled diabetes for 15 years. He was shifted from oral hypoglycaemics to insulin but has shown poor compliance to treatment. He is now beginning to have alteration in renal functions and eye changes. Which type of procedure can he benefit from?

B A 30-year-old married woman presents with a weight of 110 kg and a height of 155 cm. She has been a diabetic for the past 10 years and is on anti-hypertensives for the past 5 years with need to escalate the doses of both medications. Which surgical procedure is likely to most benefit her condition?

C A 20-year-old man, a college student, presents with a history of weight gain over the past 5 years. He has a BMI of 40 and is particularly worried about his physique. He has tried dieting and exercise and appears well motivated and wants a safe procedure and agrees for regular follow up. Which bariatric procedure should be recommended for him?

D A 35-year-old woman who underwent a sleeve gastrectomy 3 years ago, presents with regain of weight and relapse of diabetes. She presently has a BMI of 52 and is otherwise fit and healthy. Which procedure is likely to benefit her most with this history?

E A 45-year-old man presents with a BMI of 45. He has been obese for the past 10 years without any medical comorbidity except snoring during sleep for the past 1 year. Which bariatric procedure is best suited for his ailment?

Answers to multiple choice questions

1. B, C

Body mass index (BMI) is calculated by dividing weight in kilograms with square of the height in metres (kg/m^2). Normal weight ranges between 20–25 kg/m^2. Morbid obesity is defined as a body mass index (BMI) equal to or greater than 40 kg/m^2. Values between 25 and 39 kg/m^2 are classified as obesity. A number of serious medical comorbid conditions like hypertension, diabetes, obstructed sleep apnoea and chest complications are seen to develop in patients with obesity and in such patients the criteria for morbid obesity requiring treatment has been lowered to the level of 35 kg/m^2. Obesity is dangerous to health due to the excess incidence of comorbidities that obese patients often develop, especially the metabolic syndrome. Many studies have suggested that if weight loss is induced surgically this leads to improvement in various comorbidities, which translates into increased life expectancy. The rationale for doing bariatric surgery stems from the fact that there is an objective increase in life expectancy and a decrease in comorbidities and thus a decrease in the health care costs to society as a whole.

2. A, B, C, E

Selection criteria for obesity surgery (based on the International Federation for Surgery of Obesity and the National Institute for Clinical Excellence) is body mass index (BMI) >40 kg/m^2 or BMI 35–39 kg/m^2 with serious comorbid disease treatable by weight loss, minimum of 5 years obesity, failure of conservative treatment, no alcoholism or major untreated psychiatric illness, avoid if likely to get pregnant within 2 years, age limits 18–55 (relative) and an acceptable operative risk on preoperative assessment.

3. A, C, D, E

A preoperative baseline metabolic screen is desirable to determine the levels of vitamins, minerals and micronutrients, which are essential for health. It is well recognised that many bariatric patients preoperatively suffer from vitamin and micronutrient deficiencies, usually due to their poor diet. Preoperatively patients are generally put on a low carbohydrate diet for a minimum of 2 weeks to shrink the liver to allow for adequate working space to carry out the surgery and easy retraction of the left lobe of the liver to facilitate dissection around the gastro-oesophageal junction.

4. C

All the bariatric procedures are classified into one of the three types, i.e., restrictive, malabsorptive, or both.

Gastric banding involves putting an adjustable band around the upper stomach leaving a small pouch just below the cardia. The degree of restriction can be controlled by the amount of fluid injected into the subcutaneous port. This operation is especially popular in Australia, where excellent results are obtained. The perception that the band is reversible is important to some patients (although in reality it is a disadvantage). Gastric banding is certainly the least risky procedure (0.1% perioperative mortality) as it does not involve cutting any stomach or bowel and is a relatively easy operation to perform in most patients who have a BMI <50 kg/m². This is purely a restrictive procedure that is also reversible and done in almost 50% of cases worldwide. One disadvantage of the gastric band is the need for continual band adjustments in the early postoperative period and occasional long-term adjustments. It is generally considered a labour-intensive procedure that requires a lot of patient compliance to get good results. Another disadvantage of the gastric band is that when a revisional procedure is indicated it is a much higher-risk procedure due to adhesions and gastric wall thickening. However, gastric banding has a place in properly selected patients who have the correct attitude and understanding of the postoperative requirements. In selected patients a band can even be inserted as a day-case procedure. It should generally be avoided in binge-eating patients and those whose eating habits involve excessive sweets and chocolate **(see Figure 64.1)**.

Sleeve gastrectomy is a type of restrictive procedure, which is relatively new and requires less postoperative monitoring as it does not require any adjustments although it is a riskier procedure than gastric banding (0.2% operative mortality). Technically, the stomach is constructed into a sleeve by excising most of the gastric fundus and body, leaving the antrum. The long staple line can leak despite various manoeuvres to avoid leakage, such as applying reinforcing material or gluing. Another attraction of this procedure is that because it

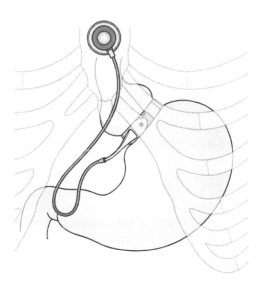

Figure 64.1   Gastric band.

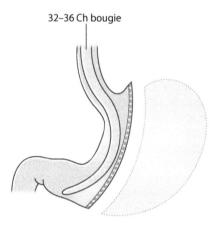

Figure 64.2 Sleeve gastrectomy.

removes most of the grehlin-secreting area of the stomach, it might have a beneficial effect on reducing appetite. The true place for sleeve gastrectomy as a primary bariatric procedure is still unclear and more long-term data are needed. Despite this, the frequency of this procedure is accelerating at a remarkable rate largely because of the relative technical ease of doing the procedure, lack of potential malabsorption problems and option of doing a relatively safe second-stage procedure if needed **(see Figure 64.2)**.

Roux-en-Y gastric bypass is a very effective weight-loss procedure but is performed with myriad technical variations, making comparisons difficult. This is a combination of restrictive and malabsorptive procedure where a small pouch of stomach is created and disconnected from the remaining stomach, and a limb of jejunum is brought to restore the continuity thus bypassing a segment of small bowel. However, overall it produces 65%–75% excess weight loss albeit at a higher risk of around 0.5% perioperative mortality. Gastric bypass is a very effective operation for alleviating and even curing type 2 diabetes – the result being almost immediate and independent of weight loss. There are two major theories as to how this happens, given that other bariatric procedures such as banding and sleeve gastrectomy are dependent on weight loss to resolve the diabetes. Over 80% of patients will have their diabetes permanently resolved. There are many variations in the actual gastric bypass technique, e.g., antecolic versus retrocolic Roux limb placement, varying alimentary and biliary limb lengths, additional banding of the gastrojejunal anastomosis to prevent dilatation, varying methods of doing the gastrojejunal anastomosis and varying methods of closing potential hernia spaces **(see Figure 64.3)**.

Biliopancreatic diversion – with or without a duodenal switch is a procedure that produces the most malabsorption of all operations, is the most effective with 75%–85% excess weight loss but at the expense of the highest perioperative mortality of 1%–2%. Additionally as time goes by, if the patient does not adhere to his or her vitamin and micronutrient supplementation regime he or she is at severe risk of many deficiency syndromes. Furthermore, due to the extreme malabsorption these operations produce there is a need for a high protein intake of around 90 g per day, which many patients find difficult. If this is not achieved, protein calorie malnutrition can be a problem. In correctly selected patients, however, the BPD can be very effective, especially in those patients with a very high BMI **(see Figure 64.4)**.

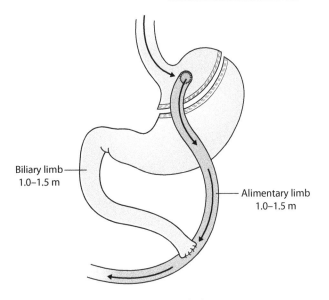

Figure 64.3 Gastric bypass.

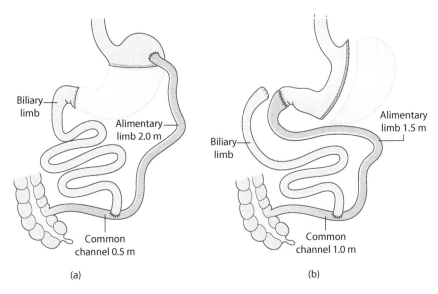

Figure 64.4 (a) Standard biliopancreatic diversion (BPD); (b) BPD with duodenal switch variation.

Ileal transposition is a malabsorptive procedure that is restricted for use in patients with metabolic syndrome such as correction of type 2 diabetes with a BMI between 30 and 34 kg/m². The procedure involves removal of a small segment of the ileum with its vascular and nervous supply and inserting it into the proximal small intestine.

5. A.B.C.E

General risks of bariatric surgery include bleeding, infection, deep vein thrombosis (± pulmonary embolism), accidental bowel perforation and perioperative mortality.

Long-term risks include protein calorie malnutrition and vitamin and micronutrient depletion syndromes. Risks of specific bariatric procedures include internal herniation (gastric bypass and BPD), staple line or anastomotic leak (gastric bypass, sleeve gastrectomy, BPD), band slippage or erosion after gastric banding and pouch dilatation after gastric band, gastric bypass or sleeve gastrectomy.

Answers to extended matching questions

1. D Bilio-pancreatic diversion

Bilio Pancreatic Division (BPD) is a procedure suited for cases of relapse after previous surgery like sleeve gastrectomy where a duodenal switch can be added to the already-done sleeve gastrectomy. The procedure has the highest percentage of resolution of comorbidities like diabetes, hypertension and dyslipidaemias.

2. C Gastric banding

Gastric banding is the safest procedure with lowest intra-operative complication and ideally suited for those requiring a reversible operation. It is best for highly motivated group of patients that are not binge eaters or addicted to sweets and that is compliant for regular band adjustments.

3. A Ileal transposition

Ileal transposition is a type of metabolic surgery being offered in the past few years for treatment of long-standing type 2 diabetics with a BMI of 30–34 kg/m^2. This procedure brings about malnutrition, and studies have shown increased levels of glucagon like peptide-1 in these patients after surgery and is a potent insulinotropic hormone that improves glucose tolerance.

4. B Roux-en-Y gastric bypass

Gastric bypass is ideally suited for patients with a BMI of 45–50 who have long-standing medical comorbidities like diabetes and hypertension. It has been seen that resolution of comorbidities like diabetes, hypertension and dyslipidaemias after this procedure is second only to BPD with a much lower intra-operative mortality.

5. E Sleeve gastrectomy

Sleeve gastrectomy is rapidly becoming one of the most common procedures performed for bariatric surgery in the world largely due to the ease of surgery and comparable results in terms of excess weight loss and resolution of comorbidities. Snoring in obesity is due to obstructed sleep apnoea (OSA) and is one of the earliest conditions to resolve after surgery.

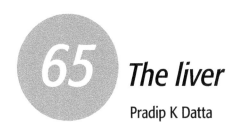

65 The liver

Pradip K Datta

Multiple choice questions

→ ## Liver anatomy

1. Which of the following statements is not true?

A The falciform ligament of the liver divides it into functional right and left units.

B The right and left triangular ligaments help to fix the liver and keep it in its place.

C The main blood supply of the liver is derived from the portal vein.

D The right hepatic vein has an extrahepatic course while the middle and left hepatic veins join the inferior vena cava within the liver.

E The left intrahepatic duct has a longer extrahepatic course than the right.

2. Which of the following statements are true?

A Cantlie's line passes through the gallbladder fossa and middle hepatic vein.

B The functional right and left units divided by Cantlie's line are further subdivided into four segments on each side.

C The free edge of the lesser omentum contains the hepatic artery, bile duct and portal vein.

D The portal vein is formed by the union of the superior and inferior mesenteric veins.

E The structures at the porta hepatis are the portal vein, bile ducts, hepatic artery and hepatic veins.

→ ## Liver function

3. Which of the following liver function tests (LFTs) are abnormal?

A Bilirubin	5–17 μmol/L
B Alkaline phosphatase (ALP)	35–130 IU/L
C Aspartate transaminase (AST)	55–80 IU/L
D Alanine transaminase (ALT)	135–240 IU/L
E Gamma-glutamyl transpeptidase (GGT)	110–148 IU/L

→ ## Liver imaging

4. Which of the following statements are true?

A Ultrasound (US) is the first-line investigation.

B Nuclear medicine scanning gives an idea of the extent of anatomical derangement.

C The 'gold standard' is contrast-enhanced computed tomographic scan (CECT).

D Magnetic resonance imaging (MRI) has advantages over CECT.

E Angiography is best reserved when embolisation is contemplated.

→ ## Acute and chronic liver disease

5. Which of the following statements are not true?

A The overall mortality from acute liver failure is about 50%.

B Chronic congestive heart failure is a terminal event in chronic liver disease.

C The most useful clinical sign is flapping tremor.

D Model for End-Stage Liver Disease (MELD) score depends upon, INR, serum bilirubin and serum creatinine.

E Liver transplantation has good short-term results in acute liver failure.

→ ## Liver trauma

6. Which of the following statements are not true?

A Liver injuries are common.

B Blunt trauma is often associated with splenic, mesenteric and renal injuries.

C Penetrating trauma is often associated with pericardial or chest injuries.

D CECT scan must be carried out in every case of liver trauma.

E Interventional radiology has a role in the management of liver injury.

7. Which of these statements are true?

A Penetrating injuries should be explored.

B Blunt injuries are usually treated conservatively.

C Exploration for a liver injury is best done by a long midline incision.

D Severe crush injury is ideally treated by packing.

E Venovenous bypass should be considered in major liver vascular injury.

→ Portal hypertension

8. The following statements are true except:

A Acute haematemesis from portal hypertension occurs most commonly from gastric varices.

B Initial endoscopic treatment of oesophageal varices with banding, as opposed to injection sclerotherapy, has less chance of oesophageal ulceration.

C Long-term beta-blocker therapy coupled with sclerotherapy regime or endoscopic banding is the mainstay of treatment of portal hypertension.

D In failed drug or endoscopic treatment, the ideal choice is the surgical shunt of portocaval anastomosis.

E Ascites in cirrhosis can be treated by a peritoneovenous shunt.

Extended matching questions

→ Diagnoses

1 Amoebic liver abscess
2 Ascending cholangitis
3 Budd–Chiari syndrome
4 Caroli's disease
5 Focal nodular hyperplasia
6 Haemangioma
7 Hepatic adenoma
8 Hepatocellular carcinoma (HCC)
9 Hydatid liver disease
10 Primary biliary cirrhosis
11 Primary sclerosing cholangitis
12 Pyogenic liver abscess
13 Secondary liver metastasis
14 Simple cystic disease
15 Viral hepatitis

Match the correct diagnosis with each of the scenarios that follow:

A A 30-year-old woman has a history of recurrent attacks of fever with rigors, right upper quadrant pain and jaundice with itching. Biochemistry shows a jaundice of obstructive nature. CT scan shows intrahepatic ductal dilatation with stones.

B A 40-year-old woman presents with recurrent episodes of right upper quadrant pain with jaundice. Biochemistry shows an obstructive pattern of the jaundice. Five years ago she underwent a panproctocolectomy for ulcerative colitis and has been well since, except for these attacks. Endoscopic retrograde cholangiopancreatography (ERCP) shows irregular narrowed intra- and extrahepatic bile ducts.

C   A 50-year-old woman complains of general malaise, lethargy, pruritus and jaundice, the latter being present over the last 3 months. The LFTs show a rise in bilirubin, transaminases and prothrombin time. She has had recurrent small haematemesis and has ascites.

D   A 30-year-old woman complains of abdominal discomfort and distension. She has had three episodes of small haematemesis in the past 6 months. On examination she has hepatomegaly and ascites. All the LFTs are deranged. CT scan of the liver shows a large congested liver.

E   A fit-looking 50-year-old man complains of recent onset of dull aching right upper quadrant pain of 3 to 4 months' duration. Examination shows no abnormality. Liver function tests are normal, as is an upper gastrointestinal endoscopy. An ultrasound of the liver shows a 6 cm solitary cystic lesion.

F   A 25-year-old man complains of generally feeling unwell with fever and weight loss. He has had bloodstained motions on and off for the last 6 weeks after he returned from the Indian subcontinent where he was working for 6 months. On examination he has a tender right upper quadrant with hepatomegaly. US shows a hypoechoic cavity in the right lobe with ill-defined borders.

G   A 50-year-old woman has had recurrent attacks of colicky right upper quadrant and epigastric pain with jaundice, high temperature with rigors and itching. 10 months ago she underwent an uneventful laparoscopic cholecystectomy. On examination she is jaundiced with scratch marks all over her body and hepatomegaly. She has raised serum bilirubin and the ALP is 1100 IU/L. US shows a dilated common bile duct with stones.

H   A 35-year-old man presents with general ill health, weight loss, anorexia and malaise for several weeks. He has developed jaundice for the last 2 weeks; he has no pruritus. Abdominal examination shows a tender hepatomegaly. Liver function tests show raised bilirubin and transaminases.

I   A 75-year-old man, an insulin-dependent diabetic for 40 years, complains of anorexia, fever, malaise and right upper quadrant discomfort. On examination there is weight loss and tender hepatomegaly. US shows a multiloculated cystic mass, a finding confirmed on CT scan.

J   A 50-year-old man, a native of Cyprus, presents with a painful mass in the right upper quadrant. The pain is a continuous dull ache and has the features of a mass arising from the right lobe of the liver. The blood count shows eosinophilia. The CT scan shows a smooth space-occupying lesion with multiple septa within it.

K   A 35-year-old woman who is on the contraceptive pill presents with right upper quadrant aching pain. She is fit without any physical findings. Her LFTs and other blood tests are normal. US of the liver shows a single well-demarcated hyperechoic mass and CT scan demonstrates a well-circumscribed vascular solid tumour.

L   A 40-year-old man presents with dull, persistent upper abdominal pain, weakness, weight loss and occasional fever. He had one episode of haematemesis. Abdominal examination shows an enlarged liver with a mass in the right lobe. Liver function tests show elevation of the transaminases and much-raised alpha-fetoprotein (AFP).

M   A 60-year-old man presents with dragging pain in the right upper quadrant for 3 months and weight loss. On examination he is slightly jaundiced. He has an enlarged liver. Three years ago he underwent a right hemicolectomy for cancer of the caecum. LFTs show elevation of all the parameters. US shows a solid mass in the right lobe, and a CECT confirms the mass with lack of enhancement.

N   In a 30-year-old woman, during laparoscopic cholecystectomy, the surgeon noticed that the under-surface of the liver has several lesions that are blue in colour.

O   A 45-year-old woman underwent an US for suspected biliary pain. The US of the biliary tract was normal but showed a solid lesion in the liver. Therefore, she had a CECT scan that showed a vascular lesion surrounding a solid mass with central scarring.

Answers to multiple choice questions

1. A

The falciform ligament does not divide the liver into functional right and left anatomical units. This is done by Cantlie's line (see the following). The falciform ligament extends from the posterior surface of the anterior abdominal wall and diaphragm on to the anterior and superior surfaces of the liver into the interlobar fissure; it divides the liver anatomically into a large right lobe and much smaller left lobe. The falciform ligament contains the ligamentum teres, which is the obliterated left umbilical vein.

The left triangular ligament is a double layer of peritoneum on the superior border of the left lobe of the liver; dividing this ligament allows the lobe to be mobilised from the diaphragm. The right triangular ligament fixes the larger right lobe of the liver to the right hemidiaphragm. To mobilize the right lobe, the right triangular ligament needs to be divided.

The main blood supply of the liver is derived from the portal vein, which supplies 80%, the remaining 20% being supplied by the hepatic artery. The right hepatic vein can be exposed outside the liver before it enters the inferior vena cava while the middle and left hepatic veins join the inferior vena cava within the liver. The left extrahepatic duct has a longer intrahepatic course. This important anatomic fact is very useful; because of its accessibility, in high common bile duct strictures, a left hepatico-jejunostomy can be carried out.

2. A, B, C

The Scottish anatomist, Sir James Cantlie, in 1897 described a line that divided the liver into two physiological halves indicating the functional midline of the liver. This is 'an extrapolated line from the posthepatic inferior vena cava across the diaphragmatic surface of the liver to the site where the fundus of the gallbladder contacts the inferior margin of the liver'. The French anatomist, Claude Couinaud, in 1957 divided these two halves of the liver into eight segments. Each of these segments are a separate functional unit with a branch of the hepatic artery, portal vein and bile duct and drained by a tributary of the hepatic vein. The physiological and functional right and left halves were thus divided into the following four segments each: segments I–IV in the left half and segments V-VIII in the right half known as the Couinaud's segments **(Figure 65.1)**.

The free edge of the lesser omentum between the stomach and liver is thin and fragile, containing the bile duct on the right, hepatic artery medially and portal vein posterior to both. The portal vein is formed by the union of the superior mesenteric and splenic veins behind

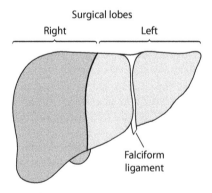

Figure 65.1   The anatomy of liver segments.

the neck of the pancreas. The inferior mesenteric vein empties into the splenic vein. At the porta hepatis the structures are the portal vein, bile ducts and hepatic artery. The hepatic veins (right, middle and left) enter separately into the inferior vena cava (see previously).

3. C, D, E

The liver has many functions chief among which are maintenance of acid-base balance; metabolism of glucose, fat and carbohydrate; urea formation from protein breakdown; manufacture of bile; maintenance of body temperature; and synthetic functions such as the manufacture of albumin and clotting factors. The normal levels of the transaminases are as follows: AST = 5-40 IU/L, ALT = 5-40 IU/L and GGT = 10-48 IU/L. Increased levels of transaminases (AST, ALT) and GGT indicate acute hepatocellular damage. Raised ALP indicates obstructive jaundice, whilst hyperbilirubinaemia indicates excessive haemoglobin breakdown, liver cell damage, or cholestasis.

For jaundice to be clinically obvious the bilirubin level needs to be almost three times the normal. For patients who are being observed for liver damage, the routine tests that are useful are serum bilirubin, albumin and prothrombin time.

4. A, C, D, E

Ultrasound is the first-line investigation, as it is safe and universally available. It detects liver tumours and biliary pathology. It is operator dependent. CECT is the 'gold standard' for liver imaging in most clinical situations – trauma, tumour, infections and inflammations. Triple-phase, multi-slice, spiral CECT provides fine detail of liver lesions. Oral contrast shows up the anatomical relationship of the stomach and duodenum to the liver hilum. Intravenous contrast gives the arterial and venous phases. MRI has the following advantages over CECT: there is no risk of allergic reaction as iodine-containing contrast is not used; there is no radiation; magnetic resonance cholangiopancreatography (MRCP) provides excellent images of the biliary tract; and magnetic resonance angiography (MRA) gives high-definition images of hepatic artery and portal vein without recourse to arterial cannulation. As vascular information can be obtained from CECT and MRI, hepatic angiography is mostly reserved when therapeutic embolisation is contemplated, as in trauma or tumour.

Radioisotope liver scanning does not show anatomical abnormalities but provides diagnostic information and is a useful noninvasive screening test in suspected bile leak or biliary obstruction. HIDA is a technetium-99m radionuclide (^{99}Tc Hydroxy Iminodiacetic Acid) administered intravenously for this purpose. A radioactive sulphur colloid liver scan allows the study of Kupffer cell activity; an adenoma or haemangioma can be diagnosed, as these do not take up sulphur colloid because they lack Kupffer cells.

5. B, E

Gradual liver failure is associated with high-output cardiac failure with hyperdynamic circulation, collapsing pulse, high systolic and low diastolic pressure (high pulse pressure) and warm extremities. Endotoxins and disordered vasomotor tone have been implicated in causing this cardiovascular problem. In acute liver failure, liver transplantation has poor short-term results.

The overall mortality from acute liver failure is about 50% in spite of the best supportive management. Management of acute liver failure should be in the ICU with meticulous fluid balance support, acid-base monitoring, adequate nutrition and organ support such as dialysis and ventilation; reducing cerebral oedema and preventing opportunistic infections are important.

Flapping tremor is the most obvious clinical sign associated with confusion, memory impairment and personality changes – all features of hepatic encephalopathy brought on by cerebral oedema. The severity of chronic liver disease is graded by the MELD score. This gives the probability of survival based on the patient's international normalised ratio (INR), serum bilirubin and serum creatinine.

6. A, D

Liver injuries are rare because of its anatomical position under the diaphragm where it is protected by the lower thoracic cage. Therefore when the liver is damaged, the overall injury is usually very severe. Blunt trauma is often associated with damage to neighbouring structures, such as the spleen, kidneys and mesentery. Stab and gunshot wounds causing penetrating injuries are associated with chest trauma.

CECT scan is not done in every case of liver trauma. If unstable, the patient needs to be taken to theatre forthwith without wasting time on a scan. On the other hand, stable patients suspected of having liver damage should undergo a CECT scan of chest and abdomen. The stable patient who has no hollow viscus damage, but continues to bleed from the liver, might well benefit from an interventional radiologist who could perform a hepatic angiogram with a view to doing embolisation.

7. A, B, D, E

A penetrating injury, such as a lower right chest and abdominal stab wound, requiring large amounts of blood replacement will need urgent exploration. The patient should be transferred to the operating theatre whilst active resuscitation is underway. Blunt injuries are mostly treated conservatively. Stable patients need to undergo a CECT scan and be treated conservatively as long as they continue to be stable. Exploration for liver injury is ideally carried out by a rooftop incision, which can be extended upward for a median sternotomy (Mercedes–Benz incision) if necessary.

Severe crush injury is treated by packing and re-exploration after 48 hours. In major liver vascular damage, the patient is put on a venovenous bypass. In this a cannula is passed from the femoral vein to the superior vena cava; this allows the IVC to be safely clamped to facilitate caval or hepatic vein repair.

Ideally these patients are best managed in a tertiary hepatobiliary unit. In the management of these patients, there should be close liaison with the blood transfusion department, as these patients will not only require large amounts of blood but also fresh frozen plasma and cryoprecipitate. These patients are prone to develop irreversible coagulopathies due to lack of fibrinogen and clotting factors. Standard intraoperative coagulation studies are inadequate and factors are given empirically. An ideal method of monitoring the coagulation status is thromboelastography (TEG), which is a dynamic form of intraoperative assessment of the coagulation profile.

8. A, D

Acute haematemesis from portal hypertension **(Figure 65.2)** most often occurs from lower oesophageal varices and not gastric varices. The initial definitive treatment is endoscopic sclerotherapy or banding, the latter having a lesser incidence of oesophageal ulceration. Long-term beta-blocker therapy with endoscopic sclerotherapy or banding is the main treatment for portal hypertension. When this fails, transjugular intrahepatic portosystemic stent shunt (TIPSS) **(Figure 65.3)** is the treatment of choice in preference to the operation of portocaval anastomosis. Ascites can be treated by insertion of a peritoneovenous shunt – either a Le Veen or Denver shunt. The latter helps to evacuate any debris blocking the shunt.

In some instances the rate of blood loss might be so severe that endoscopic evaluation by oesophagogastroduodenoscopy (OGD) might not be possible in practice. In such an extreme situation oesophageal tamponade by the use of a Sengstaken-Blakemore tube **(Figure 65.4)** might have to be carried out. The details of its use are in **Table 65.1**.

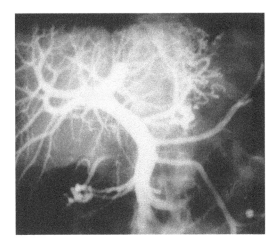

Figure 65.2 Portal venogram showing portal hypertension.

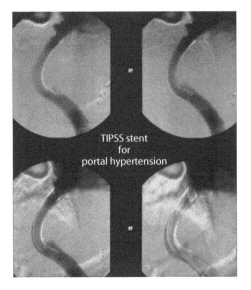

TIPSS stent
for
portal hypertension

Figure 65.3 A TIPSS in place.

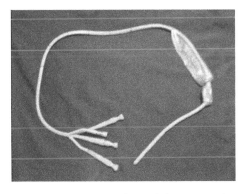

Figure 65.4 Sengstaken-Blakemore tube.

Table 65.1   The use of a Sengstaken–Blakemore tube in acute haematemesis

Insertion of Sengstaken–Blakemore tube

- Patient in ICU
- Tube kept in refrigerator to stiffen it
- Patient intubated to prevent inadvertent insertion into trachea
- Traction of 1 kg applied
- Oesophageal balloon deflated for 10 minutes every 2 hours to prevent necrosis
- Removed after 24 hours
- Complication: rupture of gastro-oesophageal junction

Answers to extended matching questions

1. F Amoebic liver abscess
Having returned from a stay in the Indian subcontinent, this patient has amoebic dysentery with an amoebic abscess. The diagnosis is confirmed by stool examination and isolation of the parasite. US of the liver followed by diagnostic aspiration of the contents are both therapeutic and diagnostic – the contents are usually sterile, the aspirate being characteristically chocolate coloured. Medical treatment with metronidazole and tinidazole should be carried out. Aspiration helps in the penetration of metronidazole and so reduces the morbidity when carried out with drug treatment in a large abscess.

Surgical treatment is reserved for rupture into the pleural, peritoneal, or pericardial cavities. Resuscitation, drainage and appropriate lavage with vigorous medical treatment are the key principles in management **(see Chapter 6, Surgery in the tropics)**.

2. G Ascending cholangitis
This patient has classical Charcot's intermittent hepatic triad (biliary colic, jaundice and high temperature with rigors) almost certainly from a retained stone as seen on the US. The LFTs show an obstructive picture, particularly the much-raised alkaline phosphatase. She needs to be resuscitated with intravenous fluids and given antibiotics to combat the sepsis and vitamin K to prevent excessive bleeding from the increase in prothrombin time. An ERCP is carried out to confirm the diagnosis and at the same time endoscopic papillotomy carried out to remove the stones **(See Chapter 67, The gallbladder and bile ducts)**.

3. D Budd-Chiari syndrome
This is Budd–Chiari syndrome where there is hepatic vein thrombosis caused by an underlying myeloproliferative disorder or procoagulant state due to antithrombin 3, protein C, or protein S deficiency. The hepatic venous outflow obstruction causes a congested liver, impaired liver function, portal hypertension, ascites and oesophageal varices. CT scan is diagnostic. Confirmation is by hepatic venography via the transjugular route, which might allow a biopsy.

Patients who present acutely in fulminant liver failure or with established cirrhosis and portal hypertension should be considered for liver transplantation. In those who do not have cirrhosis, transjugular intrahepatic portosystemic stent shunt (TIPSS) is advised. Lifelong warfarin anticoagulation is necessary.

4. A Caroli's disease
This patient has recurrent attacks of obstructive jaundice with features of sepsis – typical of bile duct stones. The CT scan confirms the diagnosis of this congenital condition. There are two types – a periportal fibrotic type occurring in childhood and a simple type that presents later in life. Treatment is with antibiotics and removal of the stones. If and when the disease is limited to one lobe of the liver, lobectomy might be carried out **(see Chapter 67, The gallbladder and bile ducts)**.

5. O Focal nodular hyperplasia

Focal nodular hyperplasia is the second most common benign liver lesion, an incidental finding, increasingly diagnosed with improvements in US and CT, which have typical images. Focal nodular hyperplasia contains hepatocytes and Kupffer cells, which are very few in tumours. Thus a sulphur colloid scan, which is taken up by Kupffer cells, would be diagnostic and differentiate it from metastasis. It is left alone.

6. N Haemangioma

Haemangioma is the most common benign liver lesion, increasingly being diagnosed with the availability of expertise in US reporting. MRI will show the classical 'light bulb' sign. Such lesions are best left alone in the vast majority, the exception being the very large 'giant' lesions that are symptomatic or show the potential for rupture.

7. K Hepatic adenoma

This woman on the contraceptive pill has a hepatic adenoma confirmed on US and CT findings. Biopsy is contraindicated because of the extreme vascularity of these tumours. Stopping the pill is known to have produced tumour regression. They are thought to have a malignant potential and therefore large symptomatic tumours are best resected.

8. L Hepatocellular carcinoma (HCC)

This male patient clinically has the features of a HCC, which is one of the world's most common cancers with the incidence set to rise because of chronic liver disease from hepatitis B virus (HBV) and hepatitis C virus (HCV). He needs to be thoroughly staged with contrast MRI, CECT, bone scan and CT scan of chest including all routine blood tests. The patient is thus assessed regarding his general condition as to his fitness for surgery and severity of the underlying liver disease. The latter is done by the MELD score (see previously) and the Child-Turcotte-Pugh (CTP) classification. Details of the CTP classification are out of the scope of this book. Once the patient is staged he is discussed in the multidisciplinary team meeting with regard to the best line of management.

If surgical treatment is a possibility, the choice is between resection and liver transplantation. The option is tailored according to the stage of liver disease, physical characteristics of the tumour, all facilities available and availability of organ (live or cadaver). Most patients are not amenable for resection because by the time of presentation the disease is beyond surgery. The choices of treatment are shown in **Figure 65.5**.

9. J Hydatid liver disease

As a native of a Mediterranean country, this patient has a hydatid cyst of the right lobe of the liver. The diagnosis is confirmed by eosinophilia, serological test for antibodies to hydatid antigen in the enzyme-linked immunosorbent assay (ELISA) and typical CT scan findings of a floating membrane within the cyst and multiple septa. This is caused by the tapeworm *Echinococcus granulosus* for which the host is the dog and the human. The cyst can rupture into the neighbouring serous cavities.

Treatment is started with albendazole and mebendazole. The acronym PAIR summarises the treatment of choice: *p*uncture of the cyst under image guidance, *a*spiration of the contents, *i*nstillation of hypertonic saline, *r*easpiration. The surgical options are liver resection, local excision and deroofing with evacuation of the contents (**see Chapter 6, Surgery in the tropics**).

10. C Primary biliary cirrhosis

Primary biliary cirrhosis is a condition of gradual onset. The liver function tests show hepatocellular dysfunction. Confirmation is by liver biopsy. The condition progresses slowly, causing portal hypertension with variceal bleeding and ascites. The treatment is supportive or liver transplantation.

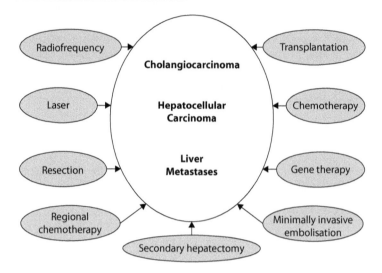

Figure 65.5 Diagrammatic representation of the choices of treatment in malignancies within the liver.

11. B Primary sclerosing cholangitis

This patient who has suffered from ulcerative colitis now has primary sclerosing cholangitis. Although her ulcerative colitis has been treated successfully by surgery, her primary sclerosing cholangitis has continued unabated. The disease causes progressive fibrous stricturing with gradual obliteration of the intra and extra-hepatic biliary tree. The ERCP is diagnostic, showing irregular narrowed biliary tree. There is no specific treatment. Death from liver failure eventually is the outcome. A close surveillance should be carried out because this patient might develop a cholangiocarcinoma. Appearance of a new or dominant stricture on repeat cholangiography should arouse this sinister suspicion.

12. I Pyogenic liver abscess

Pyogenic liver abscess usually occurs in the elderly and infirm who are immunocompromised, as is this patient who is a type 1 diabetic of long standing. The US and CT scan findings are diagnostic. The common organisms are *Streptococcus milleri* and *faecalis, E. coli, Klebsiella* and *Proteus*. The patient is treated with penicillin, aminoglycosides and metronidazole and image-guided aspiration, which might have to be repeated. A source of the infection such as the colon should be sought.

13. M Secondary liver metastasis

This patient who had a colonic cancer removed 3 years ago now has the following clinical features of secondaries in the liver: jaundice, hepatomegaly and a liver mass on imaging. He needs a thorough reassessment so that he can be considered for hepatic resection. This would consist of oral and intravenous contrast CT of the liver and abdomen, chest CT and colonoscopy to exclude recurrent or synchronous colonic cancer. As the liver secondary is being staged, at the same time the patient's general condition should be assessed with regard to his suitability for a major hepatic resection. Carcinoembryonic antigen (CEA) level is useful but has low specificity. Biopsy prior to surgery is not done, as malignant cells can seed along the biopsy track.

Macroscopically on the surface of the liver secondary a depression is felt, typically described as umbilicated. This is because with time the secondary nodule outgrows its

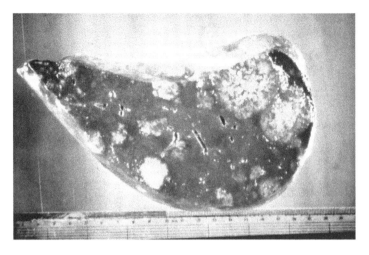

Figure 65.6 Specimen of liver showing typical multiple secondaries.

blood supply causing the central core of the secondary to necrose resulting in the surface to collapse **(Figure 65.6)**.

The longer the recurrence-free gap between the removal of the primary and appearance of the secondary, the better would be the outcome following resection of the metastasis. This patient's primary was removed 3 years ago. Therefore, he would be a good candidate for resection. As these patients have normal liver parenchyma, they could withstand removal of two-thirds of their liver parenchyma with little risk of postoperative liver failure. The resectability rate of colorectal liver metastasis is 20% to 30% whilst approximately 35% of those resected are alive after 5 years. In a selected group of patients, downstaging the metastasis with chemotherapy have enabled secondaries to be resected, which were considered 'unresectable' in the past.

14. E Simple cystic disease
This patient has a simple solitary hepatic cyst confirmed on ultrasound with the following typical findings: a regular, thin-walled unilocular space-occupying lesion without any surrounding tissue response or variation in density within the cavity. Asymptomatic cysts are left alone. Large cysts producing abdominal discomfort can be treated by laparoscopic deroofing.

15. H Viral hepatitis
Viral hepatitis can be due to hepatitis A, B and C. Hepatitis C is one of the most common causes of liver disease worldwide. Hepatitis B is the most serious and later can cause a hepatoma. Some patients might present acutely with fulminating liver failure or at a late stage with cirrhosis, variceal bleeding and ascites. Diagnosis is confirmed by the antibody titre to the infective agent. Treatment is supportive for cirrhosis and its complications. Liver transplantation can be considered. Without viral suppression, death from reinfection of the transplanted liver can occur.

66 The spleen

Pradip K Datta

Multiple choice questions

→ ### Anatomy

1. Which of the following statements are true?

A The splenic vessels are contained within the splenorenal ligament.

B The splenic artery arises from the left gastric artery.

C The short gastric branches of the splenic artery lie within the gastrosplenic ligament.

D The splenic vein and the superior mesenteric vein join to form the portal vein.

E The inferior mesenteric vein empties into the splenic vein.

2. The following statements are true except:

A The spleen lies in front of the left seventh, eighth and ninth ribs.

B The tail of the pancreas lies in the splenorenal ligament.

C The lymphatics of the spleen ultimately drain into the coeliac nodes.

D The left extremity of the lesser sac lies against the splenic hilum.

E The inner surface of the spleen has two visceral impressions for the stomach and the splenic flexure of colon.

→ ### Physiology

3. Which of the following statements is not true?

A The splenic parenchyma consists of white and red pulp.

B Pitting is a specific function of the spleen.

C The spleen is a major site of immune function.

D Haemopoiesis occurs in the foetal spleen.

E The spleen has a major reservoir function of red cell mass.

→ ### Investigations of the spleen

4. Which of the following statements are true?

A Plain abdominal x-ray is a common modality of imaging in splenomegaly.

B Splenomegaly with portal hypertension requires upper GI endoscopy (OGD).

C Lymph node biopsy may be required in some cases of splenomegaly.

D CECT is the best imaging modality.

E ^{99m}Tc–labelled colloid is useful in certain cases.

→ ### Splenectomy

5. The following statements are true except:

A Partial splenectomy can result in splenic regeneration.

B Before splenectomy for haemolytic anaemia, abdominal US is essential.

C A pancreatic or gastric fistula can occur as a post-splenectomy complication.

D In a left hemicolectomy the spleen can be in danger of iatrogenic injury.

E The risk of opportunist post-splenectomy infection (OPSI) is greatest after the first 6 months of splenectomy.

Extended matching questions

➡ Diagnoses

1. Hereditary spherocytosis
2. Idiopathic thrombocytopenic purpura (ITP)
3. Splenic artery aneurysm
4. Splenic infarction
5. Splenic rupture

Choose and match the correct diagnosis with each of the scenarios that follow:

A A male patient of 55 years, known to suffer from myelofibrosis, presents with onset of severe left upper quadrant and shoulder tip pain of 8 hours duration. On examination he has a temperature and marked tenderness over an enlarged spleen. A contrast-enhanced computed tomography scan (CECT) shows a perfusion defect in an enlarged spleen.

B An 18-year-old male presents with intermittent generalised abdominal pain, mild jaundice and anorexia. On examination he has pallor, jaundice and splenomegaly. An ultrasound of his abdomen shows multiple small gallstones and confirms splenomegaly.

C A 30-year-old female patient presents with petechial haemorrhagic spots in her skin. She suffers from menorrhagia. Abdominal examination shows no organomegaly but many areas of skin ecchymoses. The coagulation and bleeding times are normal. The blood tests show anaemia and low platelet count. Bone marrow reveals a large number of platelet-producing megakaryocytes.

D A 25-year-old male was kicked in his abdomen accidentally while playing football. He got up and continued to play for another few minutes, but then he felt dizzy with intense pain in his left upper abdomen. In the hospital he complained of pain in his left shoulder tip and had rigidity and rebound tenderness in his left hypochondrium. Until the age of 18 years, he lived in a tropical country when he had suffered from malaria.

E A 30-year-old woman during her ultrasound for pregnancy was found to have a calcified 1-cm mass in the epigastrium. A bruit was heard in the epigastric region. She does not have any symptoms.

Answers to multiple choice questions

➡ Anatomy

1. A, C, D, E

The splenic vessels travel within the two layers of the splenorenal (lienorenal) ligament, which acts as one of its two pedicles. This ligament is a part of the greater omentum that extends from the spleen to the anterior surface of the kidney. The gastrosplenic ligament, also a part of the greater omentum, extends from the hilum of the spleen to the greater curve of the stomach and contains the short gastric branches of the splenic artery. These anatomical facts are vital during splenectomy.

The splenic vein and superior mesenteric vein join to form the portal vein behind the neck of the pancreas. It enters the two layers of the lesser omentum and runs vertically upward toward the porta hepatis. The inferior mesenteric vein travels behind the lower border of the body of the pancreas in front of the left renal vein to join the splenic vein. The splenic artery arises from the coeliac axis, which also gives off the left gastric and hepatic arteries.

2. A, E

The spleen lies in front of (deep to) the left ninth, tenth and eleventh ribs. This fact is of applied importance because in fracture of these ribs the spleen is liable to be injured as a result of the broken ribs penetrating the splenic parenchyma. The inner (visceral) surface of the spleen is in contact with the flexure of the left colon, stomach, left kidney and pancreatic tail at the splenic hilum.

The tail of the pancreas lies within the two layers of the splenorenal ligament accompanied by the splenic artery, vein and lymphatics. This anatomical fact is of utmost importance in splenectomy. During the procedure the surgeon must be very careful not to damage the tail of the pancreas while ligating the splenic artery and vein. The lymphatics of the spleen drain into the splenic hilar nodes; thereafter by way of the pancreaticosplenic nodes they ultimately drain into the coeliac nodes. The left extremity of the lesser sac (omental bursa) lies against the splenic hilum.

Physiology

3. E

The spleen does not have a major reservoir function of red cell mass, containing about 8% of the total RBC mass. An enlarged spleen might contain a larger proportion.

The splenic parenchyma consists of red and white pulp within the structural framework of the trabeculae and arteriovenous bundles. The white pulp comprises of a central trabecular artery surrounded by lymphatic nodules with lymphocytes and macrophages. The lymphatic nodules (Malphigian corpuscles) are composed of lymphoid follicles rich in β-lymphocytes and lymphoid sheaths rich in T-lymphocytes. These immunoglobulins take part in the active immune response through humoral and cell-mediated pathways.

Between the white pulp and red pulp lies the marginal zone. The red pulp consists of cords (sinusoids) and sinuses. Blood passes in the trabecular artery through the centre of the white pulp into the red pulp. RBCs must elongate and become thinner to pass from the cords to the sinuses within the red pulp; this process removes abnormal red cells from the circulation. As 90% of the blood passing through the spleen flows through an open circulation, splenic pulp pressure is a reflection of the portal pressure. The remaining 10% of the splenic blood flow does not go through the cords and sinuses but travels through A-V communications. The blood flow through the spleen is about 300 mL/minute.

RBCs that contain nuclear remnants are removed by phagocytosis and the repaired RBCs then returned to the circulation – the process being called pitting. The manufacture of β-lymphocytes and T-lymphocytes is responsible for the spleen having a major immune function. Some degree of haemopoiesis occurs in the foetal spleen. To summarise, the functions of the spleen in varying degrees are the following: produce immunity, act as a filter, pitting, act as reservoir and cytopoiesis.

Investigations of the spleen

4. B, C, D, E

In patients with suspected splenic pathology, all routine haematological (including tests for haemolysis and reticulocyte count) and biochemical investigations must be done including the full gamut of liver function tests. When portal hypertension is diagnosed patients should undergo an OGD to look for gastro-oesophageal varices. As the spleen is a part of the reticuloendothelial system, in splenomegaly, enlarged lymph nodes should be sought in the neck, axilla and groins. If there is lymphadenopathy, an excision biopsy is important.

As an imaging modality CECT is the ideal investigation to determine the nature of suspected splenic pathology besides helping to exclude any other intra-abdominal pathology. A preliminary US examination might be useful and could prevent the need for a CT. Radioisotope scanning helps to determine if the spleen is the site of RBC destruction in haemolytic anaemia, thus helping to predict the response to splenectomy.

Plain abdominal x-ray is not an investigation asked for when investigating splenic pathology. However, such an x-ray taken for some other purpose might show up unsuspected splenic pathology such as calcification of a splenic artery aneurysm or old infarct, splenic cyst, hydatid disease, or multiple calcifications of tuberculosis.

5. E

The period during which a post-splenectomy patient is most susceptible to OPSI is the first 2 to 3 years after the operation because of compromised immune function. Prophylaxis should be given during this period with penicillin, erythromycin, amoxycillin, or co-amoxiclav taken orally.

If possible, partial splenectomy in trauma should always be attempted because there is rapid regeneration of lost tissue with no reduction in splenic function. When splenectomy for haemolytic anaemia is to be carried out, an abdominal US is essential to look for unsuspected pigment gallstones. If present, cholecystectomy is carried out at the same time either laparoscopically or by open operation.

A pancreatic or gastric fistula can occur following splenectomy from unrecognised inadvertent damage to the tail of the pancreas or greater curve of the stomach. The tail of the pancreas can be damaged while ligating the splenic artery and vein at the hilum. The greater curve of the stomach can be damaged during ligation and division of the short gastric vessels. The most common cause of iatrogenic injury to the spleen is a left hemicolectomy.

Answers to extended matching questions

1. B Hereditary spherocytosis

This patient has hereditary spherocytosis, an autosomal dominant disorder. As a result this patient has spherocytic RBC because of the lack of erythrocyte membrane proteins, which are necessary to maintain the normal biconcave shape of the red cell. As a result of the increased permeability of the cell membrane, sodium leaks into the cell causing a rise in the osmotic pressure and resulting in swelling and increased fragility of the cell causing RBCs to be destroyed in the spleen.

Clinically he has unconjugated hyperbilirubinaemia, splenomegaly and gallstones (almost certainly pigment stones). This patient will not have any pruritis from his jaundice because the bilirubin is unconjugated. As the bilirubin is unconjugated, it is bound to albumin and not excreted in the urine. Hence, the condition is also called acholuric (lack of bile in the urine) jaundice.

The blood picture will show anaemia, a positive fragility test and a large number of reticulocytes. During the course of the disease some patients might develop a severe crisis of RBC destruction, which presents as pyrexia, extreme pallor, abdominal pain, nausea and vomiting and increase in jaundice. Chronic leg ulcers might sometimes be present. Radioactive chromium labelling of the patient's own red cells will show the spleen to be site of red cell sequestration. Splenectomy and cholecystectomy should be carried out laparoscopically or by open surgery depending on the available expertise.

The other causes of haemolytic anaemia suitable for splenectomy are acquired autoimmune haemolytic anaemia, thalassaemia and sickle cell disease.

2. C Idiopathic thrombocytopenic purpura (ITP)

This 30-year-old female has signs of petechial haemorrhages and generalised bleeding tendency. Her low platelet count points to the diagnosis of ITP. The low platelet count is due to the development of antibodies to specific platelet glycoproteins that damage the patient's own platelets – hence it is also known as autoimmune thrombocytopenic purpura. The spleen is palpable in a minority of cases.

If the platelet count remains low and the patient has two relapses on steroid therapy, splenectomy is considered. Response to steroids indicates a good response to splenectomy. Up to two-thirds of patients will be cured by splenectomy; a further 15% will be improved, whilst in the remainder the operation will make no difference.

An enlarged spleen is not always palpable. For an enlarged spleen to be clinically palpable, the organ needs to be almost three times its normal size. A spleen enlarges toward the right iliac fossa. The classical physical findings of an enlarged spleen are that it moves with respiration and has a sharp edge with a notch.

3. E Splenic artery aneurysm

This pregnant woman has the incidental finding of a splenic artery aneurysm. These are usually silent unless they rupture. Fifty percent of cases of rupture occur in patients younger than 45 years, and 25% occur in pregnant women usually in the third trimester or during labour. Hence, a serious consideration should be given to prophylactically treating this splenic artery aneurysm by interventional radiology.

In 25% of the cases, there might be more than one aneurysm when they are usually the aftermath of pancreatic necrosis after severe acute pancreatitis. In the young patient embolisation or endovascular stenting can be considered depending upon the available expertise. Splenectomy still remains a choice.

4. A Splenic infarction

This patient has splenic infarction **(Figure 66.1)**, a condition that occurs in those with massive splenomegaly, such as in myeloproliferative disorders, portal hypertension, or splenic vein thrombosis. The infarct can be asymptomatic or give rise to left upper quadrant pain radiating to the left shoulder tip. The suspected diagnosis is confirmed by CECT showing perfusion defect in an enlarged spleen.

Conservative management is tried but if the patient continues to be septic, denoting a splenic abscess, splenectomy is carried out.

Hypersplenism is a term used to describe a combination of anaemia, leukopenia, or thrombocytopenia and compensatory bone marrow hyperplasia in the presence of splenomegaly. Almost any cause of splenomegaly can give rise to this, the mechanism being increased filtration or phagocytosis, increased pooling of cellular blood components, or reduced RBC life span. Improvement usually occurs after splenectomy.

5. D Splenic rupture

This young man has the hallmarks of a ruptured spleen. He spent the early part of his life in a tropical country where he suffered from malaria, which would have caused an enlarged spleen. Trivial trauma during contact sport caused rupture of his spleen. It is typical of a pathological organ to be badly damaged and cause bleeding after minor trauma. In a malarial spleen, blunt trauma might cause a subcapsular haematoma and the patient might be in slight discomfort to start with, only for him to collapse with severe pain and shock some time later when the haematoma ruptures.

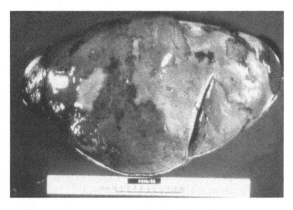

Figure 66.1 Splenic infarction.

This patient should be resuscitated immediately with two wide-bore cannulae with intravenous crystalloid, blood cross-matched and taken to theatre for an emergency laparotomy for splenectomy. If the patient is stable and time permits, a FAST or CECT can be done.

The abdomen is opened through a midline incision skirting the umbilicus. On entering the abdomen, blood will be seen coming from the left upper quadrant over the body of the stomach. The blood is sucked out, blood clots are removed, and the posterior layer of the splenorenal ligament is cut (it may be torn anyway) to deliver the shattered spleen into the wound. The splenic hilum is carefully dissected to identify the tail of the pancreas, and the splenic artery is doubly ligated and divided followed by the splenic vein. The spleen is now attached by the short gastric branches of the splenic artery. These are ligated and divided, taking care not to damage the greater curve of the stomach. The shattered spleen is now removed. A pack is placed in the splenic bed.

A thorough laparotomy is next systematically carried out to look for other injuries. If there are none, the pack is removed and the incision closed. The patient is given prophylactic anti-pneumococcal vaccine and started on an antibiotic regime to prevent OPSI.

A note about splenectomy: When doing a splenectomy in a massive spleen (electively) or for a perisplenic haematoma (as an emergency), it is a good manoeuvre to enter the lesser sac first through a window in the gastrosplenic omentum. The splenic artery is then tied in continuity at the upper border of the pancreas. Then the surgeon proceeds with splenectomy in the usual manner by approaching the splenorenal ligament as described above.

The indications for splenectomy are enumerated in **Figures 66.2 and 66.3**.

Indications for splenectomy

Trauma	Hypersplenism	Neoplasms	With other viscera	Miscellaneous
• Immediate	• Hereditary	• Lymphoma	• En bloc	• Cyst
• Delayed	spherocytosis	• Hodgkin's	resections –	• Abscess
• Iatrogenic	• ITP	• Leukaemia	gastrectomy	• Artery
• Spontaneous of	• Aids related ITP	• Massive	pancreatectomy	aneurysm
a pathological	• Sickling	haemangioma	• Spleno-renal	• Infarction
spleen	syndromes	• Secondaries	shunt	• To prevent
e.g. malaria		**(Figure 66.3)**		graft rejection

Figure 66.2 Indications for splenectomy.

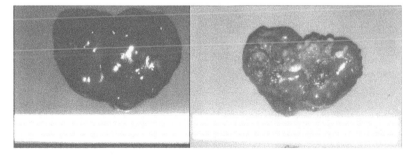

Figure 66.3 Secondaries in spleen from malignant melanoma showing typical black nodules.

67 The gall bladder and bile ducts

BV Praveen and Pradip K Datta

Multiple choice questions

→ ## Surgical anatomy and physiology

1. Which of the following statements are true?

A The common bile duct (CBD) is traditionally divided into three parts.

B The cystic duct opens into the supraduodenal part of the common hepatic duct (CHD) in 80% of cases.

C The cystic duct junction with the CHD might vary.

D The cystic artery arise from the common hepatic artery.

E The cystic artery runs across the Calot's triangle.

2. Which of the following statements are true regarding lymphatic drainage?

A The sentinel lymph node is the cystic lymph node of Lund.

B The cystic lymph node lies in the fork created by the cystic duct and the right hepatic duct.

C Efferent vessels from the cystic lymph node go to the superior mesenteric nodes.

D The lymphatics of the gall bladder also connect directly with the lymphatics of the liver.

E The lymphatic vessels are mainly in the sub-mucosal and sub-serosal layers of the wall.

3. Which of the following statements are true?

A Bile consists of 97% water.

B About 95% of bile salts are reabsorbed.

C During fasting bile is diverted into the gall bladder.

D Gall bladder concentrates the bile.

E Gall bladder secretes mucus.

→ ## Investigations of the biliary tract

4. The following statements are true except:

A Ultrasound (US) examination shows up stones and CBD dilatation.

B A HIDA scan is useful in diagnosing bile leak.

C Plain x-ray is useful to look for calcification, which is seen in 80% of gallstones.

D Endoscopic retrograde cholangiopancreatography (ERCP) is useful in showing up anatomy, stones and strictures.

E Percutaneous transhepatic cholangiogram (PTC) is ideal in high strictures.

5. Which of the following statements are true?

A Liver function tests should be routinely carried out.

B Magnetic resonance cholangiopancreatography (MRCP) images are comparable to images by ERCP and PTC.

C Peroperative cholangiography is routinely done in cholecystectomy.

D Choledochoscopy should be done in the appropriate patient to ensure complete removal of stones from CBD.

E Endoscopic and laparoscopic US are accurate techniques in staging cancers.

Extra-hepatic biliary atresia

6. Which of the following statements are true?

A Associated anomalies include situs inversus.
B Jaundice is a late feature.
C Type 1 anomaly involves the common hepatic duct.
D Kasai procedure is best done 3 to 6 months after birth.
E 70%–80% patients are alive 2 to 5 years after liver transplant.

Caroli's disease

7. Which of the following statements are true?

A It involves the intra-hepatic ducts.
B It is a hereditary condition.
C The peri-portal fibrosis type presents later in life.
D It can be associated with cholangiocarcinoma.
E The mainstay of treatments is antibiotics and removal of calculi.

Choledochal cyst

8. Which of the following statements are true?

A This only involves the extra-hepatic duct.
B 60% of cases are diagnosed before the age of 10 years.
C There is an increasing risk of developing cholangiocarcinoma.
D MRCP is useful in the definition of the anatomy.
E Cholecystectomy should be a part of the surgical treatment.

Gallstones

9. The following statements are true except:

A Cholecystectomy should be performed whenever gallstones are found.
B Types of gallstones are cholesterol, pigment and mixed.
C Gallstones can cause various complications including intestinal obstruction.

D Acute cholecystitis can occur without stones.
E In emergency presentation from biliary colic or acute cholecystitis, cholecystectomy can be performed at the index admission.

Complications of cholecystectomy

10. Which of the following statements are true?

A Complications can occur in 10%–15% of cases.
B Bile duct injury is usually recognised at the time of the operation.
C Post-cholecystectomy syndrome occurs in 15% of patients.
D Stones in the bile ducts are less often associated with infected bile than are stones in the gall bladder.
E Jaundice in the postoperative period is usually self-limiting and needs investigating only if it persists for more than 1 week.

Primary sclerosing cholangitis

11. Which of the following statements are true?

A It is more common in females.
B It involves both intra and extra biliary ducts.
C It usually starts in childhood.
D Liver biopsy is not useful.
E Liver transplantation is an option if cirrhosis is not present.

Parasitic infestation of the biliary tract

12. Which of the following statements are true?

A The round worm (Ascaris Lumbricoides) enters the biliary tact through the bloodstream.
B Clonorchiasis is endemic in Africa.
C Obstructive jaundice and cholangitis are common presentations of hydatid disease.
D Complications include bile duct carcinoma.
E Recurrent stones can be a problem.

Extended matching questions for gall bladder

→ Diagnoses

1 Acute cholecystitis
2 Biliary colic
3 Carcinoma of the gall bladder
4 Empyema of the gall bladder
5 Gallstone ileus
6 Mucocoele of the gall bladder

Match the previously listed diagnoses with the clinical features of the various conditions that follow:

→ Clinical features

A A 72-year-old woman has had dull right upper quadrant pain interspersed with occasional acute attacks for almost a year; she has lost weight. An ultrasound of the gall bladder showed uniform calcification of the gall bladder with gallstones – a porcelain gall bladder. She has raised inflammatory markers, transaminases and white cell count and is anaemic.

B A 38-year-old woman is seen as an emergency complaining of severe right upper quadrant pain radiating to the back and epigastrium of 24 hours duration. She has vomited a few times and is feverish. On examination she is febrile, and slightly jaundiced; palpation of the right upper quadrant elicits extreme tenderness, which is exacerbated by taking a deep breath (positive Murphy's sign).

C A 52-year-old woman, on the waiting list for laparoscopic cholecystectomy, has been admitted as an emergency with increasing right upper quadrant pain, swinging pyrexia and extreme tenderness over the gall bladder. She is toxic and has leucocytosis with raised inflammatory markers; ultrasound of the gall bladder shows thickened gall bladder enveloped by omentum with peri-cholecystic fluid.

D A 40-year-old woman, on the waiting list for a laparoscopic cholecystectomy, complains of recurrent right upper quadrant discomfort which is not too bad for hospital admission but bad enough to see her general practitioner (GP). The GP found that the patient has a smooth globular mass in the right upper quadrant moving with respiration and slightly tender.

E A 32-year-old woman presents as an emergency with sudden onset of severe colicky epigastric pain radiating to the right subcostal region, back and right shoulder tip. The pain makes her feel nauseated and in between attacks she is left with a dull ache on the right side where she is tender. This has been going on for 48 hours.

F A 74-year-old woman complains of intermittent generalised abdominal pain, distension and vomiting for almost 1 week. Over the past couple of days she has become much worse and has been admitted as a surgical emergency. On examination she is grossly dehydrated. Abdominal examination shows generalised distension and tenderness without any lumps or scars.

Extended matching questions for bile ducts

→ Diagnoses

1 Carcinoma of lower end of common bile duct
2 Iatrogenic damage to CBD
3 Mirrizi's syndrome
4 Post-cholecystectomy syndrome

5 Residual stone in CBD
6 Sclerosing cholangitis
7 Stone in CBD

Match the diagnoses with the clinical features of the various conditions that follow:

Clinical features

A A 36-year-old woman underwent a laparoscopic cholecystectomy. The procedure was straightforward. The following day before discharge she complained of severe itching and jaundice with generalised upper abdominal pain.

B A 60-year-old woman has been admitted as an emergency with a 4-day history of severe right upper quadrant pain, vomiting, jaundice and intense pruritis and is very toxic – high temperature with rigors and hyperdynamic circulation. She has not had any operations in the past.

C A 55-year-old woman has been admitted with jaundice, itching, right upper quadrant discomfort and a temperature of 39°C. She had similar episodes in the past that subsided with antibiotic treatment from her GP. This time the episode has lasted for more than 1 week. She is under the gastroenterologist for ulcerative colitis for which she is on regular colonoscopic surveillance.

D A 62-year-old man underwent a cholecystectomy 18 months ago, following which he remained well until 1 month ago when he developed colicky upper abdominal pain radiating to the back reminiscent of his attacks prior to his cholecystectomy. Recently he has been passing dark urine and is bothered by itching. On examination there is nothing to find except for scars of LC ports and a few scratch marks over his body.

E A 48-year-old woman underwent a cholecystectomy 4 months ago for biliary colic. She was well immediately after the operation. However, 6 weeks ago she had a recurrence of her abdominal pain, which is very similar to the pain she had prior to the removal of her gall bladder. Except for the pain she feels and looks well.

F A 45-year-old woman complains of right upper quadrant pain, jaundice with pruritis and swinging pyrexia, which at its height is 41°C. Her LFTs are deranged, with an alkaline phosphatase of 790 units. An US showed dilated common hepatic and intrahepatic ducts and an inflammatory mass in the region of the Calot's triangle.

G A 72-year-old man complains of severe itching all over his body of 6 weeks duration. He has been passing high-coloured urine and pale stools. His family noticed that he was becoming increasingly yellow in colour. On examination, besides scratch marks all over his body, he has a smooth globular nontender mass in his right upper quadrant.

Answers to multiple choice questions

Surgical anatomy and physiology

1. B, C, E

The cystic duct, about 3 cm long, opens into the CHD in 80% of cases. In the other 20% there are several variations of which the surgeon should be aware. The cystic duct might open into the CHD much lower down into the retro or infra-duodenal part while occasionally it might join the right hepatic duct. The surgeon should be aware of these variations so as not to cause inadvertent damage to the CBD during cholecystectomy. The cystic artery arises from the right hepatic artery (not common hepatic artery) and runs across the Calot's triangle where it should be identified. There are variations of the blood supply too and the surgeon must be aware of them.

The CBD, about 7.5 cm long, is divided into four parts according to its relationship to the duodenum – supraduodenal, retroduodenal, infraduodenal and intraduodenal. The infraduodenal part is intimately related to the posterior surface of the pancreas lying in a groove but sometimes in a tunnel. Cancers arising in this region in the head of the pancreas obstructs the CBD here causing obstructive jaundice.

The Calot's triangle. Readers should note that there is a distinct difference of opinion regarding this anatomical fact. Anatomy books (*Gray's Anatomy* and *Last's Anatomy*) describe the Calot's triangle as bounded by the cystic duct laterally, the CHD medially and above by the lower border of segment V of the liver. This has been traditionally taught as the Calot's Δ (also called the cystohepatic Δ in some quarters). Jean-Francois Calot, a French surgeon, described his Δ in 1891, the three sides consisting of the cystic duct, CHD and upper margin of the cystic artery, the same description as given in *Bailey and Love* and some other surgical books. This Δ is sometimes referred to as the hepatobiliary Δ. To compound the confusion further, certain quarters use the terms cystohepatic and hepatobiliary triangles synonymously. The reader is asked to make up his or her own mind from this morass of confusion. However, there is one certainty. The surgeon must be aware of the various anatomical variations and must meticulously look for the cystic artery in this region before clipping and dividing the cystic duct.

2. A, D, E
The sentinel lymph node lies in the fork created by the junction of the cystic and common hepatic ducts. It is an important landmark at lap cholecystectomy as the cystic duct is dissected at this level. The efferent vessels go to the hilum of the liver and then to the coeliac nodes. The direct connections between the lymph vessels of the gall bladder and liver can lead to early and direct spread of gall bladder cancer.

3. A, B, C, D, E
The liver produces 500–1000 mL of bile in 24 hours; 97% of bile is water, whilst the remainder consists of bile salts (cholic, chenodeoxycholic, dexoxycholic and lithocholic acids). Almost 95% of bile salts are reabsorbed in the terminal ileum through the enterohepatic circulation. Therefore, when the terminal ileum is diseased (Crohn's disease) or removed (right hemicolectomy) there is a disturbance in the enterohepatic circulation promoting the formation of gallstones.

In fasting, there is resistance of the flow of bile through the sphincter of Oddi, thus diverting bile to be stored in the gall bladder. After the ingestion of food, the sphincter relaxes and the gall bladder contracts, allowing bile to flow into the duodenum; this process is facilitated by cholecystokinin. The gall bladder has the ability to concentrate bile by absorbing water, sodium chloride and bicarbonate. It also secretes mucus, which it continues to do when a stone obstructs the cystic duct – the basis of a mucocoele.

→ Investigations of the biliary tract
4. C
Plain x-ray in biliary imaging is an obsolete investigation, as only 10% of gallstones are radio-opaque. US is the first imaging modality in suspected gall bladder disease. Besides being readily available, it is quick to perform, produces no ill effects such as radiation, inexpensive and can be repeated and accurate. It will show up stones and the diameter of the CBD. However, it is operator dependent, which is its only limitation. HIDA scan, which is radioisotope scanning, visualises the gall bladder and biliary tree. Technetium-99m (^{99m}Tc)-labelled derivative of iminodiacetic acid when injected intravenously is excreted in the bile. It is useful in diagnosing bile leak and hence useful in suspected iatrogenic biliary obstruction.

ERCP will show up the anatomy of the CBD and pancreatic ducts; it will show up strictures and stones will be seen as filling defects. US and MRCP have reduced the diagnostic use of

ERCP, which can produce acute pancreatitis. However, it has the added advantage of bile aspirates, endoluminal brushings and endoscopic papillotomy, procedures which have made ERCP into much more a therapeutic technique. PTC is particularly useful when US has shown a high stricture such as a hilar cholangiocarcinoma (Klatskin tumour). This also has the added therapeutic advantage of external biliary drainage and insertion of a stent. This procedure, as it is mostly carried out in the jaundiced patient, will require prophylactic vitamin K and antibiotics; haemorrhage and bile peritonitis are rare complications.

5. A, B, D, E

In suspected biliary tract disease liver function tests (LFTs) should be the first investigations to be carried out. This should include prothrombin time and serum amylase. In obstructive jaundice MRCP gives excellent images to determine the cause of obstruction and is fast superseding ERCP and PTC as diagnostic procedures in view of their potential complications. Once the CBD is explored for stones, laparoscopically or by open method, operative biliary endoscopy in the form of choledochoscopy should be carried out to ensure all stones have been removed.

Another technique of visualising the biliary tree and pancreas is to perform endoluminal ultrasound (EUS) using a specially designed endoscope with an ultrasound transducer at its tip. While showing stones in the CBD, it is particularly sensitive in staging pancreatic head and periampullary cancers. Laparoscopic US is another imaging technique to look at the extrahepatic biliary tree. Besides it is a very useful diagnostic procedure for pancreatic endocrine tumours and staging in oesophageal, gastric and pancreatic head cancers.

Peroperative cholangiogram (on table cholangiogram) **(Figure 67.1a** and **b)** is not routinely done in cholecystectomy. Those who routinely do it, do so to delineate the anatomy of

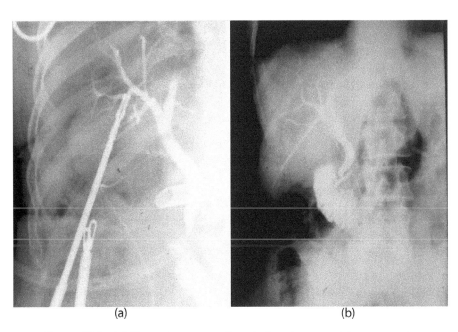

(a)   (b)

Figure 67.1   (a) Normal peroperative cholangiogram at laparoscopic. Cholecystectomy. (Courtesy of Mr Paul Fisher, Consultant Surgeon, Caithness General Hospital, Wick, UK.) (b) Normal peroperative cholangiogram at open cholecystectomy.

the biliary tree as in almost 20% there is an anatomical variation. It is also done to exclude unsuspected stones in the CBD. The advisability of doing this routinely is a highly contentious issue and discussion on the topic is beyond the scope of this book.

→ Extra-hepatic biliary atresia

6. A, E

Atresia is present in approximately 1 per 12,000 live births and affects both genders equally. About one-third of patients are jaundiced at birth, and by the end of 1st week all affected babies will have jaundice. If untreated, cirrhosis and portal hypertension will follow with eventual liver failure. Associated anomalies are seen in 20% of these patients and this includes cardiac lesions, situs inversus, absent IVC, polysplenia and preduodenal portal vein. The type 1 anomaly affects the common bile duct, the type 2 involves the common hepatic duct and the type 3 is limited to the left and right hepatic ducts. The results of Kasai procedure (porto-enterostomy) are best when done within 8 weeks after birth. Liver transplantation should be considered if Kasai procedure is unsuccessful.

→ Caroli's disease

7. A, B, D, E

The periportal fibrotic type presents early whereas the 'simple' type presents later. Biliary stasis leading to sepsis and stone formation is the typical course. Associated conditions include congenital hepatic fibrosis, polycystic liver and rarely cholangiocarcinoma. The mainstay of treatment is antibiotics and removal of the stones. If the condition is limited to one lobe, lobectomy may be a surgical option.

→ Choledochal cyst

8. B, C, D, E

It is a congenital dilatation of the bile ducts and affects the intra and extra hepatic biliary system. Jaundice, abdominal pain, fever and abdominal mass are typical symptoms. Ultrasound, MRCP and CT scan are all helpful in evaluation. Excision of the choledochal cyst and hepatico-jejunostomy to a Roux loop is the treatment of choice. Cholecystectomy is carried out at the same time because there is a high risk of development of carcinoma.

→ Gallstones

9. A

Cholecystectomy is not indicated in all cases of gallstones, the majority of which are asymptomatic. Patients with asymptomatic gallstones should only undergo a cholecystectomy in the following situations:

- They have a porcelain gall bladder, which has a high incidence of turning malignant in the long term
- If they are type 1 diabetics because they are prone to complications
- If they have a choledochal cyst (see previously)

The types of gallstones are cholesterol, pigment (black or brown) and mixed. The formation of a gallstone is explained in **Figure 67.2**. Gallstones can cause several complications as described in **Figure 67.3**. When the complication is intestinal obstruction, it is due to gallstone ileus. Acute cholecystitis can occur without stones when it is referred to as acalculous cholecystitis. Acute acalculous cholecystitis is seen in critically ill patients and those recovering from major surgery, trauma, or burns. Some of the sufferers may have one of the forms of cholecystoses (see the following).

When patients present as an emergency with acute cholecystitis or biliary colic, after full resuscitation and confirmation of the diagnosis, a cholecystectomy at the index admission has

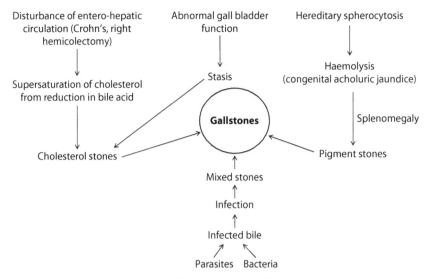

Figure 67.2 Formation of gallstones.

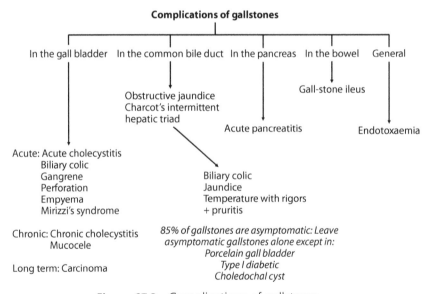

Figure 67.3 Complications of gallstones.

much to recommend it. But the ultimate definitive management depends upon the policy of the individual surgical unit. The management is described in **Figure 67.4**.

Complications of cholecystectomy

10. A, C
The operative mortality for cholecystectomy is less than 1%. Complications can occur in 10%–15% of cases. The serious complications of laparoscopic cholecystectomy fall into two areas – access-related complications and bile-duct injuries. Bile-duct injuries occur in

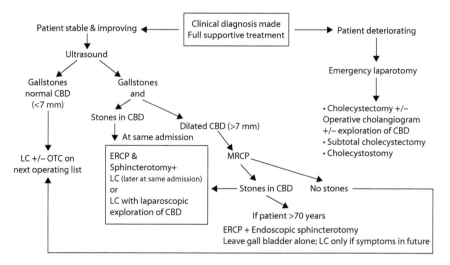

LC = Laparoscopic cholecystectomy
OTC = On table cholangiogram

Figure 67.4 Management of acute cholecystitis or biliary colic.

about 0.5% of cases, 15% of these being recognised at the time of operation whilst in the remainder postoperative problems point to the mishap.

Poor dissection and failure to identify the anatomy might contribute to this. Patients who develop jaundice should promptly undergo the full gamut of investigations – blood and imaging. Once damage to the CBD is suspected, the patient should be immediately referred to a tertiary hepatobiliary unit (see the following). The principles of management of iatrogenic damage to the CBD can be summarised as the following 4Rs:

- Recognise
- Refer
- Re-operate
- Review

Post-cholecystectomy syndrome can be defined as persistence of the same symptoms that the patient had preoperatively, which can happen in up to 15% of patients undergoing cholecystectomy. This is primarily due to performing the operation for the wrong reasons such as peptic ulcer disease, gastro-oesophageal reflux disease (GORD), or irritable bowel syndrome. Sometimes it can be due to a residual stone; 80% of stones in the CBD are due to infected bile.

Primary sclerosing cholangitis

11. B

It is an idiopathic fibrosing inflammatory condition. The majority of the patients are between 30 and 60 years, and there is a male predominance. Imaging studies and liver biopsies are all helpful in the diagnosis and in excluding cirrhosis. For patients with associated cirrhosis, liver transplantation would be the best option with 5-year survival rates in excess of 80%. There are two types – primary and secondary. (**Figure 67.5**)

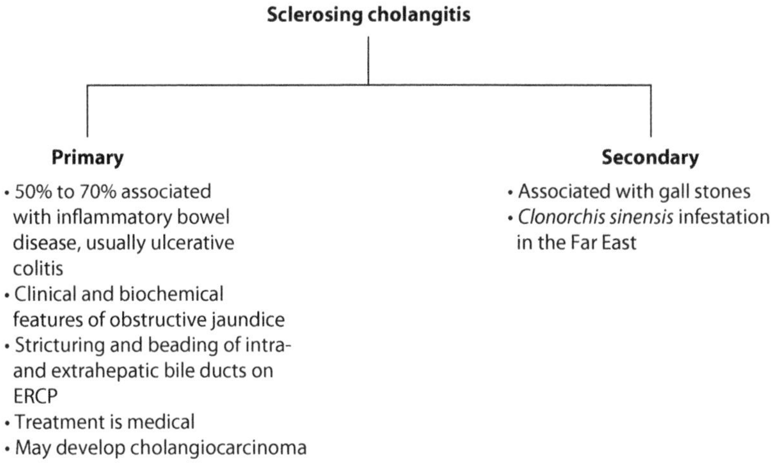

Sclerosing cholangitis

Primary	Secondary
• 50% to 70% associated with inflammatory bowel disease, usually ulcerative colitis	• Associated with gall stones
	• *Clonorchis sinensis* infestation in the Far East
• Clinical and biochemical features of obstructive jaundice	
• Stricturing and beading of intra- and extrahepatic bile ducts on ERCP	
• Treatment is medical	
• May develop cholangiocarcinoma	

Figure 67.5   Sclerosing cholangitis.

→ ## Parasitic infestation of the biliary tract (see Chapter 6)

12. C, D, E

The roundworm is commonly seen in Asia, Africa and Central America. Once it has become resident in the intestine, it enters the biliary tree through the ampulla of Vater and causes similar complications to gallstones – ascending cholangitis, biliary colic and acute pancreatitis. Hydatid disease can cause the same problems. Clonorchis sinensis is a fluke that is endemic in the Far East and occurs from eating infected fish. It can cause the same problems as described previously but with the added sinister complication of cholangiocarcinoma in the long term.

Answers to extended matching questions for gall bladder

1. B Acute cholecystitis

This patient has typical features of acute cholecystitis. However other intra-abdominal conditions must be excluded such as acute pancreatitis, retrocaecal acute appendicitis, perforated peptic ulcer, acute pyelonephritis and Curtis-Fitz-Hugh syndrome. Acute pancreatitis may co-exist when the patient is much more ill with features of shock. A serum amylase will clinch the diagnosis, although acute pancreatitis may exist in the presence of a normal amylase (**see Chapter 68, The pancreas**). Abdominal ultrasound (US) should exclude the other diagnoses; an erect chest x-ray (CXR) might show gas under the right dome of the diaphragm (although not infallible) to exclude perforated peptic ulcer. Curtiz-Fitz-Hugh syndrome is a condition that occurs in 15% to 30% of women with pelvic inflammatory disease (PID) with gonorrhoea or Chlamydia, producing flimsy adhesions (like 'violin-string') between the liver and right anterior abdominal wall causing the tenderness to simulate acute cholecystitis. US should exclude the condition or laparoscopy would confirm it (**see Chapter 65, The liver**)

The management consists of resuscitation, confirmation of diagnosis and institution of definitive treatment. Resuscitation should consist of analgesia (100 mg of pethidine), intravenous fluids and haematological and biochemical investigations including serum amylase and blood culture. This would show leucocytosis with raised liver functions tests (LFTs). Broad-spectrum antibiotics – a cephalosporin or gentamicin – are started.

Within the next 24 hours an abdominal US is done to confirm the diagnosis. If the US shows gallstones with a CBD less than 7 mm in diameter, the patient should undergo a laparoscopic cholecystectomy (LC) on the next urgent operating list at the same admission. If the CBD is not seen or dilated on US, a magnetic resonance cholangiogpancreatography (MRCP) is done to visualise the CBD; if the CBD is normal, a LC is done. If, however, the CBD contains stones, an endoscopic retrograde cholangiopancreatography (ERCP) is done with endoscopic papillotomy to remove the stones followed by LC, once again at the same admission. Endoscopic papillotomy to rid the CBD of the stones prior to LC is not universally accepted, particularly in the young patient because of long-term problems such as recurrent cholangitis from biliary-pancreatic reflux and the unproved possibility of cholangiocarcinoma. Therefore if the expertise of laparoscopic exploration of CBD is available, the procedure should be used in preference to endoscopic papillotomy **(see algorithm in Figure 67.4)**.

Should the patient not be operated upon at the index admission, she would settle down (this would happen in the majority) and discharged home to return for an interval cholecystectomy later. This management happens in some centres. This choice is unsatisfactory, as the patient would require two admissions, thus increasing the suffering; moreover, while the patient waits, she might develop another acute attack and worse still, the subsequent attack might be associated with acute pancreatitis.

2. E Biliary colic

Biliary colic occurs in up to one-quarter of patients with gallstones who present as an emergency. It is essentially an obstructive problem, whilst acute cholecystitis is an obstructive problem with superimposed infection. In biliary colic, the gall bladder contracts in trying to expel the stone into the cystic duct and CBD. This causes severe acute pain that waxes and wanes and which might last from a few minutes to hours. As it is a mechanical problem with no infection, the patient is in acute pain but not toxic. The stone drops back into the gall bladder and the patient is much better – feels almost as normal as prior to the attack. The underlying pathology in acute cholecystitis shows a red, inflamed gall bladder of varying thickness wrapped up in omentum forming an inflammatory mass. On the other hand in biliary colic, the gall bladder wall will be blue and thin-walled with minimal pericystic fluid.

The management is the same as in acute cholecystitis **(Figure 67.4)**, although the patient need not be put on antibiotics (if there is no leucocytosis and raised inflammatory markers) although some may put the patient on a short course. Technically the operation of LC is much easier because of the lack of adhesions.

3. A Carcinoma of the gall bladder (Figure 67.6)

This is a rare condition – 600 cases are diagnosed in the United Kingdom annually. Carcinoma is found as an incidental finding in 2% of patients undergoing cholecystectomy. Long-standing gallstones are regarded as a cause. However, the risk of developing cancer in those with galltones is regarded as no more than1%; hence cholecystectomy in symptomless gallstones is not recommended. However, patients with a porcelain gall bladder have a one-in-four chance of developing cancer; hence prophylactic cholecystectomy is advised in asymptomatic patients with porcelain gall bladder. Gall bladder polyp as a cause is debatable although the presence of carcinoma in adenomatous polyps larger than 1 cm has prompted some authorities to recommend prophylactic cholecystectomy in cholecystoses (see the following). The histology is adenocarcinoma. By the time the diagnosis is made it has already spread by contiguity to the liver bed (segments IV and V), the regional lymph nodes and transperitoneally; hence the poor prognosis, the 5-year survival being about 3% to 5%. Tumour markers such as CA 19-9 and CEA are elevated in the majority.

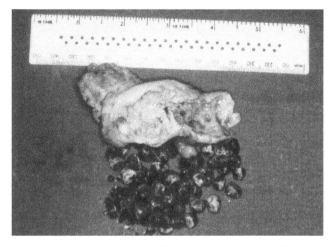

Figure 67.6 Specimen showing carcinoma of gall bladder.

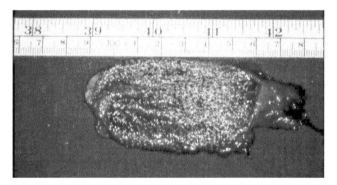

Figure 67.7 Specimen showing cholesterolosis or 'strawberry' gall bladder.

In very early disease where the cancer is diagnosed as an incidental finding and has not infiltrated beyond the muscle (T1), no further treatment is recommended. Radical surgery is considered in transmural spread without distant metastasis (T2 disease). This consists of *en bloc* resection of the gall bladder bed, including segments IV and V along with regional lymph nodes.

The term cholecystoses comprises a group of conditions that affect the gall bladder and which are often found on histological examination after LC: cholesterolosis ('strawberry' gallbladder) **(Figure 67.7)**, polyposis, cholecystitis glandularis proliferans and diverticulosis. In cholesterolosis there is accumulation of cholesterol crystals resulting from supersaturation of bile with cholesterol. All these conditions might clinically present with gallstones, which are usually pigment stones that occupy diverticula within the gall bladder wall.

4. C Empyema of the gall bladder (Figure 67.8)

If not promptly diagnosed and treated an empyema can perforate. **Perforation**, usually at the fundus, is the outcome of **gangrene**. The site might get walled off by omentum, forming a **pericholecystic abscess**. The gangrenous site might result in free perforation causing **biliary** or **purulent peritonitis** when the patient is extremely ill and toxic. Rarely the

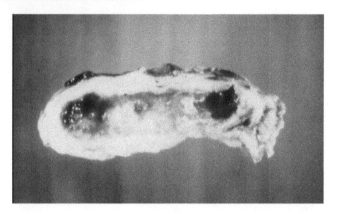

Figure 67.8 Specimen showing empyema of gall bladder.

pericholecystic abscess might get adherent to the duodenum and erode into it, forming a **cholecystoduodenal fistula** in due course.

This patient needs to be resuscitated with intravenous fluids, analgesics and broad-spectrum antibiotics. While the patient is being optimised, under US guidance percutaneous drainage of the pus is carried out and a catheter is left within the gall bladder. Once the patient has recovered, the catheter is removed and elective cholecystectomy carried out later. In this situation a 'fundus-first' approach should be done. On occasions, the gall bladder may be so densely embedded within the liver bed that a partial cholecystectomy might have to be undertaken. In this the anterior wall of the gall bladder and Hartmann's pouch are removed, leaving the posterior gall bladder wall within the liver bed; the mucosa is destroyed by diathermy leaving a drain.

5. F Gallstone ileus
Gallstone ileus accounts for almost one-fifth of all causes of acute small bowel obstruction after excluding external hernia and adhesions. Usually the diagnosis is made at laparotomy. The plain x-ray of abdomen and CT scan showing the classical radiological triad of small intestinal obstruction with a radio-opaque gallstone in the pelvis and gas in the biliary tree is an exception rather than the rule (**Figure 67.9a and b**).

A cholecystoduodenal fistula forms from long-standing chronic cholecystitis, resulting in a gallstone fistulating through into the duodenum. The stone gradually works its way down the small bowel and gets impacted in the narrow terminal ileum causing distal small bowel obstruction. The patient needs to be resuscitated with analgesics, intravenous fluids and nasogastric suction, following which a laparotomy is carried out. At operation the bowel is decompressed, the stone is removed through an enterotomy that is closed transversely, and the abdomen is closed without disturbing the site of the fistula and gall bladder.

6. D Mucocoele of the gall bladder (Figure 67.10)
After an attack of biliary colic, the gallstone remains impacted at the cystic duct, obstructing the egress of bile from the gall bladder into the CBD. This causes the bile and bile salts within the gall bladder to be reabsorbed; the gall bladder continues to secrete mucus thus becoming enlarged, tense and slightly tender, forming a mucocoele. Left untreated, infection might supervene causing an empyema with its attendant complications (see previously). The treatment is cholecystectomy. At cholecystectomy prior to starting dissection, aspiration of the gall bladder will make the procedure technically easier.

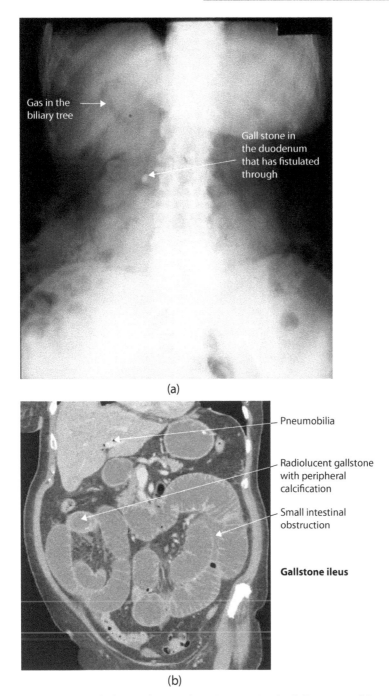

(a)

(b)

Figure 67.9 (a) Plain abdominal x-ray showing gas in the biliary tree. (b) CT scan of abdomen showing gallstone ileus. (Courtesy of Mr CR Selvasekar, consultant laparoscopic colorectal surgeon, The Christie Hospital, Manchester, UK.)

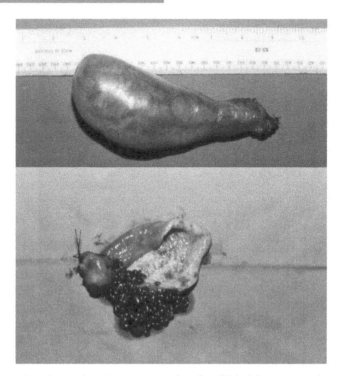

Figure 67.10 Specimen showing mucocoele of gall bladder – note absence of bile.

Answers to extended matching questions for bile ducts

1. G Carcinoma of lower end of common bile duct

This clinical picture of obstructive jaundice and an enlarged gall bladder could be from a carcinoma of the lower end of the CBD, carcinoma of the head of the pancreas or a periampullary carcinoma. However, the latter has a presentation which is slightly different in that the jaundice waxes and wanes. This is because the periampullary carcinoma in time outgrows its blood supply, which results in necrosis and sloughing of the growth allowing the egress of bile through the ampulla of Vater. This will alleviate the jaundice slightly only for the process to repeat itself as the cancer re-grows. At the same time the size of the gall bladder will also enlarge and get smaller.

This patient should have all the blood tests; LFTs will show the obstructive nature of the jaundice with possible liver derangement. Imaging should consist of US, which will show dilated intra and extra-hepatic ducts with a solid mass at the lower end of the CBD. Confirmation is done by ERCP and brush cytology of the growth; a biopsy may sometimes be possible. This is followed by CT scan of the abdomen and chest to assess local and distant spread. If there is no evidence of spread and radical resection is contemplated, laparoscopy +/– US is performed as a further staging procedure. If this is clear, a Whipple's pancreatoduodenectomy is performed. If curative resection is not possible, the patient should be palliated for the distressing symptom of pruritis by inserting a metallic stent endoscopically.

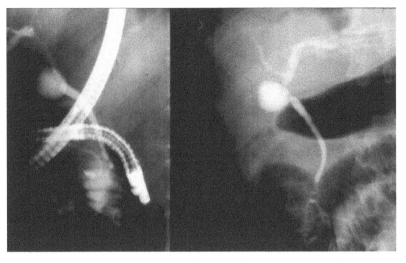

Figure 67.11   ERCP showing stricture of CBD with extravasation of contrast at site of cystic duct stump.

2. A Iatrogenic damage to CBD

This patient almost certainly has iatrogenic damage to the CBD. This happens most commonly in 'the easy cholecystectomy' where the CBD is mistaken for the cystic duct, which is then clipped and divided. The management should consist of excellent honest communication with the patient and family. All investigations – blood and imaging should be performed. US followed by the most appropriate imaging – ERCP **(Figure 67.11)**, PTC, MRCP – should be done. Once the pathology has been delineated, the patient should be referred to the tertiary hepatobiliary centre for definitive management.

The operative treatment would depend upon the classification of injury. There are several classifications, which follow:

- Bismuth 1982 Types 1 to 5
- Strasberg 1995 Types A to E – Type E re-classified according to Bismuth E1 to E5
- Bismuth and Majno 2001

Discussion of all the previously listed types of injuries is beyond the scope of this book. The lower the injury, the easier the repair. Choledochoduodenostomy (for low CBD injury), hepatico-jejunostomy to a Roux loop (CHD injury) and side-to-side left hepatico-jenunostomy to a Roux loop (for hilar injury) are the broad choices of operative repair.

The causes of CBD strictures are classified in **Figure 67.12.**

3. F Mirrizi's syndrome (Figure 67.13a and b)

This condition occurs in less than 0.5% of patients with gallstones. It results in the following situations:

- i.   The cystic duct at the neck of the gall bladder runs parallel to the common hepatic duct (CHD)
- ii. A stone is impacted at the cystic duct or neck of the gall bladder
- iii. Mechanical obstruction of the CHD by the stone or an inflammatory mass
- iv. Intermittent or progressive obstructive jaundice with recurrent ascending cholangitis

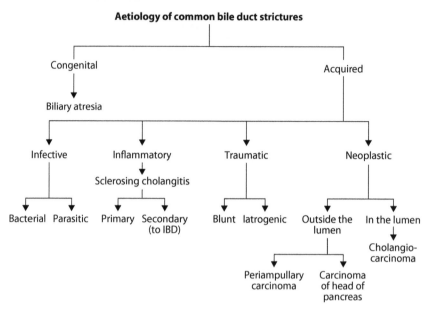

Figure 67.12   Aetiology of common bile duct strictures.

Regarding the types of this syndrome, there are 2 classifications – McSherry and Csendes. The reader is asked to look up other sources for details of this classification.

The diagnosis is suspected and confirmed by ERCP. As the patients are ill with features of septic shock, initial resuscitation (intravenous fluids, vitamin K, antibiotics) is followed by insertion of a stent into the CBD; this will relieve the patient's jaundice and improve the general condition. Once optimised, 2 to 3 weeks later, definitive surgery in the form of open cholecystectomy is carried out. Other complicated procedures might be necessary depending upon the type of the syndrome. Ideally, Mirrizi's syndrome is managed in a tertiary hepatobiliary centre.

4. E Post-cholecystectomy syndrome

Post-cholecystectomy syndrome is defined as persistence or recurrence of the same symptoms that the patient had prior to cholecystectomy. It is estimated that 5% to 40% of patients might suffer from this condition although a more realistic incidence is probably 15%. The causes can be classified as the following: (i) of biliary origin and (ii) of non-biliary origin. The incidence is about equal in both groups.

The causes of biliary origin are the following:

a. Residual stone in CBD (see the following)
b. Iatrogenic stricture of CBD (see previously)
c. Biliary dyskinesia (dysfunction of sphincter of Oddi)

The causes of non-biliary origin are the following:

d. Cholecystectomy done for the wrong reason, e.g., patient suffering from irritable bowel syndrome (IBS) and had incidental gallstones; cause of patient's abdominal pain was not properly investigated in the first instance
e. Gastro-oesophageal reflux disease (GORD)
f. Peptic ulcer disease
g. Chronic pancreatitis

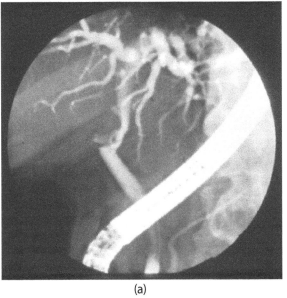

(a)

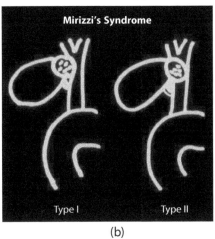

(b)

Figure 67.13   (a) ERCP showing Mirizzi's syndrome. (b) Schematic diagram showing two types of Mirizzi's syndrome.

The entire gamut of investigations is carried out: OGD, US, CT scan, MRCP and ERCP
(Figure 67.14). After thorough reinvestigation, this patient might continue to have typical
biliary pain in the absence of gallstones and pancreatic pathology. Biliary dyskinesia would
be the diagnosis in such a patient (a diagnosis by exclusion), especially in the presence
of abnormal LFTs. Such a patient should be considered for endoscopic papillotomy or
transduodenal sphincterotomy and sphincteroplasty (open operation). Prior to such a
procedure, some surgeons might consider dynamic biliary scintigraphy and sphincter of Oddi
manometry. After such operations, more than half of such patients are pain-free.

5. D Residual stone in CBD
This patient has typical features of a retained stone in the CBD. All the routine haematological
and biochemical investigations, including LFTs and prothrombin time, should be done,

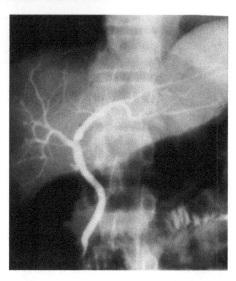

Figure 67.14   Normal ERCP in post-cholecystectomy syndrome.

followed by US and ERCP **(Figure 67.15)**. If ERCP is not possible, PTC is carried out **(Figure 67.16)** after taking the usual precautions (making sure that prothrombin time is normal and giving vitamin K if necessary). The patient is treated by endoscopic papillotomy. If the stone is larger than 1 cm, then extracorporeal shock wave lithotripsy (ESWL) through the endoscope to fragment the stone followed by extraction is carried out.

6. C Sclerosing cholangitis
Sclerosing cholangitis can be primary or secondary **(Figure 67.5)**. Primary sclerosing cholangitis is regarded as an autoimmune condition, as evidenced by elevated IgM, perinuclear anti-neutrophil cytoplasmic antibody and anti-smooth muscle antibodies. It is seen in association with ulcerative colitis in 50% to 70% of patients. The condition, when long-standing, can result in cholangiocarcinoma.

Secondary is usually due to infestation with clonorchis sinensis prevalent in the Far East, gallstones and in those who have undergone repair of CBD stricture for iatrogenic damage, particularly those having had multiple operations. The majority of patients have intra and extrahepatic ducts involvement. Delineating the anatomy of the entire biliary tree is the keystone in diagnosis. ERCP is most sensitive in showing the typical changes – irregular, beaded appearance of bile ducts with multifocal stricturing; liver biopsy shows periductal and focal fibrosis.

It is a condition that is a challenge for the hepatologist. Supportive treatment for symptoms of cholangitis, pruritis, jaundice and abdominal discomfort is the mainstay of management. In selected cases repeated ductal balloon dilatations, endoscopic stenting and hepatico-jeunostomy have been worthwhile palliative procedures. Liver transplantation, when feasible, gives good results.

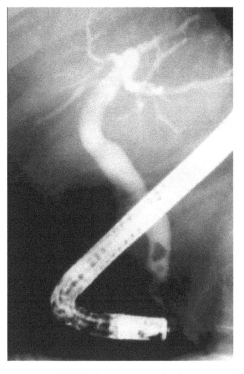

Figure 67.15   ERCP showing residual stone in CBD.

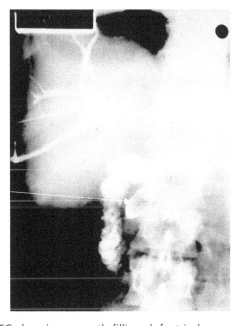

Figure 67.16   PTC showing smooth filling defect in lower end of CBD from residual stone in CBD.

7. B Stone in the CBD

This is a typical presentation called 'Charcot's intermittent hepatic triad'. The triad consists of high temperature with rigors from ascending cholangitis, biliary colic due to the stone going up and down the CBD and jaundice from obstruction to the flow of bile; in addition pruritis is a distressing symptom with the patient having scratch marks all over her body and shiny fingernails being the outcome of incessant scratching.

Her symptoms suggest that she is suffering from the effects of septic shock – toxicity with hyperdynamic circulation. She is resuscitated with analgesia, intravenous fluids, vitamin K and broad-spectrum antibiotics. All blood tests are carried out, including blood culture. An US is done to confirm the diagnosis, which will show dilated CBD with a stone and inflamed gall bladder. ERCP is next performed **(Figure 67.17)**. Once stone in the CBD is seen, an endoscopic papillotomy and stone extraction is carried out (see previously). The patient would now improve after the acute biliary obstruction has been relieved. At the same admission a laparoscopic cholecystectomy is carried out as a definitive procedure.

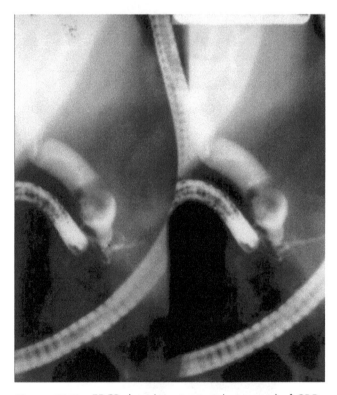

Figure 67.17 ERCP showing stone at lower end of CBD.

68 The pancreas

Pradip K Datta

Multiple choice questions

→ ## Anatomy and physiology

1. Which of the following statements are true?

A The pancreas weighs about 80 g.
B The head of the pancreas lies over the body of L2 vertebra.
C The uncinate process lies behind the superior mesenteric vessels.
D The splenic artery travels along the upper border of the pancreas.
E The potential space in front of the pancreas is called the greater sac.

2. The following statements are true except:

A The vast majority of the acinar tissue is endocrine.
B The pancreatic tail snugly fits into the splenic hilum.
C The pancreatic digestive enzymes are acidic in nature with a pH of 7.
D The islets of Langerhans have three types of cells producing hormones.
E The amount of pancreatic juice secreted is 1200 to 1500 mLs in 24 hours.

→ ## Investigations

3. Which of the following statements in biochemical investigations are true?

A Elevation of serum amylase is diagnostic.
B Estimation of serum lipase is more sensitive and specific.
C Urinary amylase and amylase-creatinine clearance is highly accurate.
D Pancreatic exocrine function can be measured.
E Serum elastase measurement is useful.

4. Which of the following statements in imaging is not true?

A Ultrasonography (US) is the initial investigation of choice in the jaundiced patient.
B When doing a computed tomography (CT) scan, initially an unenhanced scan must be done followed by a scan after intravenous contrast injection (CECT).
C While doing a magnetic resonance cholangiopancreatography (MRCP), intravenous secretin injection helps to determine any obstruction to the pancreatic duct.
D Plain abdominal x-ray showing a sentinel loop can be diagnostic.
E Endoscopic retrograde cholangiopancreatography (ERCP) should always be preceded by a plain radiograph.

→ ## Pancreatic injury

5. Which of the following statements are true?

A Pancreatic injury is common following blunt abdominal trauma.
B Pancreatic injury is often accompanied by damage to the liver, spleen and duodenum.
C The serum amylase is raised in most cases of pancreatic injury.
D A CECT scan will delineate the damage.
E In doubtful cases, urgent ERCP is helpful.

6. Which of the following statements is false?

A All patients with pancreatic trauma should undergo an exploratory laparotomy.
B Pancreatic duct disruption requires surgical exploration.

C Severe injury to the duodenum and the head of the pancreas requires a pancreatoduodenectomy.

D After conservative management for pancreatic injury, duct stricture and pseudocyst may occur as complications.

E During splenectomy, iatrogenic injury to the pancreatic tail can occur.

Acute pancreatitis

7. Which of the following statements is false?

A Acute pancreatitis accounts for 3% of hospital admissions for abdominal pain in the United Kingdom.

B Acute pancreatitis is classified into mild and severe.

C 80% of cases are mild acute pancreatitis, with a mortality rate of 1%.

D 20% are severe acute pancreatitis, with a mortality of 20%–50%.

E In all cases of acute pancreatitis, there is a marked rise in serum amylase.

Aetiology

8. Which one of the following causes of acute pancreatitis is due to a congenital anatomical variation?

A Gallstones

B Hereditary pancreatitis

C Pancreas divisum

D Autoimmune pancreatitis

E Hyperparathyroidism

9. Which of the following statements are true regarding the aetiology of postoperative acute pancreatitis?

A Following ERCP the incidence of acute pancreatitis is 10%.

B Therapeutic intervention during ERCP has a higher incidence.

C Patients after cardiothoracic surgery may develop acute pancreatitis.

D The post-gastrectomy patient might develop acute pancreatitis.

E In a post-cholecystectomy patient, acute pancreatitis may be due to a retained stone.

Severity

10. Which of the following are not parameters to assess the severity of acute pancreatitis in either Ranson or Glasgow score?

A Age

B White cell count

C Serum amylase

D Serum calcium

E Blood urea

Signs

11. Which of the following signs have been known to occur in acute pancreatitis?

A Trousseau's sign

B Courvoisier's sign

C Murphy's sign

D Grey–Turner's sign

E Cullen's sign

Pseudocysts

12. Which of the following statements are true with regard to pseudocysts?

A Pseudocysts occur within the first week of onset of acute pancreatitis.

B They can be confused with cystic neoplasms.

C The majority of them require intervention.

D They can arise after blunt trauma to the upper abdomen.

E Gastrointestinal bleeding may be a complication of a pseudocyst.

Complications

13. Which of the following statements are true with regard to complications in acute pancreatitis?

A Patients with severe acute pancreatitis require a CECT scan to detect pancreatic necrosis.

B In severe acute pancreatitis, a laparotomy must be done in all cases of pancreatic necrosis.

C Aneurysm of the superior mesenteric artery can occur.

D The vast majority of patients with peripancreatic sepsis can be treated conservatively.

E Pleural effusion is seen in 10%–20% of patients.

Extended matching questions

→ Diagnoses

1 Acute pancreatitis
2 Carcinoma of the head of the pancreas
3 Chronic pancreatitis
4 Periampullary carcinoma
5 Pseudocyst of the pancreas

Choose and match the correct diagnosis with each of the scenarios that follow:

A A 65-year-old man complains of intense itching and jaundice of 6 weeks' duration. He has upper abdominal discomfort and has noticed of late that his urine is deep yellow in colour and his stools are pale. He has some weight loss. On examination he is deeply jaundiced with scratch marks all over his body; abdominal examination reveals a globular discrete mass in the right upper quadrant.

B A 10-year-old boy presents with upper abdominal pain of 2 weeks' duration. This is associated with upper abdominal distension, nausea, intermittent vomiting and some weight loss, which his parents attribute to his loss of appetite. On abdominal examination he looks unwell, with a smooth mass in his epigastrium that is tense and does not move with respiration. There is bruising over the skin of the epigastrium and, when questioned about it, he says it was the result of his falling off his bike and the handlebar sticking into his tummy.

C A 45-year-old woman, who is on the waiting list for a laparoscopic cholecystectomy, presents as an emergency with severe epigastric pain radiating to the back and the rest of the abdomen of 3 hours duration. She has nausea, vomited a few times and has retching. On examination she is tachypnoeic, has tachycardia and a blood pressure of 110/60 mmHg. She is slightly icteric. Abdominal examination reveals a Cullen's sign, extreme tenderness all over the abdomen with rebound and rigidity.

D A 55-year-old man complains of intermittent jaundice associated with itching. This is associated with anorexia, weight loss and upper abdominal discomfort. On examination the patient is anaemic, has scratch marks over his body, is slightly jaundiced and has a gall bladder that is just palpable.

E A 50-year-old male patient presents with dull aching pain in his epigastrium and umbilical areas radiating to the back for 6 months. He has episodes of exacerbation of this pain, which last for 1 or 2 days. This is associated with nausea and occasional vomiting and diarrhoea most days. He has lost some weight over this period. Two months ago he was diagnosed with type 2 diabetes and is on oral medication. He admits to more than average alcohol consumption. Clinical examination shows no abnormality except for generalised tenderness.

Answers to multiple choice questions

→ Anatomy and physiology

1. A, B, C, D

The pancreas weighs about 80 g. The head constitutes 30% of the gland mass, whilst the remaining 70% is accounted for by the body and tail. The head of the pancreas overlies the second lumbar vertebra. This anatomical fact is important in severe blunt upper abdominal trauma where there may be a 'fracture' of the pancreas at the junction of the head and neck because of the gland being crushed between the force of injury and vertebral body.

The uncinate process is a hook-shaped projection from the head toward the left behind the superior mesenteric artery and vein and in front of the aorta. A cancer affecting the uncinate process would soon involve these vessels making the growth almost unresectable. The splenic artery travels along the upper border of the pancreas to enter the splenic hilum. The position of this artery is significant in that if there were a gastric ulcer in the posterior wall of the stomach it would penetrate into this artery causing severe haematemesis.

The space in front of the pancreas is called the lesser sac or omental bursa. The surgical importance of this is the formation of a pseudo-cyst of the pancreas, which is a collection of fluid in this space that occurs as a complication of acute pancreatitis.

2. A, C

The vast majority (80%–90%) of the pancreatic acinar tissue is exocrine. This is in the form of lobules. The pancreatic digestive enzymes, secreted in response to a meal, are a bicarbonate-rich fluid with a pH of 8.4.

The pancreatic tail fits into the splenic hilum, an important anatomical fact during the procedure of splenectomy. At the operation the surgeon needs to dissect the pancreatic tail very carefully off the hilum so as not to inadvertently damage it while ligating the main splenic vessels. The islets of Langerhans are groups of endocrine cells distributed throughout the pancreas and consist of the following different cell types: β cells producing insulin constitute 70%, α cells producing glucagon comprise 20% and δ cells producing somatostatin make up the remainder. The total amount of pancreatic juice secreted by the cells lining the ducts is about 1200 to 1500 mLs.

→ Investigations

3. B, D, E

Serum lipase is more specific and sensitive than serum amylase in the diagnosis of acute pancreatitis; unfortunately it is not readily available. Pancreatic exocrine function can be assessed by directly measuring the amount of pancreatic enzymes secreted by giving a stimulus. This can be in the form of a test meal, as in the Lundh test. The other alternative is to give an intravenous injection of secretin or cholecystokinin (CCK) and measuring the output of gastric and duodenal juices by duodenal intubation using a triple lumen tube. Measurement of the enzyme elastase in stool is specific and used widely; a low level of faecal elastase indicates pancreatic exocrine insufficiency.

Elevation of serum amylase is suggestive but not diagnostic of acute pancreatitis. It might be elevated in other causes of acute abdomen such as perforation of a hollow viscus, mesenteric vascular occlusion, retroperitoneal haematoma and sialadenitis. It therefore follows that urinary amylase and amylase-creatinine ratios are equally not diagnostic.

4. D

Plain abdominal x-ray in suspected acute pancreatitis has no role except to exclude the possibility of perforated hollow viscus (duodenal ulcer) looking for gas under the diaphragm. The presence of a sentinel loop is not specific of acute pancreatitis. It is just a loop of bowel affected by ileus and occurs in intra-abdominal infection or inflammation from any cause and is in no way diagnostic of acute pancreatitis.

Ultrasonography is always the initial investigation in the jaundiced patient. It will show gallstones, the width of the common bile duct and space-occupying lesions in the liver and pancreas. It is highly operator dependent and not effective in the obese patient and in the presence of excessive gas in the bowel.

An unenhanced CT always precedes a CECT to look for pancreatic or biliary calcification. After contrast injection, arterial and venous phases delineate accurately space-occupying lesions. During an MRCP, secretin injection will show emptying of the pancreatic duct, thereby showing the absence or presence of obstruction. A plain x-ray of the abdomen should precede an ERCP to look for calcification.

→ Pancreatic injury

5. B, C, D, E
Pancreatic injury is rare in blunt upper abdominal trauma because of the retroperitoneal position of the organ. Therefore, for the pancreas to be injured, the force of trauma has to be severe. Thus if pancreatic injury occurs, almost certainly the liver, duodenum and spleen are damaged. Penetrating injuries to the back or upper abdomen have a higher incidence of pancreatic damage. The overall damage can be from simple contusion or laceration to major parenchymal and duct destruction; in extreme cases there may be massive destruction of the pancreatic head where inevitably concomitant duodenal injury will be present. The integrity or otherwise of the pancreatic duct will decide the management.

A raised serum amylase indicates damage to the pancreas. A CECT scan will delineate the damage, failing which an urgent ERCP should be done. MRCP, whilst providing the answer in some patients, may be difficult to interpret.

6. A
All pancreatic injuries do not need a laparotomy. A stable patient following a blunt injury should be thoroughly assessed. Disruption of the main pancreatic duct is an indication for an operation. Penetrating injury in an unstable patient needs urgent surgical exploration. The procedure depends upon the type of injury. Minor parenchymal injuries are treated by haemostasis and closed drainage; a transected gland at the body and tail **(Figure 68.1)** requires a distal pancreatectomy +/- splenectomy; sometimes an end-to-side pancreatojejunostomy to a Roux loop of jejunum might be possible; finally, severe injuries to the head of the pancreas and duodenum require an emergency pancreatoduodenectomy – a procedure to be carried out by the expert hepatobiliary surgeon.

Stricture of the pancreatic duct might occur later, resulting in recurrent acute pancreatitis. Treatment in such patients is pancreatic resection distal to the strictured duct. A pseudocyst might develop in the aftermath of the injury. This is treated appropriately depending upon whether the main pancreatic duct is patent. When the duct is patent percutaneous aspiration will suffice; in the presence of a disrupted duct, cystogastrostomy is carried out. Unrecognised damage to the pancreatic tail during splenectomy may cause a pancreatic fistula or a pseudocyst.

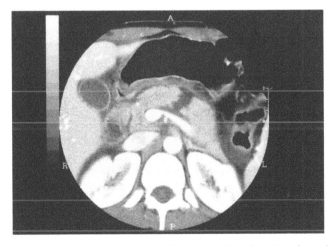

Figure 68.1 CT scan showing a pancreatic transection due to a bicycle handlebar injury. A distal pancreatectom was performed.

Acute pancreatitis

7. E

All cases of acute pancreatitis do not cause a rise in serum amylase. A normal amylase in acute pancreatitis might occur when the disease is so severe that the entire pancreas has been destroyed and there is not enough pancreatic tissue left to elaborate the enzyme. Thus, a normal amylase in the presence of acute pancreatitis indicates a poor prognosis. A normal amylase level might also be because the blood has been taken too late and the patient has recovered from the acute attack, which has been transient.

Acute pancreatitis accounts for 3% of hospital admissions for abdominal pain in the United Kingdom. Once diagnosed with the condition the patient is categorised as a mild or severe case (see the following), 80% turning out to be mild with a mortality of 1%. The remaining 20% who are severe have a mortality rate ranging from 20% to 50%.

Aetiology

8. C

During the development of the pancreas, most of the dorsal duct drains into the proximal part of the ventral duct. The proximal part of the dorsal duct persists as accessory pancreatic duct. Late in the development or in the postnatal period, the ducts fuse. Failure of fusion of the embryological dorsal and ventral parts of the pancreas results in pancreas divisum. In such a situation, which occurs in 5% to 10%, the dorsal pancreatic duct acts as the main pancreatic duct draining most of the pancreas through the minor or accessory papilla. The ventral duct drains only the uncinate process.

These papillae in pancreas divisum are smaller than the major papilla. Therefore a large volume of secretions flowing through these minor papillae cause incomplete drainage with back pressure, resulting in pancreatitis. In patients with recurrent acute pancreatitis where no cause can be found (idiopathic), pancreas divisum should be considered. It is estimated that 25% to 50% of patients who suffer from recurrent acute pancreatitis, chronic pancreatitis, or pancreatic pain have pancreas divisum as the cause.

Confirmation of the diagnosis is by MRCP, EUS, or ERCP. Treatment can range from endoscopic sphincterotomy and stenting, sphincteroplasty, pancreatojejunsotomy, or resection of the pancreatic head.

The other listed causes are not of congenital origin. Up to 70% of cases of acute pancreatitis are accounted for by gallstones, while 25% arise from alcohol abuse. The remainder are from other rare causes. A familial condition called hereditary pancreatitis seen in patients in their teens is associated with mutations of the cationic trypsinogen gene. For the aetiology of acute pancreatitis, see **Figure 68.2**.

9. B, C, D, E

The incidence of acute pancreatitis following ERCP is 1%–3%. This incidence rises if therapeutic intervention such as sphincterotomy or balloon dilatation is carried out. When cardiothoracic surgery involves cardiopulmonary bypass, acute pancreatitis is one of the postoperative complications. It is suggested that a mild subclinical injury to the pancreas occurs from cardiopulmonary bypass; if hypoperfusion follows in the postoperative period ischaemic pancreatic necrosis occurs. It has been estimated that in the postoperative period hyperamylasemia occurs in 32% whereas the incidence of acute pancreatitis is 2.7%.

Acute pancreatitis can also occur in the postoperative period following gastrectomy possibly due to manipulation in the region of the ampulla of Vater. A residual stone in the common bile duct can cause acute pancreatitis from obstruction to the pancreatic duct; this will be much more common if there is a common channel.

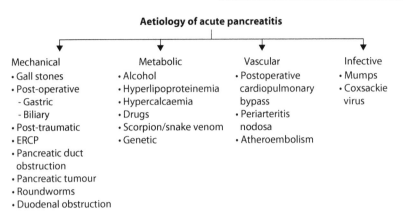

Aetiology of acute pancreatitis

Mechanical
• Gall stones
• Post-operative
  - Gastric
  - Biliary
• Post-traumatic
• ERCP
• Pancreatic duct
  obstruction
• Pancreatic tumour
• Roundworms
• Duodenal obstruction

Metabolic
• Alcohol
• Hyperlipoproteinemia
• Hypercalcaemia
• Drugs
• Scorpion/snake venom
• Genetic

Vascular
• Postoperative
  cardiopulmonary
  bypass
• Periarteritis
  nodosa
• Atheroembolism

Infective
• Mumps
• Coxsackie
  virus

Figure 68.2 Aetiology of acute pancreatitis.

Severity

10. C
Serum amylase is not one of the blood results for assessing severity. Besides the other tests mentioned in the list, serum albumin, arterial oxygen saturation, lactic dehydrogenase (LDH) and aspartate transaminase (AST) are the other important factors. The assessment of severity is very important, so much so this must be performed within 48 hours of making the diagnosis. This is because of the difference in outcome in patients with mild and severe disease and therefore the pattern of management.

In intensive care units, where the patient with severe disease should be managed, the APACHE II scoring system is used; a score of 8 or more denotes severe disease. A Glasgow score of 3 or more, C-reactive protein of >150 mm/L and worsening clinical state with organ dysfunction are indicators of severe disease and hence poor prognosis. A patient with a body mass index of >30 has a greater chance of developing complications.

Signs

11. D, E
Cullen's and Grey-Turner's signs **(Figure 59.1 in Chapter 59)** are not pathognomonic although, if present, are very suggestive of acute haemorrhagic pancreatitis. Grey–Turner's sign (originally described in leaking abdominal aortic aneurysm) is a bluish discoloration of the flanks as a result of blood tracking along the fascial planes. Cullen's sign (originally described in ruptured ectopic pregnancy) is haemorrhage around the umbilicus, the blood having tracked there through the falciform ligament. These signs can also occur in liver trauma, ruptured spleen and mesenteric vascular occlusion.

Trousseau's sign or carpal spasm is seen in tetany. It is produced by arterial occlusion of the forearm above the systolic blood pressure with a sphygmomanometer cuff. Courvoisier's sign (sometimes called law) states that a palpable, nontender gall bladder is the outcome of a malignant distal common bile duct obstruction such as a carcinoma of the head of the pancreas, common bile duct, or periampullary region and not due to stones. This is because gallstones would have rendered the gall bladder contracted from previous cholecystitis. Murphy's sign is elicited in acute cholecystitis. When a patient is asked to take a deep breath, as mild pressure is exerted in the right upper quadrant beneath the costal margin at the level of the ninth costal cartilage, the patient has a catch in the breath due to pain.

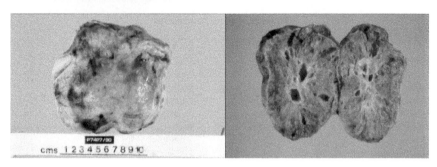

Figure 68.3 Benign cystadenoma of the head of the pancreas.

Pseudocysts

12. B, D, E

Occasionally a pseudocyst can be confused with a cystic neoplasm (Figure 68.3). This can be distinguished by aspiration under image guidance or EUS, the fluid being sent for CEA and amylase levels and cytology. High levels of CEA are seen in a mucinous neoplasm, while high amylase levels are in favour of a pseudocyst. A pseudocyst can occur after blunt abdominal trauma, which causes acute or chronic pancreatitis. This resolves in 4 to 6 weeks with the formation of a pseudocyst. Gastrointestinal bleeding might be a presenting feature as a complication of acute pancreatitis if a pseudocyst ruptures into the stomach or duodenum.

After acute pancreatitis, a pseudocyst usually takes up to 4 weeks or more to develop.

Spontaneous resolution of a pseudocyst occurs in most cases because the majority have a communication with the main pancreatic duct.

Complications

13. A, C, D, E

Patients with severe acute pancreatitis are treated in the ITU and, while they are there, a CECT is carried out at least every other day to look for pancreatic necrosis. If the CECT shows areas of reduced enhancement and peripancreatic fluid collection with pockets of gas within, it means that the necrosis is infected. Confirmation of infection is carried out by fine-needle aspiration cytology. If the fluid is purulent and obviously infected, the patient is treated with antibiotics and by insertion of the widest possible tube drains. The fluid can be viscous and the drain might require regular flushing and repeated replacement. If the sepsis worsens despite vigorous measures, a pancreatic necrosectomy should be undertaken – a challenging procedure not often encountered.

A superior mesenteric artery aneurysm can occur. The anatomical position of the superior mesenteric vessels behind the neck and between the inferior border and uncinate process of the pancreas makes these vessels vulnerable to compression and inflammation, resulting in an aneurysm (sometimes referred to as a pseudoaneurysm) of the artery and thrombosis of the vein. Rupture of such an aneurysm can be a very serious complication and challenging to treat. Pleural effusion does occur following acute pancreatitis and may require aspiration. The complications of acute pancreatitis are shown in Figure 68.4.

Answers to extended matching questions

1. C Acute pancreatitis

This patient has acute pancreatitis of biliary origin. She needs to be resuscitated forthwith with analgesia and intravenous fluids, and blood investigations need to be carried out, in particular, serum amylase. This would be elevated to well over 1000 IU. If the serum amylase is not elevated, the diagnosis of acute pancreatitis should then be confirmed by a CECT scan.

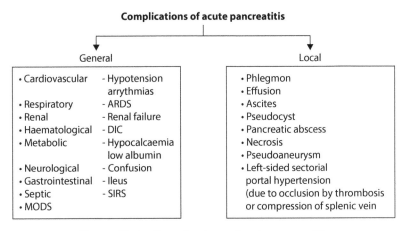

Figure 68.4   Complications of acute pancreatitis.

The patient is then stratified as mild or severe acute pancreatitis by using one of several scoring systems available – Glasgow, Ranson and APACHE II, and managed accordingly.

If the stratification shows mild acute pancreatitis the patient is treated on the surgical ward. If she has severe acute pancreatitis she is managed in the high-dependency unit (HDU) or intensive care unit (ICU) depending upon the clinical needs. In either situation full supportive therapy is instituted with analgesia, intravenous fluids and close monitoring.

An US of the biliary tract is repeated or an MRCP is done to look for a stone in the common bile duct (CBD). If there is a stone in the CBD, an ERCP and endoscopic papillotomy is carried out to remove the stone/s. At the same admission a laparoscopic cholecystectomy is carried out a few days later.

The management in severe acute pancreatitis is outlined in **Figure 68.5**.

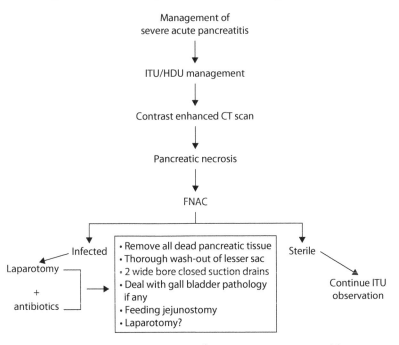

Figure 68.5   Management of severe acute pancreatitis.

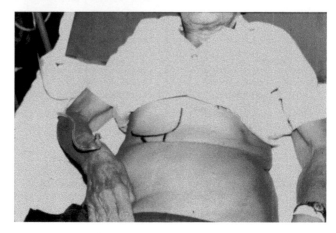

Figure 68.6   Jaundiced patient with distended gall bladder and hepatomegaly from carcinoma of head of pancreas.

2. A Carcinoma of the head of the pancreas

This patient has painless obstructive jaundice with a distended gall bladder and weight loss – classical features of a carcinoma of the head of the pancreas **(Figure 68.6)**. Clinically Courvoisier's sign (see previously) will be positive. Besides all the usual blood tests, he needs an US followed by a CT scan to see the solid mass in the head of the pancreas obstructing the lower end of the CBD. If there is evidence of secondaries in the abdomen, as there usually are, this is unresectable. After discussion in a multidisciplinary team meeting, plans for the best palliation should be made.

The patient will require palliation from itching, which is obtained by insertion of a mesh-metal stent in the common bile duct **(Figure 68.7)**. If the growth is big enough to cause gastric outlet obstruction, then at the same time mesh-metal stent is placed in the duodenum. If for any reason that palliation cannot be achieved by minimal-access surgical means described previously, then an open operation is performed. The procedure referred to as

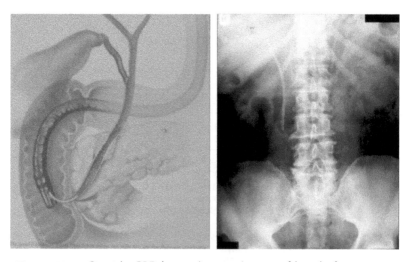

Figure 68.7   Stent in CBD bypassing carcinoma of head of pancreas.

triple bypass consists of cholecystojenunostomy, anterior gastrojejunostomy and side-to-side jejunojejunostomy.

If the patient is fit, the cancer is localised and there are no distant metastases (after thorough loco-regional staging), the patient should be considered for pancreatoduodenectomy (see the following).

3. E Chronic pancreatitis

This patient has alcoholic chronic pancreatitis with exocrine and endocrine dysfunction (diarrhoea and diabetes). He should have all the usual haematological and biochemical investigations, including estimation of 24-hours faecal fat. Confirmation is by US and CECT and ERCP to visualise the anatomy of the pancreatic duct. He should be managed by the physicians for his pancreatic insufficiency (endocrine and exocrine) and the pain clinic for analgesia.

A group of patients might have pancreatic ductal stones in a dilated duct with strictures seen on pancreatogram on ERCP, an appearance called 'chain of lakes'. Such patients could be considered for bypass surgery of side-to-side pancreato-jejunostomy to a Roux loop of jejunum. During the procedure, obviously the stones would be removed. The aetiology and pathology of chronic pancreatitis is shown in **Tables 68.1** through **68.3**.

Table 68.1   Aetiology of chronic pancreatitis

- Stricture of pancreatic duct: trauma, acute pancreatitis, pancreatic cancer
- Hereditary
- Infantile malnutrition
- Juvenile tropical chronic pancreatitis – Kerala in South India
- Hypercalcaemia
- Hyperlipidaemia
- Gall stones
- Pancreas divisum

Table 68.2   Macroscopic pathology of chronic pancreatitis

- Enlarged
- Hard from fibrosis – focal or diffuse
- Ducts: dilated, strictured and ectatic, occluded with calcified stones and gelatinous proteinaceous fluid
- Cyst formation – pseudo-cysts usually connected to the ductal system and hence unlikely to resolve spontaneously
- Splenic vein thrombosis – left-sided sectorial portal hypertension
- Cancer in those with disease for >20 years

Table 68.3   Microscopic pathology of chronic pancreatitis

- Ductular metaplasia
- Acinar atrophy
- Hyperplasia of duct epithelium
- Interlobular fibrosis

4. D Periampullary carcinoma

This patient has intermittent obstructive jaundice (where the icterus waxes and wanes) with a gall bladder that is minimally palpable. His anaemia and weight loss should point to an underlying malignant lesion in the region of the lower end of the CBD. As the jaundice is intermittent, the diagnosis is obviously a periampullary carcinoma. In this condition, as the tumour grows, the patient's jaundice gets deeper; as the carcinoma outgrows its blood supply, there is necrosis and sloughing of the cancer, resulting in alleviation of the jaundice. He needs an US, CECT, EUS and biopsy of the lesion. If the staging shows no distant spread, the patient should next undergo the final staging procedure of laparoscopy and laparoscopic US to look for small peritoneal or liver secondaries. If there are no secondaries, the patient should then be considered for radical pancreatoduodenectomy (Whipple's procedure).

This major procedure, the domain of the specialist hepatobiliary surgeon, can be done in two stages, a choice that depends on the individual surgeon. In the first stage the CBD is stented to alleviate the patient's jaundice, so as to minimise the risks of a major procedure in a jaundiced patient. The second stage of resection is carried out 10 days or so later. Following the resection, usually a pylorus-preserving reconstruction is carried out.

5. B Pseudocyst of the pancreas

This young boy has developed a pseudocyst of the pancreas. About 4 weeks ago his bicycle injury produced blunt upper abdominal trauma with transient acute pancreatitis. Although his symptoms at that time were not severe enough for him to seek help, there was a contused pancreas, which later resulted in a pseudocyst. He needs an US and CT scan for confirmation, although the latter may not be carried out to prevent undue radiation in a young boy. Moreover, the CT scan would not give much additional information that the US would not have provided.

This is to be followed by a decision as to the best method of treating him, whether by percutaneous or endoscopic drainage, or the open operation of cystogastrostomy. In an adult one would wait for 6 weeks and until the cyst is 6 cm in diameter to consider intervention by minimal access or open surgery of cystogastrostomy. The classification of pancreatic cysts is shown in **Figure 68.8**.

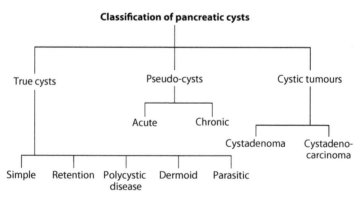

Figure 68.8 Classification of pancreatic cysts.

The small and large intestines

CR Selvasekar and Pradip K Datta

→ ## Anatomy of the small intestine

1. Which of the following statements are true?

A The proximal 40% is the jejunum.
B The arterial supply in the form of arcades distinguishes jejunum from ileum.
C The fat in the ileal mesentery is thicker.
D The small bowel has autonomic innervation from the splanchnic nerves.
E The jejunum has rich lymphoid aggregates in the form of Peyer's patches.

→ ## Anatomy of the large intestine

2. The following statements are true except:

A The taenia coli are responsible for the colonic haustrations.
B The colon on both sides are closely related to the ureters.
C The sigmoid colon has no mesentery at the back.
D The marginal artery of Drummond is the anastomosis between the superior and inferior mesenteric arteries.
E The superior mesenteric artery supplies the large bowel until the proximal two-thirds of the transverse colon.

→ ## Physiology of the small and large intestines

3. Which of the following statements are true?

A The principal function of small intestine is the digestion of food and absorption of fluid and nutrients.
B Absorption of bile salts and vitamin B12 occur in the jejunum.

C The main function of colon is to absorb water.
D 1 litre of ileal contents enter the large bowel every 24 hours.
E Faecal residue reaches the caecum 24 hours after a meal.

→ ## Ulcerative colitis (UC)

4. Which of the following statements are true in ulcerative colitis (UC)?

A In 95% of cases, the disease starts in the rectum and spreads proximally.
B Patients might present as an emergency with fulminating disease in 5% to 10%.
C It is a diffuse disease affecting all the layers of the large bowel.
D Granulomas are a typical microscopic feature.
E The transverse colon is affected in toxic megacolon.

5. Which of the following is not a complication of UC?

A Carcinoma.
B Primary sclerosing cholangitis.
C Internal fistulae.
D Ankylosing spondylitis.
E Perforation.

6. Which of the following are barium enema findings in UC?

A Loss of haustrations.
B Narrow contracted colon.
C Increase in the presacral space.
D Cobblestone appearance.
E Backwash ileitis.

7. What is colonoscopy routinely used for in UC?

A To assess the extent of the disease.
B To distinguish it from Crohn's disease.

C To monitor the response to treatment.

D To carry out surveillance for the development of cancer.

E To assess severity in acute cases.

8. Which of the following criteria indicate severe disease in UC?

A More than six motions per day.

B Pyrexia of more than 37.5°C.

C Tachycardia >90/minute.

D Tachypnoea >20/minute.

E Hypoalbuminaemia < 30 g/L.

9. Which UC patients have an enhanced risk of developing cancer?

A Those who have had the disease since childhood.

B Those who have had the disease for over 10 years.

C Those who have had a very severe first attack.

D Those who have the entire colon involved.

E Those who have another member of the family with the disease.

10. Which of the following drugs are not used in the medical treatment of UC?

A Prednisolone.

B 5-ASA compounds.

C Infliximab.

D Azathioprine.

E Isoniazid.

11. In the management of a severe attack of UC, which of the following is not true?

A Every patient needs a proctocolectomy after resuscitation.

B Daily plain abdominal x-ray is taken to assess transverse colon dilatation.

C Parenteral high-calorie alimentation is instituted.

D Intravenous hydrocortisone is given.

E Azathioprine or cyclosporin A is given.

12. What are the indications for surgery in UC?

A Severe fulminating disease not responding to vigorous medical treatment.

B Severe dysplastic change or cancer on biopsy.

C Non-compliance of medical treatment.

D Chronic steroid-dependent disease requiring large doses.

E Extraintestinal disease.

13. The following statements regarding surgery in UC are true except:

A In the emergency situation, total abdominal colectomy and ileostomy should be the procedure of choice.

B Proctocolectomy and ileostomy are associated with the lowest complication rate.

C Restorative proctocolectomy with an ileoanal pouch should be considered in all patients.

D Colectomy with ileorectal anastomosis is the most favoured procedure.

E Ileostomy with a continent intra-abdominal pouch is not often done.

14. Which of the following statements are true regarding an ileo-anal pouch procedure?

A This should be considered in any case of inflammatory bowel disease that requires surgery.

B The patient must have normal anal sphincter.

C In 15%, the pouch has to be removed.

D Small bowel obstruction as a postoperative complication occurs in 10%–15%.

E Pouchitis occurs on 30%.

➡ # Crohn's disease (Regional enteritis)

15. Which of the following statements is not true of Crohn's disease (CD)?

A The ileum is affected in 60% of cases.

B It affects the entire thickness of the bowel.

C Non-caseating granulomas are found in only 60% of patients.

D One in 10 patients have a first-degree relative with the disease.

E A patient can be cured of CD once the diseased small or large bowel is removed.

16. Which of the following pathological features is not found in CD?

A Internal fistulae.
B Serpiginous and aphthous ulcers.
C Chronic inflammation involves all layers of the bowel wall.
D Pseudopolypi.
E Cobblestone mucosa.

17. Which of the following can cause acute presentation of CD?

A Mimicking acute appendicitis.
B Perforation.
C Intestinal obstruction.
D Toxic megacolon.
E All of the above.

18. Which of the following are true of large-bowel CD?

A 50%–75% will have an anal lesion.
B Non-caseating giant-cell granulomas are most common in anorectal disease.
C In a strictured area, malignancy can occur.
D A perianal abscess or a fissure might be the first presenting feature.
E Surgery is usually indicated.

19. Which of the following is not a clinical presentation of CD?

A Bloodstained diarrhoea.
B Intermittent abdominal pain.
C Mass in the right iliac fossa.
D Typical evening rise of temperature.
E Pneumaturia and urinary tract infections.

20. Which of the following statements about imaging in CD are true?

A Small-bowel enema is the imaging of choice in small-bowel disease.
B Barium enema and colonoscopy should be done for large-bowel disease.
C MRI is the 'gold standard' for perianal fistulae.
D CT scan is used for suspected intra-abdominal abscess and internal fistulae.
E All of the above.

21. Which of the following drugs are used in the treatment of CD?

A Steroids.
B 5-ASA compounds.
C Azathioprine.
D Infliximab.
E All of the above.

22. The following operations are done in CD depending upon the indications except:

A Restorative proctocolectomy with ileoanal pouch.
B Strictureplasty.
C Proctocolectomy and ileostomy.
D Colectomy and ileorectal anastomosis.
E Segmental resections.

23. Which of the following statements about inflammatory bowel disease (UC and CD) is not true?

A Patients must be managed jointly by the physician and surgeon.
B Surgery, when indicated, must be as radical as possible.
C Patients must be given a good trial of optimum medical treatment prior to surgery.
D There is more chance of a cure after surgery in UC than in CD.
E In emergency presentation, patients must be vigorously resuscitated prior to operation and managed in the ITU postoperatively.

➔ Infections of the small and large intestine

24. Which of the following statements are true?

A *Campylobacter* is the most common cause of gastroenteritis in the United Kingdom.
B *Yersinia* can cause acute appendicitis.
C *Actinomycosis* might present as an enterocutaneous fistula.
D AIDS patients might develop opportunistic intestinal infections.
E The presence of *Clostridium difficile* might necessitate an operation.

→ ## Tumours of the small intestine

25. **Which of the following statement/s are not true?**

A Small bowel tumours account for 10% of all gastrointestinal neoplasms.

B Small bowel adenocarcinoma is more common in patients with CD.

C Carcinoid tumour of the appendix does not gives rise to carcinoid syndrome.

D Hodgkin's lymphoma is the most common type of lymphoma to affect of the small bowel.

E The ileum is the most common site for GIST (gastrointestinal stromal tumour).

26. **Which of the following statements are true of carcinoid tumour?**

A Appendicular carcinoid are most commonly found incidentally.

B The substance that causes the syndrome is 5-hydroxytryptamine (serotonin).

C The syndrome can affect the heart in the form of mitral stenosis.

D Tumours in the ileum and rectum might metastasise to the liver long after removal of the primary tumour.

E The syndrome produces features affecting the pulmonary, cardiovascular and gastrointestinal systems.

→ ## Tumours of the large intestine

27. **Which of the following statements are true about familial adenomatous polyposis (FAP)?**

A More than 80% of patients have a positive family history.

B The condition is inherited as an autosomal recessive condition.

C Family members should be screened until the age of 50 years.

D Restorative proctocolectomy with an ileal pouch is the preferred surgical treatment.

E Hereditary non-polyposis colorectal cancer (HNPCC) occurs as an autosomal dominant condition.

28. **Which of the following statements are not true?**

A Colonic adenomas occur more on the right and carcinomas in the left colon.

B Sporadic adenomas are different from those of FAP.

C The larger the adenoma the greater the chance of dysplasia.

D Colorectal cancer incidence falls with screening programmes.

E Mutations of the *APC* gene occurs in two-thirds of colonic adenomas and carcinomas.

29. **Which of the following statements are true?**

A Almost 60% occur in the rectosigmoid region.

B At the time of diagnosis, one-third will have liver metastases.

C 20% of patients present as an emergency with intestinal obstruction.

D Reduced dietary fibre is associated with an increased risk.

E All of the above.

30. **Which one of the following statements is false?**

A Right colonic cancers present with features of anaemia.

B Left colonic cancers present with rectal bleeding and obstructive symptoms.

C Even for an experienced colonoscopist, the failure rate to visualise the caecum is 10%.

D Intravenous urography (IVU) should be routinely done.

E Synchronous cancers occur in 5%.

31. **Which of the following statements are true?**

A Thorough preoperative assessment and staging should be done with colonoscopy, US and spiral CT.

B Resection is not done if the patient has liver metastases.

C If, at operation, hepatic metastases are found, biopsy should be done.

D Hepatic resection for metastases should be considered as a staged procedure.

E Left colonic carcinomas presenting with intestinal obstruction should be treated as a staged procedure.

32. The following statements are true except:

A Routine follow up after surgery for colorectal cancer is a waste of resources.

B In resectable hepatic metastases from colorectal cancer the 5-year survival is 30%.

C In Dukes' stage A the 5-year disease-free survival is 90%.

D Enhanced recovery programme (ERP) reduces hospital stay considerably.

E Preoperative chemotherapy in colonic cancer has a role in selected patients.

→ Intestinal diverticula

33. Which of the following statements are true?

A Duodenal diverticulum might result from a long-standing duodenal ulcer.

B Jejunal diverticula might give rise to malabsorption problems.

C A Meckel's diverticulum can cause severe lower gastrointestinal haemorrhage.

D A suspected Meckel's diverticulum is best imaged by a barium meal and follow through.

E Pain originating in a Meckel's diverticulum is located around the umbilicus.

34. Which of the following statements are false?

A In the Western world, 75% of the population over the age of 70 has diverticular disease.

B A low-fibre diet causes the disease.

C These diverticula consist of mucosa, muscle and serosa.

D Those with perforation have a higher mortality than those with an inflammatory mass.

E Sepsis is the principal cause of morbidity.

35. Which of the following is not a complication of diverticular disease of the colon?

A Paracolic abscess.

B Fistulae.

C Lower gastrointestinal haemorrhage.

D Carcinoma.

E Stricture.

36. Which of the following are not true in complicated diverticular disease?

A Urinary symptoms might be the predominant presentation at times.

B Profuse colonic haemorrhage might occur in 17%.

C Fistulae occur in 5% of cases.

D The most common fistula is enterocolic.

E In acute diverticulitis, CT scan is the 'gold standard' for imaging.

37. Which of the following is not a cause of colo-vesical fistula?

A Carcinoma of rectosigmoid.

B Radiation enteritis.

C Crohn's colitis.

D Diverticular disease.

E Amoebic colitis.

38. In the surgical treatment of diverticular disease, which of the following statements are true?

A Colonoscopy must be carried out in all elective cases.

B Barium enema is essential prior to elective operation.

C Primary resection and end-to-end anastomosis must be carried out in all cases.

D Hartmann's operation is the procedure of choice in perforated diverticulitis.

E In vesicolic fistula, a one-stage operation can usually be done.

→ Vascular anomalies of the intestine

39. Which of the following statements are true?

A Thrombosis most often affects the origin of superior mesenteric artery (SMA), while embolism affects the middle colic artery.

B Pain out of proportion to the physical findings is the cardinal clinical feature.

C Angiodyplasia most commonly occur in the sigmoid colon.

D Ischaemic colitis affects mostly the splenic flexure.

E Ischaemic colitis might result in a colonic stricture.

→ Intestinal stomas

40. The following statements are true except:

A A loop transverse colostomy is the ideal method to defunction an anterior resection.

B An end ileostomy is always a permanent procedure.

C A loop ileostomy is always a temporary procedure.

D An end colostomy can be a permanent or a temporary procedure.

E Stoma complications are common.

→ Enterocutaneous fistula

41. Which of the following statements are true?

A The most common cause is a surgical complication.

B In the management attention to nutrition is important.

C The 'cut-off point' between a high-output and low-output fistula is 500 mL/day.

D At operation end-to-end anastomosis should be carried out in all cases.

E Always look for a cause when a fistula does not heal spontaneously.

→ Laparoscopic colorectal surgery

42. Which of the following randomised controlled trials (RCTs) demonstrate the benefits of laparoscopic surgery over traditional surgery for colorectal cancer?

A COST.

B COLOR 1 and 2.

C CLASICC.

D LAFA.

E DREAMS.

43. Which of the following statements regarding laparoscopic colorectal surgery is not true?

A Decreased surgical site infection with minimal access technique.

B Conversion rate of >10% is considered a good outcome.

C Decreased length of stay in the hospital.

D Decreased long-term survival.

E NICE (National institute for health and clinical excellence) recommends that cancer should be suitable for laparoscopic resection and the surgeon should be experienced in performing both open and laparoscopic procedures.

44. The following statements are true except:

A Laparoscopic approach is particularly suitable for colonic resection in Crohn's disease.

B Radical lymphadenectomy in cancer is as good as in open surgery.

C Operative times are longer.

D Tattooing the lesion preoperatively is performed as per the unit policy.

E The dissection is usually performed in a medial to lateral direction.

Extended matching questions

→ Diagnoses

1 Angiodyplasia
2 Carcinoma of caecum
3 Carcinoma of descending colon
4 Colovesical fistula
5 Crohn's disease
6 Enterocutaneous fistula
7 Ischaemic colitis
8 Paracolic abscess
9 Perforated diverticulitis
10 Ulcerative colitis

Match the diagnoses with the clinical scenarios that follow:

A A 52-year-old woman complains of being 'out of sorts' for almost 3 months. During this time she has felt unduly short of breath in doing her daily household work and going up one flight of stairs. Her haemoglobin is 8.6 g/dL, and her general practitioner (GP) felt a vague mass in the right iliac fossa.

B A 75-year-old man complains of sudden onset of very severe lower abdominal pain radiating to the entire abdomen for 6 hours. On examination he is hypotensive (blood pressure of 80/60 mmHg), tachycardic (pulse rate of 120/minute) and cold and clammy; abdominal examination shows severe lower abdominal tenderness with rigidity and rebound tenderness.

C A 48-year-old man complains of altered bowel habit in the form of episodes of diarrhoea that last for few days when he has several loose stools a day with passage of mucus and sometimes blood. During the bouts of loose stools he has colicky abdominal pain mostly on the right side. A few months ago he had an acute perianal abscess drained, which has not completely healed. Examination shows vague abdominal tenderness with a discharging perianal sinus.

D An 80-year-old man complains of rectal bleeding on and off for 10 months; the blood is dark red and associated with diarrhoea off and on. He has dull left-sided abdominal pain and vague tenderness. He had a myocardial infarction 3 years ago and now is on medical treatment for angina.

E A 65-year-old man complains of frequency of micturition and passing foul-smelling urine that sometimes contains some semi-solid material. A few weeks ago he was treated as an emergency for severe bilateral loin pain diagnosed as acute bilateral pyelonephritis. Clinical examination does not show any abnormality but urine examination confirms heavy growth of *E. coli*.

F A 38-year-old woman complains of blood-stained diarrhoea with passage of slime on and off for 6 months. She passes 4 to 6 loose motions a day; this is associated with tenesmus and generalised vague abdominal pain and a feeling of ill health. She has lost some weight and recently found a raised, tender red swelling on her shin.

G A 70-year-old man complains of increasing constipation for 6 months. He has a bowel movement once in 2 or 3 days whereas previously he was regular. In spite of taking laxatives there has been no improvement. He has occasional bright-red rectal bleeding when he strains at stool. Examination reveals no abnormality.

H A 65-year-old man presents as an emergency with severe rectal bleeding that is dark red. He has features of hypovolaemia with tachycardia, with a blood pressure of 100/60 mmHg (his normal being 140/90). In the past he has had episodes of small rectal bleeds. He is known to have aortic stenosis for which he has been investigated in the past and did not need any treatment.

I A-55-year old man, a known sufferer from CD, was admitted as an emergency with high temperature with rigors and a tender mass in the right iliac fossa, which on CT scan showed an abscess. This was drained percutaneously under antibiotic cover, following which his general condition improved. However, after removal of the catheter for drainage of the pus he developed a leakage of small-bowel contents from the site.

J A 68-year-old woman, who has never been ill, presents as an emergency with temperature and rigors and generally feeling unwell for 3 days. She has not moved her bowels during this period and has vomited a few times. On examination she is pyrexial with a tender boggy mass in the left iliac fossa.

Answers to multiple choice questions

→ ### Anatomy of the small intestine

1. A, B, C, D

The jejunum is regarded as constituting two-fifths (40%) of the small bowel length. It is the distribution of the arterial supply that distinguishes the jejunum from the ileum. The jejunal arterial branches join each other in a series of anastomosing loops to form arterial arcades, which are single in the upper jejunum and double in the lower jejunum. From these arcades long straight arteries pass into the mesenteric border of the jejunum, producing narrow windows between the branches.

In the ileum the arcades are more numerous (three to five) and lie nearer to the ileal wall so that the straight arteries from the arcades are much shorter before they enter the mesenteric border of the ileum. Therefore, the windows between the arteries are broader. Another distinguishing feature is that the ileal mesentery contains much more fat. Autonomic nerves from the splanchnic nerves accompany the blood vessels. The parasympathetic augments peristaltic activity and secretion while the sympathetic inhibits and is vasoconstrictor.

Peyer's patches are aggregated lymphoid follicles concentrated in the ileum. These are sometimes visible through the muscle wall of the ileum as whitish plaques in the mucus membrane. When enlarged they form the lead point in childhood ileocaecal intussusception.

→ ### Anatomy of the large intestine

2. C

The sigmoid colon is completely invested in peritoneum and hangs free on a mesentery called the sigmoid mesocolon. Within the layers of this mesocolon travel the blood vessels and accompanying lymphatics. In resection of the sigmoid colon, the mesocolon has to be dissected with meticulous care to excise all the lymph nodes in cancer surgery.

The taenia coli, three in number, are flat bands of longitudinal muscle that extend from the base of the appendix to the rectosigmoid junction. They pull the colon to cause the haustrations. On both sides, the ascending colon on the right and descending colon on the left are very closely related to the ureters. This fact is of the utmost importance during colonic resections to identify the ureters and prevent iatrogenic damage.

The superior mesenteric artery, the artery of the midgut, supplies the large bowel until the junction of the right two-thirds and left one-third of the transverse colon. At this site is the anastomosis between the branches of the superior mesenteric and inferior mesenteric arteries (artery of the hindgut) so that there is a complete arterial supply of the entire colon along its margin referred to as 'the marginal artery of Drummond'.

Physiology of the small and large intestine

3. A, C, D
The main function of the small intestine is the digestion of food and absorption of nutrients and fluid. Carbohydrates and proteins are broken down by pancreatic enzymes and absorbed through the brush border by movements of the villi (by the 'villus pump') aided by smooth muscle contraction. Movements of the villi are regulated by Meissner's plexus of nerves stimulated by the intestinal hormones. The jejunum is the main site for absorption of water, amino acids, sugars, short chain fatty acids, vitamins, minerals and glycerol. The terminal ileum is the principal site of absorption bile salts and vitamin B12, the site being referred to as the entero-hepatic circulation.

Should a part of the jejunum be removed, the ileum will take on its function, but resection of the terminal ileum as in a right hemicolectomy or disease as in regional ileitis, will result in disturbance of the entero-hepatic circulation causing reduced bile acid pool with a greater chance of developing gallstones and deficiency of B12, and vitamins A, D and K. The small intestine is the site of synthesis of plasma lipoproteins.

Movements of the muscular coats of the small bowel is controlled by Auerbach's plexus of nerves. These two plexuses of nerves are referred to as the enteric nervous system, which controls the various intestinal hormones, abnormal secretions of which result in neuro-endocrine tumours.

The principal colonic function is to absorb water; 1 litre of ileal contents enter the caecum every 24 hours to be converted into 150 to 250 mL of faeces. The normal colonic microflora (e.g., bacteroides) cause fermentation of dietary fibre leading to the formation of short-chain fatty acids, an important metabolic fuel for the colonic mucosa. Normally faecal residue reaches the caecum 4 hours, and the rectum 24 hours, after a meal.

Ulcerative colitis

4. A, D, E
In 95% of cases the disease starts in the rectum and spreads proximally as a continuous process. If the disease does not conform to this pattern, the diagnosis of UC should be in doubt. While most patients present electively, 5% to 10% present as an emergency with acute fulminating disease. The inflammation is diffuse and continuous, being confined to the mucosa and superficial submucosa. One of the complications is toxic megacolon, which typically affects the transverse colon. If on a plain x-ray the diameter is >6 cm toxic colon should be diagnosed.

The disease does not affect all the layers of the bowel. If it does so, the diagnosis is not UC. Microscopically granulomas are not a feature. They occur in Crohn's disease and tuberculosis, in the latter they are caseating. Crypt abscesses are seen on histology, the walls of the crypts of Lieberkuhn being infiltrated by inflammatory cells which re also seen in the lamina propria.

5. C
Internal fistulae is not a complication of UC. This is because the disease process is confined to the mucosa and submucosa. Fistula tend to occur when the pathology is a transmural inflammation as in Crohn's disease. The complications in UC are carcinoma when the disease is present for longer than 10 years; primary sclerosing cholangitis is an extraintestinal

manifestation that might lead to cirrhosis and liver failure while cholangiocarcinoma might rarely occur. Ankylosing spondylitis is 20 times more common in UC than in the general population. Large-bowel perforation is a very serious complication with a mortality of 40%. The complications of ulcerative colitis are enumerated in **Tables 69.1** and **69.2**.

6. A, B, C, E

In UC the barium enema findings are lack of haustrations and a narrow contracted colon, which are the result of fibrosis **(Figure 69.1a)**. For the same reason, in long-standing disease, the rectosigmoid is pulled forward away from the sacrum thus creating an increase in the presacral or retro-rectal space **(Figure 69.1b)**. Backwash ileitis is another prominent radiological feature that can be confirmed on colonoscopy. Cobblestone appearance is not a feature seen in UC.

7. A, B, C, D

Colonoscopy has a vital role in the management of UC. Once suspected, colonoscopy is carried out to see the extent of the disease and confirm the diagnosis by taking biopsies at various levels. Macroscopically the presence of continuous disease and absence of 'skip lesions' (normal bowel between diseased bowel) will set it apart from Crohn's colitis. The procedure is also useful as a follow up to monitor response to medical treatment. Patients who have had the disease for >10 years have an increased chance of developing cancer. So such patients should undergo annual colonoscopic surveillance and biopsies to exclude dysplasia or cancer. It should not be done in the acute stage for fear of causing a perforation.

8. A, B, C, E

It is important to recognise severe disease in UC because treatment should be aggressive, otherwise the patient might go into fulminant disease or perforation. Severe UC should be diagnosed if the patient has more than six bloody stools a day, pyrexia of >37.5°C, tachycardia

Table 69.1 Local complications in ulcerative colitis

- Acute dilatation or toxic megacolon
- Perforation
- Massive haemorrhage
- Benign stricture
- Inflammatory polyposis
- Carcinoma
- Anorectal complications
  - Fissure
  - Anorectal abscess and fistula
  - Rectovaginal fistula

Table 69.2 Systemic (remote or distant) complications in ulcerative colitis

- Arthritis
- Ankylosing spondylitis
- Skin lesions: Erythema nodosum, Pyoderma gangrenosum
- Eye lesions
- Liver and biliary tract disease – sclerosing cholangitis
- Stomatitis
- Oesophagitis

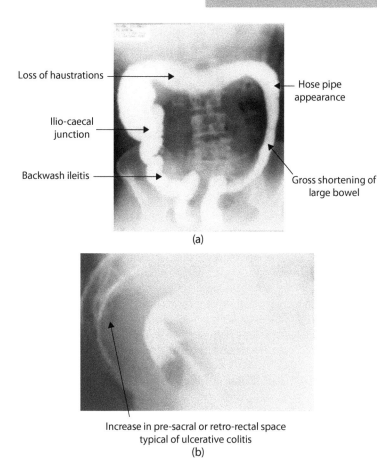

Loss of haustrations

Hose pipe appearance

Ilio-caecal junction

Backwash ileitis

Gross shortening of large bowel

(a)

Increase in pre-sacral or retro-rectal space
typical of ulcerative colitis
(b)

Figure 69.1 (a) Barium enema in ulcerative colitis. (b) Barium enema in ulcerative colitis lateral view.

of >90/minute and an albumin of <30g/L. Tachypnoea, although important, is not one of the criteria. Inflammatory markers such as ESR (>30 mm hour) and CRP are elevated. Plain abdominal x-rays are done to look for toxic megacolon.

9. A, B, C, D
Patients with inflammatory bowel disease, particularly UC, have an increased risk of developing carcinoma, the risk increasing with the duration of the disease **(Table 69.3)**. After 10 years the risk is 1% increasing to 10%–15% at 20 years and 30% at 30 years. Those who have had the disease since childhood, had a severe first attack and in whom the entire colon is involved (pancolitis) have an enhanced risk for carcinoma. Therefore patients with pancolitis of >10 years are entered into annual colonoscopic surveillance. The value of such screening programmes is questioned because most UC patients who develop cancer (3.5%) present between attendances for colonoscopic screening. Colonoscopic screening is a routine when multiple biopsies are taken to detect dysplasia, which can occur in a flat mucosa or in dysplasia-associated lesions or mass (DALMs).

10. E
Isoniazid is not a drug used in UC. It is used in tuberculosis. The other four drugs on the list are used in the medical treatment of UC. The 5-ASA (5-aminosalicylic acid) compounds are given both systemically and as enemas and can be used on a long-term basis. Prednisolone

Table 69.3 Factors associated with enhanced liability to malignant change in ulcerative colitis

- A clinically severe first attack
- Involvement of the entire colon
- Chronic continuous symptoms
- Onset in childhood or early adult life
- Long-standing disease (>10 years)

is used in acute exacerbation locally and systemically for its anti-inflammatory action. As 'steroid-sparing' drugs, azathioprine and cyclosporin are used during remission. Recently infliximab and adalimumab, as monoclonal antibodies have been used as a tumour necrosis factor α (TNF-α) antagonist that plays a central role in inflammatory cascades.

11. A
A severe case of UC is a medical emergency and occurs in about 10% of patients with UC; every patient does not require a proctocolectomy. The patient should be treated in a HDU or ICU. Daily (if necessary, twice daily) plain abdominal x-ray is taken to look for toxic dilatation of the transverse colon, presence of mucosal islands or intramural gas. Full supportive treatment is instituted in the form of intravenous fluids and alimentation, intravenous hydrocortisone and steroid enemas or suppositories. If improvement does not occur within 3–5 days, surgery should be undertaken. This should be a team decision between the surgeon and gastroenterologist to ensure that surgery is undertaken at the optimum time. Sometimes, immunosuppressive drugs and infliximab might be considered to prevent emergency surgery. As the patient is on steroids, one should be very wary of a silent perforation.

12. A, B, D, E
The indications for surgery in UC are best enumerated as those carried out as an emergency and those carried out as an elective procedure (**Tables 69.4** and **69.5**). Noncompliance by the patient should not be an indication. The patient should be educated and help from a psychologist sought if necessary.

13. D
Colectomy with ileorectal anastomosis is a rare procedure because the rectum is diseased in the vast majority. The patient needs regular rectal surveillance for malignancy. Although the

Table 69.4 Indications for emergency/urgent operations in ulcerative colitis

- Failure of medical treatment during an acute exacerbation
- Perforation
- Acute toxic megacolon
- Severe haemorrhage

Table 69.5 Indications for elective operations in ulcerative colitis

- Intractability and chronic invalidism
- Risk (or actual development) of malignant change
- Retardation of growth and development
- Local anorectal complications
- Remote or systemic complications

operation prevents a stoma and has minimal risk of sexual dysfunction, it has largely been replaced by restorative proctocolectomy.

In the emergency or urgent situation, total abdominal colectomy and terminal ileostomy should be the procedures of choice. Once the patient has fully recovered, ileoanal pouch procedure might be considered as a second stage. In the elective situation proctocolectomy and permanent terminal ileostomy does have the lowest complication rate although all patients should be considered for restorative proctocolectomy. Ileostomy with a continent intra-abdominal pouch is not often done.

14. B, C, D, E

Prior to considering a pouch procedure, the patient's anal sphincter must be normal. Some surgeons establish this by doing a rectal examination and asking the patient to tighten the anal sphincter, whilst others might do sphincter pressure studies and anal manometry. Once a pouch procedure is carried out, 15% of patients have the pouch removed for poor pouch function. Overall 50% of patients with ileoanal pouch have a very good quality of life, while 35% are less satisfied but keep their pouch.

Small-bowel obstruction as a postoperative complication occurs in about 10%–15%, while pouchitis occurs in about 30%. Pouchitis is inflammation of the pouch, which might result in increased frequency, tenesmus, bleeding, purulent discharge, malaise and fever with raised inflammatory markers. It responds to metronidazole and ciprofloxacin. Sometimes the condition might be asymptomatic.

A pouch procedure should not be done in any case of inflammatory bowel disease. It must be done only in ulcerative colitis. However, there is an entity called indeterminate colitis where after much deliberation a pouch procedure might be offered but only after warning the patient of the failure rate of 25%–30%.

Crohn's disease (Regional enteritis)

15. E

Crohn's disease is not a curable disease, let alone by resectional surgery. It can recur in other parts of the gastrointestinal tract even after removal of a diseased section of the bowel. Hence resection for CD must always be conservative, and as little bowel as possible should be sacrificed.

While CD affects any part of the gastrointestinal tract, the ileum is most commonly affected, which is in 60%, sometimes along with the right colon. Hence, when it was described by Crohn, Ginzburg and Oppenheimer in 1932, they called the disease 'Regional Ileitis'. The large bowel alone is involved in almost one-third, while in 5% the stomach and duodenum is site of the disease. Perianal disease is present in 50%–75% of sufferers. Patients with small-bowel disease have perianal involvement in 25%, whilst three-quarters of those with large bowel Crohn's have perianal disease.

The condition affects the entire thickness of the bowel in the form of transmural inflammation. Although non-caseating giant cell granulomas are regarded as the hallmark of the disease, they are found in only 60% of patients and most common in anorectal involvement. Amongst the sufferers 1 in 10 patients have a first-degree relative with the disease.

16. D

Pseudopolypi do not occur in CD. It is a feature seen in advanced chronic UC where chronic mucosal ulceration is associated with granulation tissue and regeneration of normal mucosa, also called inflammatory polyposis; this occurs in 25% of UC patients. Internal fistulae are a common complication due to the transmural inflammation, involving all layers of the bowel wall, causing the diseased bowel to penetrate into neighbouring structures – skin, urinary bladder, colon, small bowel and vagina. Macroscopically, the diseased bowel shows

Table 69.6   Local complications in Crohn's disease

- Fistulae: External-Entero-cutaneous/Colo-cutaneous
  – Entero-vaginal/Colo-vaginal
  – Perianal
- Internal–Entero-enteric
  – Entero-colic
  – Entero-vesical/Colo-vesical
- Abscesses
- Stricture
- Carcinoma
- Haemorrhage
- Perforation
- Toxic megacolon

Table 69.7   Distant (metastatic) complications in Crohn's disease

- Infected: Skin– Pyoderma gangrenosum
- Erythema nodosum
  – Eyes – Keratitis; episcleritis
  – Joints – Septic arthritis
  – Septicaemia
  – Psoas abscess
- Non-infected:
  – Polyarthropathy
  – Venous thrombosis
  – Physical retardation
  – Hepatobiliary disease
  – Ureteric strictures

serpiginous (snake-like) deep mucosal and aphthous ulcers; mucosal oedema between the ulcers gives the classical 'cobblestone' appearance. The complications of CD are enumerated in **Tables 69.6** and **69.7**.

17. E
All the previously mentioned presentations are the methods by which CD can present clinically as an acute emergency. The dilemma is obviously the management in each of these situations. When a patient has been opened as 'acute appendicitis' and the diagnosis is CD, the appendix should be removed provided the caecum and appendix are not grossly involved with an inflammatory mass. When perforation occurs, after optimum resuscitation, the bowel containing the perforation is resected with end-to-end anastomosis removing as little bowel as possible. On opening a patient with acute intestinal obstruction from structuring, after thorough optimisation, localised resection and end-to-end anastomosis is the treatment.

18. A, B, C, D
In colonic CD 50%–75% will have perianal involvement **(Figure 69.2)** in the form of fistulae-in-ano, fissures and recurrent abscesses. Non-caseating giant cell granulomas

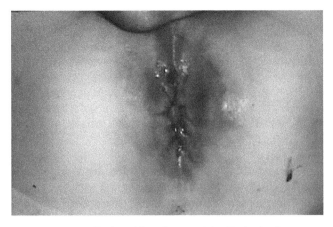

Figure 69.2 Perianal involvement in Crohn's disease.

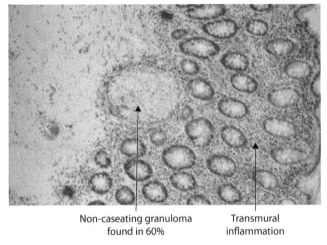

Non-caseating granuloma   Transmural
found in 60%   inflammation

Figure 69.3 Microscopic appearance in Crohn's disease.

(**Figure 69.3**), the keystone in the diagnosis, are most common in anorectal disease. When a stricture is seen in the large bowel, malignancy must be excluded by colonoscopy and biopsy as malignant transformation most often occurs in those areas. Often one of the first presentations of CD is an acute perianal abscess or a fissure that needs urgent treatment when the underlying condition of CD comes to light.

19. D
Evening pyrexia is not a clinical feature of CD. It is suggestive of tuberculosis in general and might be a typical symptom in abdominal tuberculosis (**see Chapter 6**). Patients present with blood-stained diarrhoea, particularly in colonic disease. Intermittent generalised abdominal pain, colicky in nature (denoting strictures) with a dull ache in between attacks, is common. If there is a colo-vesical or entero-vescial fistula, the patient might present with recurrent urinary infections and pneumaturia. On examination a mass might be felt in the right iliac fossa of which the patient might be unaware.

20. E

With regard to imaging in CD, all the techniques mentioned are used depending upon the clinical situation. In suspected small bowel disease when a patient presents electively, a small bowel enema **(Figure 69.4a and b)** is carried out. This would show strictures, skip lesions, string sign, fistulae, mucosal fissuring with radiating spicules and cobblestone mucosa. When large bowel disease is suspected, a barium enema would show similar features. This should be followed by colonoscopy to accurately assess the extent of the disease and biopsy to confirm the diagnosis. In perianal disease MRI is the 'gold standard', while CT scan will accurately localise abscesses and fistulae.

21. E

CD is mainly treated medically, with all the previously mentioned drugs used from time to time. Steroids (prednisolone) are the mainstay of treatment and help in remission in 70%–80%. 5-ASA compounds are particularly useful in colonic disease. Immunosuppressive agents (azathioprine) are used for their steroid-sparing effect, particularly when the disease is quiescent. Infliximab is a monoclonal antibody that is useful especially in peri-anal fistula. Metronidazole is known to control disease activity in ileocolic and colonic disease in short courses given from time to time along with the other medications.

22. A

In proven CD, restorative proctocolectomy with ileoanal pouch should never be done because of the high incidence of recurrence and pouchitis. Moreover, the ileum to be used for a pouch might be involved with the disease. Perianal disease, which is common in colonic CD, is another reason for this operation being unsuitable.

Strictureplasty, whereby a longitudinal incision is made and closed transversely (similar to the Heineke-Mikulicz pyloroplasty), is suitable for short strictures. In long strictures not suitable for the usual type of strictureplasty and where bowel preservation is vital, some surgeons have opted for a 'Finney's type' of strictureplasty. In very severe and extensive disease, proctocolectomy and ileostomy is the procedure of choice; when the rectum is free

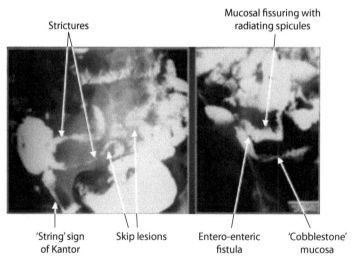

Figure 69.4 Radiological appearances in Crohn's disease.

of disease, colectomy and ileorectal anastomosis can be done. In the vast majority, however, segmental resections of diseased bowel is the procedure most often carried out.

23. B
Surgery must be as conservative as possible in inflammatory bowel disease (IBD). In CD, resections must be as limited as possible. In UC, in emergency situations such as toxic megacolon or perforation, a total abdominal colectomy and ileostomy is performed, avoiding a pelvic dissection. The rectal stump is brought out as a mucous fistula or closed as a Hartmann's procedure.

All patients with IBD must be under the joint care of the gastroenterologist and surgeon. In the elective situation, all patients must be given a very good trial of medical treatment before embarking upon surgery. When surgery is required as an emergency, ITU management is vital for preoperative optimisation and postoperative care. Overall after surgical treatment in IBD, the chances of cure are more likely after UC than CD.

Infections of small and large intestine

24. A, C, D, E
A Gram-negative rod with a spiral shape, *Campylobacter jejuni*, is the most common cause of gastroenteritis in the United Kingdom. It is due to eating infected poultry. It causes diarrhoea and acute abdominal pain; severe cases might be confused with UC. It is not easy to grow in stool culture. Treatment is supportive, the condition being notifiable. Actinomycosis is a rare infection caused by *Actinomycosis israeli*. It develops several weeks after removal of a perforated acute appendicitis. It results in an abscess that spreads across tissue planes from the retroperitoneum to the overlying skin forming a woody indurated mass that discharges thin, watery odourless material, which becomes thick and malodorous. The discharge grows sulphur granules. Treatment is long-term penicillin or cotrimoxazole in high doses.

After the development of AIDS with human immunodeficiency virus (HIV) infection, there might be opportunistic intestinal infection caused by bacteria, viruses, protozoa and fungi. Treatment is medical specifically against the organism. *Clostridium difficile* is a cause of nosocomial infection. It is caused by a Gram-positive bacillus that produces a toxin. It is a cause of antibiotic-associated diarrhoea and pseudomembranous colitis. The patient might be very ill with fever, diarrhoea and abdominal pain. Besides full supportive care, the patient is treated by vancomycin or metronidazole. In extreme cases emergency subtotal colectomy and ileostomy might be necessary.

Amoebiasis, typhoid and tuberculosis are discussed in **Chapter 6:** 'Surgery in the tropics'.

Tumours of the small intestine

25. D, E
The most common type of small bowel lymphoma is a non-Hodgkin's β-cell lymphoma. Small bowel lymphomas are classified as primary or secondary, the latter being more common and is secondary to systemic lymphoma. The condition is more common in patients with CD, immunodeficiency syndromes and coeliac disease in whom it is a T-cell lymphoma. Their elective presentation is anaemia, anorexia and weight loss; as an emergency they present with bleeding, perforation and intestinal obstruction. GISTs are stromal tumours, and most of them occur in the stomach as leiomyoma.

One in 10 gastrointestinal tumours occur in the small bowel. The benign ones are adenomas, lipomas, and Peutz–Jeghers syndrome, which is an autosomal dominant disease that has melanosis of the mouth and lips and polyps in the small bowel and colon. Adenocarcinoma of the small bowel, more often in the jejunum, occurs more commonly in patients with CD, coeliac disease, familial adenomatous polyposis and Peutz–Jeghers syndrome. A carcinoid tumour that arises from the appendix does not give rise to carcinoid syndrome. The syndrome is produced by secondaries in the liver, which are metastases from a tumour in the ileum.

26. A, B, D, E

Appendicular carcinoid is almost always found incidentally when an appendix is removed following a diagnosis of acute appendicitis. At operation no acute inflammation is found; instead a solid yellowish tumour is found usually in the distal appendix. Appendicectomy is the treatment. However, if the tumour occupies the base of the appendix or invades the caecum, a right hemicolectomy has to be done.

The cause of this syndrome is the excessive secretion of 5-hydroxytryptamine (5-HT, serotonin). These tumours arise from the gastro-entero-pancreatic part of the diffuse neuroendocrine system. Therefore this tumour is a part of the family of neuroendocrine tumours (NET). They arise from the ileum and rectum, the former being more common. They have a propensity to metastasise to the liver long after removal of the primary. It is the liver secondaries that produce the syndrome by secreting serotonin. They have a common embryological origin and cyto-chemical features which are a high amine (A) content, capacity for amine precursor uptake (APU) and the property of decarboxylation (D), hence the acronym for the tumour APUDOMA.

The clinical manifestations are protean in nature. The syndrome usually occurs in relation to malignant tumours that have metastasized, usually to the liver. The features are the following:

Vasomotor: Flushing in face and neck and sun-exposed areas; bronchial tumours can cause widespread flushes with devastating severity

Gastrointestinal: Mild to explosive diarrhoea with its effects, abdominal pain, bloating, tenesmus

Cardiopulmonary: Hypotension during flushing attacks, right-sided heart failure, pulmonary and tricuspid stenosis (not mitral stenosis), bronchospasm

Nutritional: Weight loss, features of pellagra: dementia and skin lesions from niacin deficiency

Tumours of the large intestine

27. A, C, D, E

In FAP more than 80% have a positive family history. The remaining 20% are the result of new mutations in the *adenomatous polyposis coli* (*APC*) gene. For families there should be a screening policy in place. Genetic testing should be offered in the early teens; from teenage years, annual colonoscopy should be carried out; those who get the disease would do so by the age of 20 years; those clear at the age of 20 should be offered 5-year colonoscopic surveillance until 50 years of age.

Those with the disease should be offered surgical treatment. Of the surgical options available, restorative proctocolectomy with an ileo-anal pouch is one of the choices offered. Although this removes the whole colon and rectum, in a stapled anastomosis, the small strip of rectal mucosa between the pouch and dentate line has a chance of developing cancer. Therefore some surgeons perform a complete mucosectomy of the rectal cuff; the price paid by the patient for such an immunity against cancer is a worse functional result.

HNPCC is an autosomal dominant condition caused by a mutation in one of the DNA mismatch repair genes, *MLH1* and *MSH2*. There is an 80% lifetime risk of developing colorectal cancer which is diagnosed at 45 years whilst females have an almost 50% risk of developing endometrial cancer. Genetic testing or the Amsterdam II criteria helps in diagnosing HNPCC. FAP is inherited as an autosomal dominant gene (not recessive gene).

Both sexes are equally affected and either might transmit the disease; only those with the disease can transmit the condition and half the children are likely to inherit.

28. A, B

The distribution of colonic adenomas and carcinomas is the same, 70% of them being left-sided. Sporadic adenomas are identical to those of FAP. Left untreated, cancer is inevitable, with a 100% chance of adenomas in FAP turning malignant. The larger the adenoma, the greater is the chance of it showing dysplasia; when dysplasia occurs in them, it is of a higher grade.

There is a fall in the incidence of colorectal carcinoma where screening programmes have colonoscopy and polypectomy as an integral part. In two-thirds of colonic adenomas and carcinomas, there is mutation of the *APC* gene, a process that develops early in the pathway to carcinogenesis. K-ras mutations, more common in larger lesions is associated with a poor prognosis. Mutation of the *p53* tumour suppressor gene causes the transition from the adenoma to carcinoma signalling invasion. Knowledge of certain mutations can be used to assess prognosis and target adjuvant treatment.

29. E

The most common site (60%) of colorectal cancer is the rectosigmoid region. This is thought to be due to the prolonged contact of the faeces with the mucosa in that region. It therefore follows that the majority will be within reach of the rigid sigmoidoscope so that a biopsy can be obtained in the outpatient department. At the time of diagnosis, one-third of the patients will have liver secondaries. Clinically patients might present either as electively or as an emergency; 20% of patients present as an emergency with intestinal obstruction or peritonitis, the cause of which is perforation. Emergency presentation is associated with a worse prognosis. Reduced dietary fibre is well known as a factor in the aetiology of large bowel cancer. Increased fibre in the diet causes large amount of roughage, which helps to reduce the transit time thus diminishing the exposure of mucosa to dietary carcinogens.

30. D

Intravenous urography is not a routine investigation for colorectal cancer. It is done when an US or CT shows hydronephrosis to see the function of the opposite kidney. In a patient known to have a solitary kidney, IVU is done to assess renal function. The elective clinical presentation for right and left colonic carcinomas differs. Right-sided cancers present with features of iron deficiency anaemia such as malaise or undue shortness of breath while carrying out normal daily activities due to anaemic hypoxia from microscopic bleeding; this is shown by positive faecal occult blood. Left-sided carcinomas present with altered bowel habit in the form of increasing constipation and need to use laxatives; this is because the faeces in the left colon is more formed. Rectal bleeding is another feature.

Colonoscopy is the method to confirm the diagnosis by taking a biopsy. It is also useful to exclude a synchronous carcinoma, which is present in 5% or an adenoma **(Figure 69.5)**, the latter being found in one-third of specimens resected for colonic cancer. Even in expert hands the caecum is not visualised in about 10% of colonoscopies.

31. A, D, E

Often the diagnosis can be established in the one-stop rectal bleeding clinic using a flexible sigmoidoscope, which will reach the splenic flexure. This should detect 70% of large bowel cancers. Once the diagnosis is made on colonoscopy, thorough assessment with regard to local and regional staging by spiral CECT and US is carried out.

If staging detects liver secondaries, the case is discussed in a MDT meeting as to the best way forward and considering treating the secondaries as a staged procedure. Those patients who present as acute intestinal obstruction should be considered for a staged procedure,

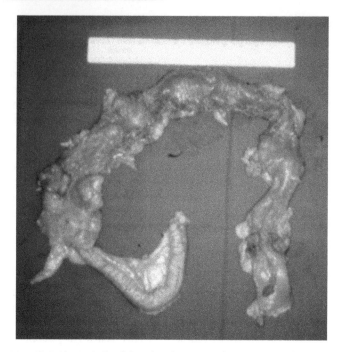

Figure 69.5 Specimen of subtotal colectomy showing synchronous cancer and a pedunculated polyp.

of which there are choices. A left colonic carcinoma causing acute closed-loop obstruction could have a stent inserted, which will get over the acute emergency. The patient can then be resuscitated and staged and then have a one-stage resection and anastomosis without a temporary stoma.

If staging shows liver secondaries, resection of the large bowel is carried out by the appropriate hemicolectomy as there is no better palliation than removal of the original cancer. Liver secondaries are never biopsied for fear of causing dissemination of the growth and bleeding.

32. A, E

Routine follow up is not a waste of resources following surgery for colonic surgery. Follow up aims to identify synchronous cancers missed during emergency surgery, metachronous cancers and liver metastases. This is done by measurement of carcinoembryonic antigen (CEA), US of liver and colonoscopic surveillance. Trials are being carried out to ascertain the optimum frequency of these follow-up methods. Preoperative chemotherapy has no role at present, although it is used in a selected group postoperatively.

After resection for hepatic metastases the 5-year survival is 30%. Hence all patients with liver secondaries should be referred to the hepatobiliary unit for consideration for surgery. In Dukes' stage A (disease confined to the bowel wall), the 5-year recurrence-free interval is 90%. Following surgery, units that have instituted the ERP have a much more rapid turnover of patients who remain in hospital for only up to 2 to 3 days after surgery.

Intestinal diverticula

33. A, B, C, E

An acquired duodenal diverticulum is always the outcome of a long-standing duodenal ulceration causing duodenal stenosis. Congenital duodenal diverticula are known to occur at the ampulla of

Vater and are most often an incidental finding. Jejunal diverticula (**Figure 69.6a** and **b**), although they might be asymptomatic, can cause malabsorption problems such as anaemia, steatorrhoea, hypoproteinaemia and vitamin B12 deficiency.

A Meckel's diverticulum can be the source of a major lower gastrointestinal bleed from a peptic ulcer arising from ectopic gastric mucosa. It can also be the source of chronic bleed presenting as anaemia. The ideal imaging method is not a barium study. Scanning after patient's own red blood cells are labelled with technetium-99 is an accurate method of identifying such a source of bleeding. As the diverticulum is part of the midgut, pain originating from it would be felt initially around the umbilicus.

34. C

Colonic diverticula are acquired. Hence, they consist of the mucosa covered by the serosa. Unlike congenital diverticula, they do not have any muscle. Because of the dietary habits, in the Western World 75% of the population of 70-year-olds has diverticular disease of the colon. A low-residue diet (consumed in the West) results in excessive segmentation of the sigmoid colon causing increased intraluminal pressure. This produces herniation of

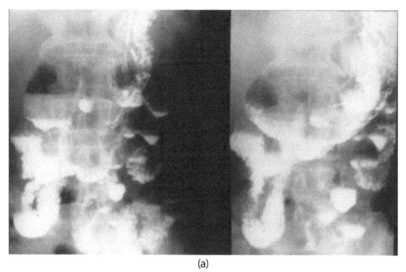
(a)

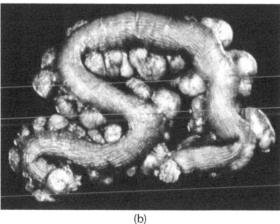
(b)

Figure 69.6   (a) Barium meal and follow through showing multiple jejunal diverticulae. (b) Specimen showing multiple jejunal diverticulae.

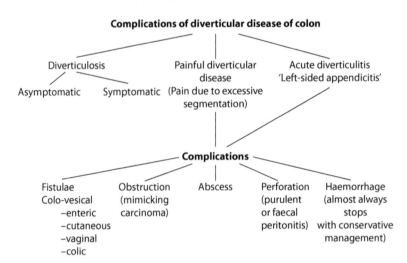

Figure 69.7 Complications of diverticular disease of colon.

the colonic mucosa at the site of maximum weakness, which is the entrance of the blood vessel; thus a diverticulum is formed. The principal cause of morbidity is sepsis, which is the underlying cause of most complications. Perforated diverticulitis causing faecal or purulent peritonitis carries a higher mortality than those with an inflammatory mass.

35. D
Carcinoma is not a complication of diverticular disease. However, as diverticular disease is so common, both can co-exist. However, paracoilic abscess, fistulae, lower gastrointestinal haemorrhage and stricture are all recognised complications. See **Figure 69.7** for a summary of the complications of diverticular disease.

36. D
Enterocolic fistula is not the most common type of fistula that occurs in complicated diverticular disease; colo-vesical fistula is the most common. Overall fistulae form in 5% of cases. Urinary symptoms might be the predominant presentation in a colo-vesical fistula. These take the form of dysuria, repeated attacks of UTI and bilateral loin pain with rigors from ascending pyelonephritis. Pneumaturia and faecaluria are symptoms that patients admit to having only when questioned.

Profuse colonic haemorrhage as a complication occurs in 17%. Typically it is painless and comes out of the blue and might be severe enough to require blood transfusion. Most often it stops by conservative management. In acute diverticulitis, the most common complication, the best investigation for confirmation is a CT scan.

37. E
Amoebic colitis does not cause colo-vesical fistula. Of the others on the list, diverticulitis, rectosigmoid cancer and Crohn's colitis are three common causes. Chronic radiation proctitis can rarely give rise to a colo-vesical fistula.

38. A, B, D, E
The imaging methods to confirm diverticular disease or one of its chronic complications are colonoscopy, barium enema, CT colonography and virtual colonoscopy. Because of narrowing of the bowel, it might not always be possible to do a full colonoscopy and biopsy,

much as it is very important to exclude any coincidental colonic cancer. A combination of all the available methods might be necessary to be sure of excluding a carcinoma.

In all cases of diverticular disease and its complications that require surgery, primary resection and anastomosis cannot be carried out, particularly the patient who presents with perforated diverticulitis where Hartmann's resection is the safest operation; only in selected cases can it be attempted in an emergency after intraoperative colonic irrigation. In a vesicocolic fistula, after thorough investigation, a one-stage resection and anastomosis can be done.

Vascular anomalies of the intestine

39. A, B, D, E

The superior mesenteric vessels is most often involved, embolisation being more common than thrombosis. Obstruction at the origin of SMA is most commonly from thrombosis, whilst embolism is the most common cause at the origin of the middle colic artery. The source of the embolus is a mural thrombus in the left ventricle adjacent to the fibrotic ventricular muscle from a recent myocardial infarction.

Patients, usually with atrial fibrillation, complain of very severe generalised abdominal pain and a paucity of signs because the pain is out of proportion to the physical findings – mild abdominal tenderness with minimal rigidity or rebound. Hypovolaemic shock of rapid onset associated with bloody diarrhoea is another feature.

Ischaemic colitis affects the left colon in the distribution of the inferior mesenteric artery with acute features similar to those affecting the SMA. The condition might also come on insidiously with left-sided abdominal pain with passage of altered blood rectally. Most of these patients recover without any treatment, the underlying pathology in due course resulting in a stricture from fibrosis.

Angiodysplasia, a vascular malformation, usually presents as an emergency with haemorrhage, occurring in the ascending colon and caecum not the sigmoid colon.

Intestinal stoma

40. A, B

A loop transverse colostomy is no longer regarded as the ideal method to defunction an anterior resection; a loop ileostomy has replaced the procedure because of the following: (1) A loop ileostomy is formed in the right iliac fossa and hence the patient finds it much easier to manage the bag; (2) Loop transverse colostomy has the potential to prolapse; (3) Proximity to the rib cage makes attachment of the bag in loop colostomy insecure; (4) Loop colostomy can sometimes compromise the blood supply to the distal anastomosis; and (5) Contents of a loop ileostomy are not malodorous. An end ileostomy is not always a permanent procedure. It is the stoma constructed in an emergency situation when a subtotal colectomy is done for acute toxic megacolon or perforation in UC or CD.

A loop ileostomy is always a temporary procedure constructed in the right iliac fossa to defunction a low anterior resection or ileo-anal pouch procedure after total colectomy for UC or FAP. Before closing it, a contrast study is always carried out to make sure that the distal anastomosis is securely intact. An end colostomy in the left iliac fossa can be permanent as after an abdomino-perineal resection for low rectal cancer or temporary as in a Hartmann's operation. To know clinically if a stoma is permanent or temporary, the patient must be turned on the side to see if the anus is still present. If it is, the stoma is temporary. Stoma complications are common and often underestimated. This is because the patient tends to put up with the inconvenience as he or she 'has had enough' and does not seek advice unless it is an emergency or making his or her life miserable.

→ Enterocutaneous fistula

41. A, B, C, E

There are several causes of an enterocutaneous fistula, the most common being a surgical complication from an anastomotic leak or an inadvertent injury to the small bowel during a difficult dissection. The other causes are CD, radiation enteritis and abdominal trauma. In the management, attention to nutrition is vital as the patient would be losing a large amount of intestinal fluid, the amount depending upon whether it is a high-output or low-output fistula. Arbitrarily, 500 mL of daily lost fluid is regarded as the 'cut-off point' – > than 500 mL/day is high-output fistula and <500 mL/day low out-put fistula.

The higher the fistula, the greater will be the loss of fluid and hence the paramount need for attention to detail regarding nutrition. Although the ideal route for nutrition is enteral, in a high-output fistula this might not be possible; hence parenteral nutrition should be instituted. When a fistula does not close spontaneously, it indicates epithelial continuity between gut and skin or underlying pathology such as an obstructing carcinoma, CD, or abscess.

→ Laparoscopic colorectal surgery

42. A, B, C, D

The COST trial from the United States, COLOR 1 trial from Europe and CLASICC trial from the United Kingdom are multi-centre RCTs that showed improved short-term benefits of laparoscopic colon surgery over conventional surgery. The benefits include less postoperative pain, less intra-operative blood loss, faster recovery of bowel function and shorter hospital stay. In addition the COST trial demonstrated there is no difference in port-site metastasis between laparoscopic and open surgery. Some of these trials have matured data at 3 and 5 years showing no difference in the oncological outcomes between laparoscopic and open surgery. The CLASICC and COLOR 2 are the two trials comparing laparoscopic and open surgery for rectal cancer. These studies similarly showed improved short-term benefits with no difference in anastomotic complications. The LAFA trial is a randomised controlled trial comparing open and laparoscopic colon surgery in the setting of the enhanced recovery programme (ERP). This has also shown a similar improved short-term benefit with minimal access surgery.

DREAMS is a randomised controlled multi-centre study to determine the use of dexamethasone at the time of induction to reduce post-operative nausea and vomiting in patients undergoing elective colorectal resections.

43. B, D

In laparoscopic colorectal surgery, one should aim for a conversion rate of <10% is aimed for. RCTs have shown increased postoperative morbidity in the converted group. Hence conversion is a bad outcome. Conversion is not a failure and nowadays it is recommended to convert early to decrease intra and postoperative complications. The large multi-centre RCTs and meta-analysis have shown similar oncological outcomes between open and laparoscopic techniques. The only long-term benefits of minimal-access techniques appear to be a tendency to demonstrate a decrease in incisional hernia and adhesion-related complications. The NICE guidance (TA 105) recommends laparoscopic colorectal surgery in patients with localised lesions and the surgeon to be experienced in performing both the procedures competently.

44. A

When resection is indicated in Crohn's colitis, laparoscopic approach is not particularly suitable for the less experienced because transmural inflammation causes the mesentery to be foreshortened and colonic disease is usually more severe. In general, benign conditions are difficult to deal with laparoscopically. However, experienced laparoscopic colorectal surgeons might consider an initial laparoscopic attempt provided there is a safe conversion threshold.

Lymph node retrieval is the same as those performed by the traditional method although the operative times are longer. In laparoscopic surgery, as the ability to palpate the lesion is not possible, tattooing the lesion at preoperative colonoscopic assessment is used according to the unit's policy; this is usually advocated as a standardised approach. Unlike in open surgery, the initial dissection is commenced medially by taking the major vascular pedicles thus freeing the mesocolon and then dividing the lateral peritoneal reflection as the lateral attachments provide retraction during early dissection.

Answers to extended matching questions

1. H Angiodysplasia

Angiodysplasia is a thin-walled arteriovenous communication located within the mucosa and submucosa of the intestine, usually the ascending colon and caecum. Sometimes it is associated with aortic stenosis, when it is called Heyde's syndrome.

The typical presentation is with lower gastrointestinal bleeding that can be overt or occult. When the bleeding is overt it might be profuse, resulting in hypovolaemic shock. Initial management is resuscitation and stabilisation. This is followed by diagnostic evaluation usually by colonoscopy. In some cases three-vessel angiogram might be done when the pathology can be seen as a vascular blush. Therapeutic embolisation can be carried out at the same time.

A CT angiogram is another diagnostic procedure; direct infusion of vasopressin will decrease or stop the bleeding. Colonoscopy could identify the bleeding site, which can then be managed by argon plasma coagulation, clips and adrenaline injection into the lesion. When bleeding cannot be controlled endoscopically, laparotomy is inevitable. On-table colonoscopy can sometimes localise the lesion when a segmental resection is carried out. If the bleeding site cannot be determined in spite of all available investigations, a subtotal colectomy might be necessary.

2. A Carcinoma of caecum

Patients with caecal carcinoma can present as an emergency or electively, the latter presentation being due to the primary tumour or metastatic disease such as liver secondaries.

In the emergency situation they can present with perforation and acute distal small bowel obstruction due to the ileocaecal valve being obstructed by the tumour and masquerading as 'acute appendicitis' as a result of the tumour causing blockage of the appendicular lumen. When an older patient presents with suspected features of acute appendicitis and preoperatively is found to be anaemic, the diagnosis is almost certainly a caecal carcinoma as genuine acute appendicitis does not cause anaemia.

In the elective situation, the presentation is from features of iron deficiency anaemia due to chronic occult bleeding or pain and lump over the right side of the abdomen. Sometimes, patients present with symptoms due to metastatic disease. This can be in the form of jaundice due to liver secondaries. A barium enema would show an irregular filling defect in the caecum (**Figures 69.8a** and **b**).

The management in the emergency situation is resuscitation and stabilisation of the patient. Electively, ideally haemoglobin close to 9 g/dL is aimed for, followed by confirmation of the diagnosis by colonoscopy and biopsy. The histology will show adenocarcinoma. This is followed by staging CT of the chest, abdomen and pelvis, and also carcinoembryonic antigen (CEA), the latter being useful in surveillance if it is elevated initially.

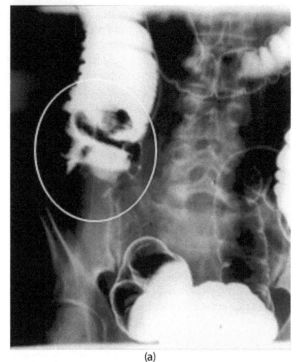

(a)

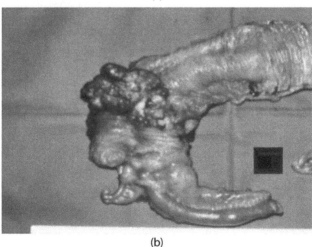

(b)

Figure 69.8 (a) Barium enema showing an irregular filling defect in the caecum typical of a carcinoma. (b) Right hemicolectomy specimen showing carcinoma of caecum (same patient as in Figure 69.8a).

Definitive treatment is radical right hemicolectomy, which can nowadays be performed using a laparoscopic approach depending upon the choice of the surgical team. Postoperatively if the growth is Dukes' C stage the patient is given adjuvant chemotherapy.

3. G Carcinoma of descending colon
Patients with descending colon carcinoma can present as an emergency or electively. As an emergency they present as acute closed-loop large-bowel obstruction or perforation

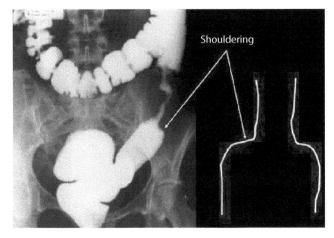

Figure 69.9   Barium enema showing long irregular stricture with 'shouldering' typical of tubular carcinoma.

and peritonitis. Elective presentation is change in bowel habit in the form of increasing constipation because the stools are formed and bowel lumen in the descending colon is narrow. Sometimes there is a history of colicky abdominal pain due to impending obstruction. A barium enema **(Figure 69.9)** would show irregular stricture and filling defect with 'shouldering'.

A colonoscopy is carried out to confirm the diagnosis by biopsy. In a stricture, it is highly unlikely that the entire colon will be visualised to exclude synchronous growths. A CT scan of the chest, abdomen and pelvis is carried out to accurately stage the disease. This is followed by discussion in a MDT meeting prior to definitive treatment. The definitive treatment is radical left hemicolectomy with end-to-end anastomosis between the transverse colon and upper rectum. Postoperatively in Dukes' stage C patients adjuvant chemotherapy is given.

All patients following large bowel surgery are placed in the enhanced recovery programme (ERP), the usual practice to reduce hospital stay and the metabolic response to the surgical insult. In this regard, patient education is commenced preoperatively by the surgical, anaesthetic and nursing teams.

4. E Colovesical fistula
Patients with colovesical fistula present primarily with urinary symptoms such as dysuria, recurrent urinary tract infections, attacks of ascending pyelonephritis, pneumaturia and passing foul-smelling urine due to faeces in the urine. On questioning patients might admit to constipation, which would point to pathology in the large bowel, most often diverticular disease. The other causes are carcinoma of the rectosigmoid and Crohn's colitis.

Management should be to confirm the diagnosis by various imaging techniques such as barium enema, which would show air **(Figure 69.10)** or barium **(Figure 69.11)** within the urinary bladder and CT scan also to confirm air in the bladder **(Figure 69.12)**. This should be followed by colonoscopy (or flexible sigmoidoscopy, as diverticular stricture would preclude a full colonoscopy) and biopsy, most importantly to exclude the possibility of a carcinoma within a segment of sigmoid diverticulitis. Once carcinoma is excluded and diverticulitis is confirmed, sigmoid colectomy is carried out. At operation the inflamed colon is pinched off the vault of the urinary bladder and the hole in the bladder closed off with interrupted absorbable sutures; sigmoid colectomy with end-to-end anastomosis is performed.

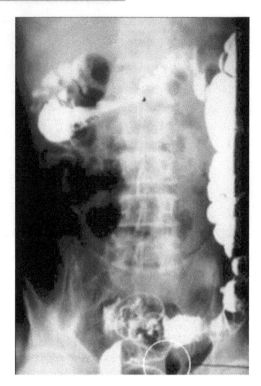

Figure 69.10 Barium enema showing air in the urinary bladder from a colovesical fistula.

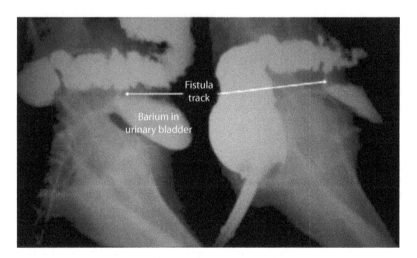

Figure 69.11 Barium enema showing barium inside the urinary bladder – colovescial fistula.

In the case of colovesical fistula due to rectosigmoid cancer, operation is performed after confirmation of the diagnosis and staging the disease. The operation will involve *en bloc* resection of the sigmoid carcinoma in the form of high anterior resection with partial cystectomy. When the fistula is due to Crohn's disease, sigmoid colectomy is performed

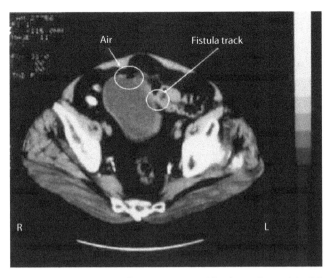

Figure 69.12   CT scan showing air inside the urinary bladder.

followed by removal of macroscopic disease from the bladder and the urinary bladder closed in two layers with catheter left in situ for 10 days.

5. C Crohn's disease

Crohn's disease was first brought to light in 1932 by Crohn, Ginzburg and Oppenheimer, from Mount Sinai Hospital in New York, who called it 'Regional ileitis'. However, it was TK Dalziell, a surgeon from Glasgow, who in 1913 described the same disease, which he called 'Chronic interstitial enteritis' and likened the macroscopic appearance of the small bowel to 'an eel in rigor mortis'.

The disease, a type of inflammatory bowel disease, is characterised by transmural inflammation that can affect the entire gastrointestinal tract from the mouth to the anus. It affects males and females equally and has a bimodal distribution with increased incidence in the twenties followed by further spike in the late sixties. The aetiology is multi-factorial, the possible causes being immunologic, infectious, genetic, and environmental.

The initial pathology is the formation of apthous and serpiginous ulcers with normal intervening mucosa that appear nodular and is referred to as cobblestone mucosa **(Figure 69.13).** Typical transmural inflammation can lead to perforation or internal fistulae or cause a stricture; there is overgrowth of fat beyond the mesentery covering the bowel wall **(Figure 69.14)** associated with regional lymphadenopathy. Diseased bowel is interspersed with normal unaffected bowel, an outcome referred to as skip lesions, which is typical of Crohn's disease. The pathology in CD is summarised in **Table 69.8**.

The most frequent site of Crohn's disease is the terminal ileum. This is followed by isolated colonic disease and then by isolated disease of the small bowel. Anal disease by itself is rare and usually accompanies colonic involvement.

On microscopy **(Figure 69.3)** the typical feature is non-caseating granuloma, which is present in about 60% of patients. The complications are local pertaining to the bowel **(Table 69.6)** and systemic or extra-intestinal **(Table 69.7)**.

Crohn's disease needs close collaboration between an aggressive physician and a conservative surgeon. The extent of the disease is established by a barium meal and follow-through showing a string sign of Kantor **(Figure 69.15)** or small bowel enema and

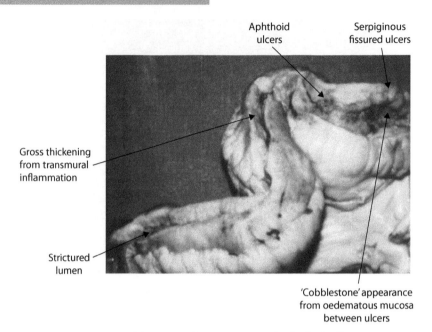

Aphthoid
ulcers

Serpiginous
fissured ulcers

Gross thickening
from transmural
inflammation

Strictured
lumen

'Cobblestone' appearance
from oedematous mucosa
between ulcers

Figure 69.13   Macroscopic appearance in Crohn's disease.

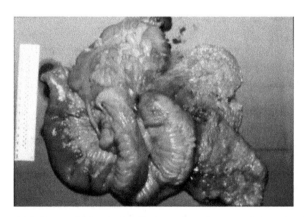

Figure 69.14   Specimen of Crohn's disease showing overgrowth of fat beyond
the mesentery covering the bowel wall.

colonoscopy and biopsy in large bowel disease. Other radiological findings are skip lesions,
cobblestone mucosa, fistulae and spiculation **(Figure 69.4)**. Treatment is mainly medical and
should be tailored for the individual patient. Drugs used are steroids, 5-aminosalicylic acid
derivatives (mainly for large bowel disease), antibiotics, immunosuppresives and tumour
necrosis factor α (TNF-α) antagonists such as infliximab and adalimumab.

The indication for surgery in Crohn's disease are shown in **Tables 69.9** and **69.10** and the
available surgical options in **Tables 69.11** and **69.12**.

Anorectal Crohn's disease **(Figure 69.2)** Perianal CD occurs most often in association with
large bowel involvement; it can, however, occur in isolation or in the presence of ileal disease.

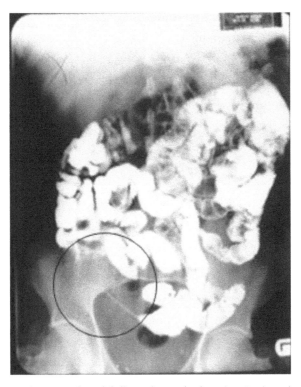

Figure 69.15 Barium meal and follow through showing 'string sign' of Kantor.

Table 69.8 Summary of pathology in Crohn's disease

- Macroscopic
  - Thickened, stenosed ileum; fibrosis
  - Discrete ulcers
  - Cobblestone appearance
  - Fissuring
  - Transmural inflammation
  - Thickened mesentery
  - lymphadenopathy
- Microscopic
  - Non-caseating grarulomata in 60%
  - Giant cells
  - Aphthous ulcers

In keeping with Crohn's disease in general, conservative approach is the first option. Perianal abscesses are drained. MRI of the pelvis is the 'gold standard' to distinguish between a high anal and a low anal fistula, a distinction that is mandatory, as the management is different. Whilst a low anal fistula can be treated by laying open, the high fistula requires the use of a seton and staged procedure to drain the sepsis and is the domain of an expert colorectal specialist.

Table 69.9 Indications for elective operation in Crohn's disease

- Failure of medical management
- Nutritional failure
- Fistulae
- Multiple strictures causing intermittent intestinal obstruction
- Malignant change

Table 69.10 Indications for emergency or urgent operation in Crohn's disease

- Perforation
- Acute intestinal obstruction
- Abscess
- Severe haemorrhage
- Toxic megacolon

Table 69.11 Elective surgical options in Crohn's disease

- Resections with primary anastomosis
- Strictureplasty
- Balloon dilatation
- Proctocolectomy and ileostomy
- Temporary loop ileostomy

Table 69.12 Emergency surgical options in Crohn's disease

- Resections: small and/or large bowel with exteriorisation procedures; primary anastomosis if safe and indicated
- Drainage of abscesses

6. I Enterocutaneous fistula

Enterocutaneous fistula (see previous multiple choice questions) is a challenging situation that requires teamwork among the surgeon, physician, radiologist, dietician and stomatherapist. The team should be prepared for a long haul. If there is no distal obstruction, or pathology, or underlying sepsis, an enetrocutaneous fistula should close by good supportive management. It is essential to find the cause; in this case it is CD. The principles of management can be summarised by the acronym SNAP which stands for the following: *S*epsis elimination and *S*kin protection; *N*utrition; *A*natomical assessment; *P*lanned surgery.

To achieve this goal, the principles of management must be instituted concurrently. ***Sepsis and skin:*** Under image guidance all sepsis must be eliminated by percutaneous drainage. Repeat CT scans, WCC count and CRP should be done. The role of the stoma nurse is very important to take care of skin excoriation, which can be very distressing for the patient.

Nutrition: In high-output fistula (> 500 mL/day) it will be necessary to establish total parenteral nutrition (TPN) as hypoproteinaemia must be combated.

Anatomy is best defined by contrast studies, which might require barium meal, and follow through, barium enema and fistulography carried out in conjunction with CT scan. This is where the radiologist's input is vital.

Planned surgical procedure, which can be most challenging, is carried out only after the aforementioned principles have been optimally established. It might be necessary to perform staged procedures of exteriorisation to be followed by anastomosis when the conditions are right.

7. D Ischaemic colitis

Patients present as an emergency with rectal bleeding with pain on the left side of the abdomen over the left colon. If the ischaemia results in complete disruption of the blood supply, infarction of the colon ensues. This manifests with full-blown peritonitis from a gangrenous colon. Elective patients present with episodes of rectal bleeding with pain in the left upper quadrant, symptoms that reflect ischaemia of the splenic flexure from atheromatous obstruction to the inferior mesenteric artery.

On examination there might be tenderness over the left side of the abdomen. Most of these patients are elderly and settle down with conservative management. In a more serious presentation there might be SIRS response in the form of hypotension, fever, oliguria and altered mental status. Patients who have settled down with conservative management might later present with features of a left colonic stricture, complaining of increasing constipation and intermittent colicky abdominal pain. This might require local resection and end-to-end anastomosis. The summary of presentations is shown in **Figure 69.16.** The various causes are shown in **Figure 69.17.**

In the elective situation colonoscopy is performed to look for mucosal ischaemia, which can be patchy. CT will show a thickened colon, while a barium enema **(Figure 69.18)** shows a narrowing of the colon confined to the distribution of the inferior mesenteric artery in the region of the splenic flexure with thumb-printing.

In the emergency presentation, initial treatment is conservative with active resuscitation in the form of bed rest, analgesia, antibiotics and appropriate treatment of hypovolaemia. The patient who presents with peritonitis from gangrenous colon needs optimisation followed by urgent laparotomy, resection of the infarcted bowel and exteriorisation as colostomy and mucus fistula. A laparostomy should be considered as these patients often have further ischaemia for which a second-look operation might be necessary.

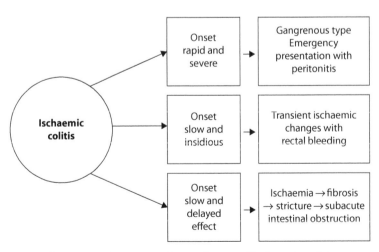

Figure 69.16   Presentation and types of ischaemic colitis.

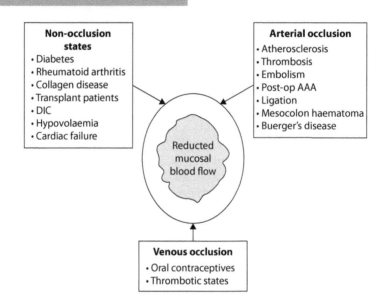

Figure 69.17   Causes of ischaemic colitis.

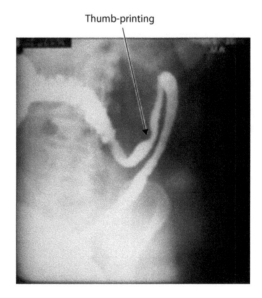

Figure 69.18   Barium enema showing ischaemic colitis.

8. J Paracolic abscess

This patient has the clinical features of a paracolic abscess, one of the complications of diverticular disease shown in **Figure 69.7**. This is an ill and septic patient who needs resuscitation, confirmation of the diagnosis and definitive treatment. The patient needs intravenous fluids with bloods having been sent for culture, haematological and biochemical investigations. Broad-spectrum antibiotics are started. The best imaging technique to confirm the diagnosis is contrast spiral CT scan.

On confirmation of the paracolic abscess the abscess is drained under CT guidance, which would result in improvement in the patient's general condition and local symptoms. Sometimes drainage of the abscess might result in a colocutaneous fistula. Once the patient has recovered from the acute episode, definitive treatment is planned after investigations in the form of a colonoscopy and contrast CT scan to exclude an unsuspected carcinoma within the diverticular segment. A sigmoid colectomy with end-to-end anastomosis is performed as an elective procedure.

Complicated diverticulitis is stratified on CT scan according to the Hinchey classification which has the following four grades: Grade I – mesenteric or pericolic abscess; Grade II – pelvic abscess; Grade III – purulent peritonitis; Grade IV – faecal peritonitis. The first two grades can be treated by minimal-access surgery in the form of image-guided drainage and laparoscopic wash-outs under antibiotic cover while the higher grades will require laparotomy. Stricture is a complication that can mimic carcinoma with the typical radiological features of shouldering on barium enema **(Figure 69.19a)**. In such patients a biopsy must be taken to exclude a carcinoma before performing a sigmoid resection **(Figure 69.19b)**.

9. B Perforated diverticulitis
A patient with perforated diverticulitis presents with generalised peritonitis with features of septic shock. The peritonitis in such patients might be purulent or faecal. The patient requires optimal resuscitation and confirmation of the diagnosis followed by definitive treatment. The patient is started on oxygen; intravenous access is obtained with bloods being sent for routine haematology, biochemistry and culture; and an indwelling urinary catheter inserted. At his age with the prospect of postoperative ITU care, a CVP line is essential as this patient could well go into SIRS or sepsis syndrome in due course. Clinical examination is followed by CT scan with oral and IV contrast, which will show extra-luminal air with CXR showing gas under the right dome of the diaphragm.

The patient with free perforation needs an emergency laparotomy after optimum resuscitation. At operation through a lower midline incision, the perforated sigmoid colon is resected with end colostomy and the rectum closed off as a Hartmann's procedure. The peritoneal cavity is thoroughly washed out with several litres of warm normal saline. The peritoneum is closed with the incision being left open for delayed primary closure a few days later. Once the patient has recovered, after 3 months consideration might be given to reversal of the Hartmann's, a procedure nowadays done laparoscopically.

10. F Ulcerative colitis
Patients with ulcerative colitis might present electively or as an emergency. The vast majority, about 95%, present electively. The usual sufferer is a female between 30 and 40 years who complains of loose stools with blood and mucus. Sometimes she has to rush to the toilet and might be caught short. Anything up to 4 to 6 trips to the lavatory per day leaves her constantly with a feeling of insufficient evacuation and tenesmus. Colicky left-sided abdominal pain usually accompanies the loose stools. On examination there is not much to find except for some left iliac fossa tenderness and blood and mucus on rectal examination. Sigmoidoscopy (rigid or flexible) in the outpatient shows evidence of proctitis – hyperaemic mucosa with purulent and mucoid exudate.

Diagnosis is by clinical assessment followed by endoscopy and histological confirmation. At endoscopy **(Figure 69.20)**, the mucosa appears reddened, oedematous and haemorrhagic; there might be tiny ulcerations. Mucosal friability with contact bleeding is a feature. Mucosal changes start in the rectum and proceed proximally to a varying extent. In left-sided colitis the proximal extent is up to the splenic flexure; when the inflammation extends proximal to this level, it is considered as extensive colitis; backwash ileitis is seen in about 10% of patients.

Barium enema shows the classical shortened pipe-stem colon **(Figure 69.1a)**, which lacks haustrations while increase in the presacral space **(Figure 69.1b)** is a typical finding in advanced disease. There might be strictures with cancer **(Figure 69.21)**. Biopsies show that inflammation is confined to the mucosa with characteristic crypt abscess **(Figure 69.22)**. A summary of the imaging procedures is shown in **Tables 69.13** and **69.14**.

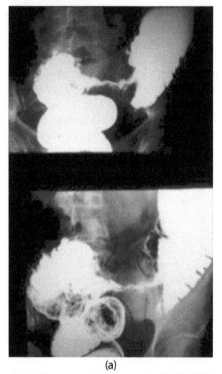

(a)

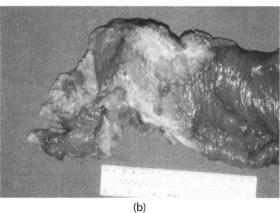

(b)

Figure 69.19   (a) Barium enema showing stricture in sigmoid colon from diverticulitis mimicking carcinoma. (b) Specimen of sigmoid colectomy showing diverticular stricture (same patient as in Figure 69.19a).

The two main differential diagnoses are Crohn's disease and indeterminate colitis. Crohn's disease is diagnosed by segmental and transmural inflammation and its propensity to affect all parts of the gastrointestinal tract from the mouth to the anus. Indeterminate colitis is diagnosed when clinical, endoscopic, radiologic and pathological features of both ulcerative colitis and Crohn's disease are present.

The emergency patient (5%) presents with cramp-like abdominal pain, tenesmus, faecal urgency, blood-stained diarrhoea and faecal incontinence. Bowel actions can be anything up to 12 times with extreme urgency. Failure to reach the toilet results in faecal incontinence.

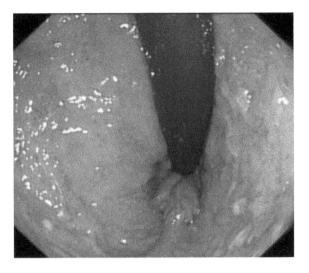

Figure 69.20 Endoscopic view of ulcerative proctitis.

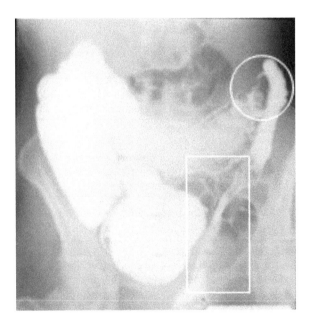

Figure 69.21 Barium enema in ulcerative colitis showing strictures due to carcinoma.

Fever, malaise, anorexia, weight loss, dehydration and anaemia will be obvious. With fulminant colitis, the patient might be suffering from acute toxic megacolon bordering on perforation. The abdomen might be distended, tympanitic and tender (see previous multiple choice questions).

The complications of ulcerative colitis are enumerated in (**Tables 69.1** and **69.2**). One of the most serious complications is dysplastic change leading to cancer. Patients most vulnerable to malignant change are shown in **Table 69.3**. The indications for surgery are shown in **Tables 69.4** and **69.5**). The surgical options, elective operations and emergency operations are shown in **Tables 69.15** and **69.16**.

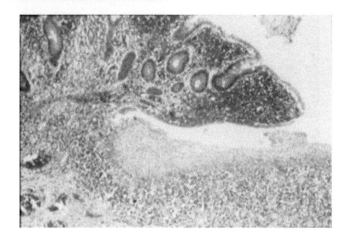

Figure 69.19   Crypt abscess in ulcerative colitis.

Table 69.13   Radiological features in elective imaging in ulcerative colitis

Barium enema
- Complete loss of haustration
- 'Pipe stem' or 'hose pipe' colon
- Increase in the presacral or retro-rectal space on lateral view
- Indium[111] labelled leucocyte scan

Table 69.14   Radiological features in emergency imaging in ulcerative colitis

- Plain x-ray abdomen (for toxic megacolon)
  - Massive dilatation of colon (>6cm)
  - No formed faeces in colon
  - Loss of haustration – Intramural air(tramlining)
- Chest-x ray – Gas under diaphragm indicating perforation

Table 69.15   Elective operations in ulcerative colitis

- Proctocolectomy with ileostomy
- Restorative proctocolectomy with an ileoanal pouch temporary (+/– loop ileostomy)
- Colectomy and ileorectal anastomosis (possible in a minority)
- Colectomy with a continent ileostomy (now rarely used)

Table 69.16   Emergency or urgent operation in ulcerative colitis

- Colectomy with terminal ileostomy and lower end brought out as a mucus fistula. The fistula can be used as a conduit for administering topical medical therapy. When the rectal stump has been closed as a Hartmann's resection the rectum is irrigated to remove the mucopurulent exudate and a catheter placed to allow decompression and prevent rectal stump blow out in the immediate postoperative period.

70 Intestinal obstruction

BV Praveen and Pradip K Datta

Multiple choice questions

➡ Pathophysiology

1. Which of the following statements are true?

A In dynamic intestinal obstruction 40% are due to adhesions.

B Proximal to an obstruction the gas is made up of 90% nitrogen and hydrogen sulphide.

C Dehydration in intestinal obstruction is solely due to vomiting.

D In dynamic obstruction the bowel distal to the obstruction initially functions normally.

E In adynamic obstruction peristalsis is absent or inadequate.

➡ Strangulation

2. The following statements are true except:

A Strangulation in intestinal obstruction is life threatening.

B In strangulation venous return is compromised before arterial supply.

C If the segment of strangulated segment of bowel is short the systemic effects will not be significant.

D Closed-loop obstruction will cause strangulation.

E The caecum might rupture in closed-loop obstruction.

➡ Special types of mechanical intestinal obstruction

3. Which of the following statements are true?

A Internal hernia is a rare cause, the diagnosis usually being made at operation.

B In the majority of internal hernia, division of the constricting agent should not be undertaken.

C Enteric strictures causing obstruction must always be resected.

D Bolus obstruction in the small bowel can be caused by stones and worms.

E Obstruction from postoperative adhesions almost never involves the large bowel.

➡ Acute intussusception

4. Which of the following statements are true?

A The condition occurs equally in children and adults.

B Intussusception in all age groups is ileocolic.

C All cases of intussusception will require an operation.

D In children the abdomen is not initially distended.

E US of abdomen has a high diagnostic sensitivity in children.

➡ Volvulus

5. Which of the following statements are true?

A The commonest type in the adult is sigmoid volvulus.

B Sigmoid volvulus can be treated by non-surgical means.

C The longer the duration of symptoms the worse the prognosis.

D Untreated the condition will result in ischaemia.

E A secondary volvulus occurs around an acquired adhesion.

Clinical features of intestinal obstruction

6. Which of the following statements are true?

A Vomiting is early and distension minimal in high small bowel obstruction.

B The vomitus is faeculent in distal small bowel obstruction.

C The more distal the obstruction in the small bowel, the greater is the abdominal distension.

D Absolute constipation is present in all cases.

E The administration of enemas can result in misleading findings.

7. The following statements are true except:

A Continuous severe pain is suggestive of strangulation.

B Tenderness over the right iliac fossa is a sinister sign.

C Fever indicates strangulation.

D Secondary polycythaemia might be a feature of dehydration.

E Normal bowel sounds excludes intestinal obstruction.

8. Which of the following statements are correct?

A The mainstay of diagnosis of strangulation is clinical.

B Shock suggests ischaemia.

C Pain is incessant in established or impending strangulation.

D Tenderness, absence of cough impulse and discoloration in an external hernia indicates strangulation.

E Generalised tenderness and rigidity requires immediate laparotomy.

Imaging in intestinal obstruction

9. The following statements are correct except:

A Erect abdominal films should be routinely carried out.

B In distal small bowel obstruction distended small bowel loops lie transversely and central in position.

C The jejunum has typical features of valvulae conniventes and the ileum is featureless.

D In colonic obstruction a water-soluble enema should be undertaken.

E Fluid levels might be seen in non-obstructive conditions.

Treatment of acute intestinal obstruction

10. Which of the following statements are not true?

A The patient must have an immediate operation.

B Antibiotic therapy is mandatory when surgery is carried out.

C In very ill patients at operation exteriorisation should be considered.

D After operation for intestinal ischaemia, reperfusion injury might occur.

E Dextrose-saline should be the fluid of choice for resuscitation.

Surgical treatment

11. Which of the following statements are true?

A Obstructed external hernia needs early operation.

B Conservative management should be considered in obstruction due to adhesions.

C On opening the abdomen, once the site of obstruction is determined, the initial step is to remove it.

D A second-look operation might sometimes be necessary.

E In obstruction without ischaemia surgery can be deferred.

Acute intestinal obstruction of the newborn

12. Which of the following statements are true?

A Congenital atresia and stenosis are the most common causes.

B Bilious vomiting is a feature of jejunal atresia.

C Perforation is never a problem.

D 'String of sausages' appearance is due to multiple atresias.

E The underlying bowel anomaly is usually an isolated finding.

→ Adynamic obstruction

13. The following statements are true except:

A In paralytic ileus colicky pain is a prominent feature.

B Metabolic abnormalities can give rise to paralytic ileus.

C CT scan should be carried out in a case that does not settle.

D Pseudo-obstruction usually affects the colon.

E Caecal perforation is a serious complication.

Extended matching questions

→ Diagnoses

1 Acute ileocolic intussusception
2 Caecal volvulus
3 Carcinoma of caecum with acute distal small bowel obstruction
4 Carcinoma of sigmoid colon with acute closed-loop obstruction
5 Colonic pseudo-obstruction
6 Faecal impaction
7 Paralytic ileus
8 Sigmoid volvulus
9 Strangulated femoral hernia
10 Strangulated umbilical hernia

Match the diagnoses with the clinical scenarios that follow:

→ Clinical scenarios

A A 45-year-old woman with a long history of intermittent right abdominal pain presents with acute onset of severe abdominal pain and distension. Examination reveals a tense tympanic lump in the left upper abdomen.

B A 62-year-old woman underwent a transperitoneal right nephrectomy for carcinoma through a transverse incision 5 days ago. She has not had a bowel action since her operation. Examination reveals a slightly tense distended abdomen with no bowel sounds. Her serum potassium is 2.4 mEq/L.

C A 74-year-old woman with a BMI of 36 presents with a painful lump around her umbilicus. She has had it for several years and it has increased in size recently. Examination reveals a large, tender, hard, lump over the umbilicus with bluish discolouration and no cough impulse.

D A 78-year-old man with chronic obstructive pulmonary disease (COPD) is an inpatient under the chest physicians. A surgical review has been requested, as he has not opened his bowels for 5 days. The abdomen is distended, which is making his chest problems worse. Examination reveals a massively distended abdomen, which is tympanic. Abdominal CT shows distended large bowel with no cut-off sign.

E A 65-year-old woman has been admitted through the Accident and Emergency Department (A&E) with abdominal pain, abdominal distension, faeculent vomiting and constipation. She has lost 20 kg in weight in 4 months. Examination reveals a patient with features of acute distal small bowel obstruction and Hb of 8 g/dL. She has never had an operation in the past.

F A 90-year-old man from the local care home was referred to A&E with abdominal pain and persistent diarrhoea. Abdominal examination reveals multiple 'masses', and rectal examination revealed a loaded rectum.

G A 78-year-old man with history of chronic constipation is brought to the A&E with a sudden onset of abdominal pain and distension. Examination reveals a distended tympanic abdomen with a 'mass' arising from the pelvis.

H A 9-month-old baby boy has been admitted to the paediatric unit with intermittent colicky abdominal with blood-stained stools and mucus in his nappy. On examination he looks unwell. Abdominal examination shows an empty right iliac fossa with a lump in the epigastrium.

I A 68-year-old man has been admitted as an emergency with colicky abdominal pain with constipation for 3 days. In between the colics he is left with a dull ache. On abdominal examination he is in some discomfort with tenderness and distension particularly in the peripheral part. Over the past 4 months he has been increasingly constipated having to take large amounts of laxatives to open his bowels.

J An 84-year-old woman has been admitted with a 12-hour history of colicky abdominal pain, distension, vomiting and constipation; the vomitus, bilious to start with, became faeculent. Clinical examination shows a small erythematous tender lump below the inguinal ligament and lateral to the pubic tubercle.

Answers to multiple choice questions

→ Pathophysiology

1. A, B, D, E

Intestinal obstruction can be dynamic where there is a mechanical obstruction or adynamic where there is no mechanical obstruction and is due to absent or diminished peristalsis. There are several causes of dynamic intestinal obstruction, 40% of which are due to adhesions; carcinoma and inflammatory conditions account for 15% each whereas obstructed hernia is a cause in 12%. Proximal to an obstruction there is distension, which is made up of gases and fluid. Overgrowth of aerobic and anaerobic organisms result in gas production, 90% of which is made up of nitrogen and hydrogen sulphide.

In dynamic obstruction, initially the bowel proximally functions normally, but if the obstruction is not relieved, peristalsis reduces and ceases resulting in paralysis. In adynamic obstruction the underlying pathology is paralysis of the Auerbach's and Meissner's plexuses resulting in stasis (see the following). Dehydration is a cardinal feature of intestinal obstruction clinically apparent by sunken eyes, dry tongue and loss of skin turgor. Vomiting is only one of the factors that cause dehydration, the others being lack of absorption, fluid sequestration within the bowel lumen (loss into third space) and transudation into the peritoneal cavity.

→ Strangulation

2. C

Strangulation denotes loss of blood supply to an obstructed bowel. The effects of strangulation do not depend upon the length of strangulated bowel. In a strangulated external hernia where the length of bowel that loses its blood supply might be short, or in a Richter's hernia where only a knuckle of bowel is strangulated, the deleterious systemic effects will still be very significant due to sepsis and proximal obstruction.

Strangulation in intestinal obstruction is life-threatening because of the loss of blood supply and the effects of ischaemia. Venous return is the first to be compromised followed by arterial supply. Strangulation can also be the outcome of a closed-loop obstruction when a loop of bowel is closed off at both ends such as a distal colonic carcinoma with a competent ileocaecal valve (which is present in a third of patients). This results in ballooning of the caecum, which distends to such an extent that it becomes gangrenous and perforates.

Special types of mechanical intestinal obstruction

3. A, B, D, E

Internal hernia is a rare cause of intestinal obstruction, almost always involving the small bowel, the diagnosis being made at laparotomy when a patient is being operated upon for unexplained intestinal obstruction. There are several potential sites of internal herniation – normal anatomical foramen such as the foramen of Winslow, paraduodenal fossae, or mesenteric defects. At operation division of the constricting agent should not be undertaken as important vessels/structures run on the edge of the constricting ring, e.g., portal vein, hepatic artery and bile duct on the edge of the epiploic foramen (of Winslow).

A gallstone can cause distal small bowel obstruction, once again the diagnosis usually made at laparotomy (see details in **Chapter 67:** The gall bladder and bile ducts). The other cause of bolus obstruction is round worms, not uncommon in developing countries (see **Chapter 6** Surgery in the tropics). Postoperative adhesive obstruction almost never involves the large bowel; it is the distal small bowel that is usually affected. When an enteric stricture is the cause, resection and end-to-end anastomosis is not always necessary such as in Crohn's disease when a strictureplasty can be done.

Acute intussusception

4. D, E

Acute intussusception, although a mechanical intestinal obstruction, when it occurs in children does not cause abdominal distension in the initial stages. There is emptiness in the right iliac fossa with a lump that is felt to be hardening in real time in 60% of cases. In children, abdominal US has a high diagnostic sensitivity showing typical doughnut appearance of concentric rings. CT scan is the most sensitive imaging showing the 'target' or 'sausage' shaped soft-tissue mass; but in view of the radiation it might not be an advisable investigation for children.

The condition mostly occurs in children between five and 10 months when 90% of cases are idiopathic. The remainder might have an underlying pathology such as a polyp, Meckel's diverticulum or Henoch-Schönlein purpura when the child is usually beyond 2 years. In children the type is ileocolic whilst in adults it is colo-colic because, in the latter group, almost always the underlying cause is a polypoid carcinoma that can be seen on barium enema as a claw-shaped deformity **(Figure 70.1)**. The condition, when it occurs in children, does not always need an operation as it can be reduced by hydrostatic decompression, the procedure being particularly successful if treated within 12 hours of onset.

Volvulus

5. A, B, D, E

Volvulus of the sigmoid colon is the commonest type that occurs in the adult. It can be primary when it occurs due to abnormal mesenteric attachments or congenital bands. When diagnosed, if the patient is not ill without any signs of ischaemia, non-surgical treatment in the form of endoscopic decompression can be successful; a flatus tube is then inserted to make sure the decompression continues and the volvulus does not recur.

If conservative measures are not successful and the patient is not promptly treated, the mechanical twisting causes the mesenteric veins to get obstructed resulting in thrombosis and ischaemia. A volvulus can be primary or secondary. The primary type is the result of congenital malrotation, abnormal mesenteric attachments, or congenital bands, for example,

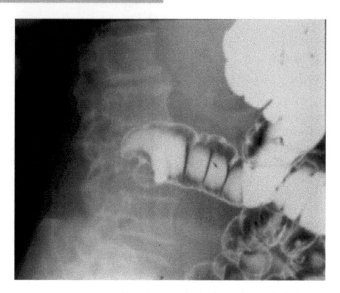

Figure 70.1　Barium enema showing typical claw-shaped deformity in adult acute colo-colic intussusception from polypoid carcinoma.

volvulus neonatorum, caecal and sigmoid volvulus. A secondary volvulus which is rotation of a bowel segment around an acquired adhesion is much more common. The prognosis of a volvulus is much better when the condition takes a slow, progressive course and is of gradual onset. On the other hand when the onset is sudden and of short duration the condition is of a fulminant variety and carries a poor prognosis.

→ Clinical features of intestinal obstruction

6. A, B, C, E

The clinical features depend upon the site of obstruction. In high small bowel obstruction vomiting occurs early; as the obstruction is high, the distal bowel is collapsed hardly causing any abdominal distension. It therefore follows that the more distal the obstruction in the ileum, the greater will be the abdominal distension. For the same reason the vomitus will be faeculent in content, which follows to bilious vomiting that occurs at the outset.

As an initial management, enemas used to be administered in days gone by. This practice gives misleading results, as there will be evacuation of faecal contents that are already present distal to the obstruction prior to the onset of the acute episode thus confusing the issue. Absolute constipation (lack of faeces and flatus), although a feature in the majority, is not always present. Diarrhoea might be present in Richter's hernia, mesenteric vascular occlusion and partial obstruction.

7. E

Normal bowel sounds do not exclude intestinal obstruction. Bowel sounds might be scanty or absent in long-standing obstruction. This is not a reliable clinical feature. Continuous severe pain is suggestive of strangulation. Pain of small bowel origin is centred on the umbilicus while pain from large bowel obstruction is in the lower abdomen. Tenderness in the right iliac fossa is a sinister sign as it signifies ischaemia and impending rupture of the caecum; this would be from a closed-loop large bowel obstruction due to a competent ileocaecal valve. Fever is a sign of toxicity and hence might indicate ischaemia from strangulation or perforation. Long-standing dehydration will result in haemoconcentration causing secondary polycythaemia.

8. A, B, C, D, E

It is essential to be able to recognise strangulation in a case of intestinal obstruction. Once strangulation (compromise of blood supply) supervenes, the mortality and morbidity rises. The mainstay of diagnosis of strangulation is clinical. The pain is incessant and severe. When an irreducible hernia (inguinal or femoral) is palpated in a case of intestinal obstruction, gentle palpation of the lump is important. If the lump is tender with no cough impulse, feels hard and looks discoloured, the picture is one of strangulation. When strangulation has been going on for some time, the patient might show features of endotoxic shock – pyrexia, hyperdynamic circulation, high pulse pressure and bounding pulse. Abdomen would show generalised tenderness, rigidity with rebound tenderness. It is time to do an urgent operation.

Imaging in intestinal obstruction

9. A

Traditionally, x-ray requests for intestinal obstruction always said 'Erect and supine'. An erect x-ray is no longer asked for because it does not give as much information as a supine film. Erect film shows only fluid levels whereas a supine film will show the pattern of abdominal distension thereby revealing the site of obstruction. Moreover, fluid levels take longer to show up because it takes longer for gas and fluid to separate; hence it is a late sign. In colonic obstruction, fluids levels are not seen when the ileocaecal valve is competent. On the other hand fluid levels might show up when there is no obstruction such as in gastroenteritis, acute pancreatitis and intra-abdominal sepsis.

In small bowel distension, the bowel loops lie centrally and are transversely placed **(Figure 70.2)** with hardly any gas in the colon. Distended jejunum has typical features – straight lines at regular intervals passing across the entire width of the dilated bowel giving the appearance of a ladder lying on its side. These are called 'valvulae conniventes'. The ileum looks like a distended tube without any features described as 'characteristically characterless'. In colonic obstruction haustrations are seen. When large bowel obstruction is suspected, a limited water-soluble enema is done to ascertain the site and cause of obstruction, particularly to exclude pseudo-obstruction. A CT colonography is the usual investigation of choice.

Treatment of acute intestinal obstruction

10. A, E

Patients should not be operated upon immediately. Every patient, even the patient with suspected ischaemic bowel, needs thorough resuscitation and anaesthetic assessment. Resuscitation must consist of nasogastric suction to decompress the distended bowel, intravenous fluids to treat dehydration and analgesia to relieve pain. Fluid used for resuscitation should be Hartmann's solution or normal saline with added potassium (depending upon the patient's urea and electrolytes) monitored by indwelling urinary catheter and a CVP line.

Prophylactic broad-spectrum antibiotics are given before the patient is taken to theatre. The very-ill patient might require planning of ICU treatment and the possible use of inotropes. Such patients undergoing bowel resection should be considered for exteriorisation of proximal and distal ends of bowel rather than primary end-to-end anastomosis. When bowel resection is done for intestinal ischaemia, one must be aware of reperfusion injury of the lung from release of inflammatory mediators. This can be prevented or the chances minimised

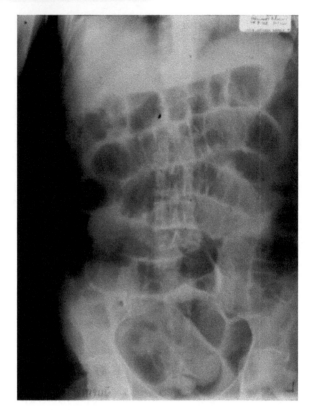

Figure 70.2 Plain x-ray of abdomen showing acute distal small bowel obstruction showing valvulae conniventes and characterless ileum.

at operation by clamping the blood vessels supplying ischaemic bowel before handling the bowel itself.

➙ Surgical treatment

11. A, B, D, E

An external hernia, femoral, inguinal or incisional, that is obstructed as diagnosed by the clinical findings of irreducibility, lack of cough impulse and pain, needs early operation before it goes on to lose its blood supply, i.e., strangulation sets in. After adequate resuscitation, the patient is taken to theatre. When obstruction is suspected to be due to adhesions and there are no signs of compromise of blood supply, a period of conservative management – analgesia, nasogastric suction and intravenous fluids – should be tried. This might help relieve the obstruction. Moreover, further operation creates more adhesions.

In mesenteric vascular occlusion with multiple ischaemic areas a second-look laparotomy is often required after 24 to 48 hours. This is to reassess the gut and perform the appropriate procedure. When intestinal obstruction is present without ischaemia, surgery can be deferred until thorough resuscitation and assessment to find the cause and site of obstruction has been made.

At operation for intestinal obstruction, once the abdomen is opened, the immediate step is not to remove the obstruction but to decompress the proximal distended bowel. This is to create room for the operation to proceed and assess the fluid loss into the third space so that it can be promptly replaced intraoperatively. To achieve this, the anaesthetist is requested to pass a large bore orogastric tube; the distended bowel contents are then milked retrogradely back into the stomach from where it is aspirated. The amount removed is replaced intravenously.

Adynamic obstruction

12. A

Colicky abdominal pain is not a feature of paralytic ileus. Pain is usually from the scar, the pain getting worse with abdominal distension. The condition is the result of lack of peristalsis from paralysis of the myenteric and submucous plexus of nerves. Although most commonly it occurs after an abdominal operation, intra-abdominal sepsis, fractures of spine or retroperitoneal haemorrhage might cause paralytic ileus; uraemia and hypokalaemia might cause or exacerbate and already existing ileus. When prolonged, CT scan to exclude intra-abdominal sepsis or a mechanical obstruction is the investigation of choice.

Pseudo-obstruction is the other cause of adynamic obstruction. Usually it affects the colon. When acute, it is called Ogilvie's syndrome. It can occur in a chronic form. It needs to be distinguished from mechanical obstruction for example from a carcinoma by a water-soluble contrast enema or CT colonography. If untreated it can give rise to caecal perforation, which is likely when the caecal diameter is 14 cm or more.

Acute intestinal obstruction of the newborn

13. A, B, D

While congenital atresia and stenosis are the most common causes of neonatal intestinal obstruction, the other causes are intestinal malrotation with midgut volvulus, meconium ileus, Hirschsprung's disease, imperforate anus, necrotising enterocolitis and an incarcerated inguinal hernia. There are four main types of jejunal or ileal atresia.

Abdominal distension is more prominent in ileal atresia and a small amount of meconium might be passed despite the atresia. The possibility of multiple atresias makes intraoperative assessment of the whole small and large bowel mandatory. Congenital anomalies and associated malformations are common and should be excluded. This is the domain of the specialist paediatric surgeon rather than the general surgeon with interest in paediatric surgery. Therefore the reader interested in this topic is asked to refer to a textbook for more details.

Answers to extended matching questions

1. H Acute ileocolic intussusception

The typical presentation is that of a little boy about to reach his first birthday who has episodes of screaming because of colicky abdominal pain. Associated with the screams the toddler pulls up his arms and legs as a reflex action to his abdominal colics. The parents might notice blood and mucus in the nappies often referred to as 'red currant jelly stools'. Vomiting is a late feature. In between the attacks the child looks unwell. Abdominal palpation when the child is pain-free, would reveal and empty right iliac fossa with the possibility of a mass in the epigastrium; the mass is sausage-shaped with the concavity towards the umbilicus. Rectal examination confirms blood-stained mucus.

The diagnosis is confirmed by an US demonstrating the typical doughnut appearance in concentric rings; a barium enema **(Figure 70.3a** and **b)** shows the classical crab-claw deformity. While CT scan is regarded as the most sensitive imaging modality which shows a 'target' or 'sausage-shaped' soft-tissue mass, exposure to the amount of radiation in a child might preclude its use. Once confirmed, reduction should be attempted using air or contrast enema under image intensifier. This is successful in 7 out of 10 patients, success being gauged by the free reflux of the contrast into the terminal ileum. Non-operative reduction

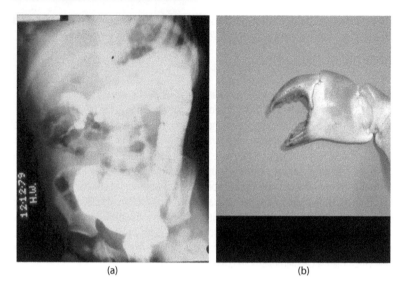

(a)   (b)

Figure 70.3 (a) and (b) Barium enema showing typical 'crab-claw' deformity in childhood ileo-colic intussusception.

should not be attempted in the presence of peritonitis. Unsuccessful reduction or peritonitis requires an urgent operation. At operation, when the bowel is viable, reduction is attempted by milking the intussusceptum out of the intussuscepiens. In the case of ischaemic bowel, limited ileocolic resection and end-to-end anastomosis is done.

2. A Caecal volvulus
This condition occurs because the caecum along with the lower part of ascending colon hangs loosely on a congenital mesentery, which is attached to the retroperitoneum in the right iliac fossa. This is called Jackson's membrane or veil and is responsible for the excessive mobility of the caecum and ascending colon making them susceptible to volvulus. Most often it is a volvulus of the caecum and ascending colon. This presents as a surgical emergency with acute abdominal pain and constipation although to start with the obstruction is partial.

Examination reveals a palpable tympanic swelling in the epigastrium or left upper quadrant. Plain abdominal x-ray might show caecal dilatation with a single air-fluid level with proximal small bowel dilatation. While ischaemia occurs early, if there are no signs of ischaemia, a barium enema or a CT scan can be done to confirm the diagnosis. The treatment is operation. At operation if the bowel is viable, the caecum and ascending colon are untwisted and the caecum is fixed by doing a caecostomy with a Foley catheter. When the bowel is gangrenous, right hemicolectomy is the treatment.

3. E Carcinoma of caecum with acute distal small bowel obstruction
Acute distal small bowel obstruction is one of the typical emergency presentations of carcinoma of the caecum. This occurs because the cancer obstructs the ileocaecal junction. The patient would complain of gradual abdominal distension associated with colicky generalised abdominal pain and vomiting. The vomitus will be bilious to start with and later it is faeculent. Examination would show an ill, dehydrated patient with sunken eyes, dry tongue and loss of skin turgor. Abdominal distension might not allow a caecal mass to be palpable.

This patient needs immediate resuscitation in the form of analgesia, nasogastric decompression and intravenous fluids. The patient is anaemic with a haemoglobin of 8 gm/dL. This might be adequate and after consultation with the anaesthetist, the patient is taken to theatre for emergency laparotomy. If time permits, a CT colonography can be carried out to confirm obstruction at the ileocaecal junction from a filling defect in the caecum – a carcinoma.

At laparotomy through a midline incision, on opening the abdomen there would be a transudate of free peritoneal fluid, which is sucked out. The distended small bowel is decompressed by milking the contents proximally into the stomach and having it aspirated by an orogastric tube. Once the bowel is decompressed, the carcinoma will be felt and assessed fully along with palpation of the liver for secondaries. A right hemicolectomy is carried out with ileotransverse anastomosis. Even if secondaries are found in the liver, the operation is still a right hemicolectomy. In the very rare instance when the growth is so far locally advanced that it cannot be resected, then a side-to-side ileotransverse anastomosis is carried out as a palliative procedure to overcome the acute bowel obstruction.

4. I Carcinoma of sigmoid colon with acute closed-loop obstruction

The typical emergency presentation is one of acute closed-loop obstruction with abdominal distention and absolute constipation. There might be nausea and vomiting depending on the patency of the ileocaecal valve. On examination, the patient is dry and dehydrated with abdominal distension and tinkling bowel sounds. A clinical diagnosis of acute closed-loop large bowel obstruction is made.

The patient is resuscitated by analgesics, maintaining airway with oxygenation, fluid resuscitation with monitoring by an indwelling urinary catheter and CVP line. Simultaneously arrangements should be made for confirmation of the diagnosis and definitive management. For confirmation plain abdominal x-ray **(Figure 70.4)** followed by CT colonography is carried out, which will show the exact site of obstruction; this will also exclude pseudo-obstruction (see the following). Some might do a flexible sigmoidoscopy, which might not be very comfortable for the patient in acute obstruction. A CXR is done.

The most common cause is left-sided carcinoma, usually the sigmoid colon; diverticular stricture and sigmoid volvulus (see the following) are other causes. In sigmoid carcinoma, after optimum resuscitation, facilities and expertise being available, colonic stenting should be considered. Stenting is an option for all left-sided malignant obstructing lesions up to

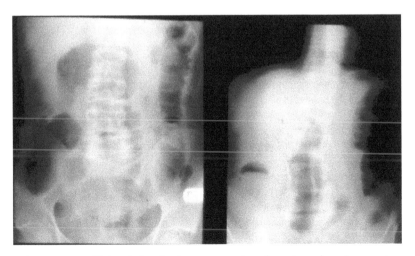

Figure 70.4 Plain abdominal x-ray, erect and supine, showing acute closed-loop large bowel obstruction with massive distension of caecum, transverse colon and descending colon.

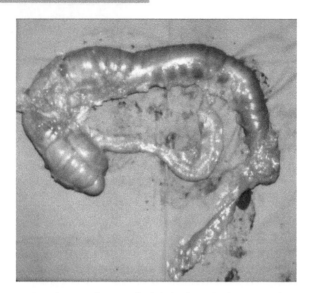

Figure 70.5 Specimen of extended right hemicolectomy showing acute closed-loop large bowel obstruction.

10 cm proximal to the anorectal junction. Sometimes more proximal lesions can be stented depending upon the expertise of the surgeon or radiologist or gastroenterologist. Successful stenting converts an emergency to a semi-elective situation. The patient can be prepared for anterior resection within the next week.

If the patient happens to be very tender over the caecum, it denotes impending caecal rupture; then stenting should not be considered. The patient should be prepared for a subtotal colectomy and ileorectal anastomosis. If the obstruction is in the region of the splenic flexure **(Figure 70.5)**, a one-stage extended right hemicolectomy is the best treatment option.

In the absence of the aforementioned facilities and expertise, the next best option is resection of the obstructing lesion followed by proximal stoma (Hartmann's procedure). If the expertise is available and the patient is a good anaesthetic risk, one-stage resection and end-to-end anastomosis with on-table colonic irrigation can be considered.

5. D Colonic pseudo-obstruction

This is due to obstruction of the large bowel without any mechanical cause. In the acute stage it is known as Ogilvie's syndrome and occurs in 10% of large bowel obstructions. While the patient has all the features of acute close-loop large bowel obstruction, imaging is essential as it is a diagnosis of exclusion. In this regard a CT colonography is carried out. Once a mechanical obstruction has been excluded, the cause has been identified and the patient treated while at the same time keeping a close watch on the patient as caecal perforation can occur.

There are several factors associated with Ogilvie's syndrome – metabolic, pelvic trauma, shock, retroperitoneal irritation or certain drugs. This particular patient who has COPD would be on various drugs, which might be the cause. After consultation with the physician colleagues, intravenous neostigmine (1 mg, repeated if needed) is given. If unsuccessful, colonoscopic decompression should be performed all the time bearing in mind the danger of impending caecal perforation. This would be suspected clinically if the patient is very tender on the right iliac fossa or if the caecum is seen to be >14 cm in diameter on the plain abdominal x-ray. Surgery is then indicated.

6. F Faecal impaction

An elderly patient, with a history of chronic constipation and long-term habitual use of laxatives, presents with abdominal pain, distension and faecal leakage (often referred to as 'diarrhoea'). The abdomen can be massively distended but is soft. Stools are usually palpable abdominally in sigmoid colon. Faecal impaction is often a cause of acute urinary retention. On rectal examination the rectum will be found to be loaded. Abdominal x-ray will confirm gross faecal loading.

The first priority is to get the stools disimpacted and rectum cleared. This is achieved by a combination of suppositories, enemas and manual evacuation under general anaesthetic. Laxatives are continued to avoid recurrence. The patient should be kept under close observation for the very serious complication of stercoral perforation.

7. B Paralytic ileus

In surgical practice this occurs most commonly postoperatively. It is due to absence of peristalsis brought on by temporary cessation of the function of the myenteric and submucous nerve plexuses. Abdominal distension without pain is the predominant clinical feature.

Other causes of paralytic ileus are recognised. This might be summarised by the acronym 'ILEUS': *I*nfection. Intra-abdominal sepsis giving rise to localised or generalised ileus; *L*ocal (reflex) causes, such as fractures of the spine or ribs, retroperitoneal haemorrhage; *E*lectrolyte abnormalities, such as hypokalaemia and hypoproteinaemia; *U*raemia and metabolic causes; *S*urgery.

The management is nasogastric decompression with close attention to fluid and electrolyte balance. Nowadays with the use of enhanced recovery programme, routine use of nasogastric tubes after abdominal surgery has been abandoned. Ileus in the postoperative period usually lasts up to a maximum of 72 hours. Beyond that period one should consider looking for a cause such as intra-abdominal sepsis or unexpected mechanical obstruction. This becomes more important when a patient relapses into ileus after a period of initial recovery in the immediate postoperative period. The ideal way of doing so is a CT scan. If no cause is found, as a last resort, gastric prokinetic agent such as domperidone or erythromycin can be tried.

8. G Sigmoid volvulus

The patient, usually elderly, presents with massively distended abdomen which might have happened over a period of several hours. There is usually a history of chronic constipation and similar previous episodes. The abdominal distension is asymmetric with a 'mass' arising from the pelvis on the left side. The abdomen is tympanic and the rectum is usually empty. The abdominal x-ray is diagnostic **(Figure 70.6)** and shows the massively dilated sigmoid loop variously described as 'coffee-bean' sign and 'bent inner-tube 'sign. Left untreated, ischaemia and perforation can occur.

After resuscitation, in the absence of signs of peritonism, conservative management in the form of endoscopic deflation should be attempted by performing a flexible sigmoidoscopy. Success in deflation is gauged by the sudden expulsion of a huge amount of gas and liquid faeces with the abdomen obviously becoming flatter and softer. A flatus tube is left in place for a few days. When there are signs of peritonism, laparotomy must be performed. Viable bowel is untwisted, a manoeuvre facilitated by the passage of a flatus tube from the anus and guided through the obstruction into the proximal colon. Once deflated, the sigmoid is fixed.

Once the patient has recovered consideration should be given to elective resection to prevent recurrence. In the younger patient this is carried out whilst in the elderly comorbidities might prevent this procedure.

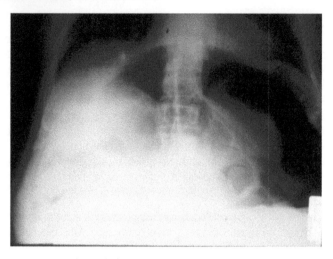

Figure 70.6 Plain abdominal x-ray showing sigmoid volvulus.

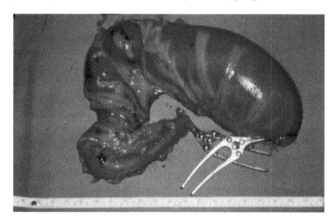

Figure 70.7 Specimen after Paul-Mickulicz resection for sigmoid volvulus.

When ischaemic sigmoid colon is found at operation, sigmoid resection is carried out with both ends being brought out in the left iliac fossa (Paul-Mickulicz operation) **(Figure 70.7)** with bowel continuity being restored at a later date. A Hartmann's operation is the other alternative, the procedure being reversed when convenient.

9. J Strangulated femoral hernia

This woman, admitted as an emergency, will be very unwell because of her distal small bowel obstruction causing dehydration, which might be compounded by toxicity if the obstructed bowel is strangulated. In such patients it can be easy to miss a small femoral hernia amidst the abdominal distension in an obese abdomen. The presence of a hernia should be sought for diligently.

The patient needs to be resuscitated with intravenous fluids, nasogastric suction and an indwelling catheter. Once fluid and electrolyte depletion has been corrected according to the blood parameters, the patient is taken to theatre. Although this is an obstructed (incarcerated) femoral hernia with the potential for strangulation, the first incision should be in the groin as for a low approach. This is because the vast majority of patients do not require a bowel resection. Should a bowel resection be necessary (and that would be necessary in a minority), it should then be carried out through a separate lower mid-line laparotomy. With this approach, the patient without an abdominal incision recovers much more quickly because of less pain from a groin incision and no paralytic ileus.

A low groin crease incision is made followed by identification and dissection of the hernial sac below the inguinal ligament. The sac is then opened and the obstructed bowel is released by incising the neck of the sac, which is the usual constricting agent. The bowel, which is usually a loop of ileum, is delivered into the wound and wrapped in hot towels with the patient being given 100% oxygen. This should make the sheen of the bowel to return with pulsations in the mesenteric arteries. The bowel is then put back into the abdomen. In some cases where the bowel was pinched by the constricting ring, there might be small dark patches. These are best invaginated with interrupted seromuscular sutures. The redundant sac is excised, the femoral ring and canal are obliterated by approximating the inguinal ligament to the pectineal ligament with interrupted prolene sutures, and the wound is closed.

In the rare instance when bowel resection has to be carried out due to gangrene, the ileal loop is held in a Babcock forceps in the groin wound. A lower midline incision is made, the ileal loop is now delivered into the laparotomy wound and resection and end-to-end anastomosis is carried out with closure of the wound. The groin wound is now dealt with as described previously after repairing the femoral ring and obliterating the canal.

10. C Strangulated umbilical hernia

Strangulation is one of the most serious consequences of intestinal obstruction and hence has to be considered when dealing with all cases of irreducible external hernia.

Shock, refractory to fluid resuscitation, especially when associated with toxicity is almost always due to impending or established strangulation. Pain is never completely absent. When strangulation occurs in an external hernia, the lump is tense, tender, hard and irreducible without a cough impulse. Skin changes such as erythema or purplish discoloration might be seen. Such a patient needs an immediate operation.

Resuscitation is carried out as previously described. A transverse incision is made below the hernia. The hernial sac is opened at the neck (not the fundus because of adhesions). Blood-stained fluid will be sucked out. The irreducible bowel is carefully held to prevent it from slipping into the peritoneal cavity, and the neck of the sac (the strangulating agent) is incised to release the bowel into the wound. The bowel is made to recover with warm moist packs and 100% oxygen. On recovery, the bowel is returned into the peritoneal cavity. The neck is now closed with interrupted non-absorbable sutures and the wound closed. It is prudent not to use any artificial mesh to reinforce the hernia in view of the infected field.

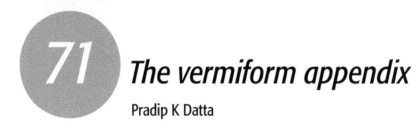

71 *The vermiform appendix*

Pradip K Datta

Multiple choice questions

→ ### Anatomy

1. The following statements are true except:

A The appendicular artery arises from the right colic artery.

B The commonest position of the appendix is retrocaecal.

C The position of the base of the appendix is constant.

D The submucosa is rich in lymphoid follicles.

E Argentaffin cells are found in the base of the crypts.

→ ### Acute appendicitis

2. Which of the following statements are true?

A The peak incidence of acute appendicitis is in the teens and early 20s.

B The incidence of acute appendicitis is lowest in those who have a high intake of dietary fibre.

C Obstruction of the appendix lumen by a caecal carcinoma might give rise to acute appendicitis.

D Aerobic and anaerobic organisms are responsible for acute appendicitis.

E A mucocele of the appendix is a clinical variation of acute appendicitis.

3. The following factors increase the chances of peritonitis and systemic sepsis except:

A Obesity

B Extremes of age

C Immunosuppression

D Pelvic position of appendix

E Previous abdominal operation

4. Which of the following are signs in acute appendicitis?

A Rovsing's sign

B Pointing sign

C Obturator sign

D Psoas sign

E Troisier's sign

5. Which of the following statements is not true in acute appendicitis?

A It carries a higher mortality in the elderly.

B Acute appendicitis in pregnancy will result in foetal loss in 30%.

C An Alvarado score of 7 or more is suggestive of the diagnosis.

D A decision to operate based on clinical suspicion alone will result in removal of a normal appendix in 15%–30%

E Cancer of the caecum might masquerade as acute appendicitis.

→ ### Differential diagnosis

6. In children the following could be confused with acute appendicitis except:

A Gastroenteritis

B Mesenteric adenitis

C Henoch-Schönlein purpura

D Urinary tract infection (UTI)

E Lobar pneumonia

7. In the adult male, which of the following conditions are differential diagnosis of acute appendicitis?

A Mesenteric cyst

B Right ureteric colic

C Perforated peptic ulcer

D Crohn's disease

E Right testicular torsion

8. In the adult female, which of the following is not part of the differential diagnosis of acute appendicitis?
A Mittelschmerz
B Pelvic inflammatory disease (PID)
C Acute cholecystitis
D Ruptured ectopic pregnancy or right tubal abortion
E Torsion or ruptured ovarian cyst

9. In the elderly, which of the following is not part of the differential diagnosis of acute appendicitis?
A Diverticulitis
B Intestinal obstruction
C Mesenteric infarction
D Bladder calculus
E Carcinoma of the caecum

Extended matching questions

→ Diagnoses

1 Acute appendicitis
2 Carcinoid tumour
3 Carcinoma of caecum
4 Crohn's disease
5 Mittelschmerz
6 Perforated duodenal ulcer
7 Pseudomyxoma peritonei
8 Right ureteric colic
9 Ruptured ectopic pregnancy

→ Clinical scenarios

Match the diagnoses with each of the scenarios that follow:

A A 25-year-old female complains of severe pain in her central lower abdomen of 4 hours duration. She feels faint, is very thirsty and is unsure about her last menstrual period. On examination she is in agony, looks pale and is cold, clammy and sweaty. She is apyrexial with marked tenderness, rigidity and rebound tenderness over her entire lower abdomen. She has a Cullen's sign.

B A 35-year-old male complains of colicky pain in the right iliac fossa for the last 6 hours. In between the attacks he is left with a dull ache. He has vomited a few times and feels feverish. In the past he has had diarrhoea on and off for almost 1 year. On examination he has a temperature of 38°C, is in discomfort from his pain and has tenderness, rigidity and minimal rebound tenderness in the right iliac fossa.

C A 40-year-old male complains of pain in his right iliac fossa over the past 2 days. His pain in the right iliac fossa was preceded by a bout of sudden onset of severe epigastric and right upper quadrant pain 3 days ago that lasted for a few hours. This initial pain subsided with some antacids, which he has been taking on and off for 'indigestion' for almost 18 months. On examination he is pyrexial (39°C) and very tender and rigid over the right iliac fossa.

D An 18-year-old male complains of generalised colicky abdominal pain for about 6 hours. He feels unwell, has vomited a couple of times and is anorexic. The pain has shifted to the right iliac fossa. On examination he has pyrexia of 38°C, is tender over the right iliac fossa with rigidity and rebound tenderness.

E A 28-year-old male complains of sudden onset of severe right-sided abdominal pain, which started in his loin. He is in agony, writhing around and cannot find a comfortable position to get any relief from his pain, which is radiating to his groin. He has some strangury. On examination he is tender all over the right side of his abdomen with some rigidity but no rebound. On percussion there is a tympanic note.

F A 22-year-old female patient complains of pain in the right iliac fossa. The pain started suddenly and has spread all over the lower abdomen. Her last menstrual period was 2 weeks ago. On examination she looks slightly pale and apyrexial and is tender with rigidity and rebound tenderness in the right iliac fossa.

G A 60-year-old male patient complains of pain in his right iliac fossa of 24-hour duration. The pain has been constant in the right iliac fossa. He has felt unwell for a few months, being unduly short of breath during his normal activities. On examination he looks pale and is tender with rigidity and rebound tenderness in the right iliac fossa.

H A 35-year-old woman underwent an emergency appendicectomy for suspected 'acute appendicitis'. At operation the appendix looked normal with a bulbous solid yellowish coloured mass at its tip.

I A 42-year-old woman complains of generalised lower abdominal pain, abdominal distension and generally feeling unwell and putting on weight. On examination she has a distended abdomen with a feeling of ascites without shifting dullness. She has been unsuccessfully trying for a baby for a few years.

Answers to multiple choice questions

→ Anatomy

1. A

The appendicular artery arises from the lower branch of the ileo-colic artery and enters the mesoappendix behind the terminal ileum lying in its free border. The appendicular artery is an end artery so that when it is thrombosed in acute appendicitis gangrene and perforation are inevitable. The positions of the appendix are as follows: retrocaecal 74%, pelvic 21%, paracaecal 2%, subcaecal 1.5%, preileal 1% and postileal 0.5%.

The position of the base of the appendix is constant. It is found at the confluence of the three taeniae coli, an anatomical fact often used to find the appendix during an operation for acute appendicitis. Histologically the submucosa of the appendix is rich in lymphoid follicles. In the base of the appendicular crypts argentaffin (Kulschitsky) cells, the source of carcinoid tumours, are present.

→ Acute appendicitis

2. A, B, C, D

The peak incidence of acute appendicitis is in the teens and early twenties. The incidence is lowest in societies that have a high-residue diet similar to that of colonic diverticular disease. Obstruction of the lumen of the appendix might trigger the onset of acute inflammation. This obstruction in the older age group might be caused by a caecal carcinoma, which therefore in some cases presents as acute appendicitis. The cause is usually a mixture of aerobic and anaerobic organisms.

When the appendicular lumen at the base is obstructed initiating infection and inflammation, rarely the pathology resolves. In due course the appendix distends over a period of time due to the lumen filling with mucus causing the formation of a mucocele. This is not a variation of acute appendicitis.

3. A

The obese patient who would be endowed with ample greater omentum will be protected from perforation and its sinister effects. Once there is an inflamed appendix, the greater omentum will help to localise the infection by enveloping the inflamed appendix preventing perforation and its ill effects.

At the extremes of age the amount of greater omentum is less; therefore there is less likelihood of the peritonitis being localised causing greater risk of perforation. The immunosuppressed patient and diabetics are more susceptible to perforation and its ill effects. Pelvic position of the appendix causing it to hang freely over the pelvic brim results in free perforation and spread of peritonitis without a chance of localisation. The situation is similar if the patient has had a previous abdominal operation; adhesions would limit the ability of the greater omentum to wall off the infection. In all these situations generalised peritonitis will occur quickly and if it is not diagnosed and treated promptly systemic inflammatory response syndrome would supervene.

4. A, B, C, D
Rovsing's sign is pain in the right iliac fossa elicited on deep palpation of the left iliac fossa. Rovsing's original description was to distend the caecum by pushing the bowel contents (gas) in an anti-peristaltic manoeuvre toward the ileocaecal valve increasing pressure around the appendix. Others believe that the pain in the right iliac fossa is a mere reflection of local peritoneal irritation. **'Pointing sign'** is merely asking the patient to point with one finger where the pain began and where it settled. When an inflamed appendix lies against the psoas muscle, the patient finds that the pain eases on flexing the hip – the **'psoas sign'**. If an inflamed appendix is in contact with the obturator internus, contracting it by flexing and internally rotating the hip will elicit pain in the suprapubic area – **'obturator test' of Cope**.

Troisier's sign is a palpable left supraclavicular lymph node due to a metastasis from cancer stomach that has spread through the thoracic duct.

5. B
Acute appendicitis is the most common extrauterine abdominal emergency in pregnancy. Foetal loss occurs in 3% to 5% of cases, increasing to 20% in perforated appendicitis. Diagnosis is sometimes delayed because early symptoms might be nonspecific and attributed to the pregnancy.

The condition carries a higher mortality in the elderly for the following reasons: They often have comorbidities; and they might harbour gangrenous appendicitis without obvious clinical features that might mimic subacute intestinal obstruction. Operating on clinical grounds alone results in the removal of a normal appendix in 15% to 30% of cases. Therefore scoring systems have been devised based on the clinical criteria and laboratory investigations to be certain as much as possible about the diagnosis. An Alvarado score of >7 strongly points to a diagnosis of acute appendicitis.

In the elderly, sometimes carcinoma of the caecum can present as acute appendicitis when the growth encroaches into the appendicular lumen. Any patient beyond middle age who is anaemic and presents with features of 'acute appendicitis' has almost certainly a caecal carcinoma because anaemia is not a feature of genuine acute appendicitis.

Differential diagnosis
6. D
In children UTI is not commonly confused with acute appendicitis. UTI is a rare cause of acute abdominal pain; urinary symptoms, vomiting and fever are common features. Urinalysis and microscopy are helpful although sterile pyuria might be present in acute appendicitis. In **acute gastroenteritis** abdominal pain, diarrhoea and vomiting usually start at the same time and rebound is uncommon. In **mesenteric adenitis**, high fever and upper-respiratory symptoms predominate besides abdominal pain. **Henoch-Schonlein purpura** often starts with sore throat and is associated with ecchymosis of the limbs and buttocks. In **right lobar pneumonia** there is high temperature with minimal right upper quadrant tenderness.

In spite of the awareness of these conditions, at times it might be impossible to exclude acute appendicitis in children and to be on the safe side, appendicectomy has to be carried out.

7. B, C, D, E

Right ureteric colic can be confused with acute appendicitis if the history is atypical. Presence of RBCs in urine should help in diagnosing ureteric calculus although a spiral CT should clinch the diagnosis. **Perforated duodenal ulcer** can be confused with acute appendicitis when the contents have tracked down the right paracolic gutter to produce signs in the right iliac fossa. A careful history with an erect CXR to look for gas under the right dome of the diaphragm should help. Previous history of altered bowel habit should suggest **Crohn's disease**. Pain starting in the suprapubic area radiating to the right groin with red and tender scrotum should alert one to the diagnosis of **torsion of testis**. In **mesenteric cyst** a lump should be palpable in the umbilical region with typical mobility.

8. C

Acute cholecystitis does not often cause diagnostic confusion if a good history is taken and Murphy's sign can be elicited. **Mittelschmerz**, midcycle pain from rupture of a follicular cyst, can easily be mistaken for acute appendicitis. A good history helps and there are no constitutional symptoms. **PID** can be confused, particularly as the term includes salpingitis, endometriosis and tubo-ovarian sepsis. Usually the pain is supra-pubic with bilateral signs and vaginal discharge. A **ruptured ectopic pregnancy** would be more obvious with features of hypovolaemic shock, but a right **tubal abortion** might be more difficult to differentiate. History is helpful as would be a pregnancy test. **Torsion or rupture of an ovarian cyst** might be difficult to diagnose from acute appendicitis. Fever and toxic features are uncommon. In the female whenever a doubt exists about the diagnosis, a pelvic ultrasound should be carried out. If that does not help then laparoscopy should be the ultimate investigation, which can also be therapeutic in treating the pathology by minimal- access surgery if the expertise is available.

9. D

A **urinary bladder stone** is unlikely to be confused with acute appendicitis as the patient usually has symptoms of dysuria with haematuria, the symptoms being present over a period of time. **Acute diverticulitis** might mimic acute appendicitis in a patient who has a redundant sigmoid colon the loop of which lies over to the right side. In case of doubt a CT scan will clinch the diagnosis. **Intestinal obstruction** might sometimes confuse the issue because acute appendicitis might mimic the condition. A trial period of conservative management might be helpful with close observation with an option for early laparotomy if there is no improvement. **Mesenteric infarction** would have signs of quite severe peritonitis with a toxic patient who might have cardiac irregularities. A laparotomy might be the safest option. **Cancer caecum** can masquerade as acute appendicitis when the cancer impinges into the appendicular lumen. However, if the patient is found to be anaemic with features of right iliac fossa peritonism, it is almost certainly a case of caecal carcinoma as anaemia is a classical feature of right colonic malignancy, whereas acute appendicitis does not produce anaemia.

Answers to extended matching questions

1. D Acute appendicitis

This 18-year-old boy has the classical features of acute appendicitis. The clinical examination is in keeping with his history of visceral-somatic sequence of pain. When asked to point to the site of his pain, he would almost certainly point to where the pain started (periumbilical) and where it subsequently moved (right iliac fossa) – 'pointing sign'. He does not need any investigations. In doubtful cases, an Alvarado scoring system can be used. He needs an emergency appendicectomy, which should be covered by antibiotics according to the hospital protocol.

2. H Carcinoid tumour

This patient has a carcinoid tumour of the appendix, the incidence of which is one in 300–400 histologically examined appendices. The tumour most commonly occurs in the distal third. Macroscopically the tumour is yellow and hard and lies between the intact mucosa and the peritoneum. Microscopically small tumour cells are arranged within the muscle as small nests. They hardly ever metastasise unless the tumour is larger than 1.5 cm. Appendicectomy as a treatment is all that is necessary. If the tumour involves the base of the appendix involving the caecum, right hemicolectomy should be carried out.

3. G Carcinoma of caecum

This 60-year-old patient has pain and signs of an acute abdominal episode in the right iliac fossa. A diagnosis of acute appendicitis would naturally cross one's mind. After eliciting a good history it is apparent that he has felt short of breath in his daily routine and looks pale – features of anaemic hypoxia. He has signs in the right iliac fossa. The scenario of anaemia with signs in the right iliac fossa is very typical of a carcinoma of the caecum masquerading as acute appendicitis. It important to remember that true acute appendicitis will not cause anaemia.

This patient should be given analgesia and investigated to confirm the diagnosis and stage the disease by a contrast CT scan and colonoscopy and biopsy. This should be followed by the definitive treatment of right hemicolectomy on an urgent basis at the same admission. While these investigations are being arranged, a close watch must be kept so as not miss an impending or definite perforation of the cancer. In such a situation, he will need an emergency right hemicolectomy.

4. B Crohn's disease

This male patient complains of colicky right-sided abdominal pain from the start, denoting an obstructive feature. His past history of diarrhoea should alert one to the possibility of primary bowel pathology. He is generally feeling unwell with acute signs in the right iliac fossa. These features should point to a diagnosis of acute terminal ileitis from Crohn's disease.

His immediate treatment requires analgesia and supportive therapy in the form of intravenous fluids. He needs to be thoroughly investigated with routine haematological and biochemical investigations, including ESR and CRP. This should be followed by contrast CT scan to look for features of Crohn's disease in the form of small bowel strictures with skip lesions, 'string sign' in the terminal ileum, and cobblestone mucosa. A colonoscopy and biopsy should follow. Thereafter the patient should be under the combined care of the gastroenterologist and surgeon and treated medically.

In the rare instance when a patient has been operated upon for a diagnosis of 'acute appendicitis' through a gridiron incision in the right iliac fossa and found to have acute terminal ileitis from Crohn's disease, the appendix should be removed. This would prevent any confusion in diagnosis if and when the patient returns with attacks of abdominal pain.

5. F Mittelschmerz

This young woman has developed pain in the right iliac fossa halfway through her menstrual period. She has signs in her lower abdomen of bleeding from a ruptured lutein cyst. The diagnosis is Mittelschmerz. She is treated with analgesics. In case of doubt, a laparoscopy is carried out. Occasionally retrograde menstruation might present in a similar manner.

6. C Perforated duodenal ulcer

This patient who has suffered from indigestion in the past, for which he has taken antacids, has had a sudden attack of epigastric and right hypochondrial pain from a leaking duodenal ulcer. This pain was thought by the patient to be an acute episode of his indigestion, for which he tried to get relief by taking some more antacids. However, he did not get better and has come in with signs of peritonitis in the right iliac fossa. This scenario is typical of a leaking duodenal ulcer that has been closed off by omentum and the leaked contents have gravitated to the right iliac fossa along the right paracolic gutter, mimicking acute appendicitis.

The patient needs to be resuscitated with analgesia, intravenous fluids and antibiotics. A CXR might show gas under the right dome of the diaphragm. He needs a laparotomy, formal closure of the perforation, thorough peritoneal toilet and postoperative antibiotics. He is given a course of anti *H. pylori* medication.

7. I Pseudomyxoma peritonei

Awareness of this condition is one of the secrets of suspecting this diagnosis. The diagnosis is confirmed by CT scan or ultrasound. Sometimes the diagnosis is made at operation when the abdomen is found to be full of jelly-like material (hence the name 'jelly belly'). Previously it was thought that the tumour was the result of spread from a mucinous adenocarcinoma of the ovaries; it is now understood that it is derived from mucus-producing adenocarcinoma of the appendix. When diagnosed, ideally it should be managed in a specialised unit. Treatment is in the form of radical resection of all involved parietal peritoneal surfaces and aggressive intraperitoneal chemotherapy. Recurrence is inevitable, but repeated laparotomies for further excision gives good palliation (see **Chapter 61**).

8. E Right ureteric colic

This young man has sudden onset of severe right-sided abdominal pain that started in his loin and radiated to the groin. The fact that he is in agony and writhing around in pain, unable to find a position of comfort, is typical of ureteric colic. Abdominal examination shows a tympanic abdomen, which is due to ileus, a common accompaniment of ureteric colic.

He should be given intravenous morphine immediately. The diagnosis should be confirmed by a spiral CT scan, failing which an emergency IVU is done. On confirmation, analgesia is continued with diclofenac suppositories. If the stone is <5 mm in diameter, expectant treatment is continued and the patient imaged in about 6 weeks. If there is urinary infection or the stone is >5 mm, intervention by minimal-access surgery is carried out.

9. A Ruptured ectopic pregnancy

This young woman who is unsure about her menstrual periods has had sudden onset of very severe lower abdominal pain and has presented with features of hypovolaemic shock and peritonism. The clinical picture is typical, particularly with Cullen's sign (blood-stained discoloration around the umbilicus), of a ruptured ectopic pregnancy. Pelvic ultrasound is carried out followed by referral to a gynaecologist as an emergency for definitive treatment.

72 The rectum

CR Selvasekar and Pradip K Datta

Multiple choice questions

→ Anatomy

1. Which of the following statements are true?

A The rectum is completely enveloped by peritoneum.

B The rectovesical pouch in the male is 7.5 cm and rectouterine pouch is 5.5 cm from the anal verge.

C The fascia in front of the rectum is the Denonvilliers' fascia and behind is the Waldeyer's fascia.

D The mesorectum contains the superior rectal vessels and lymphatics.

E The lymphatics from the rectum mainly drain upwards.

→ Clinical features and examination for rectal disease

2. The following statements are true except:

A Patients with rectal disease might present with extra-rectal symptoms and signs.

B Rectal bleeding is always a sinister symptom.

C Altered bowel habit of recent onset should be of concern.

D Flexible sigmoidoscopy can visualise a maximum distance of 40 cm of the colon.

E Examination of the rectum by finger or endoscope is best carried out in the left lateral position.

→ Injuries and foreign bodies in the rectum

3. Which of the following statements are true?

A Impalement injury is the usual accidental cause.

B Intraperitoneal rectal injuries might require a staged procedure.

C A temporary colostomy is usually necessary.

D In severe injuries, faecal incontinence might be the long-term outcome.

E When a patient arrives with a self-introduced foreign body (FB), it should be removed immediately.

→ Rectal prolapse

4. The following statements are true except:

A In children it is usually a mucosal prolapse.

B In children the differential diagnosis is ileocaecal intussusception.

C In adults it is usually a full-thickness prolapse.

D Majority of children will need an operation.

E Majority of adults can be managed conservatively.

→ Proctitis

5. Which of the following statements are true?

A The diagnosis is made on sigmoidoscopy followed by colonoscopy.

B Crohn's disease is a common cause.

C Specific infections as a cause must be excluded.

D It is present in majority of patients with ulcerative colitis.

E AIDS due to HIV infection can cause the condition.

→ Rectal polyps

6. Which of the following statements are true?

A A polyp >1 cm is likely to be malignant.

B When a rectal polyp is found a full colonoscopy should be performed.

C In certain cases a patient might present with the effects of hypokalaemia.

D In villous adenoma abdomino-perineal excision is the operation of choice.

E In familial adenomatous polyposis the patient should be treated according to the prescribed protocol.

→ Carcinoma of the rectum

7. The following statements are true except:

A Most patients with rectal cancer will require an abdomino-perineal resection (APR).

B Early-morning spurious diarrhoea is a typical symptom.

C In locally advanced tumours preoperative chemoradiotherapy makes curative surgery possible.

D Following an anterior resection, a defunctioning loop ileostomy is usually performed.

E Endoluminal stenting can be done as a temporary or permanent procedure.

Extended matching questions

→ Diagnoses

1 Adenomatous polyp
2 Carcinoma of rectum
3 Radiation proctitis
4 Rectal prolapse
5 Solitary rectal ulcer
6 Villous adenoma

Match the diagnoses with the clinical features of the various conditions that follow:

→ Clinical scenarios

A An 80-year-old woman complains of a large lump protruding from her back passage for few years. This is associated with mucus discharge and faecal incontinence.

B A 65-year-old man, having been invited for bowel cancer screening, went through the process diligently. His result came back as abnormal; therefore a colonoscopy was performed. At colonoscopy two polyps less than 1 cm were found and removed.

C A 78-year-old woman complains of difficulty in evacuating her bowels for many years. Sometimes she has to digitally remove the stools or apply pressure in the vagina to facilitate bowel movement. While straining during her bowel movement, she noticed bright-red rectal bleeding and mucus. She has some pain on defecation but is otherwise well.

D An 86-year-old man complains of fresh rectal bleeding and loose stools with mucus for few weeks. He had prostate cancer treated many years ago with radiotherapy. He has atrial fibrillation and is on warfarin. He is otherwise well.

E A 55-year-old man saw his general practitioner with a history of rectal bleeding for a few months. Recently, his symptoms were getting worse and he has also started passing mucus per rectum. He has been otherwise well without any significant past medical and family history. His GP sent him to be assessed at the rectal bleeding clinic.

F A 52-year-old man complains of watery diarrhoea for several months. Recently the diarrhoea has become so profuse that he feels quite weak, with some loss of power in his muscles. On his blood tests done by his GP he has a serum potassium of 2.1 mmol/L. On rectal examination, a frond-like growth is felt.

Answers to multiple choice questions

Anatomy

1. B, C, D, E

The rectovesical pouch in the male is formed by the peritoneal reflection from the front of the lower part of the middle one-third of the rectum on to the bladder; this is 7.5 cm from the anus. In the female this peritoneal reflection from the rectum goes on to the posterior vaginal wall forming the rectouterine pouch of Douglas, which is 5.5 cm from the anal verge. Both points should be within reach on rectal examination by the average index finger.

The lower one-third of rectum is separated from the prostate or vagina in front by a condensation of mesorectal fascia called the rectovescial fascia of Denonvilliers. At the back there is another fascial layer that extends from the coccyx and the lower two sacral vertebrae called the presacral fascia (of Waldeyer). These fascial layers are a barrier to the spread of cancer. In mesorectal excision for rectal cancer, the surgeon posteriorly should dissect in the plane between the rectum and mesorectum and presacral fascia – called the 'holy plane' (Heald). The mesorectum is intimately related to the rectum down to the levator ani and contains the superior rectal artery (continuation of the inferior mesenteric artery), accompanying veins, lymphatics and nodes. These should be excised in total mesorectal excision during surgery for cancer.

The rectal lymphatics drain upwards along the superior rectal vessels to the nodes at the origin of the inferior mesenteric artery. This fact is important because in low rectal cancer, leaving a small amount of uninvolved tumour-free margin is adequate to perform a curative resection.

The rectum is not completely enveloped by peritoneum. The upper one-third is covered by peritoneum in front and both sides; the middle one-third has peritoneum only anteriorly while the lower one-third is completely extraperitoneal.

Clinical features and examination for rectal disease

2. B, D

Rectal bleeding, while alarming for the patient, is not always a symptom from a sinister cause. Painless bright-red rectal bleeding in the young is almost always from haemorrhoids. However, the symptom should never be dismissed as a cause of 'haemorrhoids' without thorough history and examination. The flexible sigmoidoscope reaches to a distance of 60 cm, usually up to the splenic flexure.

Patients with rectal disease might present with extra-rectal symptoms such as weight loss, abdominal pain and jaundice. The patient might be aware of an abdominal lump, which can turn out to be hepatomegaly from liver secondaries. When a patient complains of altered bowel habit of recent onset it should be of concern. This might take the form of diarrhoea, constipation, or alternating constipation and diarrhoea. A patient who is constipated might not complain of alteration in bowel habit because he or she routinely started taking laxatives in increasing amounts.

An integral part of clinical examination is rectal examination, which should be followed by sigmoidoscopy. This examination is carried out in the left lateral position. This is because of the three anatomical lateral curves of the rectum – the upper and lower are convex to the right and the middle convex to the left. Having the patient in left lateral position allows easier visualisation. Depending upon the surgical unit, if the patient is seen in a 'one-stop rectal bleeding clinic', flexible sigmoidoscopy might be a routine. Otherwise rigid sigmoidoscopy with a plastic disposable instrument, which visualises up to 25 cm, should be routine.

→ Injuries and foreign bodies in the rectum

3. A, B, C, D, E

While most rectal injuries are accidental, foreign bodies in the rectum are usually self-inflicted. Injuries occur as a result of a fall on a sharp metal object, or a gardening injury from impalement on a garden tool. Other causes might be gunshot injury or prolonged obstructed labour. When a patient is seen with an impalement injury (**Figures 72.1** and **72.2a** and **b**) usually the patient will arrive with the impaled object in place, as the paramedics giving first-aid would have been instructed not to remove the impaled object for fear of worsening the effects of the injury.

After resuscitation and x-rays, in intraperitoneal injuries the patient is taken to theatre. The abdomen is opened, under controlled conditions, and the impaled object is removed. Depending upon the extent of damage, the rectum is repaired with a proximal defunctioning ileostomy; alternatively the damaged area might be transected, the edges freshened and brought out as an end colostomy with the distal end closed off as a Hartmann's procedure or brought out as a mucus fistula.

In extraperitoneal lower one-third rectal injuries, a defunctioning double-barrel left iliac colostomy is done with debridement of the perineal wound. Prophylactic broad-spectrum antibiotics against aerobic and anaerobic organisms are mandatory. In severe injuries after repair and recovery, the patient might experience faecal incontinence from damage to the levator ani.

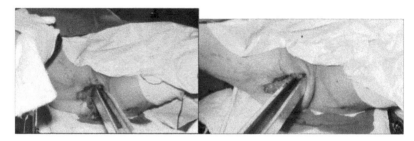

Figure 72.1   Impalement injury of the rectum – impalement with a metal girder.

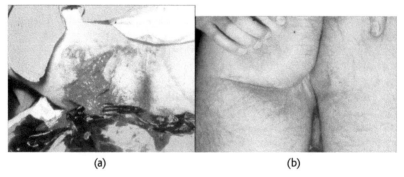

(a)   (b)

Figure 72.2   (a) and (b) Same patient as in Figure 72.1 showing (a) immediately after removal of the metal girder and (b) 14 months later.

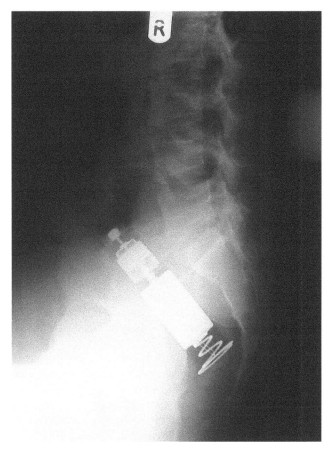

Figure 72.3 Foreign body (vibrator) in rectum.

In a case of foreign body (FB) in the rectum (**Figure 72.3**), the object is removed under general anaesthetic. It might be necessary to do a laparotomy to push the foreign body out to be retrieved through the anal canal. Prior to the laparotomy, an x-ray to rule out intraperitoneal air is advisable.

Rectal prolapse

4. D, E

In the management of rectal prolapse in children the vast majority, if not all, are treated conservatively by digital repositioning. If this is not successful after a 6-week period, submucosal injection usually cures the condition. In adults as it is usually a full-thickness (complete) prolapse, an operation is most often required. There are several procedures, including laparoscopic approach.

In children it is a mucosal prolapse (partial prolapse), the cause usually being diarrhoea and weight loss resulting in loss of fat in the ischio-rectal fossa. It might be confused with an ileocaecal intussusception. In a prolapse the finger cannot be insinuated between the mucosa and anal verge whereas in intussusception the finger will enter a gap between the bowel and anus. In adults, women are six times more often affected than men. It is almost always a full-thickness or complete prolapse, and in 50% there is faecal incontinence. There are several choices of surgical treatment, the option taken depending upon the age of the patient and presence of comorbidities.

→ ## Proctitis

5. A, C, D, E

The condition is diagnosed by sigmoidoscopy when inflammation is seen confined to the rectum; there is pus, blood, mucus and red mucosa. Once suspected, colonoscopy with multiple biopsies is essential to find out the extent of the disease. Specific infections as a cause must be excluded by histology, bacteriology, stool culture, serological tests and examination of scrapings or swabs from ulcers.

Patients known to suffer from ulcerative colitis (UC) will almost certainly have proctitis. Those who are not suffering from UC, specific infections as a cause must be excluded. Such infections are *C. difficile*, bacillary dysentery, amoebic dysentery, tuberculosis, gonococcal infection, lymphogranuloma venereum, AIDS and bilharziasis. While some of these conditions are rare, a good history and proper patient profile should help make the diagnosis. Crohn's disease is not a common cause of proctitis. Although the rectum might be involved, it is patchy. There might be other perianal manifestations such as fistulae.

→ ## Rectal polyps

6. A, B, C, E

When, on sigmoidoscopy, a patient is found to have a rectal polyp >1 cm there is a high chance of it being malignant. Therefore it should be removed by endoscopic hot biopsy or snare polypectomy. However, before this is done, a full colonoscopy should be carried out to exclude a proximal colonic cancer. This is to prevent implantation of cancer cells in the polypectomy wound should a cancer be found.

Villous adenomas are usually very large with a typical frond-like appearance often occupying the entire rectum. These might present with profuse watery mucoid diarrhoea, making the patient very weak because of loss of large amount of potassium. They have a propensity to malignant change, something that can be strongly suspected on digital examination. If the tumour is not malignant, and the vast majority are benign, abdomino-perineal excision is not required. They can be treated by trans-anal endoscopic microsurgery (TEM). Those with FAP should undergo the whole gamut of genetic counselling and profiling followed by radical surgery (see Chapter 69).

→ ## Carcinoma of the rectum

7. A

Most patients with carcinoma of the rectum do not require an APR. The vast majority (almost 90%) can have a sphincter-saving resection (anterior resection) because of increased refinements of surgical techniques such as use of the stapler and the understanding that spread occurs proximally upwards. This has enabled restorative procedures, anterior resection and abdominotransanal-coloanal anastomosis to be performed in patients with a carcinoma where the lower margin is 2 cm above the anal canal. Surgery for rectal carcinoma is being carried out laparoscopically in certain centres.

Patients with rectal carcinoma typically complain of 'early-morning spurious diarrhoea'. The patient typically complains of having to wake up in the morning earlier than usual because of an intense desire to defecate only to rush to the lavatory to pass 'wind and water', which the patient refers to as 'diarrhoea'; this is 'spurious' because it is false as there are no faeces but really just pent-up mucus secretion proximal to an obstruction. The patient has to make several such trips being left with a constant desire to defecate – a symptom called tenesmus.

In locally advanced tumours preoperative neoadjuvant chemoradiotherapy over 6 weeks will downstage the tumour making curative surgery feasible. Following low anterior resection for growths in the middle and lower thirds of rectum, a defunctioning ileostomy is usually carried out and left in place for about 6 weeks. A contrast study is carried out 6 weeks later to confirm the integrity of the anastomosis, after which the ileostomy is closed and bowel continuity restored.

In patients with low rectal growths that are inoperable, a self-expanding metallic endoluminal stent is inserted as a means of palliation. This procedure is also done when a patient presents with acute intestinal obstruction. This will get the patient over the acute episode. Over the subsequent week the patient is optimised, the growth is staged and a definitive sphincter-saving operation carried out +/− defunctioning ileostomy.

Answers to extended matching questions

1. B Adenomatous polyp

All polyps detected at screening are removed for histology. If the polyp is over 1 cm in size, the area is marked with a tattoo and the polyp removed. Tattoo assists with identification of the polyp site for surveillance or if the removed polyp comes back as cancer. The surveillance for adenomatous polyps removed at colonoscopy is based on the British Society of Gastroenterology's (BSG) guidelines, which are based on the number and size of the adenomatous polyps. Hyperplastic or metaplastic polyps do not need surveillance. Patients with multiple polyps should be considered for assessment in a family history clinic for detailed evaluation to exclude FAP when the whole gamut of genetic investigations, assessment and family counselling should be carried out.

2. E Carcinoma of rectum

A detailed history is taken with regard to recent change in bowel habit such as constipation, early-morning spurious diarrhoea, rectal bleeding with mucus, pain, tenesmus and a feeling of insufficient evacuation. Examination would reveal a palpable indurated mass in the rectum; this is followed by sigmoidoscopy and biopsy. Thereafter the patient needs the full gamut of investigations. A barium enema will show a 'napkin-ring' appearance **(Figure 72.4)**; as an imaging modality it has now been replaced by a CT colonography. A full colonoscopy is done to exclude synchronous carcinoma proximally. Sometimes a colonoscopy might not be possible because of the nature of the lesion; in such a case, CT colonography is done. Besides all routine blood investigations, staging is carried out by CT scan of the abdomen and chest and MRI of the pelvis.

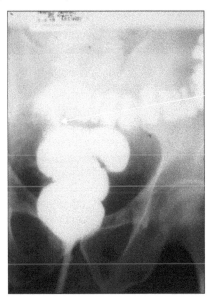

Figure 72.4 Barium enema showing a typical 'napkin-ring' appearance of an annular carcinoma of the upper rectum.

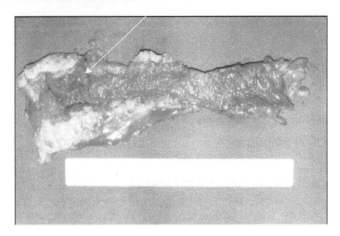

Figure 72.5 Specimen of an anterior resection for a carcinoma of the upper one-third of rectum.

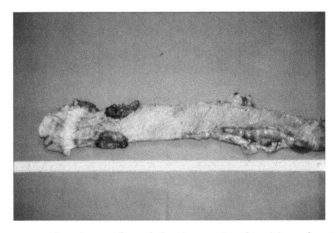

Figure 72.6 Specimen of an abdomino-perineal excision of rectum.

Once all investigations are available, the patient is discussed in the colorectal MDT as to the best way to proceed. The decision will depend upon the stage of the disease. The option taken will be from a choice of the following: primary surgical treatment in the form of an anterior resection (**Figure 72.5**) or preoperative chemoradiotherapy followed by surgery and palliation. Surgery, in the vast majority will be in the form of a sphincter-saving procedure with total mesorectal excision (TME) +/– a defunctioning ileostomy. A minority will require APR with permanent colostomy (**Figure 72.6**). Palliation can take one of several options, including stenting, interstitial radiation, laser ablation, or a Hartmann's operation (Also see previously).

3. D Radiation proctitis

Diagnosis is confirmed at endoscopic examination of the rectum. Macroscopically there will be telangiectasia and fibrosis over the anterior rectal wall in the middle and the low one-third of rectum. Biopsies will confirm radiation proctitis, chronic inflammation, ulceration, submucosal fibrosis and crypt abscesses.

The treatment involves topical administration of anti-inflammatories such as 5-aminosalicylic acid preparations in the form of enemas or suppositories. Usually a 6-week course is enough to alleviate the symptoms. Sometimes there is a long-term need for anti-inflammtories and occasionally steroid enemas have to be used. If the proctitis is extensive, argon plasma coagulation is performed to gain initial control followed by medical treatment.

4. A Rectal prolapse

Full-thickness rectal prolapse (complete prolapse) is six times more common in women. The complications are bleeding, incarceration and small-bowel evisceration. The management consists of colonoscopy or a flexible sigmoidoscopy to exclude any mucosal lesions. Surgery is the mainstay of treatment, the options being abdominal or perineal approach, the former being open or laparoscopic. There are several operations all having their own protagonists, a sure indication that most procedures have some limitation or other. Details of these operations are beyond the scope of this book.

5. C Solitary rectal ulcer

Also called solitary rectal ulcer syndrome (SRUS), this condition is often associated with other pelvic floor disorders. Despite the name, sometimes there might be no ulcer while at times there might be multiple ulcers or erosions. Typically there is an ulcer in the anterior rectal wall when a carcinoma or inflammatory bowel disease must be excluded. It might heal by itself, leaving a polypoid-looking lesion. The cause can be explained as follows: chronic constipation → straining at stool → increase in intra-rectal pressure → prolapse of anterior rectal wall → internal intussusception → ulceration → bleeding.

The diagnosis is confirmed by endoscopy, which reveals a red, oedematous mucosa of varying length over the anterior rectal wall 7–10 cm from the anal verge. Biopsies are done to exclude malignancy. The hallmark of SRUS is smooth muscle proliferation from the muscularis mucosa into the lamina propria. Although a benign condition, it is difficult to treat. Treatment is conservative aimed at symptomatic relief. As a last resort, laparoscopic ventral mesh rectopexy is offered.

6. F Villous adenoma

This is usually a large tumour that secretes potassium-rich mucus, causing profuse watery diarrhoea. Patients are hypokalaemic on two counts – diarrhoea and the secretion of potassium from the tumour. This makes the patient clinically ill both from dehydration and muscle weakness. On rectal examination a frond-like, soft, tumour is felt; a hard indurated area might denote malignancy. Endoscopy confirms the diagnosis when a large, broad-based, elevated lesion with shaggy cauliflower-like surface occupying a section of the bowel wall like a carpet is seen.

Multiple biopsies are taken, as there is a high chance of invasive cancer. Histologically, they are composed of finger-like processes with fibrovascular cores with hyperchromatic nuclei. When they are larger than 2 cm, 50% will have invasive cancer. Considering that most villous adenomas are >2 cm in diameter, exclusion of invasive cancer is paramount as the surgical treatment would be different. If cancer is excluded, TEM can be carried out. If cancer is confirmed, anterior resection (see previously) will be the treatment.

73 The anus and anal canal

BV Praveen and Pradip K Datta

Multiple choice questions

→ Anatomy and physiology

1. Which of the following statements are true?

A The junction between the rectum and anal canal is the anorectal ring.

B The puborectalis muscle is an important component of the continence mechanism.

C The external sphincter forms the bulk of the anal sphincter complex.

D The longitudinal muscle is a direct continuation of the smooth muscle of the outer muscle coat of the rectum.

E The internal anal sphincter is the continuation of the circular muscle coat of the rectum.

2. The following statements are true except:

A The dentate line (pectinate line) divides the anal canal into an upper two-thirds and lower one-third.

B The mucosa and submucosa above the dentate line form anal cushions.

C The anal glands drain into the anal sinuses and are the source of anal sepsis.

D The lymphatics from the anal canal drain into the inguinal group of lymph nodes.

E The lower part of the anal canal is lined by stratified squamous epithelium.

→ Special investigations on the ano-rectum

3. Which of the following statements are true?

A The resting tone is a reflection of internal sphincter activity.

B A maximal anal pressure of 60 cm of water is abnormal.

C Pelvic dyssynergia can be identified by evacuatory proctogram.

D Megarectum might be a finding in rectal hyposensitivity.

E Perineal position and descent reflects pelvic floor and pudendal nerve function.

→ Imperforate anus

4. Which of the following statements are true?

A Imperforate anus are classified into high and low types.

B Fistula with the urethra is uncommon.

C The most common abnormality in girls is a fistula into the vagina.

D The finding of a single perineal orifice suggests a persistent cloaca.

E Meconium on the perineum indicates a low defect.

→ Pilonidal sinus

5. The following statements are true except:

A The condition always occurs in the natal cleft.

B It is a disease of the elderly.

C The condition predominantly affects males.

D Recurrent abscesses are common.

E Treatment is always surgical excision.

→ Anal incontinence

6. Which of the following statements are true?

A Neurological pathways must be intact to maintain anal continence.

B Structural integrity of the gastrointestinal tract and pelvic floor musculature is essential to maintain continence.

C History and clinical examination might be enough to determine aetiology.

D Surgical treatment is tailored to the cause.

E A permanent stoma is a choice.

Anal fissure

7. Which of the following statement(s) is/are false?

A Anal fissure occurs most commonly on the anterior midline at 12 o'clock position.

B Acute anal fissure results from trauma from the passage of a hard stool.

C A fissure at an unusual site might have an underlying cause.

D Operation is the treatment of choice.

E Anal dilatation should be tried as the first surgical procedure.

Haemorrhoids

8. Which of the following statements are true?

A Haemorrhoids are symptomatic anal cushions.

B Traditionally, four degrees are recognised.

C Conservative treatment should be the first line of management.

D Urgent surgery is justified in certain complications.

E Operation when indicated is usually carried out by the 'open technique'.

Pruritis ani

9. Which of the following statements are not true?

A Usually there is an underlying cause.

B Diabetes must be excluded.

C Treat the cause of pruritis ani.

D Surgical treatment is required in the majority.

E Hydrocortisone should be the first line of conservative treatment.

Anorectal abscesses

10. Which of the following statements are true?

A Anorectal abscesses might be a manifestation of a generalised disease.

B Primary colorectal disease might be a cause.

C The main cause is infection of the anal glands.

D Presentation is always as a very tender, fluctuant lump in the perianal region.

E Immediate fistulotomy should be performed if a fistula is present.

Fistula-in-ano

11. The following statements are true except:

A There is always an underlying associated specific cause.

B The most common cause is persistent infection of the anal glands.

C MRI is an essential investigation in all cases.

D Classification is into high and low-anal fistula.

E The majority can be treated by fistulotomy.

12. Which of the following statements are true?

A MRI and EUS should be undertaken before surgical treatment.

B Fistulotomy is the treatment for intersphincteric and trans-sphincteric types.

C Setons are used in the treatment of high and complicated fistulae.

D Anal advancement flaps aims to preserve anatomy and function.

E Biological agents have been used with variable results.

Extended matching questions

Diagnoses

1 Anal fissure
2 Anal incontinence
3 Anal intraepithelial neoplasia (AIN)

4 Anal stenosis
5 Condylomata accuminata (anal warts)
6 Fistula-in-ano
7 Haemorrhoids
8 Hydradenitis suppurativa
9 Perianal abscess
10 Pilonidal sinus
11 Pruritis ani
12 Squamous cell carcinoma

Match the diagnoses with the clinical scenarios that follow:

→ Clinical scenarios

A A 25-year-old woman complains of bright-red rectal bleeding for 6 weeks. This is not mixed with her stools and comes on every time she opens her bowels. It started toward the end of her pregnancy and got worse after the birth of her baby 2 months ago. She has no other symptoms.

B A 38-year-old man complains of severe pain on defecation for a week. He has seen streaks of blood every time he has a bowel action. He has been very constipated ever since he has been on strong analgesia for his fractured ankle, which is in plaster.

C A 32-year-old woman complains of severe perianal itching, which she finds very distressing. She has also had foul-smelling vaginal discharge for which she is taking antibiotics.

D A 26-year-old man complains of recurrent discharge from his natal cleft. It started 6 months ago with an abscess that burst on its own.

E A 42-year-old man who is on medical treatment for Crohn's disease complains of severe pain in his left perianal area. On examination he has a very tender, shiny, fluctuant mass.

F A 32-year-old man complains of serosanguinous discharge from his right perianal area. He had a tender lump about 1 week ago that burst on its own, after which he felt much better but has been left with a smelly discharge.

G A 35-year-old woman complains of recurrent abscesses in her buttocks. On examination she has several tender, raised, discharging lesions with fibrosis and scarring.

H A 27-year-old man complains of perianal itching, bleeding, discharge, pain and lumps for a few months. On examination he has pinkish-white excrescences outside and inside the anal canal, partially obscuring the anal orifice.

I A 56-year-old man complains of pruritis, pain intermittent bleeding and discharge from the perianal area for several weeks. On examination there is a raised, greyish-white, irregular plaque-like lesion.

J A 66-year-old man complains of pain and bleeding from the perianal area where he has felt a lump for 6 weeks. On examination there is an irreducible lump protruding from the anus that is indurated, and the edge looks everted.

K A 47-year-old man complains of difficulty in passing stools for 2 months in spite of using increasing amounts of laxatives. The stools are 'tape-like'. About 3 months ago, he underwent an urgent haemorrhoidectomy for prolapsed, thrombosed, strangulated piles.

L A 72-year-old woman complains of continuous faecal leak for 6 weeks. Prior to this the problem was intermittent. She gradually developed constipation and has not had a proper bowel action for almost the same period. On examination she has faecal incontinence with soiled underwear. Rectal examination reveals a rectum completely loaded with hard stools.

Answers to multiple choice questions

→ Anatomy and physiology

1. A, B, C, D, E

The region where the puborectalis (part of the levator ani) fuses with the external sphincter and the upper end of the internal sphincter is called the anorectal ring. It is the junction between the rectum and the anal canal, the last 4 cm of the alimentary tract. Clinically on rectal examination the anorectal ring can be felt posteriorly as a shelf over which the fingertip can be hooked when the patient is asked to strain.

The understanding of the anatomy of the anorectal muscles has been studied by endoanal US and MRI in recent years. The puborectalis is part of the pubococcygeus section of the levator ani. It clasps the gut, forming a U-shaped sling which angles the anorectal junction forward. It blends with the external anal sphincter, the two becoming one single component, which plays an important role in maintaining continence. The external anal sphincter (previously described as consisting of deep, superficial and subcutaneous parts) is an oval muscular tube of striated skeletal muscle well suited to prolonged contraction, forming the major part of the anal sphincter. It is supplied by the pudendal nerve (S2–S4).

The longitudinal muscle is a continuation of the outer muscle coat of the rectum strengthened in the upper part by fibres from the puborectalis. It extends distally dividing into several septa, which divide the external sphincter terminating in the perianal skin. It has an important role in defecation in widening the anal lumen and subsequently forming an airtight seal.

The internal anal sphincter is an involuntary muscle which is a thickened downward continuation of the inner circular muscle coat of the rectum; the muscle is in a tonic state of contraction. It extends from the pelvic diaphragm to the anal orifice. It is innervated by the autonomic nervous system. It receives non-adrenergic and non-cholinergic fibres, which release the nitric oxide that induces internal sphincter relaxation – a principle used for the treatment of anal fissure with glyceryl trinitrate (GTN) and diltiazem application to relax the internal sphincter.

2. D

The lymphatics of the anal canal drain to two different sites. Those from the upper end of the anal canal drain upward to join the epicolic nodes of the rectum and then on to the pararectal nodes in the mesorectum. The upward drainage is via nodes along the inferior mesenteric vessels to the preaortic nodes. From the lower half of the anal canal, the lymphatics drain to the superficial and then the deep inguinal group of nodes.

The dentate line, an important landmark, divides the rectum into an upper two-thirds and lower one-third developmentally, anatomically and clinically. Embryologically it is the junction between the postallantoic gut above and the proctodeum below. Anatomically it is the site of the crypts of Morgagni (anal crypts, anal sinuses). Anal glands drain through ducts into the crypts, the junction of columnar epithelium above with stratified squamous epithelium below. The clinical significance lies in the fact that the mucosa proximal to the dentate line is not very pain sensitive whereas the distal mucosa is extremely pain sensitive. This means injection of piles higher up will be relatively painless, while the same carried out distally will be very painful.

The mucosa and submucosa above the dentate line is in folds or columns containing a radicle of the superior rectal artery and vein. The numbers of these columns vary but they are largest in the left lateral, right anterior and right posterior quadrants of the anal canal where they are called anal cushions – the traditionally described sites of haemorrhoids, which are in effect abnormal enlargement of anal cushions.

The anal glands, found in the submucosa and intersphincteric space, is the source of cryptoglandular anal sepsis and fistula-in-ano. The infection drains downward between the internal and external sphincters, appearing as a perianal abscess which on rupturing will form a fistula. The lower part of the anal canal is lined by stratified squamous epithelium and hence extremely sensitive to any minor surgical procedures or surgical conditions; malignancies in this area can take the form of any of those occurring in the skin anywhere else – squamous cell cancer or a malignant melanoma.

→ Special investigations on the ano-rectum

3. A, C, D, E

The resting tone reflects the internal sphincter activity, whereas squeeze increment reflects the external sphincter activity. Perineal position and degree of descent on straining are parameters to gauge function of the pelvic floor and pudendal nerve. These can be quantified, and functional anal length can be measured by manometric techniques.

The structural integrity of the sphincters can be visualised by endoanal ultrasonography (EUS) to detect external anal sphincter defects by obstetric injury or internal anal sphincter defects after sphincterotomy. Electromyogram (EMG) studies or pudendal nerve-conduction velocity will assess the structural integrity of the sphincters.

MRI evacuation proctography is a method of assessing the dynamics of defecation. In this procedure radio-opaque pseudo-stool is inserted into the rectum and the patient is asked to rest, squeeze and bear down to evacuate the contents (simulate defecation) under real-time imaging. Pelvic dyssynergia can thus be identified. Rectal hyposensitivity is a diminished perception of rectal distension and might result in megarectum.

→ Imperforate anus

4. A, D, E

The condition is divided into high and low depending on whether the rectum terminates above or below the pelvic floor. The management will obviously be different in each category. Low defects are relatively easier to correct than high ones. In both sexes low defects include rectoperineal fistula, covered anus and anal membrane. In boys the most common abnormality is where the distal rectum is sited within the puborectalis sling but has a fistula with the urethra. In girls the most common abnormality is a rectovestibular fistula where the fistula opens into the posterior vestibule and not the vagina. A single perineal orifice indicates a persistent cloaca where the rectum, vagina and urethra form a confluence.

In both sexes, low defects embrace rectoperineal fistula and covered anus and anal membrane. The most frequent defect in boys with imperforate anus is one in which the distal rectum is sited within the puborectalis sling, but terminates as a fistula into the bulbar urethra or prostatic urethra above the main anal sphincter complex. The most common defect in girls is a rectovestibular fistula, in which the fistula opens into the posterior vestibule and not the vagina.

Clinically meconium on the perineum indicates a low defect; when mixed with urine it confirms a urinary fistula. This condition is the domain of the specialist paediatric surgeon. The reader, if interested, is advised to refer to relevant textbooks.

→ Pilonidal sinus

5. A, B, E

While the natal cleft is the most common site of this condition, pilonidal sinus does not always occur on the natal cleft. It is an occupational hazard amongst hairdressers who suffer from the condition in their interdigital cleft. It is thought that the customers' hair grows into an opening in the skin. It is also known to occur in the axilla and umbilicus.

Almost exclusively young men are affected by this condition. More than 80% of sufferers are men in their third decade. They have hairy buttocks where friction causes hair that has been shed to burrow through the midline skin, forming a track and an abscess. Therefore recurrent abscesses are common which will require incision and drainage with curettage of the granulation tissue and hair. Surgical excision of the track is not always necessary. Conservative management in the form of cleaning of the tracks, removal of all hair and regular shaving of the buttocks with good hygiene might suffice. Various surgical procedures are described, a sure indication that none of them are universally successful.

Anal incontinence

6. A, B, C, D, E
Normal anal continence is maintained by the pressure within the anal canal being higher than in the rectum. Therefore any damage to the neurological pathways such as multiple sclerosis, spinal cord injury, cerebrovascular accident and Parkinson's disease might result in incontinence. Loss of integrity of the musculature of the pelvic floor for reasons such as obstetric injury or surgical damage might account for this problem. In the vast majority a good history covering all aspects of psychobehavioural factors, previous surgery and thorough clinical examination should be enough to come to a decision with regard to the cause.

Once the cause is determined, treatment is tailored to the needs of the individual patient. Management of these patients will require a team effort between medical and other non-medical professionals. Any surgical treatment should be the domain of the specialist colorectal and pelvic floor surgeon. In general, operations, to be considered by the specialist, are procedures to reunite divided sphincter muscles, procedures to reef the external sphincter and puborectalis muscle and procedures to augment the anal sphincters. As a last resort, a left iliac end colostomy provides some relief.

Anal fissure

7. A, D, E
The most common site of an anal fissure is posterior midline at 6 o'clock position, probably because of the excessive shearing force acting at that part during defecation. The usual cause is trauma caused by the passage of a constipated hard stool. Anterior fissure is more commonly seen in women probably as a result of a vaginal delivery. In women 10% of fissures are anterior, whereas in men it is 1%.

When a fissure occurs at a site away from the usual point in the anus, almost always there is an underlying cause such as Crohn's disease, tuberculosis, HIV-related ulcers, or a squamous cell carcinoma. In such a situation, the patient should be examined under anaesthetic (EUA) and relevant biopsies taken. After confirmation of the diagnosis, if necessary after EUA, if there is no underlying cause, conservative measures should be instituted first as they are successful in almost all of acute fissures and most of chronic fissures. This consists of stool-bulking agents, topical application of glyceryl trinitrate (GTN) and diltiazem.

Surgery should not be the first-line management. In recurrent or indolent cases only, surgery should be considered. Anal dilatation is an obsolete procedure and might result in incontinence. Lateral anal sphincterotomy or anal advancement flap are the choice of procedures for anal fissure when less invasive methods have failed.

Haemorrhoids

8. A, B, C, D, E
Anal cushions (see previously on anatomy) are normal anatomical anal mucosal and submucosal vascular folds just above the dentate line. Haemorrhoids occur when these

cushions enlarge, become symptomatic, bleeding being the main feature for which the patient seeks advice. Typically it is bright-red blood separate from the motion, painless, sometimes associated with mucous discharge and prolapse. Symptoms are worse when there is any cause producing raised intra-abdominal pressure. While theories abound in their development, it is accepted that forces causing increased pressure on the anus (for various reasons) cause the anal cushions to descend with trauma to the overlying mucosa resulting in bleeding. Prolonged straining at defecation due to constipation is the initiating trauma.

Traditionally four degrees are described: First, only bleeding; second, rectal bleeding + prolapse that reduces spontaneously; third, rectal bleeding + prolapse that requires manual reduction; fourth, rectal bleeding + prolapse that cannot be reduced. Since these vascular anal cushions form a continuous venous plexus, the differentiation of haemorrhoids into external and internal is rather artificial. Normally the higher internal haemorrhoids merge with their lower counterparts to form what is commonly called 'interno-external piles'. They should be regarded as external extensions of internal haemorrhoids.

In the management, in the vast majority, reassurance that there is no serious underlying condition such as colorectal cancer, along with conservative measures is all that is necessary. When complications such as strangulation, thrombosis and gangrene occur, some advocate urgent surgery. Under antibiotic cover, open haemorrhoidectomy can be carried out although conservative management with analgesics, bed rest, hot baths, or cold compresses will cure the problem in almost all cases. Moreover, late anal stenosis might be one of the complications associated with early operation.

When operation is decided upon (for third and fourth degree), open haemorrhoidectomy is the usual procedure. There are various surgical procedures, minor and operative, details of which are beyond the scope of this book. However, less-invasive measures such as injections and banding should be tried first. These measures will be relatively painless when it is carried out in the upper anal canal, because it is lined with insensate columnar epithelium; the same treatment in the lower anal canal is very painful because the stratified squamous mucosa is rich in sensory nerve endings.

→ Pruritis ani

9. D, E

In the management, surgery is not the treatment. Conservative management is the treatment, which should be directed toward the cause. Hydrocortisone ointment should not be used universally. It should only be used as 0.5% or 1% prednisolone cream when the cause is dermatitis.

Pruritis ani, intractable perianal itching, is a very distressing condition, not to mention the embarrassment it causes. There almost always is a cause. Lack of hygiene, parasites (particularly in children), allergic skin condition, bacterial infection and psychoneurosis are but a few. The last cause should not be assumed unless all other causes have been excluded. Diabetes should be excluded. Treatment is to find the cause and treat it. The letter 'P' is a useful reminder of possible causes: polyp, pus, parasites, piles, psyche.

→ Anorectal abscesses

10. A, B, C

An anorectal abscess might be a local manifestation of a generalised disease, such as diabetes or acquired immunodeficiency syndrome (AIDS), when the presentation can be fulminating. It is also important to exclude a colorectal disease such as inflammatory bowel disease (Crohn's disease) or rectal cancer. A good history and clinical examination would make such an aetiology obvious.

Infection of the anal glands is the main cause that results in cryptoglandular sepsis, which spreads readily into the intersphincteric tissue plane; the most common route taken is between the internal and external anal sphincters to point beneath the skin at the anal verge. Rupture of the abscess before treatment might result in a fistula-in-ano. The presentation is usually a short history of severe perianal pain with swinging pyrexia. Examination shows an excruciatingly tender, hot, indurated lump.

However, in cases where the infection is high within the pelvis, the presentation might not be as obvious. The patient might complain of fever or vague anorectal discomfort with urinary symptoms with nothing obvious externally; rectal examination might reveal painful induration above the anorectal junction. As treatment, immediate fistulotomy should not be performed. Under general anaesthetic, immediate drainage with a cruciate incision and deroofing of the abscess is the treatment. EUA and biopsy of the abscess walls and sigmoidoscopy is carried out to exclude underlying colorectal disease.

Fistula-in-ano

11. A, C

An underlying specific cause is not present in all cases; it is the exception rather than the rule. Nonetheless underlying conditions as a primary cause must be excluded when the condition is recurrent, indolent, or unusual. Crohn's disease and colloid carcinoma of the rectum should be excluded when there are multiple external openings; rare causes are tuberculosis, lymphogranuloma venerum (LGV) and actniomycosis. A clinical axiom called Goodsall's rule, which follows, is worth remembering: When an external opening is anterior to a transverse mid-anal line, the fistula usually runs radially into the anal canal; when the opening is posterior to this imaginary line, the track is usually curvilinear opening into the anal canal in the posterior midline.

MRI, whilst being regarded as the 'gold standard' for imaging, is not essential in all cases. It is mandatory in Crohn's disease and complicated fistulae with multiple tracks to distinguish the high from the low fistula. EUS and manometry are other useful investigations in these situations.

The underlying pathology is a cryptogenic fistula as a result of persistent infection of the anal glands in the intersphincteric space. Fistulae are classified as the following: trans-sphincteric (40%) where the primary track passes through the external sphincter at varying levels into the ischiorectal fossa; intersphincteric (45%) when the track passes from the anal canal across the internal sphincter into the perianal skin; and suprasphincteric and extrasphincteric, which are rare.

Ideally they are classified into high-anal and low-anal depending upon whether the internal opening is above or below the external sphincter. The surgical management is completely different in the two types. The majority can be treated by fistulotomy as they are uncomplicated and below the sphincter.

12. B, C, D, E

As trans-sphincteric and intersphincteric fistulae constitute 85% of all fistulae and the majority are uncomplicated, fistulotomy is the surgical treatment in the vast majority. The procedure involves division and laying open all the structures between the internal and external openings. Although it involves division of a small part of the voluntary musculature, there still might be some compromise of continence. Secondary tracks are also laid open and curetted and the wound marsupialised. High and complicated fistula need to be treated in a staged manner by using a seton. These are of two types – loose and cutting. Different types of seton materials are used, all non-absorbable. Surgery involving the use of a seton is the domain of a specialist colorectal surgeon and the reader interested in the procedures should refer to specialised sources. Anal advancement flap procedure, an operation for the expert, is indicated where the sphincter-complex is not too indurated with adequate intra-anal access. It should be done after elimination of all sepsis and secondary tracks.

Specialised investigations such as MRI and EUS are not necessary before surgery in all cases. It is mandatory only in complicated cases and where there is an underlying colorectal pathology. Because of the incidence of recurrence following sphincter-saving techniques, biological agents to plug and seal the track have been tried. Fibrin glue, porcine small intestinal submucosa and cross-linked porcine dermal collagen have all been tried, with variable results.

Answers to extended matching questions

1. B Anal fissure

This young man has an acute fissure-in-ano. The history suggests that constipation is the cause in this patient brought about by the ingestion of analgesics. Clinical examination would confirm the diagnosis. If clinical examination in the clinic is too painful, EUA would confirm the presence of a hypertrophied anal papilla and sentinel pile – both being tell-tale evidence of healing and breakdown. He needs to be given stool-bulking agents and stool softeners to treat his constipation. As his analgesic intake reduces, his constipation should improve. In the interim he could be given GTN for local application.

2. L Anal incontinence

In most patients history and clinical examination would elucidate the cause. In this patient incontinence is due to faecal impaction arising from a disorder of rectal evacuation. A plain abdominal x-ray will confirm that the entire large bowel is loaded with hard faeces. At the outset the patient will require manual evacuation under general anaesthetic. This should be followed by regulation of bowel habit by drugs and diet.

3. I Anal intraepithelial neoplasia (AIN)

AIN is the result of HPV infection and is encountered in the HIV-positive patients. It exhibits multifocal dysplasia. The disease is classified as AIN I, AIN II and AIN III, depending upon the extent of dysplasia. Left untreated it would become anal cancer. The condition should be treated in specialised centres. Local excision suffices where less than 30% of the anal circumference is involved. In extensive disease wide local excision with closure of the defect by flap or skin graft is carried out. The procedure and immediate postoperative period might have to be covered by a temporary stoma.

4. K Anal stenosis

While there are several causes of anal strictures, in this patient it is the result of complication following haemorrhoidectomy. This has resulted from removal of too much anoderm and mucosa without adequate skin bridges, causing scarring and stricture. This is treated initially by dilatation under general anaesthetic followed by self-dilatation by an anal dilator. In intractable or severe cases anoplasty using an advancement flap can be done.

5. H Condylomata accuminata

This patient should undergo a thorough clinical examination and, if necessary, EUA for complete evaluation of the extent of the warts as there might be extension into the genitalia. Careful application of 25% podophyllin to external warts and surgical excision is the treatment. Complete long-term cure is a problem unless there is a change in the patient's lifestyle.

6. F Fistula-in-ano

This patient's history is suggestive of a fistula-in-ano, which has resulted from a perianal abscess that burst on its own a while ago. Besides clinical examination, which should include a proctosigmoidoscopy, complete assessment is best carried out by EUA. While under the anaesthetic a flexible sigmoidoscopy is performed to make sure that there is no colorectal pathology and ascertain the position of the internal opening. It is then treated by fistulotomy.

7. A Haemorrhoids

This young woman's history is suggestive of piles, resulting from pregnancy. After a history, she is examined by proctosigmoidoscopy to confirm and ascertain the degree of piles. The history is suggestive of first-degree piles. At the outset, she is given advice regarding conservative management – normalising bowel habits, stool-softening agents and minimising straining. If after a period of conservative management, matters do not improve, injection sclerotherapy with 5% phenol in almond oil or banding is considered.

8. G Hydradenitis suppurativa

This condition is a difficult condition to treat mainly because of its intractability. The lesions start as multiple raised boils, which are recurrent leading to discharge, sinus formation and scarring. It also occurs in the axilla, groin, neck and perineum giving rise to physical and psychological morbidity.

Treatment includes general measures such as antiseptic soaps and antibiotics which keep the condition at bay only to recur. Surgical interventions consist of incision and drainage of abscesses in the acute stage. In a quiescent phase, consideration should be given to radical excision of all apocrine gland-bearing skin. This might require closure by skin graft or rotation flap.

9. E Perianal abscess

This patient has a typical perianal abscess (see **Figure 69.2** in **Chapter 69**) from his underlying Crohn's disease. It is almost certain he will have colorectal involvement with the disease. At the outset, the emergency management would be to give him analgesia and antibiotics and drain the abscess immediately. During drainage, EUA should be carried out, including a sigmoidoscopy, biopsy of tissue from the abscess cavity and biopsy of suspicious colonic mucosa.

Once the patient has recovered, a thorough assessment of the extent of the patient's disease must be carried out (if it has not already been done) with the gastroenterologist. This patient will almost certainly develop a fistula-in-ano. When that happens an MRI is mandatory and the patient is treated according to the findings. Patients with perianal Crohn's disease might need to be treated with infliximab (a tumour necrosis factor-α, TNF-α antagonist).

10. D Pilonidal sinus

This patient has developed a post-anal pilonidal sinus after initially suffering from an abscess. After thorough examination of the original tract and any openings on the skin, the condition is assessed and the options of treatment discussed with the patient. The fact that there are several surgical treatment options means that they all have a rate of failure.

Therefore, as the condition has a history of regression, conservative measures such as cleaning out of the tracks, removal of all hair with regular shaving of the buttocks and strict hygiene are advised.

11. C Pruritis ani

While there are many causes of pruritis ani, in this patient it is highly likely that it is the result of the patient's vaginal discharge. In this regard she needs a gynaecological opinion; a vaginal swab is taken to exclude *Trichomonas vaginalis* infection, and she is started on the appropriate antibiotics. This should be supplemented by strict measures of hygiene and cleanliness.

12. J Squamous cell carcinoma (SCC)

SCC of the anus is associated with HPV and is more common in those with HIV infection. This patient has the hallmarks of a squamous cell carcinoma of the anus with an indurated mass with everted edges at the anal verge. The inguinal group of lymph nodes need to be palpated for evidence of secondaries although enlargement might be due to infection. The diagnosis has to be confirmed, the carcinoma staged and then definitive treatment instituted. The condition should be managed in a specialised centre.

Confirmation is by biopsy best carried out under general anaesthetic so that at the same time EUA can be performed for local staging. This can be complemented by MRI and PET/CT, the latter helping to seek inguinal node involvement if present; this can also be done by FNAC. CT of chest and abdomen would complete the staging.

Definitive treatment is chemoradiotherapy (combined modality therapy, CMT) using 5-fluorouracil (5-FU) with mitomycin C or cisplatin. Local control is the mainstay of treatment because only 5% have distant metastasis at diagnosis. Small, marginal tumours are best treated by local excision. In spite of good results with CMT, almost one-quarter will have a relapse. Such patients will need an abdominoperineal resection.

PART 12

Genitourinary

74 Urinary symptoms and investigations

Pradip K Datta

Multiple choice questions

→ ## Haematuria

1. The following statements are true except:

A Microscopic haematuria is not always abnormal.

B Haematuria at the start of urinary stream indicates a cause in the lower urinary tract.

C Haematuria where the urine is uniformly mixed with the urine points to a cause in the upper urinary tract.

D Terminal haematuria is caused by bladder irritation or infection.

E Painful haematuria indicates malignant pathology.

→ ## Pain of urological origin

2. Which of the following statements are true?

A Pain of renal origin is a deep-seated sickening ache and 'bursting' in nature.

B Pain from a ureteric stone is colicky and radiates to the groin, scrotum, or labium.

C Pain from the urinary bladder is a suprapubic discomfort.

D Perineal pain is a penetrating ache and can be referred to the rectum.

E Large, slow-growing, space-occupying lesions produce a constant ache.

→ ## Preliminary investigations of the urinary tract

3. The following statements are true except:

A If 30% of kidney function is lost, renal failure becomes evident by blood results.

B Negative dipstick usually indicates a negative urine culture.

C Organisms of >10^5/mL on a midstream specimen of urine (MSU) is due to contamination.

D Biochemical examination of urine helps in calculus disease.

E Cytological examination of urine is sensitive and specific for poorly differentiated transitional cell cancer.

→ ## Imaging in urological conditions

4. Which of the following statements are true?

A All urinary calculi are radiodense.

B Pelvic phleboliths cannot be distinguished from lower ureteric calculi on a plain x-ray.

C Ultrasound scanning (US) provides the same information as an intravenous urogram (IVU).

D IVU can be dangerous.

E The procedure of antegrade pyelography can be used therapeutically.

5. The following statements are true except:

A Retrograde ureteropyelography can cause septicaemia.

B Venography should be used when tumour invasion into the inferior vena cava (IVC) is suspected.

C Non-contrast spiral CT should be routine for diagnosis of urinary calculi.

D CT scan is crucial in the staging of renal carcinoma.

E Radioisotope scanning has a role to ascertain selective renal function.

→ Renal failure

6. Which of the following statements is false?

A Anuria is defined as complete absence of urine production.

B Oliguria is defined as urinary output of less than 300 mL in 24 hours.

C Certain drugs can cause renal failure.

D All patients with renal failure will require renal replacement therapy.

E Indwelling stents can be used to relieve ureteric obstruction.

Extended matching questions

→ Imaging techniques

1 Antegrade pyelogram
2 CT scan of urinary bladder
3 Cystogram
4 Intravenous urogram
5 Plain x-ray
6 Renal angiogram
7 Retrograde ureterogram

Match the imaging techniques with the illustrations (Figures 74.1 through 74.7) shown:

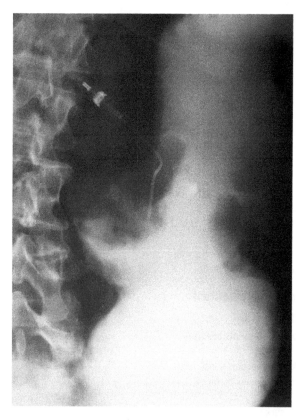

Figure 74.1

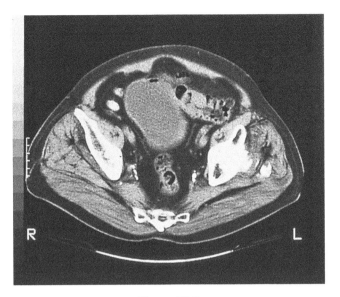

Figure 74.2

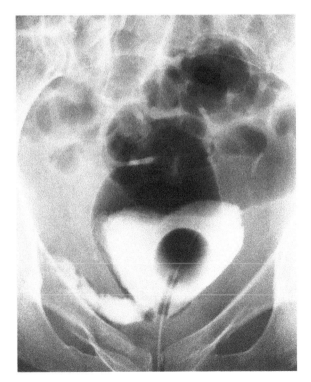

Figure 74.3

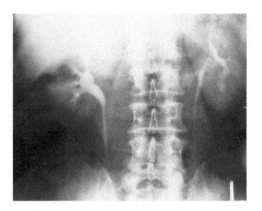

Figure 74.4

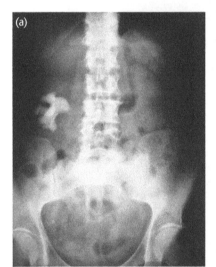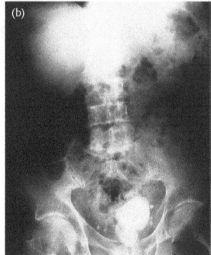

Figure 74.5

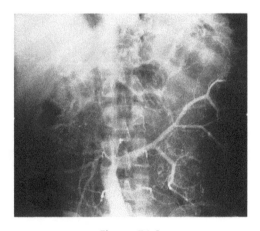

Figure 74.6

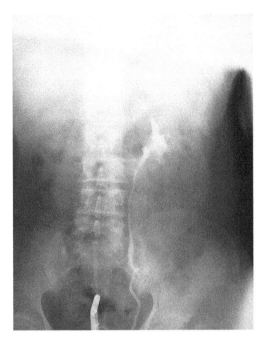

Figure 74.7

Answers to multiple choice questions

1. A, E
Haematuria, whether macroscopic or microscopic, is always abnormal and therefore should always be investigated. Haematuria from a malignant cause is usually painless as in bladder cancer when it is typically painless, profuse and periodic. It must be borne in mind that renal cell carcinoma presents with loin pain.

Haematuria at the commencement of the urinary stream indicates a cause in the bladder such as cancer or prostatic urethra. When the urine is uniformly mixed with blood, the cause is usually in the kidney. Haematuria at the end of micturition is caused by bladder irritation or infection. When it occurs in young women, the usual cause is urinary infection.

When haematuria is the presenting urinary symptom, the patient is placed on the urgent 'one-stop haematuria clinic'. Here the patient undergoes an ultrasound of the genito-urinary tract and flexible cystoscopy and further imaging if indicated.

2. A, B, C, D
Renal pain is a deep ache in the loin caused by stretching of the renal capsule. When the cause is inflammatory, there might be deep local tenderness with psoas spasm causing flexion of the hip. If the cause is a hydronephrosis the patient describes the pain as 'bursting'. Ureteric calculus causes one of the most severe pains ever, with the patient writhing around unable to find a comfortable position, and the pain radiates to the groin and genitalia. Pain originating from a cause in the urinary bladder, such as a stone, takes the form of wrenching discomfort at the end of micturition referred to as strangury. Pain in the perineum is a penetrating ache radiating to the rectum with inguinal discomfort. Although usually of prostatic origin when it is called 'prostadynia', it is also known to occur in women.

Large, slow-growing, space-occupying lesions are silent and do not cause pain. Hence some of the tumours or cysts grow to a large size before they are discovered.

3. A, C

More than 70% of kidney function must be lost before renal failure becomes evident on blood tests, because the kidneys have a large functional reserve. Renal damage must be quite severe before this is reflected in the serum biochemistry with a raised urea and creatinine. Renal damage can be from reduction in blood flow as in renal artery stenosis or severe hypertension; it can be from acute cortical necrosis with loss of glomeruli as in glomerulonephritis; or when tubular function is impaired as in pyelonephritis. When culture shows organisms of >10^5/mL on a midstream specimen of urine (MSU), it indicates infection and not contamination.

Negative dipstick means that there is no blood, protein, or nitrates in the urine. Organisms produce them, and hence their absence indicates no infection. Biochemical examination of urine in a 24-hour sample for calcium, oxalate and uric acid is useful in investigation of calculus disease. Cytology of urinary sediment can be sensitive and specific in identifying poorly differentiated transitional cell carcinoma whereas false negatives are common in well differentiated tumours.

4. B, D, E

Pelvic phleboliths, a common occurrence, cannot be distinguished from ureteric calculus in the lower one-third; only an intravenous urogram (IVU) will help distinguish them. An IVU can be dangerous because of allergic reactions. This is much more common in patients with a history of allergy, atopy and eczema; rarely severe reactions might occur without warning. Hence, the patient should be observed very closely after the injection of a small amount of the contrast medium. Antegrade pyelography done through direct puncture of the renal pelvis (usually dilated) can be used therapeutically to decompress the kidney in obstructive uropathy.

Most, but not all, urinary calculi are radiodense. Uric acid calculi are radiolucent and hence not visible on a plain x-ray. US does not provide the same information as an IVU. IVU has the advantage of showing renal function. The IVU images show up tumours, calculi and details of abnormal anatomy better than US.

5. B

Venography is an obsolete investigation to look for extension of growth in renal carcinoma into the IVC. Ultrasound and CT scan can obtain this information. Retrograde ureteropyelography (retrograde ureterogram) entails cystoscopy and ureteric catheterisation. The procedure can be done through a flexible cystoscope under topical anaesthesia. Therefore it has the potential to introduce infection and if carried out in the presence of obstruction, the procedure carries a real risk of septicaemia.

Non-contrast spiral CT is used routinely for the diagnosis of urinary calculi, particularly for ureteric stone that presents as an emergency with ureteric colic. Contrast CT is essential for staging in renal cancer – site, size, invasion of adjacent structures, hilar lymphadenopathy and extension into renal vein and IVC. It is equally mandatory in the staging and follow-up of testicular tumours. Radioisotope scanning gives useful information about selective renal function. In this diethyltriaminepentaacetic acid (DTPA) labelled with technetium-99 is used to give a dynamic renal function of individual kidneys. It is also of use in hydronephrosis from pelvi-ureteric junction obstruction.

→ ## Renal failure

6. D

All patients with renal failure will not require renal replacement therapy. The cause of renal failure should be established – prerenal, renal, or postrenal **(Figure 74.8)**. Patients in renal failure must be managed by a team involving the nephrologist and intensive care specialist. The patient is treated depending on the cause **(Figure 74.9)**.

Drugs such as aminoglycosides, cephalosporins, diuretics, NSAIDs (long-term use) and ACE inhibitors might damage the kidneys.

Anuria is complete absence of urine production while oliguria is <300 mL of urine excretion in 24 hours. If the cause has been established as obstructive (post-renal) stent insertion into the ureter/s is the treatment of choice. Obstruction at the bladder outlet is treated by urethral catheterisation, failing which suprapubic cystostomy is carried out.

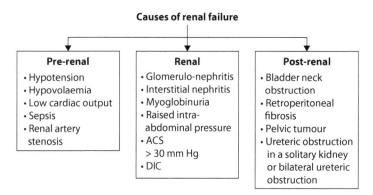

Figure 74.8 Causes of renal failure.

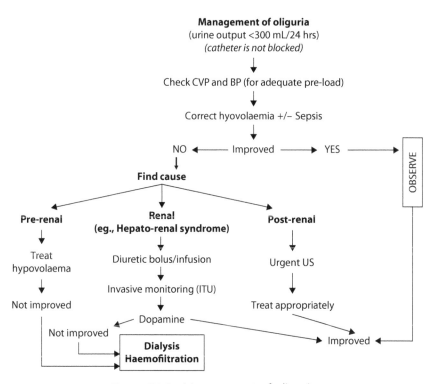

Figure 74.9 Management of oliguria.

Answers to extended matching questions

1. Antegrade pyelogram, Figure 74.1

This investigation is done in obstructive uropathy to see the site and cause of obstruction. It is also useful therapeutically to insert a nephrostomy tube to drain the urine. This patient has several filling defects in his grossly dilated renal pelvis from transitional cell carcinoma of the renal pelvis.

2. CT scan of urinary bladder, Figure 74.2

This is a CT scan of the urinary bladder showing air in the vault of the bladder with loop of sigmoid colon adherent to the bladder denoting a colo-vesical fistula from diverticulitis.

3. Cystogram, Figure 74.3

This is a cystogram carried out by injecting contrast through the indwelling catheter. It shows extravasation of contrast at the bladder neck due to extra-peritoneal rupture of the urinary bladder.

4. Intravenous urogram, Figure 74.4

This is an intravenous urogram showing an irregular filling defect in the left renal pelvis from a transitional cell carcinoma.

5. Plain x-ray KUB area, Figure 74.5a

This plain x-ray of KUB (kidney, ureter, bladder) area shows a typical stag-horn calculus of the right kidney.

Plain x-ray pelvis **Figure 74.5b**.

This plain x-ray of pelvis shows a stone in the urinary bladder.

6. Renal angiogram, Figure 74.6

This is a left renal angiogram showing a large vascular renal cell carcinoma. As an investigation this is obsolete, as a contrast-enhanced CT scan would give the same information. However, it is still carried out only when renal artery embolisation is contemplated in a very vascular tumour.

7. Retrograde ureterogram, Figure 74.7

This is a left retrograde ureterogram showing cystoscope in place. The image shows an irregular filling defect in the upper part of the renal pelvis typical of a transitional cell carcinoma.

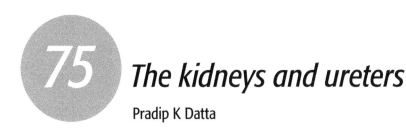

The kidneys and ureters

Pradip K Datta

Multiple choice questions

Congenital abnormalities of the kidney, renal pelvis and ureters

1. **Which of the following statements are true?**

A The incidence of horseshoe kidney is one in 1000.

B A horseshoe kidney is liable to pelviureteric junction obstruction.

C Once the diagnosis of a horseshoe kidney is made the isthmus should be divided.

D Polycystic kidneys can be transmitted by either parent as an autosomal dominant trait.

E Polycystic kidneys present in childhood as renal failure.

2. **The following statements are true except:**

A Duplication of the renal pelvis is found in 4% and ureter in 3% of patients.

B The previoiusly mentioned abnormalities are usually incidental findings.

C Retrocaval ureter cause bilateral hydronephrosis.

D Ureterocele is a cystic enlargement of the intramural ureter.

E All ureteroceles must be treated by endoscopic diathermy incision.

Renal injury

3. **Which of the following statements are true?**

A Haematuria following trivial injury to the kidney indicates damage to a pathological kidney.

B Closed renal injury is usually extraperitoneal.

C In closed renal injury, surgical exploration is necessary in the majority.

D Intravenous urography or contrast-enhanced computed tomography (CECT) scan should be performed urgently in suspected renal injury.

E Hypertension might be a long-term complication of renal injury.

Ureteric injury

4. **Which of the following statements are false?**

A Most ureteric injuries are due to surgical trauma during pelvic surgery.

B Preoperative ureteric catheterisation helps to protect them from injury during operation.

C When recognised during operation, an injured ureter should be repaired immediately.

D When ureteric injury is diagnosed postoperatively, delayed repair is undertaken.

E Urinary fistula through an abdominal or vaginal wound indicates a damaged ureter.

Hydronephrosis

5. **In pelviureteric junction (PUJ) obstruction (idiopathic or congenital hydronephrosis) the following statements are true except:**

A The condition might be asymptomatic.

B It can be diagnosed in utero.

C Ultrasound scanning is the least invasive method of imaging.

D An intravenous urogram (IVU) is the ideal imaging.

E The kidney should be preserved if it has more than 5% of renal function.

→ Renal calculi

6. Which of the following statements are true?

A The common bacteria found as a nidus for urinary stones are staphylococci, streptococci and *Proteus*.

B Hyperparathyroidism is found in 5% or less of those presenting with radio-opaque calculi.

C If a parathyroid adenoma is found to be the cause of renal calculi, it should be removed before treatment of the calculus.

D Pure uric acid stones are radio-opaque.

E A staghorn calculus is composed of calcium-ammonium-magnesium phosphate.

7. Which of the following statements are false?

A Renal stones are usually visible on a plain x-ray.

B The severity of pain of ureteric colic is related to the size of stone.

C Hydronephrosis or pyonephrosis with a palpable loin swelling is a common clinical presentation

D Haematuria is common.

E There are very few physical signs.

→ Imaging for calculus disease

8. Which of the following imaging techniques are used for urinary calculus disease?

A Plain kidney, ureter and bladder (KUB) x-ray

B Spiral CT scan

C IVU

D Ultrasound (US)

E Retrograde pyelography

→ Management of urinary calculi

9. The following statements are true except:

A Ureteric calculi smaller than 1 cm will pass spontaneously.

B Infection in the presence of upper urinary tract obstruction due to a stone requires surgical intervention.

C Most urinary calculi can be treated by minimal-access surgical techniques.

D In bilateral renal stones, the kidney with poorer function is treated first.

E Open operations for renal stones are performed through an extraperitoneal loin approach.

10. Which of the following statements are true in ureteric stones?

A The majority pass spontaneously.

B If a stone has not passed after 6 weeks, intervention is required.

C Stones are commonly arrested at the two sites of ureteric narrowing.

D Most stones are treated by ureteroscopic electrohydraulic fragmentation.

E Severe renal pain subsiding after a day or two suggests that the stone has passed.

→ Infections

11. The following statements are true except:

A Ascending infection in the urinary tract is the most common route.

B *E. coli* and other Gram-negative organisms are most commonly responsible.

C *Proteus* and staphylococci thrive in acidic urine.

D Up to 50% of children with urinary infection have an underlying abnormality.

E All patients present electively with dysuria and frequency of micturition.

12. Which of the following statements are true?

A Sterile pyuria should alert one to the possibility of renal tuberculosis.

B Chronic pyelonephritis is often associated with vesicoureteric reflux.

C Pyonephrosis is an infected hydronephrosis and is most commonly due to a stone-causing obstruction.

D Renal carbuncle is most commonly seen in the immunocompromised.

E Perinephric abscess might occur from extension of a retrocaecal appendix abscess.

Renal neoplasms

13. Which of the following statements about Wilms' tumour is false?

A It is a tumour of embryonic nephrogenic tissue occurring below the age of 5 years.

B Haematuria and fever are the most common presentations.

C Lymphatic spread is rare.

D Imaging modalities are US, CT and MRI.

E Treatment is by chemotherapy, surgery and radiotherapy.

14. Which of the following statements are true about hypernephroma?

A In 25% of patients there are no local symptoms.

B A left-sided varicocele might be a presenting feature in a male.

C Haematuria and clot colic are the most common presentations.

D IVU, US and CECT are the imaging methods of choice.

E Following nephrectomy, chemotherapy and radiotherapy should be given.

Extended matching questions

Diagnoses

1 Carcinoma of kidney
2 Carcinoma of ureter
3 Congenital hydronephrosis
4 Horse-shoe kidney
5 Pyonephrosis
6 Staghorn calculus
7 Transitional cell carcinoma (TCC) of renal pelvis
8 Trauma to kidney
9 Ureteric calculus
10 Wilm's tumour

Match the following scenarios with the diagnoses:

Clinical scenarios

A A 40-year-old man has come to A&E complaining of a sudden onset of very severe pain in his left loin of 4 hours duration, radiating to the front of the lumbar area and groin and the left testis. He has vomited a couple of times and has urinary frequency. On examination he is writhing in pain and cannot find a comfortable position.

B A 60-year-old man complains of haematuria associated with pain in his left loin radiating to the lower abdomen for about 2 months. He passes clots that are 'worm-like'. On examination he has an enlarged left kidney, and scrotal examination reveals a varicocele of which he was unaware.

C A 45-year-old female patient complains of nagging pain in her right loin and urinary frequency for several months. On examination she has tenderness in her loin over the kidney. Urine examination shows red blood cells and a growth of *Proteus* and staphylococci.

D A fit 20-year-old young man had a game of rugby, following which he passed frank blood in his urine in the changing room. He felt some discomfort in his left loin. After returning home, his haematuria became worse and he noticed some fullness in his left loin. He then came to A&E. His blood pressure was 110/60 mmHg, his pulse was 110/minute and he had fullness in his left loin.

E A 60-year-old female patient was seen as an emergency with high temperature, rigors, and pain in her right loin. She had a blood pressure of 160/70 mmHg, bounding pulse of 90/minute, and extreme tenderness in her right loin.

F A 62-year-old man complains of left loin ache with intermittent painless haematuria in the form of clots, occasional high temperature and rigors, some dysuria, and frequency for 6 months. An

IVU shows an irregular filling defect in the lower one-third of the left ureter. There is nothing to find on clinical examination. His Hb is 10.2 gm/dL.

G A 35-year-old woman presents with recurrent attacks of urinary tract infection. On every occasion this was successfully treated with antibiotics. In view of several such episodes in the past, she underwent an IVU, which showed the renal calyces to be pointing toward the vertebrae.

H A male child of 3 years has been brought by his mother, who noticed while bathing him that the right side of his abdomen felt larger than the left and was asymmetrical; she thought that there was probably a lump in his abdomen.

I A 10-year-old boy has been brought in as an emergency by his parents as they noticed that he had bright red haematuria for the past 24 hours or so. About 6 hours prior to that he was climbing a tree and accidentally fell on his left side.

J A 72-year-old woman complains of intermittent haematuria associated with a dull ache in her left loin. She has some dysuria and urine specimen showed *E. coli* infection. She has no physical findings. An IVU showed a persistent irregular filling defect in the left renal pelvis.

Answers to multiple choice questions

→ Congenital abnormalities of the kidney, renal pelvis, and ureters

1. A, B, D

The incidence of horseshoe kidney is 1:1000. The two kidneys are usually fused by its isthmus at the lower pole. The two ureters pass in front of the isthmus and are therefore angulated. Diagnosis is made on ultrasound or IVU, which shows the calyces pointing medially toward the vertebral bodies **(Figure 75.1)**. This causes pelviureteric junction obstruction with resultant inefficient drainage of urine causing stasis, inevitably the outcome being infection

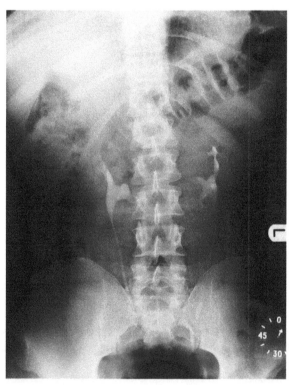

Figure 75.1   IVU showing horseshoe kidney.

and stone formation. Most of the time, however, they are an incidental finding and therefore best left alone. The isthmus does not need to be divided except when operating for an abdominal aortic aneurysm (AAA). If the AAA is being repaired by endovascular method, then the horseshoe kidney can be left alone.

Polycystic kidneys are hereditary and transmitted by either parent as an autosomal dominant trait. The condition does not manifest itself clinically before the age of 30 years and therefore does not present in childhood as renal failure.

2. C, E
Retrocaval or postcaval ureter only causes right-sided hydronephrosis and hydroureter. This is because the abnormality lies in the development of the inferior vena cava (IVC). The latter develops from various sources. Persistence of the posterior cardinal vein with high confluence of the right and left iliac veins or a double inferior vena cava results in retrocaval ureter. This passes behind the IVC before it emerges in front of it to pass from medial to lateral. The incidence is 1:1500. It is often an incidental finding, rarely causing symptoms from right ureteric obstruction.

The majority of ureteroceles are incidental findings and hence do not need surgical treatment. An ureterocele is a cystic dilatation of the lower end of the ureter, the ureteric orifice being covered by a membrane that expands and deflates as it is filled with urine, a finding seen on cystoscopy. IVU shows the typical 'adder-head' appearance. Treatment, in the form of endoscopic diathermy incision, is carried out only if there is recurrent infection, obstruction, or stone formation.

Duplication of a renal pelvis occurs in 4% of patients, whereas the ureter is duplicated in 3%. The latter join up in the lower third of their course so that they have a single orifice in the bladder. These are incidental findings.

3. A, B, D, E
Haematuria following trivial blunt abdominal or loin trauma indicates a pathological kidney such as congenital hydronephrosis or calculus disease. The kidney tends to get injured from a fall, blow, or crushing from a road-traffic accident. Closed renal injury is usually extraperitoneal, particularly in adults. However, in children, because they have very little extraperitoneal fat, the peritoneum, which is closely adherent to the kidney, can tear with the renal capsule and cause urine and blood to leak into the peritoneum.

After resuscitation according to the ATLS protocol, an urgent IVU and contrast-enhanced CT must be carried out; this is to make sure that the contralateral kidney is normal while ascertaining the extent of damage of the injured kidney. After recovery, in the long term, hypertension due to renal fibrosis, is a complication.

The mainstay of management of renal injury is conservative, surgical exploration being necessary in less than one-tenth of patients with closed renal injury.

4. D
When ureteric injury is diagnosed postoperatively, early repair should be undertaken as delayed repair can be difficult due to fibrosis. If diagnosed at the time of injury, immediate repair is carried out. The ureter is a well-protected deep retroperitoneal tube and hence most causes of injury are iatrogenic (Table 75.1). Preoperative ureteric stenting helps to protect or instantly recognise damage should it occur during operations such as retroperitoneal lymph node dissection in testicular tumours, excision of retroperitoneal liposarcoma, or open repair of inflammatory abdominal aortic aneurysm.

Damaged ureter manifests itself as a urinary fistula through the abdominal or vaginal wound. Sometimes loin pain and fever might be a presenting feature of an unrecognised

Table 75.1 Causes of iatrogenic ureteric injury

- Large bowel operations: right and left hemicolectomy
  - Anterior resection
  - Abdomino-perineal resection
- Vascular operations: Resection of AAA
- Gynaecological operations: Hysterectomy
- Retroperitoneal operations: Lymph node dissection in teratoma
  - Excision of sarcoma

ureteric injury. There are various methods of repair that must be undertaken by the urologist. The procedure chosen will depend upon the type of injury, time of diagnosis, and whether a segment of ureter is missing. The choices are end-to-end anastomosis with spatulation, ureteric re-implantation, Boari operation, and ileal ureteric replacement.

5. D, E

IVU is not the ideal imaging method. Isotope renography is the best test to establish that dilatation is caused by obstruction. It would also determine the percentage function of the kidney. DTPA labelled with technetium-99 is injected and its progress through the kidneys is monitored by a gamma camera. In hydronephrosis the isotope remains in the renal pelvis and does so in spite of frusemide. A procedure to preserve the kidney is carried out when a renogram shows that there is more than 20% (not 5%) of renal function.

Hydronephrosis is defined as an aseptic dilatation of the pelvi-calyceal system from an obstruction. The condition caused by PUJ obstruction **(Figure 75.2)**, although congenital in

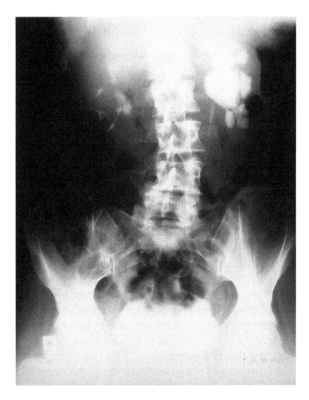

Figure 75.2 IVU showing left hydronephrosis from PUJ obstruction.

origin, might remain relatively asymptomatic until adulthood. Clinically the condition might present as loin pain exacerbated by excessive fluid intake. It can be diagnosed in utero by ante-natal ultrasound.

The operation of choice is Anderson–Hynes pyeloplasty, a procedure that can be carried out laparoscopically. Minimal-access surgical techniques such as endoscopic pyelotomy with balloon dilatation and temporary stenting are the alternative procedures.

6. A, B, C, E

Infected urine acts as a culture medium for urinary stones. Staphylococci, streptococci, and *Proteus* species have the ability to split urea, causing alkaline urine that is conducive to the formation of stones. Primary hyperparathyroidism causing hypercalcaemia and hypercalciuria is found in 5% of patients who present with radio-opaque calculi. This metabolic disturbance must be excluded in patients who present with recurrent urinary calculi (see **Chapter 51**, dealing with section on hyperparathyroidism). If a parathyroid adenoma is found in the presence of renal calculi, it must be removed first before treating the kidney stones.

A staghorn calculus is composed of calcium ammonium magnesium phosphate. Because of its composition it is smooth and dirty white growing in alkaline urine, is radio-opaque, and grows to occupy the entire renal pelvis. It might be asymptomatic and found incidentally. When symptomatic it might cause haematuria, infection, and renal failure in bilateral calculi.

Pure uric acid stones (hard, smooth, multiple, multifaceted) are radiolucent and show up as a filling defect on an IVU, mimicking a transitional cell carcinoma of the renal pelvis. Some might cast a faint shadow on plain x-ray by virtue of containing some calcium. Confirmation is done by a CT scan.

7. B, C

The severity of ureteric colic is not related to the size of the stone. The pain is agonising, typically passing from the loin to the groin and then to the genitalia with the patient writhing and unable to find a comfortable position. The pain from a renal stone is fixed in the renal angle and hypochondrium. Haematuria, macroscopic or microscopic, is common. Physical signs are few. Hydronephrosis or pyonephrosis as a palpable loin swelling is rare. Renal stones are usually visible on a plain abdominal x-ray.

8. A, B, C, D

Plain radiography has a limited place as opacities from calcified mesenteric lymph nodes, gallstones, foreign bodies, phleboliths and calcified adrenal gland might cause confusion. In suspected renal stone, a lateral view is helpful. A kidney stone will be seen superimposed on the vertebral body while the others would be in front.

Spiral CT scan is the gold standard of investigation in acute ureteric colic. IVU has a role if CT is not available. It would show delayed excretion from the affected kidney; repeated pictures at delayed intervals might show the exact site of stone in the ureter. It would also help to confirm that the opposite kidney is normal. Ultrasound is essential for treatment with extracorporeal shock wave lithotripsy (ESWL). Retrograde pyelography has no role as the information obtained from it would be available from the above methods; moreover it can introduce infection.

9. A, D

Ureteric calculi smaller than 0.5 cm will pass spontaneously, larger stones requiring surgical intervention **(Figures 75.3a** and **b)**. Presence of infection in an obstructed upper urinary tract requires urgent surgical intervention under antibiotic cover. In bilateral renal stones, the kidney with better function is treated first. The exception is that the kidney with pain or pyonephrosis is treated first by decompression through a nephrostomy.

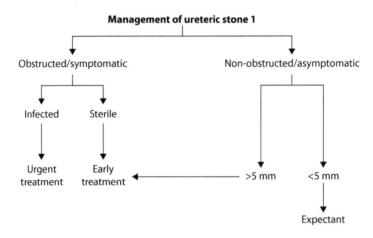

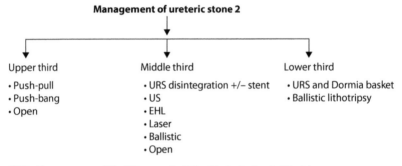

URS = Ureteroscopy   US = Ultrasound   EHL = Electrohydraulic lithotripsy

Figure 75.3   Management of ureteric stones.

The vast majority of stones in the genito-urinary tract are treated by minimal access surgery. Stone in the renal pelvis is removed by percutaneous nephrolithotomy. A cannula is placed in the renal pelvis; a balloon catheter is passed to stop stone fragments migrating into the ureter. The stone is then fragmented by contact lithotripsy; the fragments are then removed by forceps or washed out. Finally a nephrostogram is done to make sure of the integrity of the renal pelvis.

When extracorporeal shockwave lithotripsy (ESWL) is used, preliminary ureteric stent is placed to prevent ureteric obstruction from stone fragments ('steinstrasse' = stone street). The patient is then given ESWL, the number of sessions depending upon the size of the stone. In the rare instance when an open procedure is to be done, the approach is extraperitoneal through the loin.

10. A, D

The vast majority of ureteric stones pass spontaneously as they are <5 mm in diameter. Stones that require surgical intervention (those > 5mm or presence of infection) are treated by minimal access surgical methods in the vast majority. The most common method is electrohydraulic fragmentation, washout +/− stent insertion through an ureteroscope.

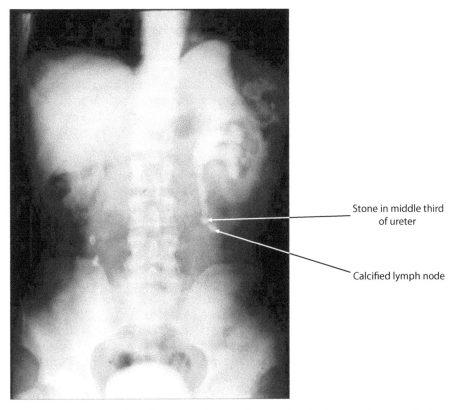

Stone in middle third
of ureter

Calcified lymph node

Figure 75.4 IVU showing stone in middle one-third of ureter that needed surgical removal.

If obstruction from a ureteric stone persists after 1 or 2 weeks **(Figure 75.4)**, the stone should be removed; one should never wait for 6 weeks because it might cause renal atrophy and loss of function. In the ureter, stones are commonly arrested at one of the following five (not two) anatomical sites of narrowing: pelviureteric junction, crossing of the iliac vessels, proximity of vas deferens or broad ligament, entrance to the bladder wall, and ureteric orifice. Severe renal pain subsiding after 1 day or so is a sinister symptom and denotes complete ureteric obstruction, a situation that requires immediate decompression by percutaneous nephrostomy followed by definitive treatment.

11. C, E

Proteus and staphylococci thrive in alkaline urine. They are urea-splitting organisms and form ammonia, which makes the urine alkaline, predisposing to stone formation. *E. coli* and other Gram-negative organisms are commonly responsible for kidney infections. In *E. coli* and streptococcal infections the urine is acidic.

Patients might present either as an emergency with acute pyelonephritis or electively as chronic pyelonephritis. Acute pyelonephritis is more common in females at all ages and presents with lassitude, nausea and vomiting, loin pain with rigors and high temperature and scalding micturition. Septicaemia might occur. The elective patient with chronic pyelonephritis is usually a woman who presents with dull lumbar non-specific pain and generally feeling unwell over a period of time.

The most common route is ascending infection. When it occurs in children, 50% have an underlying abnormality such as vesicoureteric reflux or obstruction. In 35% of them vesicoureteric reflux is the cause and in extreme cases reflux nephropathy might result in end-stage renal failure.

12. A, B, C, D, E

Sterile pyuria, when there are abundant white cells in the urine without any growth of organisms, is typical in renal tuberculosis. Frequency of micturition is often the only symptom; suprapubic pain might be present with minimal loin ache. Haematuria might occur in a minority. The diagnosis should be suspected when symptoms of cystitis persist in spite of prolonged antibiotic therapy. Other clinical features of TB should be sought.

Vesico-ureteric reflux is often the cause of chronic pyelonephritis that results in renal scarring in the long term ultimately causing end-stage renal failure. Pyonephrosis is infected hydronephrosis and is caused by a stone obstructing the ureter. This is a surgical emergency. The patient should be resuscitated, started on antibiotics and the diagnosis confirmed by US. The renal pelvis is drained by a nephrostomy. Once the patient has recovered, the function of the kidney is determined and appropriate definitive treatment instituted.

Renal carbuncle is an abscess within the renal parenchyma that results from blood-borne infection. It is commonly seen in the immunocompromised—diabetic, drug abusers, chronic debilitating diseases, and acquired immunodeficiency. The patient has an ill-defined tender loin swelling. Diagnosis is confirmed by US or CT scan. The abscess is drained by open surgery, as the pus is usually too thick for percutaneous aspiration.

Perinephric abscess might result from a retrocaecal appendix abscess, extension from a cortical abscess or by haematogenous spread. The patient presents as a surgical emergency with swinging pyrexia and tender loin mass. The diagnosis is confirmed by US or CT scan. The patient is treated by open incision and drainage.

→ Renal neoplasms

13. B

The most common presentation is an abdominal mass noticed by the mother when bathing the child. Haematuria is a late symptom and denotes extension of the tumour into the renal pelvis and therefore a poor prognosis. Pyrexia is another late presentation. Failure to thrive is often noticed by the parents. Besides a lump, on examination there might be hemi-hypertrophy of the body and absence of the iris.

Once suspected, the patient should be referred to the paediatric surgeon with special interest in oncology. An IVU should be done to make sure that the other kidney is normal. This is followed by staging of the tumour by US, CT scan, MRI, and CXR. Depending upon the staging the management is discussed in a multidisciplinary team meeting followed by treatment that would consist of a combination of surgery, chemotherapy, and radiotherapy. The exact order of the modalities of treatment depends upon the staging.

14. A, B, C, D

One in four patients presents with features of secondaries such as bone pain, pathological fracture, or haemoptysis. A left-sided varicocele of recent onset in the male patient might indicate a renal cell carcinoma. This is because growth has extended along the left renal vein obstructing the left testicular vein. Therefore, any middle-aged patient presenting with a recent left-sided varicocele should have the left renal area felt and investigated for a space-occupying lesion.

Haematuria and clot colic are the most common clinical symptoms, the clots are often worm-like taking the shape of the ureter. The disease is staged by IVU, US, and CECT and management discussed in a multidisciplinary team meeting.

Chemotherapy and radiotherapy have no role in adjuvant treatment. The cytokine interleukin-2 has had some encouraging outcomes.

Answers to extended matching questions

1. B Hypernephroma (Grawitz's tumour, clear cell, or adenocarcinoma of kidney)

This male patient has the classical presentation of a left hypernephroma: haematuria, loin pain and clot colic and an enlarged kidney. He also has a left varicocele caused by growth extending into the left renal vein, obstructing the entry of left testicular vein. The atypical presentations are the following: hypertension of recent onset, polycythaemia, pyrexia of unknown origin, and features of anaemia and nephrotic syndrome. Symptoms from secondaries might be the presenting features in 25% of patients, including haemoptysis from lung secondaries, bone pain, or pathological fracture from skeletal secondaries that are typically very vascular and cause a hot pulsatile swelling with throbbing pain in a long bone.

He needs an IVU **(Figure 75.5)**, which would show calyceal splaying, irregular excretion of contrast with soft-tissue shadow. Staging is done by CECT and a chest x-ray (CXR). The CT scan might show invasion of the renal vein and inferior vena cava with growth. Selective renal angiogram **(Figure 75.6)** is an investigation rarely done nowadays; however, it is carried out when embolisation is contemplated in very large growths and in small growths or in a solitary kidney where partial nephrectomy is considered.

Macroscopically the cancer is yellowish in colour (because of lipid content), with cystic areas and lobules with haemorrhage and necrosis **(Figure 75.7)**. Microscopically it is a clear cell carcinoma due to abundant lipid and glycogen. It spreads to the hilar lymph nodes and has a propensity to spread by bloodstream to lungs and bone.

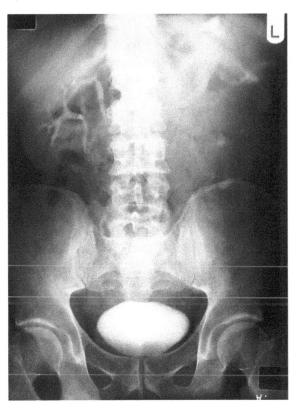

Figure 75.5   IVU showing irregular excretion of contrast in left kidney with large soft tissue shadow – renal cell carcinoma.

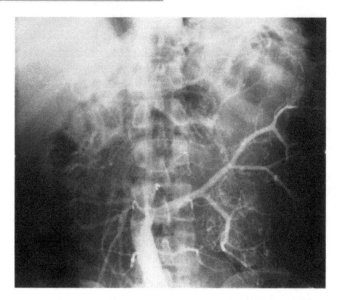

Figure 75.6   Left renal angiogram showing abnormal tumour circulation in a large renal cell carcinoma (same patient as in Figure 75.5).

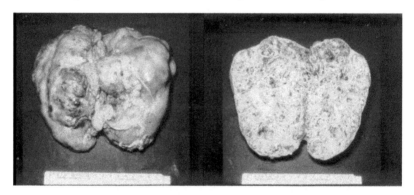

Figure 75.7   Pathological specimen of a renal cell carcinoma.

Treatment is radical nephrectomy often carried out transperitoneally because of the anatomical position of the renal vein. Sometimes the nephrectomy is carried out laparoscopically. In rare instances where there is tumour extension into the inferior vena cava and right atrium, the nephrectomy can be carried out with tumour excision in continuity by enlisting the help of the cardiac surgeon with the patient on cardio-pulmonary bypass.

2. F Carcinoma of ureter
This patient has macroscopic haematuria with attacks of bacteraemia from UTI. The IVU (**Figure 75.8**) shows an irregular filling defect in the lower one-third of left ureter, producing back pressure accounting for his left loin ache. This is a transitional cell carcinoma (TCC) of the ureter.

He needs staging by CT scan and CXR. A cystoscopy should follow to exclude a TCC in the bladder. The treatment is nephrourterectomy with excision of a cuff of the urinary bladder. The patient should have regular check cystoscopies thereafter to look for recurrence within the urinary bladder.

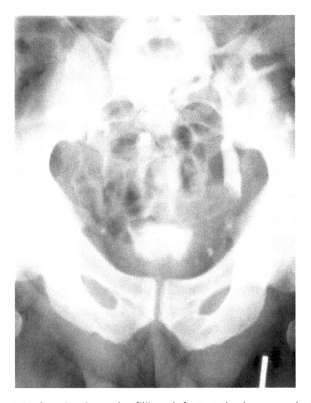

Figure 75.8 IVU showing irregular filling defect at the lower end of left ureter with proximal dilatation – transitional cell carcinoma (TCC) of the ureter.

3. D Congenital hydronephrosis
This 20-year-old man developed haematuria following minor trauma while playing rugby. He was completely unaware of the trauma and surprised to have haematuria. He did notice some left loin discomfort. Haematuria following minor trauma occurs typically in a pathological kidney. In a fit young man this would be a congenital hydronephrosis (sometimes called idiopathic hydronephrosis) from a pelvi-ureteric junction (PUJ) obstruction that has ruptured with urinary extravasation, the cause of fullness in his left loin.

This patient needs resuscitation, although he is probably stable from the cardiovascular point of view but for his tachycardia. He needs an IVU to make sure that the other kidney is normal; it will also show urinary extravasation. A CECT is also done to accurately assess the damage. This should be followed by urgent exploration and possible Anderson–Hynes operation.

4. G Horseshoe kidney
This young woman has had recurrent attacks of UTI successfully treated on each occasion with antibiotics. In view of recurrent attacks, an IVU was carried out that showed the typical features of a horseshoe kidney with the calyces facing medially toward the vertebrae, the appearance often likened to a 'flower vase' **(Figure 75.1)**.

Patients with horseshoe kidney (incidence 1:1000) are often found incidentally when an ultrasound has been done for some other purpose. If they produce symptoms it is due to infections and stone formation. This is because the pelves and ureters have to travel over the isthmus as a result of which there is stasis. The condition very rarely needs an operation.

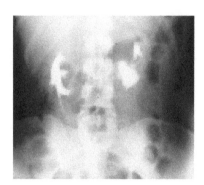

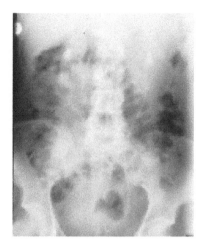

Figure 75.9 Postoperative pyeloplasty in a horseshoe kidney. (Courtesy of Mr S Bramwell, Former Consultant Urological Surgeon, Raigmore Hospital, Inverness, UK.)

The reason for surgical treatment would be PUJ obstruction **(Figure 75.9)** or prior to open operation for abdominal aortic aneurysm.

5. E Pyonephrosis
This woman has all the features of septicaemia, which include shock and hyperdynamic circulation (large pulse pressure) and bounding pulse. Marked loin tenderness points to a diagnosis of pyonephrosis. She needs urgent resuscitation with intravenous fluids, oxygen, and bloods sent for cultures, haematology, and biochemistry. The appropriate antibiotics are started and the diagnosis confirmed.

An urgent IVU is carried out to make sure that the other kidney is normal; the affected kidney will be seen to be non-functioning. Once stabilised, further imaging is done by US and CECT. During imaging, the interventional radiologist would insert a nephrostomy under image guidance. In a few days the patient would recover. An ante-grade pyelogram is done to find out the cause such as a stone. Once the cause is determined, the patient is appropriately treated.

If the kidney function is in doubt, an isotope renogram is performed to assess the exact amount of functioning renal tissue. If this found to be minimal, a subcapsular nephrectomy **(Figure 75.10)** is carried out as a definitive procedure.

6. C Staghorn calculus
This patient with nagging pain in her right loin and urinary frequency has symptoms suggestive of a kidney stone. The growth of urea-splitting organisms of *Proteus* and staphylococci indicate alkaline urine, which is conducive to the formation of phosphate calculi **(Figure 75.11)**. An IVU is carried out to assess the function of the opposite kidney. An isotope renogram would be appropriate to see the amount of function in the affected kidney. If the function is good enough to preserve the kidney then the stone is treated by minimal access surgical techniques.

As the stone is quite large, this will need to be treated by a combination of percutaneous nephrolithotomy (PCNL) and extracorporeal shockwave lithotripsy (ESWL). Under general anaesthetic, a track is made under US guidance through the loin into the renal pelvis and the stone shattered by ultrasound. Stone fragments are removed by PCNL thereby de-bulking the stone. The parts of the stone that cannot be removed are then treated by ESWL in due course as an outpatient procedure. A ureteric stent is inserted prior to starting ESWL to prevent ureteric obstruction.

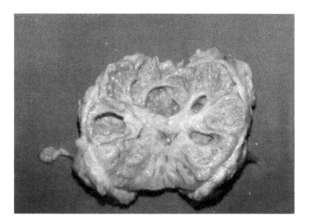

Figure 75.10   Kidney after subcapsular nephrectomy for pyonephrosis.

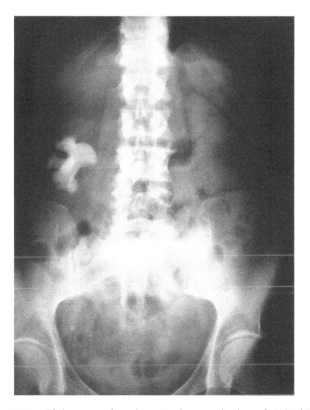

Figure 75.11   Plain x-ray showing staghorn calculus of right kidney.

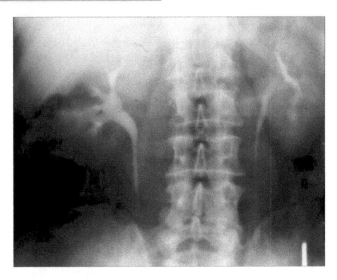

Figure 75.12   IVU showing irregular filling defect in left renal pelvis from TCC.

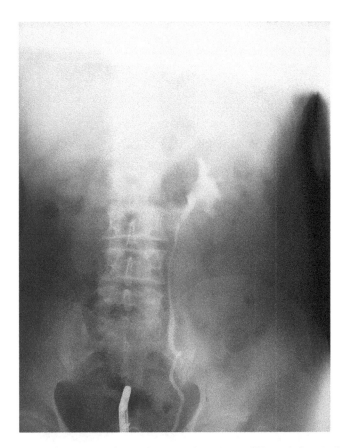

Figure 75.13   Left retrograde pyelogram showing a filling defect in left renal pelvis (same patient as in Figure 75.12).

7. J Transitional cell carcinoma (TCC) of the renal pelvis

This patient presents with haematuria and UTI with dull ache in her left loin – typical presenting features of a TCC. The presence of an irregular filling defect in the left renal pelvis on IVU (**Figure 75.12**) strongly supports the diagnosis, which is confirmed by a CT scan; urine is sent for cytology although a negative cytology has no significance. Further confirmation can be achieved by a retrograde pyelogram (**Figure 75.13**).

The treatment is cystoscopy followed by nephroureterectomy with excision of a cuff of the urinary bladder (**Figure 75.14**). The operation is done extraperitoneally with two separate incisions – one through the loin for approaching the kidney and another through a lower midline incision for the lower ureter. However, this can also be approached through an oblique abdominal extraperitoneal incision, the lower end being carried out through a transurethral resection ('pluck operation'). The procedure can also be done by laparoscopically.

8. I Trauma to kidney

This young boy has had a blunt injury to his left kidney, the cardinal feature of presentation being haematuria. He should be resuscitated with intravenous access and oxygen is administered through a mask, while his airway is expected to be normal. His kidney damage should be assessed by a limited IVU so as to minimise the radiation. The IVU (**Figure 75.15**) is primarily to make sure that the other kidney is normal while also showing the extent of damage and urinary extravasation. An US is done to see the size of the perirenal haematoma.

Treatment is conservative and expectant. Every time the patient passes urine, a specimen is saved and the time noted. This serial inspection of urine passed will determine if the haematuria is getting less. The vast majority settle down. A repeat US is done

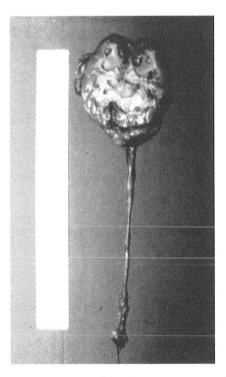

Figure 75.14   Specimen of nephroureterectomy for TCC (same patient as in Figures 75.12 and 75.13).

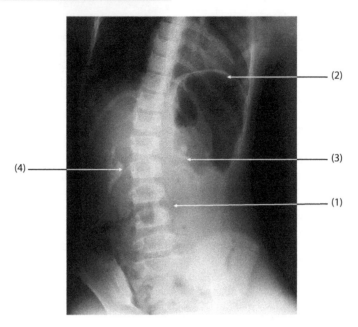

Figure 75.15 IVU in left renal trauma showing: (1) scoliosis with concavity to left from a perinephric haematoma (2) elevation of left dome of diaphragm (3) extravasation of contrast from left kidney (4) normal right kidney.

before discharge to make sure that the haematoma, which is naturally contained in the retroperitoneum is receding in size.

9. A Ureteric calculus

This patient has typical ureteric colic, which is one of the most painful conditions ever. He needs immediate analgesia with intravenous morphine, which is subsequently supplemented with diclofenac and indomethacin suppositories. Confirmation of the diagnosis is made by spiral CT scan. If this is not readily available, a limited IVU with delayed films will give the exact site and size of the stone. In the vast majority expectant treatment with analgesia suffices. If the stone is >5 mm, then surgical intervention will be required. The overall management is shown in **Figures 75.3a and b**.

10. H Wilms' tumour

This young boy has been brought by his parents with features of an abdominal mass. With a suspicion of a Wilms' tumour, one should look for absence of the iris (aniridia) and hemihypertrophy of the body – features that are sometimes associated with this condition. Haematuria is a sinister symptom as it denotes that the growth has invaded the renal pelvis.

Occurring in 1 in 10,000 this is the most common solid tumour in children and 85% of paediatric renal neoplasms. The tumour resembles normal foetal renal tissue and consists of undifferentiated blastema, immature stroma, and immature epithelial elements **(Figure 75.16)**.

An IVU will show irregular calyceal splaying within a soft tissue mass besides confirming a normal opposite kidney **(Figures 75.17a and b)**. The tumour can be bilateral in 5%. It is staged by CT scan and MRI (Stages 1 to 5). Management consists of chemotherapy, radiotherapy, and surgery, and must be managed in a paediatric oncology unit.

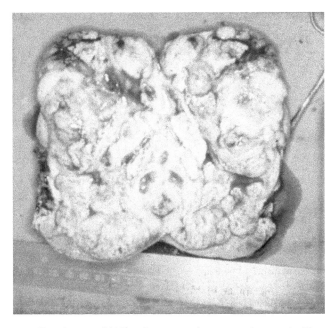

Figure 75.16 Specimen of Wilms' tumour (same patient as in Figure 75.17).

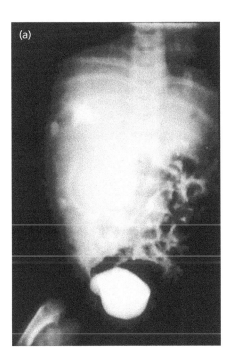

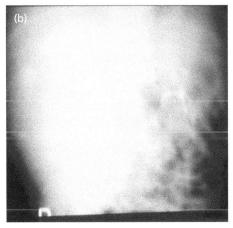

Figure 75.17 IVU (a) and nephrotomogram (b) showing large soft tissue shadow of right kidney with irregularity of calyces with displacement of intestines to the left and normal excretion of contrast from left kidney.

The urinary bladder

Pradip K Datta

Multiple choice questions

→ ## Anatomy

1. Which of the following statements are true?

A The bladder is lined by transitional epithelium.

B Hypertrophy of the detrusor muscle results in bladder trabeculation.

C The epithelium of the trigone extends into the lower ends of ureters and proximal urethra.

D The internal sphincter prevents urinary incontinence.

E The distal urethral sphincter is supplied by S2–S4 fibres via the pudendal nerves.

2. The following statements are true except:

A Pubovesical ligaments anchor the bladder neck to the pubis.

B The bladder is supplied to a minor extent by the obturator and inferior gluteal arteries.

C The principal lymphatic drainage is to the external iliac nodes.

D Parasympathetic fibres provide the main motor innervation.

E The sympathetic input is from L1 to L4 segments.

→ ## Bladder injury

3. Which of the following statements are true?

A Extraperitoneal rupture is more common than intraperitoneal rupture.

B Extraperitoneal rupture mimics rupture of membranous urethra.

C CT scan is the investigation of choice.

D Retrograde cystography is useful in making a diagnosis.

E Laparotomy is required in all cases of bladder rupture.

→ ## Retention of urine

4. In acute retention the following statements are true except:

A Bladder outlet obstruction is the most common cause in the male.

B Retroverted gravid uterus is a cause in the female.

C Non-urological conditions might cause acute retention.

D Suprapubic puncture should be done if urethral catheterisation fails.

E Once urine drains on passing the catheter, the balloon should be immediately inflated.

5. In chronic retention which of the following statements are true?

A The patient complains of very severe pain from his distended bladder.

B Diuresis might follow catheterisation.

C Spinal cord injury might result in acute neuropathic bladder.

D Intermittent self-catheterisation is a form of treatment for patients with spinal cord injury.

E Bladder dysfunction can occur after radical rectal excision.

→ ## Incontinence of urine

6. Which of the following statements is false?

A Urodynamic studies are essential in the investigation of urinary incontinence.

B In men with bladder outflow obstruction, 50% have detrusor instability.

C Genuine stress incontinence (GSI) is from increased true detrusor pressure.

D Vesicourethral fistula might be a cause in the female.

E Intravesical Botox injection has a role in treatment.

Bladder stones

7. Which of the following statements are true?

A Men are more often affected than women.

B An oxalate calculus develops in sterile urine.

C A cystine calculus is radio-opaque.

D Treatment is crushing with an optical lithotrite in all cases.

E In men with stones and outflow obstruction from enlarged prostate, both can be dealt with at the same time.

Bladder diverticula

8. Which of the following statements are true?

A They are diagnosed when they produce double micturition and repeated urinary tract infections.

B All bladder diverticula must be excised.

C Trabeculation and sacculation precede diverticula formation.

D The normal intravesical pressure during voiding is 35–50 cm H_2O.

E Haematuria is a symptom in 30%.

Urinary fistulae

9. Which of the following statements is not true?

A Most urinary fistulae are vesicovaginal.

B A combined ureterovaginal fistula might be present in 10% of patients.

C Examination under anaesthesia (EUA), intravenous urogram (IVU) and cystoscopy are necessary to evaluate them.

D When there are multiple tracts, the causes might be radiation, malignancy, or sepsis.

E Conservative management by catheter drainage of the bladder is usually successful in a post-hysterectomy fistula.

Lower urinary tract infection (UTI) and cystitis

10. Which of the following statements are true?

A The condition is more common in women.

B In recurrent infections, haematuria and rigors, cystoscopy and imaging are essential.

C Sterile pyuria is a sinister finding.

D In tuberculous cystitis, the route of infection is usually haematogenous or lymphogenous

E Carcinoma in situ might present as recurrent abacterial cystitis.

Carcinoma of the bladder

11. Which of the following statements are true?

A More than 90% of primary bladder cancers are transitional cell carcinomas.

B Painful haematuria is the most significant symptom.

C In newly diagnosed patients, 70% do not invade muscle.

D In a quarter of new patients, the muscle is invaded.

E Depth of invasion (T) in TNM classification and grade (WHO classification I, II, III) are important factors in planning treatment.

12. Which of the following investigations are routinely carried out?

A Urine cytology

B IVU and US

C Contrast-enhanced computed tomography (CECT) and MRI

D Bone scan

E Cystourethroscopy and bimanual examination

13. In the treatment of bladder cancers, which of the following statements are true?

A Non-muscle invasive (superficial) tumours are treated by endoscopic resection and a single dose of mitomycin instillation.

B Grade 3 superficial disease is best managed by BCG immunotherapy.

C External beam radiotherapy should be the first-line treatment in muscle-invasive disease.

D When the cancer has invaded muscle (pT2 and pT3) radical cystectomy and lymphadenectomy is the treatment of choice.

E Neoadjuvant cisplatin-based chemotherapy improves survival in muscle-invasive tumours.

Extended matching questions

→ Diagnose

1 Bladder calculus
2 Bladder carcinoma
3 Bladder diverticulum
4 Schistosomiasis of bladder
5 Tuberculosis of the bladder

→ Clinical scenarios

Match the diagnoses with the clinical scenarios that follow:

A A 35-year-old male, a recent visitor from Egypt, attended the emergency department with painless terminal haematuria. He had a few similar episodes while at home in Egypt. Clinical examination revealed no abnormality. On flexible cystoscopy at the one-stop haematuria clinic, he was found to have scattered tubercles and islands of pale patches resembling sand.

B A 70-year-old male, a heavy smoker for more than 50 years, complains of painless, profuse and periodic haematuria for 6 weeks. The blood is uniformly mixed with the urine. He has frequency of micturition and some retropubic discomfort. Clinical examination reveals no abnormality.

C A 70-year-old male complains of poor micturition stream, post-micturition dribbling and a feeling of insufficient emptying of his bladder. He has some dysuria. On occasions he has found that shortly after micturition he again passes a large amount of urine. Clinical examination reveals no abnormality.

D A 60-year-old man complains of haematuria and painful micturition, and he occasionally finds that his micturition stream suddenly stops. He has learned to re-start his stream by changing position. Clinical examination reveals no abnormality.

E A 35-year-old female patient, a recent visitor from the Indian subcontinent, complains of frequency of micturition and bilateral loin discomfort. She has evening pyrexia, general malaise and weight loss. Clinical examination reveals no abnormality. Urine examination carried out by her doctor shows sterile pyuria.

Answers to multiple choice questions

1. A, B, C, E

The bladder is lined by transitional epithelium as is the entire urinary tract, extending from the renal pelvis down to the distal urethra (in the male), to the tip of the glans, called the navicular fossa, where the lining is stratified squamous epithelium. In the female the transitional epithelium extends down until the proximal two-thirds of the urethra. The epithelium of the trigone does extend proximally to lower ends of ureters and distally down to the proximal urethra.

Hypertrophy of the detrusor muscle results in trabeculation of the bladder, the outcome of bladder outflow obstruction. Trabeculation later leads to sacculation and diverticula formation. The distal urethral sphincter is supplied by the S2–S4 fibres via the pudendal nerves. The internal sphincter is the smooth muscle around the male bladder neck, which prevents retrograde ejaculation and has no role in urinary continence.

2. E

The sympathetic input is from the T10 to L2 segments passing via the presacral hypogastric nerves to the inferior hypogastric plexus. They convey afferents from the fundus responding to touch, temperature, pain and stretch information. The parasympathetic fibres derived from the S2 to S4 are the pelvic splanchnic nerves, which are motor helping to empty the bladder. Aspects of micturition are controlled centrally in the pons where detrusor activity is coordinated.

Mean bladder capacity is about 400 mL although micturition occurs at smaller volumes; up to 500 mL of urine within the bladder might be tolerated but beyond that pain results in urgency.

The pubovesical ligaments are stout bands of fibromuscular tissue extending from the bladder neck to the lower part of the pubic bones. They constitute the pubouretheral ligaments in the female and puboprostatic ligaments in the male. The bladder derives its blood supply to a minor extent from the obturator and inferior gluteal arteries, while its principal blood supply comes from the anterior branch of the internal iliac arteries through the superior and inferior vesical arteries. The lymphatic drainage is mainly to the external iliac and obturator lymph nodes.

3. A, B, C, D

Extraperitoneal rupture is much more common, occurring in about 80%. The causes are usually blunt trauma or iatrogenic injury, the latter occurring during inguinal hernia repair, hysterectomy, or operations on the rectosigmoid. This can mimic rupture of membranous urethra, particularly when it is associated with fracture pelvis. Intraperitoneal rupture occurs in a distended bladder when the patient, due to inebriation, is unaware of a full bladder and sustains blunt lower abdominal injury usually from an assault.

The ideal imaging is a CT scan although retrograde cystogram will also give the diagnosis **(Figure 76.1)**.

A laparotomy is not necessary in all cases of bladder rupture. Laparotomy is the treatment in intraperitoneal rupture. Here the torn edges are freshened, the rent closed with interrupted absorbable sutures and a urethral catheter left for about 10 days. In extraperitoneal injury, suprapubic or urethral drainage of the bladder for 10 days under antibiotic cover is the treatment.

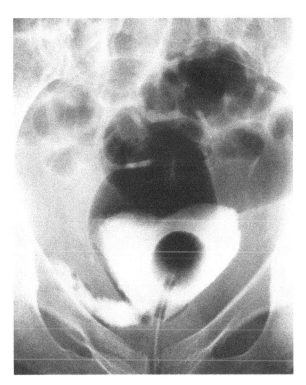

Figure 76.1 Retrograde cystogram showing extraperitoneal rupture of bladder.

4. E

Once the catheter has been successfully passed as evidenced by the passage of urine, the balloon should not be immediately inflated. The catheter should be further pushed into the bladder before the balloon is inflated to prevent the balloon being inflated within the prostatic urethra.

In the male the most common cause for acute urinary retention is bladder outlet obstruction, the causes of which might be benign prostatic hypertrophy (BPH) or carcinoma of the prostate. Patients who suffer from lower urinary tract symptoms (LUTS) might go into acute retention under the following circumstances: not able to void when necessary due to social reasons, having had too much alcohol and having had certain drugs such as diuretics, antihistamines, anti-cholinergics and tricyclic antidepressants.

In the female a retroverted gravid uterus might result in acute retention. Besides, there are non-urological conditions that might cause acute retention. This might be the first sign of certain neurological conditions such a spinal cord compression or multiple sclerosis; bladder or urethral calculus, acute perianal conditions, faecal impaction and following spinal anaesthesia.

5. B, C, D, E

Once a patient with chronic retention is catheterised, he develops post-obstructive diuresis and might go into hypovolaemic shock. The patient should be closely monitored and volume loss is combated by intravenous normal saline. The patient will have bilateral hydronephrosis and hydroureter and require urgent urological management. Occasionally relief of the chronic retention might result in haematuria, because the distended urinary tract is decompressed. Once catheterised the catheter is connected to a closed drainage system and the patient started on prophylactic antibiotics.

Spinal-cord injury produces spinal shock. This results in the inability of the detrusor to contract, resulting in bladder distension with overflow incontinence. This is treated by intermittent catheterisation and full urodynamic assessment undertaken once the patient is stable in a few weeks hence. The long-term aim would be to promote good bladder emptying to prevent upper-tract damage. One of the methods of achieving this is clean intermittent self-catheterisation (CISC). Those with poor emptying and low-bladder capacity might benefit from endoscopic sphincterotomy and condom drainage.

Up to 15% of patients undergoing anterior resection or abdomino-perineal resection for cancer might fail to pass urine after removal of the urinary catheter. This is due to neurogenic bladder dysfunction from damage to inferior hypogastric plexus of nerves. The treatment is catheterisation, followed by thorough urodynamic investigation once the patient has fully recovered from the original operation.

Patients with chronic urinary retention never have pain, so much so that the majority are unaware of the problem. Others might have incontinence due to retention with overflow.

6. C

When there is increased intra-abdominal pressure as in coughing, sneezing and laughing, pressure within the urinary bladder is increased. This causes urinary leakage and is referred to as genuine stress incontinence. This is not due to true detrusor pressure.

Incontinence of urine is a major part of lower urinary tract dysfunction. Urodynamic testing needs to be carried out in most of these patients and is essential in all patients who might proceed to an operation. In this investigation bladder filling and emptying is artificially simulated while measuring the pressure and taking tracings. In men, half the patients who have bladder outflow obstruction, detrusor instability is present. In men the normal voiding pressure should be less than 60 cm of H_2O and less than 40 cm H_2O in women with a flow rate of 20–25 mL/sec.

In certain parts of the world, due to neglected and difficult labour, vesicourethral fistula is a cause of incontinence and managing such a patient is extremely challenging. Various modalities of treatment are available – drugs, physiotherapy, surgical procedures and insertion of artificial urinary sphincter. Intravesical injection of Botox has had a limited success and is useful in postponing major surgery.

7. A, B, C, E

Bladder stones occur eight times more often in men. A primary bladder calculus is one that develops in sterile urine and an oxalate calculus is one of them. It grows slowly, is of moderate size and is solitary with an uneven surface. Although calcium oxalate is white, the stone is often dark-brown or black because it is impregnated with blood pigment. A cystine calculus occurs in cystinuria and is radio-opaque because of its high sulphur content. A triple phosphate calculus is composed of ammonium, calcium and magnesium phosphate and might occur around a foreign body **(Figure 76.2)**.

When a stone occurs in a male patient due to stasis from bladder outflow obstruction from an enlarged prostate, both the cause and the effect can be treated at the same time. An open prostatectomy can be carried out; during the procedure the stone is also removed. Obviously the condition can also be treated by minimal access surgery by the transurethral route.

While most bladder stones can be treated by minimal-access surgery by litholapaxy using an optical lithotrite, the procedure is contraindicated in patients below 10 years for fear of damaging the urethra and causing a stricture.

8. C, D, E

As a result of long-standing obstruction there is a rise in intra-vesical pressure, which might go up to 150 cm of H_2O (normal voiding pressure is 35–50 cm H_2O). This initially causes hypertrophy of the bladder musculature, resulting in trabeculation; as the pressure continues, this causes the inner layer of the hypertrophied muscle to protrude causing sacculation. Ultimately, a diverticula (consisting of only the mucosa) forms at the site of maximum weakness, which is the ureteric orifice **(Figure 76.3)**.

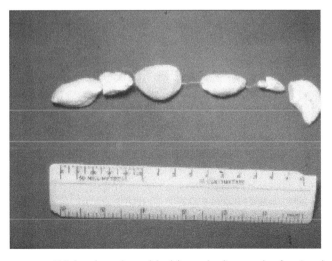

Figure 76.2 Triple phosphate bladder calculi round a foreign body (piece of nylon).

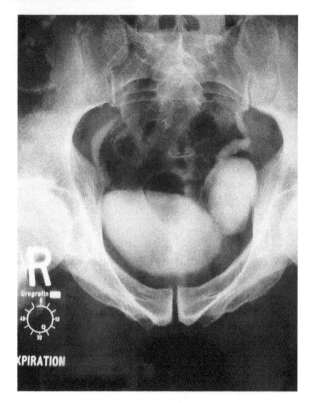

Figure 76.3 IVU showing left-sided bladder diverticulum.

Most often a diverticulum is an incidental finding found on imaging or cystoscopy. It produces symptoms of UTI and associated bladder outflow obstruction; haematuria occurs in 30% due to a stone, tumour, or infection within the diverticulum. The majority of them do not need any treatment. Transurethral resection of the prostate is carried out to treat the bladder outflow obstruction. The diverticulum is excised only if it has created any complications such as stone, tumour or recurrent infections.

9. E
Conservative management of a vesicovaginal fistula by urethral bladder drainage is rarely successful in a fistula following hysterectomy. Most urinary fistula are vesicovaginal and the result of prolonged or neglected labour – the result of ischaemic necrosis of the bladder from prolonged pressure of the foetal head in obstructed labour. In one in 10 patients there might be an associated ureterovaginal fistula.

Thorough evaluation is necessary for successful management. The diagnosis is established by the 'three swab test', EUA (examination under anaesthesia), vaginoscopy, cystoscopy, IVU and, sometimes, retrograde pyelography.

When there are multiple fistulous tracks the situation is quite complex and the cause can be malignancy, post-radiation, or sepsis. An intractable fistula indicates distal obstruction, chronic infection such as TB, a foreign body such as a stone, or non-absorbable sutures. A combined team effort between the gynaecologist and urologist yields the best outcome, the principles of surgery being good exposure, excision of diseased tissue and tension-free anatomical repair with good blood supply.

10. A, B, C, E

Lower UTIs are much more common in women. They are usually associated with pyelonephritis and present with loin pain, fever, rigors and malaise, and might present with septicaemia. Recurrent infection in both sexes should be treated promptly with empirical antibiotics and thoroughly investigated with urine microscopy, IVU, US, CT scan and a cystoscopy, the latter being mandatory in haematuria. Urodynamic studies should be initiated in incomplete emptying.

Predisposing causes are bladder outflow obstruction, neurogenic bladder dysfunction, stones, neoplasm, vesico-ureteric reflux and immunosuppression. Carcinoma in situ of the urinary bladder might often present as abacterial cystitis – hence the importance of cystoscopy. Sterile pyuria should always be looked upon as sinister as it is a feature of genitourinary TB.

Tuberculous cystitis is secondary to renal tuberculosis and not due to haematogenous or lymphogenous spread. Therefore, changes commence around the ureteric orifices and trigone in the form of pallor of the mucosa and submucosal oedema with tubercles appearing subsequently. Fibrosis causes the ureteric orifices to be indrawn and hence called 'golf-hole' ureter; the bladder is small and contracted and referred to as 'thimble' bladder, also the result of fibrosis.

11. A, C, D, E

More than 90% of primary bladder cancers are urothelial in origin being transitional cell cancers. Squamous cancers account for about 5%, although this is higher in countries where bilharzia is endemic. Adenocarcinoma occurs in 1% to 2% arising from the urachal remnant or from glandular metaplasia.

When new patients are diagnosed 70% do not invade the muscle and are hence pTa and pT1 tumours. In 25% of new patients, muscle-invasive disease pT2 is seen. In 5% carcinoma in situ (CIS) is seen as a flat noninvasive lesion. In planning treatment, accurate staging of the tumour is paramount. Depth of invasion (T) in TNM classification and WHO classification (grade I, II, III) are important in planning treatment and determining prognosis.

In the clinical presentation, bladder cancers classically produce painless, profuse, progressive and periodic haematuria; pain is conspicuous by its absence. If haematuria is painful in bladder cancer it denotes extravesical spread.

12. A, B, C, E

Urine cytology is only useful when positive; such a result is very specific and is particularly useful in high-grade disease and CIS. A negative result has no significance. Thorough urinary tract assessment is mandatory. IVU, still carried out in many centres, is fast becoming an obsolete investigation, being replaced by CECT and MRI. US will help in delineating irregularity of the bladder wall, hydronephrosis and show obstructive uropathy. Muscle invasion and lymph node metastasis are better demonstrated by cross-sectional MRI.

Cystourethroscopy supplemented by bimanual palpation and EUA is the keystone in the assessment. This manoeuvre should be carried out with the bladder empty before and after endoscopic resection of the tumour. It is bimanual palpability that will differentiate between a pT2 and pT3 tumour, the latter being palpable. Invasion into the prostate or vagina is pT4a and when fixed is pT4b. Bone scan, not a routine investigation, is carried out only if there is a strong suspicion of skeletal spread.

13. A, B, D, E

Non-muscle invasive tumours are treated by endoscopic resection. A single dose of intravesical mitomycin decreases the risk of recurrence in pTa and pT1 grade 1 and 2 disease. In patients with high-grade pT1 tumour, when multiple or accompanied by CIS, immediate cystectomy is offered by some; others would treat the condition with endoscopic resection with BCG immunotherapy.

In muscle-invasive tumours, the treatment is debatable. Primary surgical treatment in the form of radical cystectomy and pelvic lymphadenectomy is regarded as the standard treatment. Preoperative systemic chemotherapy with a combination of cisplatin, methotrexate, doxorubicin and vinblastine has been shown to be beneficial. External-beam radiotherapy is not regarded as the best first-line treatment for muscle-invasive tumours, as some patients do not respond, others respond partially, whilst some others have very troublesome side effects. It is to be considered as an option in those who decline or are unfit for surgery.

Answers to extended matching questions

1. D Bladder calculus

Most bladder calculi are mixed. A primary calculus is one that develops in sterile urine such as an oxalate calculus. This is usually solitary, spiky and dark brown in colour as the white calcium oxalate is incorporated with blood pigment. A triple phosphate calculus, dirty white and chalky, is one that is composed of ammonium, magnesium and calcium and grows in urine infected with urea-splitting organisms. When there is a large intravesical prostate, urine stagnates in the retroprostatic pouch; infection supervenes and silent stones tend to form. It might also occur around a foreign body (**Figure 76.2**, see previously).

The incidence between the sexes is M:F 8:1. Pain in the form of strangury, dysuria, haematuria and sudden cessation of the urinary stream are the presenting features. Young boys pull on the prepuce or penis during micturition screaming with pain, a typical symptom of bladder calculus. When lodged within a bladder diverticulum, a stone is usually silent. A plain x-ray (**Figure 76.4**) followed by cystoscopy confirms the diagnosis.

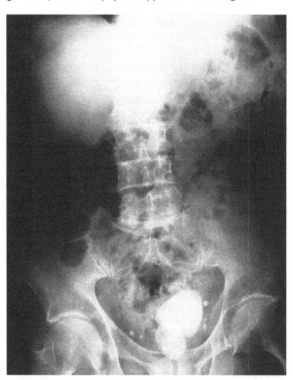

Figure 76.4   Plain x-ray showing large bladder stone.

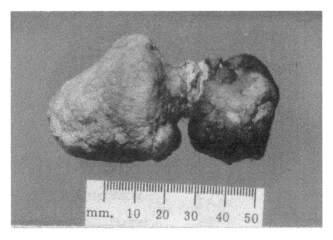

Figure 76.5 Large bladder stone treated by open cystolithotomy (same patient as in Figure 76.4).

Treatment is by litholapaxy using an optical lithotrite. A very large stone **(Figure 76.5)** is ideally removed by suprapubic cystolithotomy, a procedure that takes a few minutes under general anaesthetic compared to minimal access surgical techniques.

2. B Bladder carcinoma

Carcinoma of the bladder is the fourth most common non-dermatological malignancy in men who are affected three times more than women. Smoking is the principal cause although exposure to urothelial carcinogens of a chemical nature might occur as an occupational hazard. Painless, progressive, profuse and periodic haematuria is the classical presentation and physical signs are few except for anaemia. The diagnosis is made by cystoscopy in a one-stop haematuria clinic.

Once diagnosed the patient should be accurately staged by CECT, MRI, US and IVU followed by cystourethroscopy and EUA with bimanual palpation, the latter also carried out after endoscopic resection. Management depends upon staging. An IVU **(Figure 76.6)** might be particularly useful when there is obstruction to a ureter with hydronephrosis and hydroureter. When bladder cancer is first diagnosed, 70% will be non-muscle invasive tumours (pTa and pT1), 25% will be muscle invasive (pT2 or pT3) while 5% will be CIS. Histologically more than 90% are TCC.

Transurethral resection of bladder tumour (TURBT) is the treatment in pTa and pT1 tumours with a dose of mitomycin instillation. Treatment of muscle-invasive disease (pT2 and pT3) is debatable. TURBT is one choice; the other is radical cystectomy and pelvic lymphadenectomy. Those undergoing TURBT are kept under regular cystoscopic surveillance. In advanced cases such as pT4a or pT4b external-beam radiotherapy is the option.

3. C Bladder diverticulum

This is the outcome of bladder outflow obstruction (BOO). In the vast majority of patients, the symptoms are related to BOO and the diverticulum happens to be an incidental finding seen on cystoscopy or US. Trabeculation and sacculation precede the formation of a diverticulum. They arise next to the ureter (para-ureteric), the site of maximum weakness. Rarely a large diverticulum might cause ureteric obstruction from peridiverticular inflammation.

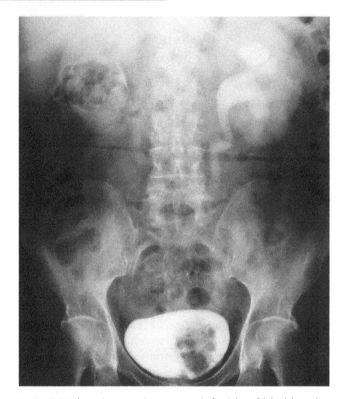

Figure 76.6   IVU showing carcinoma on left side of bladder obstructing left ureter.

In the majority these do not require any treatment. Tending to the BOO by transurtheral resection of the prostate (TURP) is all that is necessary. However, prior to doing a TURP, it is prudent to visualise the inside of the diverticulum to make sure that there is no pathology inside such as an unsuspected stone or cancer. The diverticulum needs to be excised if there are complications such as stone formation, tumour or persistent infection. Excision is carried out by the open procedure of intra and extravesical diverticulectomy after cannulating the ureter on the affected site to safeguard it from injury or instantly recognise any injury that might occur inadvertently.

4. A Schistosomiasis

The condition is endemic in parts of the Middle East. It is caused by the trematode *Schistosoma haematobium*. The snail is the intermediate host for this parasite, which penetrates the human skin, while man, the definitive host, bathes in infected freshwater. The male and female worms, having attained sexual maturity in the liver, leave the hepatic circulation through the portosystemic anastomoses to enter the systemic circulation, where they have an affinity for the vesical venous circulation ultimately entering the urinary bladder.

After the incubation period of 4 to 12 weeks patients might develop high evening temperature, sweating and asthma-like attacks. After several months of quiescence, patients develop intermittent, painless, terminal haematuria. There is eosinophilia. An early-morning specimen of the patient's urine is used to perform the ELISA test (enzyme-linked immunoabsorbent assay) using *Schistosoma masnsoni* microsomal antigen. A positive test is specific.

A high index of suspicion helps in making the diagnosis, which is confirmed by cystoscopy. The findings on cystoscopy depend on the stage of the disease. From the earliest to the most advanced the appearances are pseudotubercles, nodules, 'sandy patches', ulceration, fibrosis, granulomas and papillomas. In very late cases the end result might be a squamous carcinoma, bladder and bladder neck fibrosis and urethral strictures. Drug treatment in the form of a course of praziquantel is effective in the early stages.

5. E Tuberculosis

This condition is still rife in developing countries. The infection spreads from the kidneys. The patient might also have pulmonary TB. Clinical features of weight loss, malaise, evening rise of temperature, dysuria, urinary frequency and painless haematuria might be present. Sterile pyuria is a typical finding on urine examination. Early morning urine (EMU) specimen should be sent for culture, which might take several weeks to obtain an answer.

Cystoscopic findings are typical. Tubercles might be seen in early stages; undermined ulcer, a small contracted bladder and 'golf-hole' ureteric orifices due to fibrosis may be the other findings. The patient is treated with anti-tuberculous chemotherapy. Depending upon the extent of the disease, the patient might require nephro-ureterectomy. A permanently contracted bladder ('thimble' bladder) will require bladder augmentation procedures such as ileocystoplasty or caecocystoplasty.

The prostate and seminal vesicles

Pradip K Datta

Multiple choice questions

→ Anatomy and physiology

1. The following statements are true except:

A The prostate is anatomically divided into a peripheral zone, a central zone and a transitional zone.

B The glands of the peripheral zone are lined by transitional epithelium.

C Benign prostatic hypertrophy occurs in the transitional zone.

D Most carcinomas arise in the peripheral zone.

E Denonvilliers' fascia separates the prostate from the rectum.

2. Which of the following statements are true?

A Luteinising hormone (LH) from the anterior pituitary controls the secretion of testosterone.

B Leydig cells from the testes secrete 90% of the testosterone.

C The enzyme 5α-reductase type II is found in high concentration in the prostate.

D 5α-reductase converts testosterone into 1.5-dihydrotestosterone (DHT).

E Prostate-specific antigen (PSA) is both specific and sensitive in the diagnosis of prostate cancer.

→ Benign prostatic hyperplasia (BPH)

3. Which of the following statements are true?

A It is the most common cause of bladder outflow obstruction (BOO) in men >70 years of age.

B Decrease in serum testosterone levels and therefore relative increase in serum oestrogens cause BPH.

C The condition affects the transitional zone and the central zone.

D All lower urinary tract symptoms (LUTS) in men >70 years are due to BPH.

E The prostatic urethra is elongated in BPH.

4. In urodynamic studies, which of the following statements are true?

A A voided volume >200 mL with a peak flow rate >15 mL/s is normal.

B A voiding pressure of <60 cm H_2O is normal.

C Increase in voiding pressures with a low flow rate is diagnostic of BOO.

D In patients with a residual volume of 250 mL or more, bilateral hydronephrosis will result.

E Urodynamically proven BOO only occurs from BPH.

5. In assessing LUTS in men, which of the following statements are false?

A Charting a patient's symptoms according to the International Prostate Symptom Score (IPSS) is routinely used.

B Flow-rate measurement studies and pressure-flow urodynamic studies are done.

C Thorough nervous system examination is mandatory.

D The upper urinary tract should always be imaged.

E Cystourethroscopy is a good guide as an indication for surgery.

→ Management of BPH causing BOO

6. Which of the following statements are true?

A All patients with acute retention ultimately require prostatectomy.

B Chronic retention accounts for 15% of prostatectomies.

C Severe symptoms account for 60% of prostatectomies.

D Drug therapy is with α-blockers and/or 5α-reductase inhibitor.

E A low maximum flow rate of <10 mL/s and a residual volume of 100–250 mL are indications for surgery.

7. The following statements are true except:

A α-adrenergic blocking agents inhibit the contraction of prostatic smooth muscle.

B 5α-reductase inhibitors inhibit the conversion of testosterone to DHT.

C Drug therapy results in 20% improvement in symptom scores.

D Transurethral resection of the prostate (TURP) results in 75% improvement in the symptom scores.

E Retrograde ejaculation occurs in all patients after TURP.

→ Carcinoma of the prostate

8. Which of the following statements are true in carcinoma of the prostate?

A It is the most common cancer in men over the age of 65 years.

B In the younger age group who develop prostate cancer, 10%–15% have a positive family history.

C A patient who has had a prostatectomy for BPH can develop prostate cancer.

D Carcinoma mostly originates in the peripheral zone of the prostate.

E Prostate-specific antigen (PSA) is an extremely reliable method of screening.

9. The following statements are true except:

A The histological type is an adenocarcinoma.

B Gleason scoring system is based on the degree of glandular differentiation.

C The Gleason score correlates well with spread and prognosis.

D Prostate is the most common site of origin for skeletal metastasis.

E Skeletal metastases from prostate cancer are mostly osteolytic.

10. On rectal examination, which of the following features does not suggest carcinoma?

A Nodules within the prostate.

B Obliteration of the median sulcus.

C Irregular stony hard induration.

D Mobile rectal mucosa over the prostate.

E Extension of a hard nodule beyond the capsule into the bladder base.

11. In the assessment of prostate cancer which of the following investigations are necessary?

A Transrectal ultrasound-guided biopsy (TRUS)

B Cross-sectional MRI

C Bone scan

D General blood tests, PSA and liver function tests

E IVU

12. Regarding treatment, the following statements are true except:

A Radical prostatectomy is only suitable for T1 and T2 disease (early cancer).

B Radical external-beam radiotherapy is an alternative to radical prostatectomy.

C T3 patients are treated by surgery, radical radiotherapy, or androgen ablation.

D Incidentally diagnosed disease is treated by radical prostatectomy.

E The incidence of severe stress incontinence after radical prostatectomy is about 2%.

Extended matching questions

→ ## Diagnoses

1 Acute prostatitis
2 Acute retention of urine
3 Benign prostatic hypertrophy (BPH) causing BOO
4 Carcinoma of prostate
5 Chronic urinary retention with overflow

→ ## Clinical scenarios

Match the diagnoses with the clinical scenarios that follow:

A A 40-year-old man complains of feeling ill with pyrexia of 39°C, rigors with aches all over his body, and flu-like symptoms in general. He has rectal irritation, pain on defecation and perineal discomfort. He has pain on micturition and passes threads in his urine. Rectal examination reveals a tender, swollen prostate.

B A 70-year-old man complains of poor stream, frequency of micturition both in the day and at night, hesitancy and intermittent stream, a feeling of incomplete emptying and terminal haematuria for about 4 months; recently he has had backache. Clinical examination shows no abnormality. On rectal examination he has a hard, nodular prostate with overlying fixed rectal mucosa.

C A 72-year-old man has come to the emergency department with severe acute pain in his lower abdomen not having passed urine for almost 10 hours. He has been on some medicines, which he bought across the counter for cold and flu. This has also made him constipated. On examination he is in severe pain from a large mass in his suprapubic region arising from the pelvis. The mass is dull to percussion.

D A 70-year-old man complains of urgency, frequency and hesitancy of micturition with a feeling of incomplete emptying. He also has poor flow, intermittent stream and post-micturition dribbling. These symptoms have been going on for 2 years and are gradually getting worse. Clinical examination reveals no abnormality. On rectal examination he has an enlarged smooth prostate with overlying mobile rectal mucosa, and the median vertical groove is easily felt.

E A 75-year-old male complains of general malaise, lethargy, abdominal distension and urinary incontinence. On examination he has a large painless mass in his suprapubic region arising from the pelvis and has continuous urinary dribbling. The mass is dull on percussion. He is a type 2 diabetic on oral medication.

Answers to multiple choice questions

→ ## Anatomy and physiology

1. B

The glands of the peripheral zone are not lined by transitional epithelium but by columnar epithelium. It is the peripheral zone that is the site where cancer originates and hence prostate carcinomas are adenocarcinomas. In the past, the prostate was described as divided into lobes. Now the prostate gland is considered to consist of a peripheral zone (PZ, 70% of the glandular substance), central zone (CZ, 25%) and transitional zone (TZ, 5%). The CZ is wedge-shaped, forming the base of the gland with its apex at the verumontanum, and surrounds the ejaculatory ducts. The verumontanum is an important anatomical landmark; in transurethral resection of the prostate (TURP) all resection must be confined proximal to the verumontanum to prevent incontinence. The TZ lies around the distal part of the pre-prostatic urethra proximal to the apex of the central zone.

The zonal anatomy is clinically important in that most cancers arise from the PZ and benign prostatic hypertrophy (BPH) affects the TZ. The CZ is rarely involved in any disease process. MRI in T2-weighted images can distinguish the zonal anatomy. The PZ and verumontanum have high-signal intensity (looking intensely white), while the CZ and TZ have low signal (looking grey). The rectovesical fascia of Denonvillier's separates the posterior surface of the gland covered by the capsule, bladder base and seminal vesicles from the rectum anteriorly.

2. A, B, C, D
Testosterone is the main hormone acting on the prostate. This hormone (90%) is secreted by the Leydig cells of the testes under the control of the luteinising hormone (LH) of the anterior pituitary. LH is under the control of hypothalamic luteinising hormone-releasing hormone (LHRH). The use of LHRH analogues forms the physiological basis of androgen-deprivation therapy in prostate cancer. The enzyme 5α-reductase type II is found abundantly in the prostate. This enzyme converts testosterone into 1,5-dihydrotestosterone (DHT), which is five times as potent as testosterone. The adrenals contribute 5% to 10% of the testosterone output.

Prostate specific antigen (PSA) is neither specific nor sensitive in diagnosing prostate cancer. Although normal values might vary a little in different laboratories, a value of <3 ng/mL is regarded as normal. Both BPH and prostate cancer might show a PSA in the range of 3 to 15 ng/mL. Almost 25% of men with a PSA of 4–10 ng/mL have prostate cancer (hence not very specific) whilst 15%–20% of men with a prostate cancer have a PSA of 1 to 4 ng/mL (hence not very sensitive). In general, men aged 50–69 years with a PSA of >3 ng/mL would be advised to undergo a prostatic biopsy, although the threshold would be lower in the younger age group with a strong family history of prostate cancer.

Benign prostatic hyperplasia (BPH)
3. A, B, C, E
BPH is the most common cause of BOO in men >70 years of age. It is a condition that occurs in men over the age of 50 years; 50% of those >60 years will have histological evidence of BPH. It affects the submucous group of glands and connective-tissue stroma in the TZ; this forms a nodular enlargement which, as it grows, compresses the PZ into a false capsule giving rise to the 'lateral lobes'. When the condition affects the CZ glands (rarely), a 'middle lobe' forms. When BPH affects two lateral lobes and a middle lobe, an intravesical 'prostatic collar' forms. With advancing age there is an unequal reduction in the serum testosterone compared with oestrogen levels; thus BPH occurs from increased effects of oestrogen.

Anatomically, as the lateral lobes enlarge, the prostatic urethra elongates – the larger the lobes the longer the urethra becomes with exaggeration of the posterior curve. If only one lateral lobe enlarges, distortion of the urethra occurs. In clinical practice this might result in difficulty in passing a Foley catheter should the patient present with acute urinary retention. In that case a curved (*coudé*) catheter might have to be used.

All lower urinary tract symptoms (LUTS) in men over the age of 70 years are not always the result of BPH causing BOO. The other conditions that can give rise to LUTS are idiopathic detrusor overactivity or instability, neuropathic bladder and degeneration of bladder smooth muscle with impaired voiding.

4. A, B, C, D
In urodynamic studies a decrease in urinary flow rates is a feature of BPH. For a voided volume of 200 mL or more with a peak flow rate of more than 15 mL/second is normal. A flow of 10–15 mL/second is equivocal and one of < 10mL/second is low. Decreased flow rate is caused by BOO, urethral stricture, or a weak detrusor. Increase in voiding pressures is a feature of BOO. Pressures of <60 cm H_2O are normal; a pressure of >80 cm H_2O is high, and anything in between is equivocal. Increase in voiding pressure with a low flow rate is diagnostic of BOO.

Chronic retention is one of the complications of BOO. As a result of inefficient bladder emptying, over a period, urine tends to stagnate in the bladder producing residual urine. If this amount reaches 250 mL, high-pressure chronic retention results; this causes back pressure to the upper urinary tract with bilateral hydronephrosis. Urodynamically proven BOO not only occurs from BPH but also from bladder neck stenosis, bladder neck hypertrophy, prostate cancer, urethral stricture and neuropathic bladder.

5. D, E

In patients with routine symptoms of BPH, the upper urinary tract does not need to be imaged unless infection or haematuria is present. In that case, the upper tract is imaged by US or IVU. Cystourethroscopy is not a good guide as to the indication for surgical intervention. The decision whether to perform prostatectomy is based on the patient's symptoms, signs and investigations. Cystourethroscopy, however, is mandatory immediately prior to a prostatectomy, either open or transurethrally, to make sure there is no incidental intravesical pathology. It also provides information on the size of the intravesical prostate, length of the prostatic urethra and presence of trabeculation, sacculation or unsuspected diverticula.

In assessing men with LUTS, the IPSS score and a frequency-volume diary from the patient is very important before the patient attends the clinic to complement clinical examination and relevant investigations. These should include flow-rate measurement studies and pressure-flow urodynamic studies. Transrectal US scanning is not routine unless, on rectal examination, a carcinoma is suspected. Some surgeons do this investigation, nevertheless, for accurate assessment of the size of the prostatic adenoma.

Comprehensive assessment of BPH or BOO should include abdominal and rectal examination and neurological examination to exclude multiple sclerosis, Parkinson's disease and spinal-cord compression. Investigations such as serum PSA, serum biochemistry, full blood count and urine culture are done besides urodynamic studies. The importance of thorough assessment prior to surgery cannot be overstated because surgical treatment in the wrong patient will make the patient worse.

→ Management of BPH causing BOO

6. B, C, D, E

Chronic retention accounts for 15% of prostatectomies. These patients with a residual urine of >200 mL have a degree of renal impairment with features of back pressure. Once the renal impairment has been stabilised and the diagnosis confirmed, prostatectomy is carried out. Severe symptoms, as seen from a high IPSS score in the form of poor stream, hesitancy, marked frequency and a feeling of insufficient evacuation, are strong indications for surgery. A maximum flow rate of <10 mL/second and an increasing residual volume (100–250 mL) as seen on repeated US strengthens the case for surgery. Such a picture accounts for 60% of prostatectomies.

A period of drug treatment with α-blockers with a combination of α-reductase inhibitors (in those with an adenoma of >50 g), taken for a period of 6 months or so is worthwhile after full discussion between the patient and urologist. Only 25% of fit male patients with acute retention, where no cause for the retention has been found (e.g., constipation, drugs, recent operation) need a prostatectomy. In some patients after initial catheterisation, drug therapy is used for a while followed by trial without catheter. Such management is sometimes successful. The same is true of patients with chronic retention of urine, provided renal function has been stabilised by catheterisation.

7. E

Retrograde ejaculation causing spermaturia occurs in about 65% of patients after prostatectomy because of damage to the internal sphincter, causing disruption of the bladder neck mechanism. This is important to mention when counselling men for TURP.

The following two types of drugs are available: α-adrenergic-blocking agents that inhibit the contraction of smooth muscle in the prostate and 5α-reductase inhibitors that inhibit the conversion of testosterone to DHT (the most active form of androgen). α-blockers are more quick-acting, while the 5α-reductase inhibitors need to be taken for a longer period, have fewer side effects and work better in patients with glands >50 g. Drug therapy over 1 year produces a 25% shrinkage of the prostate gland. Drugs result in 20% improvement in symptom scores, while TURP results in 75% improvement.

Carcinoma of the prostate

8. A, B, C, D

Carcinoma of the prostate is the most common cancer in men over the age of 65 years. When serial histological sections of the prostate gland is performed at routine autopsy, foci of cancer can be found although their progression to metastatic disease is uncertain. When prostate cancer occurs in younger men, 10%–15% have a family history.

At the operation of prostatectomy for BPH, the prostatic adenoma is removed. This arises from the TZ of the prostate whereas cancer arises from the PZ. Therefore after the operation of 'prostatectomy' for BPH, there is no immunity toward carcinoma of the prostate that can therefore occur.

PSA is not a reliable method of screening for prostate cancer. There is no consensus about its use as a screening procedure. Detection of cancer using PSA is 2%–4%. About 30% of men with a raised PSA will have proven prostate cancer. A normal PSA will be found in 20% of men with proven prostate cancer. Population-based screening for prostate cancer is carried out within clinical trials and it remains unclear whether national screening programmes should be established.

9. E

Skeletal metastases from prostate cancer are mostly osteosclerotic (osteoblastic) where they form new bone. The spread occurs mainly into the pelvis and lumbar vertebrae (**Figure 77.1**) through the vertebral venous system of Batson, which are a plexus of valveless veins, the latter fact encouraging the formation of secondaries.

It is an adenocarcinoma. A scoring system devised by Donald Gleason is based on the degree of glandular de-differentiation and its relationship to stroma. The score ranges from 2 to 10 and correlates well with the prognosis and possibility of spread. Haematogenous spread occurs to the skeleton, the prostate being the most common site for such metastases. Whilst the pelvis and lumbar vertebrae are the most common sties, the femoral head, rib cage and skull follow closely in incidence (**Figure 77.2**).

10. D

Mobile rectal mucosa over the prostate is a normal finding of BPH. In prostate carcinoma the rectal mucosa will be adherent to the prostate or nodules might be felt within the gland. Obliteration of the median sulcus with irregular, stony hard induration is a typical feature. In advanced cases extension beyond the capsule infiltrating the bladder base and the seminal vesicles might occur, while in extreme cases the rectum is known to be stenosed from external compression.

11. A, B, C, D

Once suspected, the diagnosis has to be confirmed and staged. Confirmation is obtained by TRUS (trans-rectal ultrasound-guided) core biopsy. TRUS is very useful in local staging supplemented by cross-sectional MR imaging. Having confirmed the diagnosis, bone scan is performed as a part of the staging procedure; CXR and abdominal x-rays for obvious lung and skeletal metastasis are carried out. All the general blood tests, including LFTs, are done and might be normal unless there are skeletal secondaries with bone-marrow infiltration. PSA, although not specific or sensitive, is used for diagnosis and monitoring the effects of

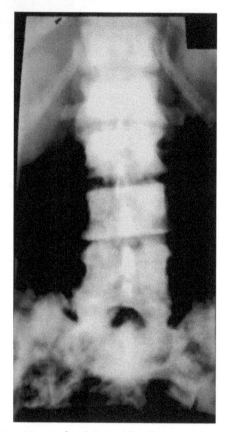

Figure 77.1   X-ray of pelvis and lumbar vertebrae showing sclerotic skeletal secondaries from prostate carcinoma.

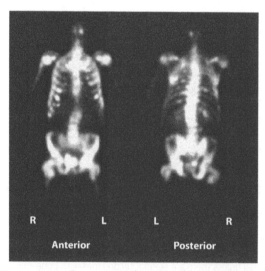

Figure 77.2   Bone scan showing 'hot spots' from secondaries from prostate carcinoma.

treatment. IVU is not routinely carried out unless there is haematuria. US gives a good idea of any back pressure of the kidneys and ureters.

12. D

Incidentally discovered disease at TURP (T1a and T1b) for clinically diagnosed BPH is managed by active surveillance with regular digital rectal examination (DRE) and PSA estimation. Radical prostatectomy might be considered in this group in patients below the age of 70 years although some will elect to pursue a conservative approach. T1c tumour, diagnosed after investigations for a raised PSA and T2 tumours (2a is suspicious nodule confined within prostatic capsule in one lobe and 2b involving both lobes) are suitable for radical prostatectomy particularly below the age of 70 years.

Radical external-beam radiotherapy (ERBT) is an alternative for early cancer where survival rates is almost similar to radical prostatectomy; in 30% though, persistent tumour is found histologically in treated patients. In T3 disease where the cancer has extended through the capsule, surgery, radiotherapy and androgen ablation or a combination are used. Following radical prostatectomy, carried out by the expert, stress incontinence is <2%.

Answers to extended matching questions

1. A Acute prostatitis

This young male has features of acute prostatitis where the general features are far more predominant than the local. The findings on rectal examination give the diagnosis. The usual causative organism is *E. coli*; *Staphylococcus aureus* and *albus*, *Streptoccocus faecalis*, *Neisseria gonorrhoea* and *Chlamydia* are also the causative organisms. The seminal vesicles and posterior urethra are also usually affected.

This is a clinical diagnosis and must be treated vigorously and over long term. After urine has been sent for culture, the patient must be started on trimethoprim or ciprofloxacin. In due course epidydimo-orchitis might occur. Analgesia on a long-term basis in the form of NSAIDs or stronger might be necessary.

Rarely this might proceed on to an abscess when the patient has constant perineal and rectal pain with tenesmus. The prostate will be felt as an enlarged, hot, very tender and fluctuant mass; acute urinary retention might occur when suprapubic catheterisation would be the ideal approach. Under antibiotic cover the abscess should be drained by transurethral resection and unroofing of the cavity.

Inadequately treated acute prostatitis might lead to chronic prostatitis, the symptoms of which are sometimes loosely referred to as 'prostatodynia'. This is a combination of perigenital pain and testicular and perineal pain. *Chlamydia* might be responsible. The diagnosis can be very difficult to make with certainty. Presence of prostatic threads in the urine is confirmatory. Urethroscopy might reveal inflamed prostatic urethra with an enlarged oedematous verumontanum. Long-term treatment with trimethoprim and metronidazole for 1 week helps when anaerobes are involved. Doxycycline is the antibiotic if *Chlamydia* is suspected. Pain relief might be such a challenge that a referral to the pain clinic might be warranted.

2. C Acute retention of urine

This patient has acute urinary retention almost certainly precipitated by the use of proprietary cough and flu medicines. Constipation might be a contributory factor too. The patient, who will be in agony, needs strong analgesia followed by immediate decompression of his bladder by the passage of a Foley catheter. Even when urine comes out, the catheter should be pushed further into the bladder before inflating the balloon so as not to inflate the balloon within the prostatic urethra, which might be elongated and distorted. If urethral catheterisation is not successful, suprapubic puncture under local analgesia is carried out using a commercially available pack.

Once the urine has been drained into a close system of catheter drainage and the patient is comfortable, a detailed history and examination is undertaken. If the patient did not have any LUTS prior this episode of acute retention, a trial without catheter a few days later is likely to be successful. Some units might give the patient a course of α-adrenergic drugs prior to 'trial without catheter'. If the patient does not succeed in passing urine, then after urodynamic studies TURP is carried out. Acute retention of urine accounts for 25% of prostatectomies.

3. D Benign prostatic hypertrophy causing BOO

This patient has typical LUTS from BOO due to BPH. These symptoms used to be referred to as prostatism. The patient's symptoms would have been stratified according to the IPSS as mild, moderate and severe before he comes to the outpatient clinic. The patient should be fully examined, although there will be very little to find on clinical examination except for a benign enlarged prostate on rectal examination. A neurological examination is essential.

The patient should undergo all of the following routine investigations: urine culture, blood tests including serum biochemistry, PSA and full blood count. Special investigation would be pressure-flow urodynamic studies and imaging of the upper tract if indicated because of infection or haematuria. This is done by ultrasound or IVU. In large benign prostates, the typical appearance is that of 'fish-hook' deformities of the lower ends of ureters **(Figure 77.3)**. This sort of a picture is an extreme rarity, because IVU is not carried out by most urologists for BOO.

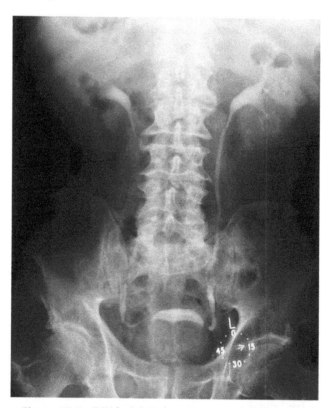

Figure 77.3   IVU in BOO showing typical 'fish-hook' deformities of lower ends of both ureters.

Once the patient assessment has been completed, a full discussion between the patient and urologist about the best line of management should take place. The choice is between expectant management, drug therapy and surgery. Expectant management consists of fluid and caffeine restriction in the evening or at night. Drug treatment would consist of α-blockers or 5α-reductase inhibitors (for large prostates). While the patient is under observation during these two modalities of treatment, he should undergo US of the bladder just to make sure that there is no significant residual urine. If the patient opts for an operation, TURP is the ideal operation. However, if the prostate is very large (>80–100 g), then the urologist might choose to do an open prostatectomy. The size of the prostate for which an open procedure (Millin's retropubic prostatectomy) will be done is entirely dependent upon the individual urologist.

4. B Carcinoma of prostate

This patient has typical LUTS from BOO of short duration. The findings on rectal examination are very suggestive of a carcinoma of the prostate. The backache also of recent onset might indicate skeletal secondaries. After thorough clinical examination, the diagnosis should be confirmed followed by staging and then instituting definitive treatment.

After all blood tests (see above) a trans-rectal ultrasound guided (TRUS) biopsy using an automated gun is carried out. The biopsy is scored according to the Gleason system. An MR cross-sectional imaging, bone scan and CXR are essential in the staging process; x-ray of the pelvis might also be done. Now the patient's management is discussed at the urological multidisciplinary team meeting with a major input from the patient with regard to his wishes.

Radical prostatectomy is suitable for T1 and T2 disease and carried out in men with a life expectancy of >10 years. The procedure should be a nerve-sparing operation, the choice of approaches being the traditional open procedure, laparoscopic procedure or robotic procedure depending upon the available expertise. An alternative is radical radiotherapy bearing in mind that in 30% of treated patients persistent tumour is found within the prostate. Brachytherapy is another form of radiation treatment in which radioisotopes iodine-125 and palladium-103 are implanted as seeds directly into the prostate through the transperineal route.

In advanced disease the treatment is palliative. Those with BOO undergo TURP ('channel TURP'), which might need to be repeated. Patients with bone secondaries are offered bilateral subcapsular orchidectomy (or zoladex) + local radiotherapy to the bones.

5. E Chronic urinary retention with overflow

This patient has chronic retention with overflow, an aftermath of neglected retention. The patient needs immediate catheterisation. This might result in the following: (i) haematuria as the distended bladder veins collapse as the pressure is released and (ii) post-obstructive diuresis, which needs to be monitored carefully with fluid replacement by intravenous saline. US of the upper urinary tract will show hydronephrosis and hydroureter and serum biochemistry will reveal chronic renal failure with metabolic acidosis. This will take several days to stabilise, during which time the patient's electrolytes are closely monitored.

Whilst the patient is being stabilised and his renal failure being brought under control, he should be seen by a neurologist for a thorough neurological examination to exclude neurogenic bladder dysfunction as in multiple sclerosis, Parkinson's disease or spinal cord abnormalities. In these conditions chronic urinary retention might be an early sign. Once stabilised, the patient might be found to be anaemic. If the haemoglobin is <9 g/L the patient might need blood transfusion.

After pressure-flow urodynamic assessment and excluding any neurological problem and uncontrolled diabetes causing neuropathy, this patient will need an operation in the form of TURP, as trial without catheter and medical treatment is highly unlikely to succeed.

Multiple choice questions

→ Anatomy

1. Which of the following statements are true?

A The verumontanum is situated in the membranous urethra.

B The membranous urethra is the primary location of continence.

C The anterior urethra is composed of a bulbar and a penile part.

D The posterior urethra comprises of preprostatic, prostatic and membranous segments.

E The major portion of the female urethra is lined by stratified squamous epithelium.

→ Congenital abnormalities

2. Which of the following statements is false?

A Posterior urethral valves causing obstruction can be diagnosed antenatally.

B The incidence of hypospadias is 1 in 200–300.

C Hypospadias is the most common congenital urethral anomaly.

D Glandular hypospadias should be surgically treated early in life.

E Circumcision must be avoided in boys with hypospadias.

→ Urethral rupture

3. In bulbous urethral rupture, which of the following statements are true?

A Urethral rupture is caused by direct blow to perineum.

B Acute retention occurs.

C There is perineal haematoma with blood at the urethral meatus.

D In a full bladder, suprapubic catheterisation is carried out.

E Urethral catheterisation might be attempted as an alternative.

4. In rupture of the membranous urethra, the following statements are true except:

A It is almost always associated with a pelvic fracture.

B In fractured pelvis 5% will have associated urethral injury.

C It is usually a part of multiple trauma.

D The prostate might be high-riding and out of reach on rectal examination.

E A urethral catheter is inserted as a part of initial resuscitation.

→ Inflammation of the urethra

5. Which of the following statements are true?

A Meatal ulcer occurs in middle-aged men from sexually-transmitted disease.

B Gonorrhoeal urethritis might lead to urethral stricture.

C The causative agent in nonspecific urethritis (NSU) is unknown in 50% of patients.

D In Reiter's disease conjunctivitis is a feature in 50% of patients.

E Bulbar periurethral abscess might cause urinary extravasation.

→ Urethral stricture

6. The following statements are true except:

A Urinary flow trace will show a prolonged flow with a plateau-shaped curve.

B In acute retention suprapubic catheterisation is required.

C Causes are inflammatory, traumatic and iatrogenic.

D Traumatic strictures are best treated by urethroplasty.

E The ideal treatment in the majority is urethral dilatation.

Female urethra

7. Which of the following statements are true?

A The bladder neck is the most important entity for urinary continence.

B Urethral prolapse occurs as a result of childbirth.

C Fowler's syndrome is best treated by urethral dilatation.

D Urethral caruncle is premalignant.

E Urethral diverticulum is more common in women than men.

Surgical conditions of the foreskin

8. The following statements are true except:

A The most common indication for circumcision is cultural reasons.

B In children circumcision is the treatment for non-retractile foreskin due to adhesions.

C Circumcision is indicated in true phimosis with balanoposthitis.

D Balanoposthitis is precancerous.

E Monopolar diathermy should never be used during a circumcision.

Extended matching questions

Diagnoses

1 Balanitis xerotica obliterans (BXO)
2 Balanoposthitis
3 Carcinoma of penis
4 Chordee
5 Persistent priapism
6 Peyronie's disease
7 Rupture of bulbous urethra
8 Rupture of membranous urethra

Clinical scenarios

Match the diagnoses with the scenarios that follow:

A A 35-year-old man complains of deformity of his penis during erection. He has increasing difficulty in sexual intercourse. In the past he had urethritis, which was treated successfully with antibiotics.

B A 68-year-old man complains of bloody, foul-smelling discharge from his penis. He has a hard ulcerated lesion under his prepuce (**Figure 78.1**). He also complains of lumps in his groin.

C A 45-year-old man complains of progressive deformity of his penis, which is very pronounced during erection; this has been going on for the past 2 years. On examination, indurated plaques can be palpated around the penile shaft. On questioning he has thickening of his palmar fascia on both hands.

D A 60-year-old man who is under treatment for leukaemia recently started developing penile erection without any reason. This is prolonged and painful and is now distressing him.

E A 22-year-old man complains of itching around his glans penis and prepuce. Recently, he has developed purulent discharge from the subpreputial area. His glans and foreskin look red and inflamed. He is a type I diabetic on insulin.

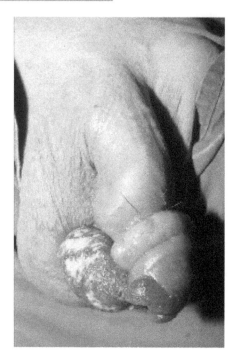

Figure 78.1 Carcinoma of penis.

F A 32-year-old man was involved in a road-traffic accident in which he sustained polytrauma, chief among which was fracture of pelvis with fractured femoral shaft. After stabilisation according to the ATLS protocol, it became apparent that he has a distended bladder and unable to pass urine.

G A 24-year-old man while performing on a Pommel Horse in a gymnastics competition, slipped and fell astride on the Pommel Horse. He complains of severe perineal pain in the peno-scrotal junction where there is a haematoma. He has blood in his external urinary meatus.

H A 52-year-old man complains of thickening of his foreskin over a period of 2 years. During this period he has had difficulty in retracting his foreskin, as a result of which he has been having difficulty in maintaining good hygiene. He finds that his urinary stream tends to spray around.

Answers to multiple choice questions

→ Anatomy

1. B, C, D, E

The membranous urethra, about 1.5 cm long, lies distal to the verumontanum and is the primary site of urinary continence. The urethral sphincter mechanism consists of the intrinsic striated and smooth muscle of the urethra and the pubourethralis component of the levator ani, which surrounds the membranous urethra in the male and the middle and lower thirds of the female urethra. In the female, it blends proximally with the smooth muscle of the bladder neck and distally with the lower urethra and vagina.

The anterior urethra is subdivided into a proximal bulbar part that is surrounded by the bulbospongiosus and situated within the perineum and a distal penile part, the tip of which is the navicular fossa. The posterior urethra is constituted by the preprostatic, prostatic and membranous segments. The female urethra, about 4 cm long, is lined proximally by transitional epithelium whereas the major portion is lined by stratified squamous epithelium distally. In pregnancy, the urethra is considerably elongated.

The verumontanum (colliculus seminalis) is an important endoscopic landmark situated in the prostatic urethra that is 3 to 4 cm long; this is much elongated in benign prostatic hypertrophy when there is a considerable intravesical projection of the prostate. The verumontanum is a midline-rounded eminence that marks the proximal extent of the external urethral sphincter and is a very important landmark for the urologist performing transurethral resection of the prostate; all resection must be proximal to this vital landmark.

Congenital abnormalities

2. D
Glandular hypospadias does not need surgical treatment unless the meatus is stenosed, in which case a meatotomy is performed. Posterior urethral valves can be diagnosed at antenatal US when proximal urinary tract dilatation will be seen. Treatment is endoscopic valve destruction and treatment of any concomitant infection or renal impairment.

The incidence of hypospadias is 1 in 200–300 live male births and is the most common congenital abnormality of the urethra. Once diagnosed the baby must be referred to a paediatric urologist. According to the position of the meatus, the condition is classified in order of severity as glandular, coronal, penile and perineal. Surgery is undertaken before the age of 1 year. Circumcision should be avoided in these boys, as the prepuce would be invaluable in the repair of the deformity.

Urethral rupture

3. A, B, C, D
A fall astride a projecting object, such as might occur in scaffolders, gymnasium accidents caused by a fall across a beam, or cycling accidents, are the usual causes of direct blow to the perineum. Recently skateboarding injuries have become a recognised cause of rupture of the bulbar urethra. (**Figure 78.2**). The clinical triad is acute urinary retention, blood at the external meatus and perineal haematoma. In delayed cases, urinary extravasation occurs. The anatomical attachments of the Colles' fascia to the triangular ligament and Scarpa's fascia just below the inguinal ligament cause the extravasated urine to collect in the scrotum and penis and beneath the deep layer of the superficial fascia of the abdominal wall.

Diagnosis is confirmed by retrograde cystourethrogram. A suprapubic cystostomy is carried out to divert the urine and allow the damaged urethra to heal. Significant urinary extravasation is drained. The patient is placed on an antibiotic and referred to the urologist for definitive treatment. This would be delayed urethroplasty in complete rupture. In partial rupture the patient will require treatment for a stricture, which would be internal visual urethrotomy or dilatation. Urethral catheterisation, rarely advocated, is best avoided for fear of converting a partial tear into a complete tear.

4. E
In a fractured pelvis as seen on a plain x-ray, a urethral catheter should not be passed as more damage might be created by converting a partial rupture into a complete one; in the majority it is a complete rupture to start with. When a patient has not passed urine and there is blood at the meatus, ruptured urethra should be suspected unless otherwise proved. The diagnosis is confirmed by an ascending urethrogram. A suprapubic catheter is inserted.

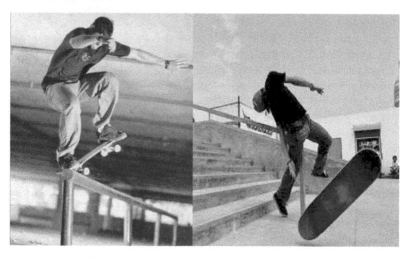

Figure 78.2 Skateboarding injuries can cause bulbar urethral rupture. (Courtesy of Dr Yeznen Sheena, SHO in Plastic Surgery, Oxford, UK.)

As the membranous urethra passes through the bony pelvis, a fracture more often results in complete tear with an interposed haematoma. It is almost always a part of multiple trauma, the most common cause being a road-traffic accident.

Rectal examination will reveal a high-riding prostate, which would not be felt. Treatment is suprapubic cystostomy, the procedure being straightforward in a distended bladder; if a distended bladder cannot be felt, ultrasound guidance will be required. If there is coincidental extraperitoneal rupture of the bladder, emergency surgical repair is carried out along with suprapubic catheter drainage and drainage of the retropubic space. Delayed urethroplasty is carried out by the urologist 3 to 6 months later.

→ Inflammation of the urethra
5. B, C, D, E
Gonorrhoeal urethritis, a sexually-transmitted disease caused by *Neisseria gonorrhoea*, which is a Gram-negative diplococcus, infects the anterior urethra in men and the urethra and cervix in women. Men complain of urethral discomfort, urethral discharge and burning dysuria; it might be asymptomatic in women. Diagnosis is confirmed by identifying the organism in a urethral smear or better still in polymerase chain reaction (PCR)-based techniques. Besides urethritis it can cause prostatitis, epidydimo-orchitis and periurethral abscess. Ceftriaxone is the antibiotic of choice as there is increasing resistance to penicillin and ciprofloxacin. Strictures are treated with dilatation.

In NSU the causative organism is not identified in 50%; in 40% it is caused by *Chlamydia* and caused by sexual transmission. Dysuria and mucopurulent urethral discharge are the symptoms. Diagnosis is confirmed by PCR techniques on a urethral swab or urine sample. Oxytetracycline, doxycycline, or azithromycin are the antibiotics of choice.

Reiter's disease, also sexually transmitted, is an autoimmune condition that presents with urethritis or diarrhoea, conjunctivitis and polyarthritis. Conjunctivitis occurs in 50% of sufferers, the causative organisms being *Chlamydia*, gonococci, *Salmonella*, *Shigella*, or *Campylobacter*. Treatment is with the appropriate antibiotics and analgesia.

Periurethral abscesses can be penile or bulbar, the latter presents as spreading cellulitis as a result of infection form streptococci and anaerobic organisms. It might be associated with a stricture and urinary extravasation might occur. Under antibiotic cover pus is drained and the urethra bypassed by a suprapubic cystostomy.

Meatal ulcer does not occur in middle-aged men, but is a complication of neonatal circumcision. This is the result of friction from clothing and ammoniacal dermatitis due to lack of protection of the glans because of the absent prepuce. Measures to soften the scab and alkalinise the urine cure the condition, although rarely meatotomy of an acquired pinhole meatus might be necessary.

Urethral stricture

6. E
In the majority the ideal treatment is not urethral dilatation, a mode of treatment reserved for the elderly man with a short stricture that needs infrequent dilatation. It is also used for a bladder neck stricture following radical prostatectomy.

The usual sufferer is a young man with features of BOO with prolonged micturition and post-micturition dribbling. Urinary flow rate shows a decrease in the maximum and average rate of <10 mL/second, with the trace showing a prolonged flow with a typical plateau-shaped curve. Rarely the patient might present with acute retention when attempts at urethral catheterisation will result in a false passage; hence suprapubic catheterisation should be done.

Causes of urethral strictures are inflammatory, such as secondary to urethritis, traumatic as after external trauma as in fractured pelvis, or blunt perineal trauma and iatrogenic secondary to TURP or radical prostatectomy. When the cause is due to external trauma, urethroplasty should be the treatment of choice.

Female urethra

7. B, E
Urethral prolapse, also called urethrocele, often occurs with cystoceles. The condition occurs in later life and is partly due to trauma at childbirth. Weakening of the tissue that hold the urethra in place cause it to move, producing pressure on the vagina and resulting in prolapse of the anterior vaginal wall.

Urethral diverticulum is much more common in women. It occurs due to rupture of a distended urethral gland or urethral injury during labour. It causes local pain and repeated cystitis. Diagnosis is by MRI or transvaginal US. Excision is the treatment that should be carried out with great caution, as it might damage the urethral sphincter.

Bladder neck has hardly any role in maintaining urinary continence, which is maintained by the external urethral sphincter, which consists of striated muscle that envelops the whole length of the female urethra. Fowler's syndrome causes urinary retention. It is caused by abnormal myotonic discharge in the striated urethral sphincter. Treatment is by intermittent self-catheterisation, as urethral dilatation is ineffective. Urethral caruncle is a pedunculated granuloma and is not premalignant.

Surgical conditions of the foreskin

8. B
Circumcision is not indicated in children with non-retractile foreskin due to preputial adhesions; no treatment is necessary. The most common indication for circumcision worldwide is for cultural reasons. Medical indications are true phimosis and balanoposthitis and infection of the prepuce and glans that results in phimosis. Balanoposthitis is a precancerous condition. When performing circumcision, monopolar diathermy should never be used for fear of causing burns.

Answers to extended matching questions

1. H Balanitis xerotica obliterans (BXO)

BXO is a chronic inflammatory condition of the foreskin of unknown aetiology in which the foreskin becomes thickened by fibrosis and sclerosis of subepithelial connective tissue. The glans is white and indurated. Fibrosis constricts the urethral meatus, causing phimosis and meatal stenosis. The foreskin forms a constricting band; recurrent balanitis causes problems in hygiene. The condition is precancerous.

Circumcision is the treatment. When the glans is affected, topical steroid cream in the early stages helps. In late cases, meatotomy or meatoplasty might be necessary.

2. E Balanoposthitis

Balanitis is inflammation of the glans, whereas posthitis is inflammation of the prepuce. The two anatomical parts are almost always involved together, hence the term. The condition can be mild with itching with some discharge; in severe cases the glans and foreskin would look red and raw with purulent discharge. This young man has balanoposthitis and needs to be treated with the appropriate broad-spectrum antibiotics. One should make sure that his diabetes is under good control. He should be given advice with regard to local hygiene. Monilial infections are a common accompaniment. The condition is associated with penile cancer. In advanced cases circumcision should be considered, particularly if phimosis is present.

3. B Carcinoma of penis

This patient has a carcinoma of the penis with probable secondaries in his inguinal lymph nodes. The following usual principles of cancer management should be followed: confirmation of diagnosis, staging of the disease and definitive treatment. In 50% of patients the inguinal lymph node enlargement is from sepsis. He needs confirmation by a biopsy of the lesion, staging by fine-needle aspiration of his groin nodes, CT of pelvis and groin, liver ultrasound and chest X-ray. Thereafter, discussion in a multidisciplinary meeting is followed by the appropriate definitive treatment.

It is a squamous cell carcinoma. For the original tumour, treatment will be partial or total amputation of the penis, in the latter situation with a perineal urethrostomy. Involved groin nodes are subjected to bilateral groin dissection, carried out at a second stage. Uninvolved nodes might be treated by prophylactic block dissection for T2 and poorly differentiated tumours. When the growth is confined to the penis the 5-year survival rate is 80%, but it drops to 40% with nodal involvement.

When the condition occurs as a red cutaneous patch on the glans, it is regarded as a carcinoma in situ, also called Bowen's disease or erythroplasia of Queryat. After confirmation by biopsy it is treated by topical 5-FU cream, CO_2 laser ablation, or excision.

4. A Chordee

This patient suffers from chordee, which is a fixed bowing of his penis resulting in deformed erection. This can be the result of hypospadias. In this patient it is the aftermath of chronic urethritis. Treatment would be to treat the cause and hence surgical.

5. D Persistent priapism

This patient, who suffers from leukaemia, has persistent priapism. It can also occur due to sickle cell disease or any hypercoagulable blood disorder. He can be treated by aspiration of the sludged blood in the corpora cavernosa or injection of phenylephrine solution (α-adrenoreceptor agonist). Failure of such treatment might require decompression of the penis by creating a shunt between the corpus cavernosum and the corpus spongiosum.

6. C Peyronie's disease

This patient has Peyronie's disease, which is often accompanied by Dupuytren's contracture, as in this case. A plain X-ray of the penis might show up calcification of plaques that might be palpable. The aetiology is unknown, the condition being characterised by focal asymmetric fibrosis of the penile shaft. The condition is self-limiting but surgery might be indicated when the condition interferes with sexual function, some 25% opting for surgical treatment, which is the domain of the specialist.

7. G Rupture of bulbous urethra

Blunt perineal trauma is the cause of rupture of the bulbar urethra. This might happen for various reasons such as assault from a kick in the perineum, gymnasium injury, contact-sport injuries (football, rugby) and fall astride firm or hard objects. The diagnostic triad consists of blood at the external urethral meatus, perineal bruising and inability to pass urine. Undiagnosed late cases present with urinary extravasation. Confirmation is by ascending urethrogram. The emergency treatment is suprapubic cystostomy. The patient is then referred to an urologist for urethroplasty at a later date.

For details please see multiple choice question answer 3 previously.

8. F Rupture of membranous urethra

Membranous urethral rupture is almost always associated with a fractured pelvis, except when it simulates an extra-peritoneal rupture of the bladder (**Figure 76.1** in **Chapter 76**). The diagnosis is suspected by the history and confirmed by an ascending urethrogram. The immediate treatment is a suprapubic cystostomy. At times a retropubic haematoma and extravasation might need to be drained. Definitive treatment must always be by the urologist who will do a delayed repair and urethroplasty.

For details please see multiple choice question answer 4 previously.

79 Testis and scrotum

Pradip K Datta

Extended matching questions

→ **Embryology and anatomy**

1. Which of the following statements are true?

A The processus vaginalis accompanies the testis as it descends.

B The testis is at the deep inguinal ring by the seventh month of fetal life.

C The testicular veins drain into the inferior vena cava.

D The lymphatics of the testes drain into the para-aortic lymph nodes.

E The testicular arteries arise from the abdominal aorta.

→ **Incompletely descended testis**

2. The following statements are true except:

A The incidence is 4%.

B A testis absent from the scrotum after 3 months is unlikely to descend.

C An incompletely descended testis tends to atrophy as puberty approaches.

D Retractile testis is best treated by orchidopexy.

E Orchidopexy reduces the chances of developing a testicular tumour.

3. The hazards of incomplete descent of testis are the following:

A Impaired fertility

B Hernia

C Torsion

D Increased liability to malignant change in later life

E Epididymo-orchitis

→ **Testicular torsion**

4. Which of the following statements are true?

A The typical symptom is sudden agonising pain in the scrotum.

B It is most common between 10 and 25 years of age.

C Inversion of the testis and a transverse lie are the most common causes.

D Doppler ultrasound (US) scan should be done to confirm the diagnosis

E The emergency operation of fixation of the testis to the tunica albuginea with non-absorbable sutures should be carried out on the affected side.

→ **Varicocele**

5. Which of the following statements are false?

A The usual cause is absence or incompetence of valves in the testicular vein.

B The vast majority occur on the right side.

C When it occurs on the left side it might indicate a left renal carcinoma.

D In a person with a varicocele and reduced sperm count, the latter can be improved by an operation on the varicocele.

E In symptomatic patients, the first line treatment should be embolisation.

→ **Hydrocele**

6. The following statements are true except:

A A hydrocele is a collection of fluid within the tunica vaginalis.

B A congenital hydrocele causes an intermittent swelling.

C An acute hydrocele in a young man might be a sinister finding.

D Testicular pathology might cause a hydrocele.

E Aspiration is an effective treatment.

→ Epididymo-orchitis

7. Which of the following statements are true?

A The causes are *Chlamydia* and gonococci as sexually-transmitted infections.

B The initial symptoms are those of urinary tract infection (UTI).

C In mumps, 18% of men might develop this condition.

D It is a common postoperative complication after prostatectomy.

E Treatment is doxycycline for *Chlamydia* or a broad-spectrum antibiotic.

→ Testicular tumour

8. Which of the following statements are false?

A A testicular lump that is inseparable from the testis is likely to be a tumour.

B Lymphatic spread is usually to the inguinal lymph nodes.

C Teratomas occur in the third decade and seminomas in the fourth decade.

D Seminomas usually spread via the lymphatics.

E Diagnosis is confirmed by US-guided fine-needle aspiration cytology (FNAC).

9. Which of the following statements are true with regard to the management of testicular tumours?

A Tumour markers are measured and a chest x-ray carried out.

B Initial surgical treatment is orchidectomy through the groin.

C Staging is done by CT scan of the abdomen and chest.

D Seminomas are radiosensitive.

E Secondaries from teratoma are always treated by surgery, as they are radio-resistant.

Extended matching questions

→ Diagnoses

1 Acute epidydimo-orchitis
2 Encysted hydrocele of the cord
3 Epidydimal cyst
4 Idiopathic oedema of the scrotum
5 Spermatocele
6 Testicular tumour
7 Torsion of the hydatid of Morgagni
8 Torsion of the testis
9 Vaginal hydrocele
10 Varicocele

Match the diagnoses with the clinical scenarios that follow:

→ Clinical scenarios

A A 22-year-old man complains of acute pain in the top of his left testis for 16 hours. On examination the scrotum looks normal and the testis can be felt with care without undue tenderness. There is a small, blue, pea-sized tender mass on top of the testis.

B A 30-year-old man complains of a swollen scrotum for almost 1 year. This is not painful but recently has caused discomfort. On examination he has a tense fluctuant lump in his right scrotum where the testis cannot be felt separately. The swelling transilluminates.

C A 45-year-old man complains of a painful left testis of 4 days' duration. This is associated with fever and rigors. He has painful micturition and considerable frequency. On examination he looks unwell, has pyrexia of 39°C and has a swollen, red, oedematous and shiny left hemiscrotum; the testis and epididymis feel indurated and tender.

D An 18-year-old man complains of sudden onset of agonising pain in his right groin and suprapubic area of 6 hours' duration. He has no urinary symptoms. On examination he is in agony, the right testis is drawn up and the scrotum is red. The testis is impossible to feel because of pain.

E A 25-year-old man complains of feeling heavy in his left scrotum where he noticed a lump while in the shower. A few days before, he felt a lump in the periumbilical region of his abdomen. At the same time he noticed another lump on the left side of his neck. The abdominal and neck lumps do not give him any symptoms. On questioning he admits to coughing up some blood in his sputum 1 month ago. On examination he has a 2 cm irregular lump over his left supraclavicular area and a 5-cm irregular firm lump in his umbilical region. Examination of the left testis reveals a large lump, which is hard and heavy.

F A 50-year-old man complains of a lump in his right scrotum of 1 year's duration. This is gradually growing larger in size and gives him some discomfort. Examination of his scrotum reveals a cystic lump, about 7 cm in diameter, above and behind the left testis, which is minimally tender. Transillumination is positive and shows septa within the lump. There is a smaller similar lump on the other side of which he is unaware.

G A 4-year-old boy has been brought by his parents to A&E with a red, swollen scrotum. On examination the child is not in any pain and there is redness and oedema around the penis and perineum.

H A 40-year-old man presents with a swelling in his right scrotum, which he says feels like 'a third testis'. He noticed it in the shower and is worried that he has got cancer. He has no symptoms. On examination he has a lax, cystic swelling on top of his right testis. It is not tender and transillumination is hazy.

I A 30-year-old man presents with a swelling in his left hemiscrotum, which he discovered by chance in the bath. On examination the testis feel separate from the swelling, which is about 2 cm in diameter and above the testis. It transilluminates and comes down on traction to the testis.

J A 45-year-old man complains of a dragging discomfort in the left side of his scrotum. He noticed an irregular lump in his scrotum separate from the testis. He thinks he has had this for many years but only recently he noticed discomfort in the lump. On examination he has a bunch of veins in the scrotum and the testis feels normal. On lying down the veins disappear. Abdominal examination in the left renal area does not show any abnormality.

Answers to multiple choice questions

→ Embryology and anatomy

1. A, B, D, E

The processus vaginalis is a sac of peritoneum that accompanies the testis as it proceeds down the inguinal canal. By the seventh month of fetal life the testis is at the level of the deep inguinal ring from where it progresses rapidly into the scrotum by the time of birth when it projects into the processus vaginalis which normally gets obliterated. Persistence of the processus vaginalis in whole or in part when continuous with the peritoneal cavity results in a hernia. Persistence of an intervening segment of the processus leads to an encysted hydrocele of the cord. Accumulation of serous fluid constitutes a hydrocele.

The lymphatics of the testes drain to the para-aortic nodes lying alongside the aorta at the origin of the testicular arteries, which arise from the abdominal aorta at the level of T10 vertebrae. Hence lymphatic spread from a testicular tumour will from a periumbilical mass.

Both testicular veins do not drain into the inferior vena cava (IVC); the right vein drains into the IVC at an acute angle whereas the left vein drains into the left renal vein at a right angle. This fact is clinically important because a recent varicocele in a middle-aged patient should arouse suspicion of a left renal carcinoma that has locally spread along the renal vein obstructing the testicular vein.

Incompletely descended testis

2. D, E

Retractile testis require no treatment. An incompletely descended testis has a much greater chance of developing a tumour in later life. Correcting the abnormality by orchidopexy does not reduce the incidence of a tumour but greatly enhances the chances of early detection. This is because young men will notice changes in the size, weight and feel of a testis much more readily when it is in the scrotum.

Incomplete descent, so called when it is arrested in its normal path to the scrotum, occurs in 4%. If an undescended testis (UDT) has not come down to the scrotum within 3 months of birth, it is unlikely to do so thereafter. As puberty approaches an UDT will atrophy. While early orchidopexy is regarded to help preserve function, evidence to show that this benefits fertility is lacking. However, in UDT from the age of 1 to 2 years, there is loss of Leydig cells, degeneration of Sertoli cells and reduced spermatogenesis.

3. A, B, C, D

There is no increased risk of epididymo-orchitis. However, should it occur in an incompletely descended testis on the right side, it can be confused with acute appendicitis. Impaired fertility is a recognised hazard of testicular maldescent. A hernia is present in 90% of cases, although most of them are not clinically apparent. There is a higher incidence of testicular torsion because of a congenital abnormality between the testis and its mesentery. The risk of testicular tumour is 5 to 10 times greater than normal, the most common tumour being a seminoma. Whether an orchidopexy in early childhood reduces the chance of developing a cancer is uncertain. However, a testis within the scrotum enhances the chances of early detection because any change in the size or weight of the testis (as happens in a testicular tumour) will be much more readily felt.

Testicular torsion

4. B, C

The typical symptom in testicular torsion, most common in men between 10 and 25 years, is sudden agonising pain in the groin and suprapubic area and not the testis. The causes are anatomical abnormalities such as a rotated testis that lies transversely or upside down, high investment of the tunica vaginalis causing the testis to lie transversely like a clapper-bell and separation of the epididymis from the body of the testis and a pedicle that connects them.

Doppler US might show lack of blood supply although false-positive results can occur. It should not be done routinely as precious time might be lost. In case of doubt, the scrotum should be explored. At operation the twisted and viable testis is untwisted and the tunica vaginalis is fixed to the tunica albugenia with interrupted unabsorbable sutures. The same procedure must be carried out in all cases on the other non-affected side, as the congenital anatomical abnormality that caused the condition in the first place is usually bilateral.

→ Varicocele
5. B, D

90% of varicoceles occur on the left side, perhaps because the left testicular vein drains at right angles into the renal vein (an orthogonal junction). There is no evidence that operating on a varicocele improves the semen quality or raises sperm count. The reason to operate on a varicocele is pain and discomfort and not subfertility.

The usual cause is absence or incompetence of the valves in the testicular vein. In a middle-aged man with a left-sided varicocele, particularly if it is of recent onset, his abdomen must be examined for the possibility of a left renal mass because a renal cell carcinoma might extend into the left renal vein blocking the ostium of the left testicular vein causing the varicocele. When intervention is considered for a symptomatic varicocele, the first-line treatment should be therapeutic embolisation.

→ Hydrocele
6. E

Drainage is not an effective treatment for hydrocele. Following such treatment it recurs or might get infected. Refusal to have an operation is the indication for repeated aspiration. A congenital hydrocele is due to a patent processus vaginalis, within which is a collection of serous fluid, and usually does not need an operation. An acute hydrocele that appears within a short time might indicate an underlying testicular tumour, a sinister finding. Other testicular pathology such as acute or chronic epididymo-orchitis might cause a secondary hydrocele; it is also seen when the scrotum is explored for a testicular torsion.

→ Epididymo-orchitis
7. A, B, C, E

The most common cause in sexually active young men is *Chlamydia* followed by gonococci. In older men the cause is UTI from BOO. As a result of outflow obstruction, infected urine from the prostatic urethra travels up the vas causing epididymitis. For those who have had a vasectomy, the infection would be blood-borne when the causative organisms are *E. coli, Streptococcus, Staphylococcus* and *Proteus*. Acute infection might occur following instrumentation such as catheterisation, cystoscopy, or urethral dilatation. The initial symptoms are dysuria and frequency followed by tender, red, swollen epididymis and testis. Ache in the groin and fever are the initial symptoms. Confirmation, if necessary, is done by ultrasound.

Treatment is with doxacycline or a broad-spectrum antibiotic. Epididymo-orchitis is almost unknown nowadays following prostatectomy because of closed catheter drainage and prophylactic antibiotics.

→ Testicular tumour
8. B, E

The lymphatic drainage of the testis is alongside the blood vessels draining to the para-aortic group of lymph nodes. Metastasis to inguinal lymph nodes does not occur unless the scrotal skin is involved, which is rare. Diagnosis is confirmed by US where the homogenous tumour tissue produces multiple tumour reflections. FNAC should never be done, as it would disseminate tumour cells along the needle track. In case of any doubt about the diagnosis, frozen section during inguinal orchidectomy should be arranged.

Clinically a testicular lump that cannot be felt separately from the testis is a sinister finding and almost certainly a malignant tumour. Seminomas occur in the fourth decade of life whereas teratomas or non-seminomatous germ cell tumours (NSGCT) occur in the third decade. Seminomas predominantly spread via the lymphatics to the para-aortic nodes and hence clinically an irregular hard periumbilical mass might be felt.

9. A, B, C, D
Once a testicular tumour is diagnosed on clinical grounds, it is mandatory to measure tumour markers – beta-human chorionic gonadotrophin (β-HCG), alpha-fetoprotein (α-FP) and lactate dehydrogenase (LDH). In 30% of seminomas β-HCG is raised. In NSGCTs α-fetoprotein (AFP) is raised in 50%–70% and β-HCG in 40%–60%. These tumour markers are used to reassess following orchidectomy as the half-lives of AFP and HCG are 5–7 days and 2–3 days, respectively. On confirmation by US and after a CT scan of chest, a high inguinal orchidectomy is performed through a groin incision.

Once orchidectomy has been performed, staging is carried out by CT scan of the abdomen and chest. Treatment is according to the stage, of which there are four (1 to 4). Early stages of seminoma (Stages 1 and 2) have excellent results following radiotherapy; later stages are treated by chemotherapy. Secondaries from NSGCT (teratoma) are not always treated by surgery. Stage 1 is monitored, whilst stages 2–4 are treated by chemotherapy. Surgery in the form of retroperitoneal lymph node dissection is only carried out if secondary lymph nodal masses are still present following chemotherapy.

Answers to extended matching questions

1. C Acute epididymo-orchitis
This patient has acute epididymo-orchitis. In the young male it is usually the aftermath of genital infection from *Chlamydia trachomatis* and gonococcus. Clinically there is thickening, swelling and tenderness and swelling of the epididymis with red and shiny adherent scrotum. US will confirm the diagnosis. Urine is sent for culture and the patient is treated with doxycycline or a quinolone for 2 weeks. It can take up to 8 weeks to subside. Rarely an abscess might need draining.

2. I Encysted hydrocele of the cord
This is a small cystic swelling felt well above the testis in line with the spermatic cord. It is the result of a part of the processus vaginalis not becoming completely obliterated where the proximal and distal parts become closed off and fibrotic and the middle part remains as a fluid-filled sac, i.e., persistence of an intervening part of the processus. It is a clinical diagnosis confirmed by the cyst moving downward and immobile when the testis is subjected to gentle traction. Usually they are small, and reassurance about their benign nature is enough. It is removed if the patient requests.

3. F Epididymal cyst
This is a cystic degeneration of the epididymis, which is often bilateral. They are present above, behind and separate from the upper pole of the testis. Usually tense with several septa, they brilliantly transilluminate. This is a clinical diagnosis that can be confirmed by US. The treatment is excision, which might interfere with transmission of sperm from the testis on the affected side; this should be a part of informed consent.

4. G Idiopathic oedema of the scrotum
Idiopathic oedema of the scrotum, often confused for torsion, is distinguished by absence of pain or tenderness. The condition is usually bilateral affecting the perineal region and the genitalia. Allergy is regarded as the cause, which is supported by eosinophilia. No active treatment is necessary, as it subsides by itself. In case of doubt when a torsion cannot be excluded, a colour Doppler is useful to prevent an unnecessary operation in a child.

5. H Spermatocele

This is a cystic swelling and hence exhibiting fluctuation (as all cystic swellings do). It is a retention cyst from a part of the epididymis. It lies above the epididymis behind the upper pole of the testis. Like other scrotal cystic swellings, it transilluminates but unlike them it is softer. It is not large and resembles and feels like a testis – hence, most patients complain of a 'third testicle'. On aspiration the fluid is barley-coloured because of the presence of dead spermatozoa. Confirmation, if necessary, like all scrotal swellings is by US. It is removed if the patient requests.

6. E Testicular tumour

This young man has the hallmarks of a metastatic testicular teratoma – hard enlarged testis, abdominal and supraclavicular lumps from metastatic lymph nodes and haemoptysis from pulmonary secondaries. Testicular tumours constitute 1% to 2% of all male cancers. The vast majority (90%) complain of an enlarged testis, most of them being painless. Sometimes trauma at sport draws the attention of the patient to the presence of the lump. Heaviness of the testis and feeling a testicular lump while in the shower brings the patient to consultation. Rarely, unresolving epididymo-orchitis might be a presentation.

Examination reveals a hard, heavy, non-tender lump. Once a tumour is suspected, repeated palpation of the lump should be desisted to prevent dissemination. It is said that testicular sensation is lost. However, eliciting such a physical finding is bad doctoring as it would encourage tumour spread. On similar grounds repeated clinical examination, for example, by medical students, should be discouraged.

This patient needs bloods to be sent for tumour markers, AFP (α-fetoprotein), β-HCG (β-human chorionic gonadotropin) and LDH (lactic dehydrogenase). A testicular and abdominal US and a CT scan of his chest is done. A high inguinal orchidectomy is then undertaken, followed by a repeat of the tumour markers and CT scanning of his abdomen and neck. The multidisciplinary team then discusses the patient and decides upon the treatment for his secondaries. This would be intensive chemotherapy. However, prior to starting chemotherapy, he should have sperm freezing for future. Once his chemotherapy is completed, further assessment of his secondaries is done after about 6 weeks. If they are still obvious, he is considered for retroperitoneal lymph node dissection (RPLND) and pulmonary metastasectomy.

Germ cell tumours constitute 90%–95% of all testicular tumours. These are seminoma, teratoma (NSGCT), embryonal cell carcinoma, yolk-sac tumour and choriocarcinoma. Of these, the first two are most common. While TNM staging is the most commonly used to stage testicular tumours, the Royal Marsden staging of I to IV **(Figure 79.1)** is followed for treatment:

Stage I – Tumour confined to testis
Stage II – Sub-diaphragmatic involved nodes
Stage III – Supra-diaphragmatic involved nodes
Stage IV – Non-lymphatic metastatic disease (pulmonary)

Testicular tumours are very sensitive to platinum-based chemotherapy, which has revolutionised the survival rates over the past couple of decades especially when management has been carried out in specialised cancer centres. The details of such treatment are beyond the scope of this book.

Staging for testicular tumours

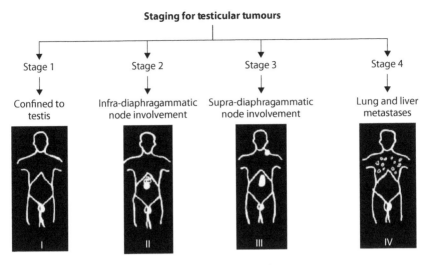

Stage 1	Stage 2	Stage 3	Stage 4
Confined to testis	Infra-diaphragammatic node involvement	Supra-diaphragammatic node involvement	Lung and liver metastases

Figure 79.1   Staging of testicular tumour.

7. A Torsion of the hydatid of Morgagni
This 22-year-old man complains of acute pain in his scrotum. On examination the testis is not tender, but there is tenderness over a small swelling at the top of the testis. The small lump, blue-black in colour, is the twisted hydatid of Morgagni, a remnant of the Mullerian duct. The symptoms, although similar to testicular torsion, is much less severe. Removal of the lump cures the condition.

8. D Torsion of the testis
This 18-year-old male has testicular torsion. Pain, which is sudden and excruciating, starts typically in the groin and lower abdomen and the testis is pulled up. The diagnosis can be difficult to be certain. In case of doubt, immediate exploration should be carried out. It is better surgical practice to explore unnecessarily an epididymo-orchtis than to observe and miss testicular torsion resulting in a gangrenous testis.

Although a colour Doppler might be helpful in excluding a torsion, the investigation is not infallible. The patient should be explored through a scrotal incision and the testis should be fixed on both sides to the tunica albuginea with non-absorbable sutures.

9. B Vaginal hydrocele
This patient has a vaginal hydrocele **(Figure 79.2)** – a tense cystic swelling in his scrotum where the testis is not separately palpable and the swelling transilluminates. Typically the swelling lies in front of and surrounds the testis. It is a clinical diagnosis and can be confirmed by US if desired.

Rarely a small hydrocele might be secondary to epididymo-orchitis or a tumour. It can also occur from infestation with the filarial parasite. When treatment is asked for by the patient in primary hydroceles, the option is an operation or aspiration with injection of tetracycline as a scelrosant.

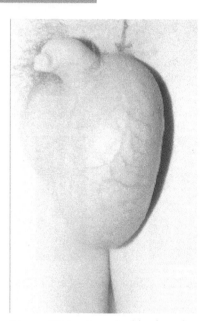

Figure 79.2 A vaginal hydrocele.

10. J Varicocele

This patient has a left varicocele. As it is on the left side, it is important to exclude a left renal carcinoma. Rarely a tumour thrombus might spread along the left renal vein, blocking the left testicular vein causing the varicocele. Abdominal examination of the left lumbar area and loin is mandatory. In the vast majority the cause is not known and 90% occur on the left side, probably because of the termination of the left testicular vein into the left renal vein at right angles.

The association of a varicocele with subfertility or oligospermia is anything but proven and improvement of semen quality is not an indication for surgical intervention. Indication for intervention for a varicocele is significant discomfort. Under the circumstances embolisation of the testicular veins is the treatment of choice. If that fails, operation by an extraperitoneal route for surgical ligation of the testicular vein through an incision in the iliac fossa is undertaken. Recurrence does occur even after surgical ligation.

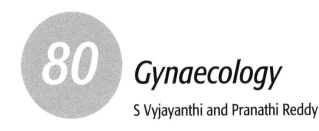

80 Gynaecology

S Vyjayanthi and Pranathi Reddy

Multiple choice questions

→ ## Anatomy and physiology

1. Which of the following statements are true?

A Broad ligament provides the main support for the uterus.

B The ovarian artery arises from the anterior branch of internal iliac artery.

C Gonadotrophin hormones, follicle-stimulating hormones (FSH) and Luteinising hormones (LH) are produced by the pituitary.

D Under the influence of FSH and LH, ovary undergoes cyclical changes leading to the development and release of mature oocyte.

E The ovary produces hormones oestrogen and progesterone that prepare the endometrial lining for implantation.

→ ## Abnormal or excessive vaginal bleeding

2. Which of the following statements are true regarding performing endometrial biopsy?

A All women more than 40 years old with excessively heavy or irregular or frequent bleeding.

B Thirty-year-old woman presenting with menorrhagia.

C Younger women with polycystic ovarian syndrome (PCOS).

D Women taking tamoxifen.

E Eighteen-year-old presenting with heavy irregular periods.

→ ## Acute pelvic pain in pregnancy

3. Regarding ectopic pregnancy, which of the following statements are false?

A Ectopic pregnancy accounts for 1% of all maternal deaths in the United Kingdom.

B Transvaginal ultrasound is the gold-standard diagnostic test.

C In equivocal cases, measuring serum levels of β-hCG can help to establish the diagnosis.

D It can mimic acute urinary tract infection in early pregnancy.

E Smoking increases the risk of ectopic pregnancy.

4. Regarding management of ectopic pregnancy, which of the following statements are true?

A Salpingostomy is preferred if a woman has had a previous ectopic pregnancy or tubal surgery in the same tube.

B The principal disadvantage of salpingostomy is that some residual trophoblastic tissue can be left inside the tube.

C An immediate laparotomy might be required if the woman has lost a great deal of blood.

D Methotrexate, is toxic to trophoblastic tissue and hence does not carry any risks associated with residual trophoblastic tissue.

E After treatment, the patient who still has one or both tubes should be warned that she is at increased risk of another ectopic pregnancy.

→ Infection

5. **Regarding management of acute pelvic inflammatory disease (PID), which of the following statements are true?**

A Single therapy with azithromycin is effective if given for 7 days.

B In hospital, antibiotics should be given intravenously until 24 hours after clinical improvement.

C Where the woman has an intrauterine contraceptive device in situ, removal is recommended along with administration of appropriate antibiotics.

D It is recommended that tubo-ovarian abscesses be managed conservatively unless the patient fails to respond to intravenous antibiotics and systemic support.

E Concomitant use of hormonal contraception reduces the efficacy of antibiotics.

→ Utero-vaginal prolapse

6. **Which of the following statements are true regarding rectocele?**

A Urinary frequency.

B Difficulties with defecation.

C Sensation of incomplete defecation.

D Recurrent urinary tract infections.

E A sensation of a lump in the vagina.

→ Endometriosis

7. **Which of the following statements are true in the diagnosis of endometriosis?**

A The symptom complex of dysmenorrhea, deep dyspareunia and infertility is diagnostic of endometriosis.

B Ultrasound scanning can reliably detect only severe forms of the disease, i.e., endometriomas.

C CA-125 levels are typically >1000 u.

D Visual inspection of the pelvis at laparoscopy is a reliable method of diagnosis.

E Magnetic Resonance Imaging (MRI) is helpful in differentiating endometriomas from other ovarian cysts such as dermoid.

→ Ovarian cancer

8. **Which of the following statements regarding ovarian cancer are false?**

A It is the leading cause of malignancy in women.

B Approximately two thirds of women present in an advanced stage.

C Can present with persistent non-specific abdominal symptoms.

D The peak age of incidence is 40 to 50 years.

E Overall five-year survival rate is above 60%.

9. **Which of the following statements are true in relation to ovarian cancer?**

A The use of combined oral contraceptive pill reduces the risk of developing ovarian cancer in later life.

B About 50% of ovarian cancers are clearly associated with specific genetic factors.

C In stage I of ovarian cancer, the tumour is confined to the ovary.

D Stage 1 grade 1 epithelial adenocarcinoma requires no postoperative therapy.

E Ovarian stimulation with embryo preservation is a fertility-preserving option in women with all grades of ovarian cancer.

Extended matching questions

→ Diagnoses

1 Adenomyosis
2 Benign ovarian cyst
3 Chronic PID
4 Endometriosis
5 Residual ovary syndrome

6 Ruptured ectopic pregnancy
7 Twisted ovarian cyst
8 Uterine fibroid

Match the diagnoses with the clinical scenarios that follow:

→ Clinical scenarios

A A 34-year-old mother of 3 children with a 10-year history of menorrhagia underwent a total abdominal hysterectomy with conservation of the ovaries 2 years earlier. She now complains of persistent pelvic pain that is worse when her period would have been due and deep dyspareunia. Pelvic ultrasound scan shows small bilateral ovarian cysts 2–3cm in diameter but no other abnormalities.

B A 35-year-old woman complains of a 10-month history of pelvic pain, dysmenorrhoea and deep dyspareunia since discontinuing the combined oral contraceptive pill. She also complains of rectal bleeding during menstruation but has a regular bowel habit and there is no recent weight loss. Clinical examination showed a bulky tender uterus with decreased mobility and palpable nodules within the pouch of Douglas. Rectal examination was normal.

C A 35-year-old woman has been admitted with sudden onset of severe lower abdominal pain of few hours duration. She has a 3-year-old child. She had an intrauterine contraceptive device inserted 2 years ago. She gives history of irregular menstrual cycles and her last menstrual period was about 6 weeks ago. On examination she looks pale, her blood pressure is 80/50 mmHg and pulse is 120/minute; she is extremely tender over the entire lower abdomen. On vaginal examination there is cervical excitation and the os is closed.

D A 30-year-old woman has been admitted with severe right-sided lower abdominal pain and vomiting. The pain was colicky to start with but has now settled to a continuous agonising pain. Her last menstrual period was 10 days ago. She is apyrexial, sweaty, with a blood pressure of 110/60 mmHg and a pulse of 120/minute. Abdomen examination reveals tenderness, rigidity and rebound tenderness over the entire lower abdomen.

E A 28 year old woman has been trying for a pregnancy for 18 months and complains of severe dysmenorrhea and heavy periods with a constant feeling of pelvic pressure. Clinical examination reveals the presence of a 15 weeks size irregularly enlarged firm pelvic mass. The uterus could not be palpated separately from the mass.

F A 34-year-old woman with one previous ectopic pregnancy complains of a 3-year history of progressive pelvic and lower abdominal pain, dysmenorrhoea and deep dyspareunia. She has no bowel symptoms but has two previous laparoscopies for drainage of tubo-ovarian abscesses. Endocervical swabs for Chlamydia are negative and her white cell count and CRP are within normal limits. Pelvic ultrasound scan shows a normal size anteverted uterus with normal ovaries and a small amount of free fluid in the Pouch of Douglas.

G A 30-year-old mother of 2 children who has undergone tubectomy presents with a 2-year history of menorrhagia and severe dysmenorrhea with flooding. Pelvic examination reveals a uniformly enlarged uterus of 8 weeks size, which is mobile and non-tender. She did not show any response to a prescription of the combined oral contraceptive pill but responded well to a combination therapy of tranexamic acid and mefenamic acid.

H A 32-year-old mother of 2 children presented with a dull ache and dragging sensation in the lower abdomen of few months duration. Her cycles are regular and flow normal. On examination, she has a mass in the right iliac fossa and the lower edge of the mass is not felt per abdomen. Bimanual examination reveals a cystic swelling felt through the right and anterior fornices, and it is non-tender and mobile. The uterus is felt separately from the mass.

Answers to multiple choice questions

→ Anatomy and physiology

1. C, D, E

The broad ligaments are simply folds of peritoneum and provide no support. The parametrium, composed of the cardinal and uterosacral ligaments, attaches the cervix and upper vagina to the pelvic sidewall and provides the main support to the uterus. The ovarian artery arises from the abdominal aorta and the uterine artery arises from the anterior branch of the internal iliac artery.

The gonadotrophin-releasing hormone (GnRH) is produced by the hypothalamus in a pulsatile fashion, which acts on the pituitary to release the reproductive hormones FSH and LH. The coordinated secretion of FSH and LH is responsible for follicle growth, ovulation and maintenance of corpus luteum. The growing follicle produces oestrogen in the proliferative phase of the cycle and progesterone by the corpus luteum after ovulation in the luteal phase of the cycle.

→ Abnormal or excessive vaginal bleeding

2. A, C, D

The mainstay of management when women more than 40 years of age present with heavy or irregular bleeding is to identify and treat pathology which usually involves ultrasound and an endometrial biopsy either under direct vision at hysteroscopy or with a Pipelle. Women taking tamoxifen are at high risk of developing endometrial polyps, hyperplasia and cancer and hence the need to perform endometrial biopsy when these women present with irregular vaginal bleeding. Young women with PCOS are also at high risk of developing endometrial hyperplasia and cancer and hence biopsy is indicated in these women.

Menstrual bleeding might be excessively heavy or irregular in women less than 40 years of age in whom pathology is very rarely found which is known as dysfunctional uterine bleeding. These women can be treated symptomatically and there is no need to perform endometrial biopsy initially in these women.

→ Ectopic pregnancy

3. A, B

An ectopic pregnancy is one that grows outside the uterine cavity and is the most common cause of maternal death in the first trimester accounting for 9% of maternal deaths in the United Kingdom. The complete absence of an intrauterine gestational sac on transvaginal ultrasound with a positive pregnancy test increases the probability of an ectopic pregnancy but is not diagnostic since the pregnancy might not be advanced enough for the sac to be seen on ultrasound.

In equivocal cases where ultrasound is inconclusive, measuring serum levels of β-hCG can help to establish the diagnosis. A single level above approximately 1500 IU/L in association with an empty uterus on ultrasound is highly suggestive of an ectopic pregnancy. The most common presentation of an ectopic pregnancy is with acute pain. It might be associated with urinary frequency and can be confused with urinary tract infection. Cigarette smoking increases the risk by affecting fallopian tube function.

4. B, C, E

Salpingostomy is a conservative surgery whereby only the ectopic pregnancy is removed by making an incision in the tube. The principal disadvantage is that some residual trophoblastic tissue can be left inside the tube. If the woman is haemodynamically unstable and has already lost a lot of blood an immediate laparotomy is needed because it is the quicker option. Since the primary cause of ectopic is tubal pathology, after treatment the patient who still has one or both tubes should be warned that she is at increased risk of another ectopic pregnancy.

Multiple surgeries on the tube increase the risk of subsequent ectopic and hence a salpingectomy should be performed if a woman has already had surgery on the tube. Methotrexate has to be administered in well-chosen cases to avoid failure. Methotrexate treatment carries the risk associated with residual trophoblastic tissue namely internal bleeding and the eventual need for a laparoscopy.

Acute pelvic inflammatory disease (PID)

5. B, C, D

Inpatient antibiotic treatment should be based on intravenous therapy, which should be continued until 24 hours after clinical improvement followed by oral therapy. Consideration should be given to removing an intrauterine contraceptive device in women presenting with PID, especially if symptoms have not resolved within 72 hours. Women with tubo-ovarian abscess can be treated with intravenous antibiotic regimes in order to maximise antimicrobial dosing and surgical intervention be considered only in cases of leaking or rupture of the abscess or failure to respond to antibiotics.

Broad-spectrum antibiotic therapy is generally required to cover *N. gonorrhoeae, C. trachomatis* and anaerobic infection. The recommended regime is oral ofloxacin 400 mg twice daily plus oral metronidazole 400 mg twice daily for 14 days. Data supporting azithromycin monotherapy for PID is limited at present. Use of combined oral contraceptive pill has usually been regarded as protective against symptomatic PID. Concomitant use does not reduce efficacy.

Utero-vaginal prolapse

6. B, C, E

A rectocele (prolapse of the rectum into the vagina) might cause difficulties with defecation or a sensation of incomplete defecation, which is relieved by digital reduction of the prolapse. It is also associated with a feeling of lump in the vagina. It might cause sexual concerns, such as feeling embarrassed or sensing looseness in the tone of vaginal tissue.

However, since the urinary bladder is not involved a rectocele by itself does not cause urinary symptoms in the form of urinary frequency or recurrent urinary tract infections.

Endometriosis

7. B, D, E

The diagnosis of endometriosis is usually made on visual inspection of the pelvis at laparoscopy; non-invasive diagnostic tools, such as ultrasound scanning, can reliably detect only severe forms of the disease, i.e., endometriomas.

The symptoms associated with the disease include severe dysmenorrhoea, chronic pelvic pain, ovulation pain, deep dyspareunia, cyclical symptoms related to the involvement of other organs (e.g., bowel or bladder) with or without abnormal bleeding, infertility and chronic fatigue. However, the predictive value of any one symptom or set of symptoms remains uncertain as each can have other causes (e.g., irritable bowel syndrome or interstitial cystitis) and a significant proportion of affected women are asymptomatic. Serologic testing for CA-125 has been widely used for detection of endometriosis and monitoring of progressive disease. Typically in endometriosis the values are over 35. Very high values in the range of 1000 u are typically associated with epithelial ovarian cancers. Endometriomas have a classic appearance on MRI because of the signal characteristics of blood and hence serves as an additional diagnostic modality.

→ # Ovarian cancer

8. A, D, E

Ovarian cancer is the sixth most common malignancy among women worldwide and the leading gynaecological cause of death in the developing world. The peak incidence is in the age range of 60–70 years. The overall 5-year survival rate is less than 50%.

Approximately two-thirds of women present with advanced disease. The usual presenting symptoms are abdominal distension or pain. However, more than half of all women present initially with vague symptoms caused by metastatic disease such as shortness of breath or gastrointestinal disturbance. Consequently, it is important to include ovarian cancer in the differential diagnosis of any woman presenting with recent onset of persistent, nonspecific, abdominal symptoms including those whose abdomen and pelvis appears normal on clinical examination.

9. A, C, D

Women who use oral contraceptives have reduced risks of ovarian and endometrial cancer. This protective effect increases with the length of time oral contraceptives are used. In Stage 1, the cancer is confined to ovaries only. Surgery is the mainstay of treatment for ovarian cancer. Staging laparotomy and histological findings provide accurate information about prognosis and the need for additional postoperative therapy. The general principle is cytoreductive surgery followed by combination chemotherapy. However, Stage I/grade 1 epithelial adenocarcinoma requires no postoperative therapy.

About 10% to 30% of ovarian cancers are associated with some genetic mutations. There are still no effective screening methods for ovarian cancer in the general population. Ovarian stimulation with oocyte or embryo freezing has been reported in patients with low-grade tumours (and not all grades of tumours) who wish to preserve fertility, but the effect of this on the underlying disease is as yet unknown and it must therefore be carried out with caution.

Answers to extended matching questions

1. G Adenomyosis

Adenomyosis is defined as the ectopic location of endometrial glands within the uterine myometrium, usually the inner one-third, with surrounding smooth muscle hyperplasia. Most patients with adenomyosis typically present with menorrhagia and dysmenorrhea, which becomes severe as the disease progresses. It is more common in women who have had children. It is often called endometriosis externa, however, both endometriosis and adenomyosis are present simultaneously in fewer than one in four patients. Adenomyosis is a difficult diagnosis to make clinically because the signs and symptoms are nonspecific and often mimic endometriosis or leiomyomas. In adenomyosis, the uterus is enlarged asymmetrically up to a maximum of three times its normal size (less than 14 weeks gestation). The uterus is usually irregularly enlarged with leiomyomas and can attain bigger sizes.

Both transvaginal and transabdominal ultrasound have been used to diagnose adenomyosis. Magnetic Resonance Imaging (MRI) is more sensitive and can differentiate adenomyosis from the presence of fibroids.

Medical management of adenomyosis includes prostaglandin synthetase inhibitors, Danazol and GnRH agonists. Diffuse adenomyosis shows good therapeutic response to a combination therapy of tranexamic acid and mefenamic acid to control pain and menorrhagia. Levonorgesttel-IUS is also another therapeutic option. Hysterectomy is the definitive treatment and is ideal for patients who have completed their family or if the conservative measures have failed in controlling the symptoms.

2. H Benign ovarian cyst

Most women with benign ovarian cysts are asymptomatic. Dull ache or feeling of heaviness and abdominal swelling are noticed with larger tumours. Conversely, they might also present with pain and pressure effects. The pain might be the result of complications such as torsion or bleeding inside the cysts. Benign ovarian cysts apart from the functional cysts do not affect the menstrual cycles. Pressure symptoms due to ovarian cysts such as urinary frequency or retention are seen if the tumour or cyst is impacted in the Pouch of Douglas or if they are present in the anterior uterovesical pouch.

Evaluation of a woman who presents with an ovarian mass should be systematic and thorough in order to exclude ovarian malignancy. Transvaginal or trans-abdominal ultrasonography can usually confirm the diagnosis. If results are indeterminate, magnetic resonance imaging or computed tomography scanning might help. Tumour markers might help in the diagnosis of specific tumours.

In women of reproductive age, simple, thin-walled cystic adnexal masses of 5–8 cm without characteristics of cancer do not require further investigation unless they persist for more than three menstrual cycles. Many ovarian cysts resolve without treatment; serial ultrasonography is carried out to document resolution. Cyst removal (ovarian cystectomy) via laparoscopy or laparotomy might be necessary for cysts ≥ 8 cm, cysts that persist for more than three menstrual cycles and haemorrhagic corpus luteum cysts with signs of peritonitis. Cystic teratomas require removal via cystectomy if possible. Oophorectomy is carried out for fibromas, cystadenomas, cystic teratomas >10 cm and cysts that cannot be surgically removed from the ovary.

3. F Chronic PID

PID is an infection of the female pelvic organs, typically caused by ascending polymicrobial infection with an inciting sexually transmitted pathogen, such as gonorrhea or *Chlamydia*. Chronic PID is usually due to inadequate treatment of acute infection or due to reinfection. Symptoms often include chronic pelvic pain, dyspareunia, dysmenorrheal and menstrual abnormalities. Clinical examination might reveal fixed tender retroverted uterus, adnexal tenderness, or adnexal masses such as hydrosalpinges or tubo-ovarian masses.

Ultrasonography might reveal a hydrosalpinx or tubo-ovarian mass. Laparoscopy is often required when women present with dysmenorrhea or dyspareunia and chronic pelvic pain to confirm the diagnosis and rule out endometriosis.

The complications of chronic or recurrent pelvic infection are hydrosalpinx, pyosalpinx, tubo-ovarian abscess, or long-term consequences of untreated disease, including infertility, ectopic pregnancy and chronic pelvic pain. Prompt and adequate treatment of acute PID is the essential preventive measure. Health care professionals should have a high index of suspicion for diagnosing acute PID in young, sexually active women and a low threshold for treatment to prevent chronic PID. Total abdominal hysterectomy with bilateral salpingo-oophorectomy is indicated in chronic PID if the disease is very advanced and the patient is symptomatic. However in young patients with low parity, laparoscopy or laparotomy to remove adnexal masses could be performed as a conservative option. However, assisted reproductive techniques such as in vitro fertilisation (IVF) are needed if the patient wishes to conceive, as most patients have bilateral tubal damage.

4. B Endometriosis

Endometriosis – defined as the presence of endometrial-like tissue in extra uterine sites. The symptoms associated with the disease include severe dysmenorrhoea, chronic pelvic pain, ovulation pain, deep dyspareunia, cyclical symptoms related to the involvement of other organs (e.g., bowel or bladder) with or without abnormal bleeding, infertility and chronic fatigue.

Finding pelvic tenderness, a fixed retroverted uterus, tender uterosacral ligaments, or enlarged ovaries on examination is suggestive of endometriosis. The diagnosis is more certain if deeply infiltrating nodules are found on the uterosacral ligaments or in the Pouch of Douglas or visible lesions are seen in the vagina or on the cervix. However, the definitive diagnosis of endometriosis is usually made on visual inspection of the pelvis at laparoscopy. Noninvasive diagnostic tools, such as ultrasound scanning, can reliably detect only severe forms of the disease, i.e., endometriomas.

The treatment options are limited and these include hormonal drugs to suppress ovarian function, the levonorgestrel-IUS and surgical ablation of endometriotic lesions. For a woman who has completed her family, hysterectomy plus bilateral salpingo-oophorectomy and removal of all the endometriosis present offers a good chance of cure. However, surgical treatment in a woman who wishes to conceive in the future aims to be as conservative as possible, ensuring in particular that ovarian function is preserved. The aim is to remove all of the endometriotic tissue and restore anatomy to normal by lysing adhesions. The standard (preferably laparoscopic) methods used are ovarian cystectomy and tissue excision or ablation with electrodiathermy.

5. A Residual ovary syndrome

One or both ovaries if retained at the time of hysterectomy can be buried in adhesions and give rise to chronic pelvic pain and dyspareunia. This is called residual ovary syndrome. The residual ovary syndrome usually occurs within 5 years after hysterectomy. The probable incidence of the residual ovary syndrome is 2.3%.

Diagnosis is most often made from the history and localisation of pelvic pain. The most common symptom of these patients is chronic pelvic pain. In addition, patients characterise the pain as dull and aching to sharp and stabbing. They might also experience low back pain, variable bowel symptoms and dyspareunia. In severe endometriosis or PID a small amount of ovarian tissue that might be left behind during oophorectomy might cause symptoms of chronic pelvic pain and this condition is called remnant ovary syndrome. Imaging studies, including vaginal ultrasound, CT and MRI, aid in the diagnosis.

As definitive treatment, surgical excision of the ovary is the best choice in the majority of cases. Extensive pelvic adhesions were the typical operative findings, while follicular cysts and corpus luteum hematoma were the common pathological findings of the residual ovaries. The incidence of malignant neoplastic change in these patients was 3.0%, related to whether hysterectomy was performed before or after the age of 40. In view of the incidence of the residual ovary syndrome and the risk of malignant neoplastic change when hysterectomy is performed after the age of 40, serious consideration of total ovarian ablation at the time of hysterectomy should be weighed against any temporary physiologic or psychologic benefits to be gained from conservation.

6. C Ruptured ectopic pregnancy

The clinical features are suggestive of ruptured ectopic pregnancy – hypovolaemic shock, sudden onset of lower abdominal pain and signs of peritonism in the pelvis. Current or previous use of an intrauterine contraceptive device is a high risk factor for ectopic pregnancy.

Clinicians should have a high index of suspicion of the diagnosis of ectopic pregnancy in any woman in the reproductive age group presenting with severe lower abdominal pain and hypotension or tachycardia irrespective of the last menstrual period. Urine pregnancy test should be carried out, and an ultrasound is required to confirm the presence of haemoperitoneum. Bleeding or rupture of haemorrhagic corpus luteum might also produce acute pelvic pain and on rare occasions shock, thus simulating ruptured ectopic pregnancy. However, pregnancy test helps in the differentiation of these two conditions.

Ruptured ectopic pregnancy is a surgical emergency that requires prompt resuscitation and immediate surgery by laparotomy. Laparotomy remains the mainstay of management of ruptured ectopic pregnancy if the patient is hypotensive, tachycardic, or otherwise in a haemodynamically unstable condition. Laparoscopic approach of managing ectopic pregnancy has become the gold standard in hemodynamically stable patients. However, in an acute situation, laparoscopy might be performed prior to laparotomy, or the definitive procedure can be carried out by the laparoscopic route if expertise permits.

7. D Twisted ovarian cyst

Torsion of ovarian cyst is a common complication of an ovarian cyst and is a surgical emergency. The usual presenting symptoms are sudden onset of acute abdominal pain. The cyst, if palpable, is tender and signs of acute abdomen such as rigidity and rebound tenderness are usually present. Confirmation is by ultrasound and this should be followed by emergency laparoscopy or laparotomy. Ovarian cystectomy might be possible after untwisting the ovary or adnexa, however, if the twisted ovary is gangrenous oophorectomy is indicated.

Torsion of an ovarian cyst is a very common complication and occurs in about 12%. In most cases, the cyst is about 10 cm or more when it undergoes torsion. The tumour rotates through several complete circles, causing the veins in the pedicle to be occluded and the tumour becomes congested. The increased tension inside the tumour causes severe abdominal pain and signs of peritoneal irritation. Torsion of ovarian cyst is seen more commonly with benign cysts, such as dermoid or mucinous cystadenomas, whereas malignant ovarian tumour or endometriotic cysts are unlikely to undergo torsion.

8. E Uterine fibroid

Fibroids are benign, well-circumscribed, smooth muscle tumors of the uterus. Women with uterine fibroids will present with heavy or irregular menstrual bleeding, pressure symptoms, or problems conceiving, especially if there is a fibroid in the uterine cavity. The pressure symptoms include pelvic discomfort, urinary incontinence, frequency and retention, constipation and backache.

The diagnosis is usually apparent on bimanual or abdominal examination, on the basis of finding an enlarged uterus with attached swellings. The principal differential diagnosis is an ovarian tumour. As a general rule, the uterus is felt separately on vaginal examination if an ovarian tumour is present, although not if the structures are adherent to each other. Ultrasound can usually establish diagnosis and distinguish fibroids from ovarian tumors.

Treatment options include shrinkage of the fibroids by inducing a hypo-oestrogenic state with a GnRH agonist, uterine artery embolisation (UAE), myomectomy (removal of the individual fibroids) and hysterectomy. The choice depends upon the woman's age and fertility intentions and size and number of fibroids and their location. It is also important to know whether there are fibroids in the uterine cavity, especially if the woman is trying to conceive.

Transplantation

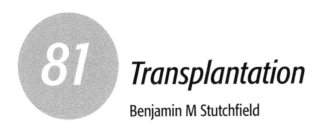

Transplantation

Benjamin M Stutchfield

Multiple choice questions

Transplantation terms

1. Which of the following statements are true?

A An allograft occurs between individuals of the same species.

B A xenograft is defined as a graft performed between humans of different sex.

C Renal transplantation is usually defined as an orthotopic graft.

D An alloantibody is formed in a recipient in response to transplantation of an organ.

E A heterotopic graft is placed in its normal anatomical location.

Graft rejection

2. The following statements are true except:

A In ABO blood grouping, a group A donor can donate to group A or AB recipients.

B Rhesus antigen compatibility is crucial to successful graft outcomes.

C HLA antigens are highly polymorphic and are the most common cause of rejection.

D HLA antigens activate T cells, which play a central role in graft rejection.

E CD4 and CD8 T cells are the main effector cells.

3. Which of the following statements are false?

A Hyperacute rejection is powerful, immediate allograft rejection following transplantation.

B Acute rejection is defined as graft rejection occurring within the first month.

C Chronic rejection is the least common form of rejection.

D Acute rejection invariably leads to loss of the graft.

E Chronic rejection is readily reversible with appropriate treatment.

Immunosuppressive therapy

4. The following statements are true except:

A Corticosteroids have broad-spectrum anti-inflammatory properties.

B Calcineurin inhibitors block transcription of the Il-2 gene.

C Azathioprine prevents proliferation of neutrophils.

D Mycophenolic acid preparations prevent proliferation of lymphocytes.

E mTOR inhibitors block signal transduction from the IL-2.

Immunosuppressive agents

5. Which of the following statements are false?

A Immunosupressive agents can aid wound healing and reduce risk of wound infection.

B mTOR inhibitors are a major cause of avascular necrosis.

C Nephrotoxicity can occur with tacrolimus.

D Corticosteroids can cause gingival hyperplasia.

E Cyclosporin typically results in a Cushingoid appearance.

→ ## Organ donation

6. Which of the following statements are true?

A Living donation provides the majority of liver grafts for transplantation.

B Deceased donors are by definition non-heart-beating donors.

C An adult liver can be split to provide a liver graft for two recipients.

D Warm ischaemia leads to more organ damage than cold ischaemia.

E Age of donor is the most important factor in predicting graft outcome.

Extended matching questions

→ ## Post-transplantation complications

1 Acute rejection
2 Arterial stenosis
3 Haemorrhage
4 Malignancy
5 Venous thrombosis
6 Viral infection

Match the diagnoses with the clinical scenarios that follow:

→ ## Clinical scenarios

A A 59-year-old woman presents with a 2-day history of intermittent fever, cough and lethargy. 6 weeks previously she had undergone renal transplantation. On examination she has is pyrexial and tachycardic with evidence of consolidation at the right lung base. The surgical wound is well healed and there is not tenderness at the site.

B A 67-year-old man presents with a 2-week history of firm swellings in both groins, which have gradually increased in size. He complains of general fatigue but is otherwise well. The patient had undergone kidney pancreas transplantation 2 years previously and had required an aggressive immunosuppressive regimen over the first 18 months post-transplant. Examination confirms firm, rubbery swellings in both groins.

C A 70-year-old man is found by his general practitioner to have persistent high blood pressure, which has proved refractory to antihypertensive therapy. He had undergone renal transplantation 3 years previously. Postoperatively he has progressed very well, and immunosuppressive regimen has been stable for a number of years.

D A 58-year-old woman develops pain and swelling at the site of renal transplantation 2 days postoperatively. She otherwise appears well, haemodynamically stable and apyrexial. Blood tests show that renal function has deteriorated.

E A 52-year-old woman has undergone liver transplantation 12 hours previously. She is being monitored closely in the intensive care unit when her blood pressure abruptly falls and heart rate rises rapidly. She appears pale, and her peripheries are cool and clammy to the touch.

F A 58-year-old woman has undergone simultaneous kidney pancreas transplantation 1 week previously and has been progressing well on the surgical ward. However blood tests show that serum creatinine has increased rapidly over the past 48 hours, with both lipase and amylase also elevated.

→ Transplantation terms

1. A, D

An allograft refers to organ transplantation between members of the same species, resulting in the formation of alloantibodies in the recipient as part of the strong immune response the allograft can induce.

Xenotransplantation (xenograft) occurs between members of different species. An orthotopic graft is placed in its usual anatomical location, as is generally the case with liver transplantation. A heterotopic graft is placed in a non-anatomical position, such as occurs with renal transplantation where the renal vessels are anastomosed to the iliac vessels.

→ Graft rejection

2. B

Rhesus antigen compatibility is of little concern in organ transplantation, as rhesus factor is present on the surface of red blood cells rather than viscera.

ABO blood grouping is crucial for any allograft, and a mismatch will result in an immediate robust rejection response. Group A can donate to Group A or AB, Group B can donate to Group B or AB, Group AB only to AB and Group O can donate to any group. HLA antigens serve to aid recognition of foreign pathogens by T lymphocytes, are highly polymorphic and are the main target in allograft rejection. CD4 T cells drive many of the effector mechanisms in graft rejection, after activation by HLA antigens. CD8 T cells can lead to targeted cell death by releasing substances such as perforin and granzyme, which promote cell lysis.

→ Graft rejection

3. B, C, D, E

Acute rejection can generally occur up to 6 months following transplantation, but can occur later. Acute rejection is predominantly due to HLA mismatch and subsequent T-cell mediated graft injury. A mononuclear cell infiltrate is evident, including T cells, B cells, NK cells and activated macrophages. An acute rejection episode can generally be reversed by additional immunosuppression. Chronic rejection is a major cause of allograft loss, generally occurring after 6 months. Some of the main risk factors for chronic rejection include previous acute rejection, poor HLA matching and long cold ischemia time. Histological changes of chronic rejection are characterised by ischaemia and fibrosis.

Hyperacute rejection is generally due to ABO mismatch or presence of preformed anti-HLA antibodies. The graft can rapidly develop thrombotic occlusions, with haemorrhage of the graft vasculature within minutes to hours following perfusion.

→ Immunosuppressive therapy

4. C

Azathioprines (and mycophenolates) are termed antiproliferative agents and act against lymphocytes. Neutrophils are terminally differentiated cells and not capable of proliferation.

Corticosteroids have wide-ranging effects, including the inhibition of proinflammatory cytokines and chemokines. They can be used for management of episodes of acute rejection as well as for induction and maintenance of immunosuppression. The calcineurin inhibitors ciclosporin and tacrolimus form the cornerstone of most immunosuppression protocols in organ transplantation. Both of these drugs block the activity of calcineurin within the T cell by binding to cyclophilin (cyclosporine) or FK-binding protein (tacrolimus). Calcineurin is involved with transcription of IL-2, which is the main T-cell growth factor.

mTOR (mammalian target of rapamcin) inhibitors, such as tacrolimus and everolimus, affect IL-2 receptor intracellular signalling, stopping T-cell proliferation in the G1 phase.

→ Immunosuppressive agents

5. A, B, E

Inflammation is a central part of wound healing, in terms of tissue repair and minimising risk of infection. Immunosuppression impairs the inflammatory response and can lead to impaired wound healing and increased risk of infection. mTOR (mammalian target of rapamycin) inhibitors block IL-2 receptor signal transduction, which is a major T-cell growth factor. Side effects of mTOR inhibitors can include thrombocytopenia, dyslipidaemia and impaired wound healing. Corticosteroids are a well-recognised cause of avascular necrosis. Ciclosporin can lead to hirsuitism and gingival hyperplasia, while corticosteroids can lead to a Cushingoid appearance.

Tacrolimus use risks hypertension, diabetes, neurotoxicity and nephrotoxicity among others. Gingival hyperplasia (increase in gum size) can be caused by a number of immunosuppressants, typically corticosteroids, mycophenolic acid derivatives and ciclosporin.

→ Organ donation

6. C, D

A donated liver can be split to potentially provide a liver graft for both an adult (right lobe) and child (left lateral segment). Minimising ischaemic time is crucial for successful graft outcome. Warm ischaemia is the most damaging period, which is more of an issue with circulatory death donors given the practicalities of rapid cooling in this group.

The majority of liver grafts are performed from deceased donors, however, increasingly living donor liver transplantation is performed. Deceased donors can either be brainstem-dead heart-beating donors (DBD) or donation-after-circulatory death (DCD) donors. While age of the donor is important, underlying quality of the organ is one of the most important determinants of outcome.

Answers to extended matching questions

1. F Acute rejection

Recognising acute rejection in simultaneous kidney pancreas transplantation involved tends to rely on monitoring parameters related to renal function. Bladder-drained pancreas transplantation enables monitoring of urinary amylase levels, a fall in which could indicate impaired function and rejection. However, most centres now prefer primary enteric drainage following SKP transplantation. Serum amylase and lipase levels can give an indication of pancreatic graft inflammation, which might be caused by acute rejection (among other causes of pancreatitis postoperatively). A rise in blood glucose level is generally a late feature of rejection, indicating a high likelihood of graft loss.

Acute rejection can occur in 10%–20% of SPK transplants, but if identified early can be reversed with steroid treatment. Rejection generally involves both organs with renal functional parameters the most sensitive indicators of impaired function and possible rejection.

2. C Arterial stenosis

Stenosis of the renal artery is generally a late complication, which can occur many years following renal transplantation. It can be recognised by rising blood pressure and reduction in renal function. Doppler ultrasonography and magnetic resonance angiography can provide a detailed assessment of vascular flow.

This is a readily reversible cause of graft dysfunction, which untreated can lead to progressive impairment and eventual graft loss. The treatment of choice is percutaneous transluminal angioplasty, which can restore graft function in the majority of cases. A stent can also be placed using the endovascular approach to maintain blood pressure. Surgery might be required if angioplasty fails or is not appropriate.

3. E Haemorrhage

This patient shows clear signs of circulatory collapse. Any surgical procedure carries the risk of postoperative haemorrhage. Liver transplantation involves multiple anastomoses with major vessels in patients who might have coagulation abnormalities relating to impaired hepatic function. Meticulous surgical technique is central to minimising risks of bleeding from the site of vessel anastomosis or aberrant anatomy. Maximising haemostatic function by optimising fibrinolytic function, platelet function and coagulation factors also plays an important role in the prevention of postoperative haemorrhage.

While hyperacute rejection can lead to circulatory instability, and graft destruction, this is usually apparent immediately. The liver is relatively resistant to hyperacute rejection although the reason for this is not clear. Acute rejection generally occurs within the first 6 months following transplantation and would not lead to the sudden deterioration seen in this patient.

4. B Malignancy

This patient presents with a clear history of lymphadenopathy in both groins. Post-transplant lymphoproliferative disorder is characterised by widespread proliferation of lymphoid cells, in particular, B lymphocytes. Presentation can vary widely, from general, nonspecific symptoms such as weight loss and malaise to lymphadenopathy. The lymphadenopathy can lead to secondary effects related to increasing size, such as abdominal pain, respiratory difficulty and even seizures. Neurological features are associated with the worst prognosis, with the condition carrying an overall mortality rate up to 50%.

If diagnosed early enough reduction in immunosuppression can improve the condition. However, a multimodal treatment strategy might be required, involving surgery to reduce pressure effects, and radiotherapy and antiviral therapy.

There is a general increased risk of malignancy following transplantation, related to the strong immunosuppression required to prevent rejection. Skin cancer is a particular concern, including squamous cell carcinoma, basal cell carcinoma and malignant melanoma. Patients must be made aware of this risk and take appropriate precautions to protect themselves from excessive sunlight.

5. D Venous thrombosis

The main venous complication following renal transplantation is renal vein thrombosis. This typically presents during the first week, particularly within the first 2 days following transplantation with pain and swelling at the graft site. Surgical exploration is indicated, although renal vein thrombosis usually leads to loss of the graft. Heparinisation and thrombectomy might be successful in selected cases.

The aetiology of venous thrombosis might relate to poor surgical technique, compression of the renal vein, coagulopathy, or hypovolaemia. This necessitates a multifactorial approach to minimise this complication.

6. A Viral infection

Following transplantation there is a risk of viral infection, which most frequently occurs within the first 6 months. Cytomegalovirus is the most common viral infection and can arise due to reactivation of latent infection or be transmitted via the organ of a CMV-positive donor. CMV is related to the herpes virus family and affects approximately 50% of all donors from the United Kingdom. The infection generally only becomes an issue when the immune system is compromised, such as with immunosuppressive therapies following transplantation. Matching negative donors and recipients is impractical, so routine prophylaxis involves the use of nucleoside analogues that inhibit DNA synthesis.

Without prophylaxis, patients most commonly present between 4 and 8 weeks with fever, fatigue and leukopenia. Organs affected can be variable, with consequences including pneumonia, hepatitis, retinitis or colitis.

Appendix

Common instruments used in general surgery

Pradip K Datta

This chapter is written purely as extended matching questions and does not lend itself to multiple-choice questions. First, certain operations have been listed in alphabetical order. Below there are the pictures of certain instruments with their names. You are expected to match the operations with the specific instruments, bearing in mind that a particular instrument can be used in more than one of the operations listed. Also more than one instrument may be used in a single operation, for example, a pair of scissors. All operations described are open procedures.

→ List of operations

1 Abdomino-perineal resection (upper end)
2 Abdomino-perineal resection (lower end)
3 Anterior resection
4 Appendicectomy
5 Groin dissection in varicose vein surgery
6 Laparotomy
7 Lymph node biopsy
8 Open cholecystectomy/right hemicolectomy
9 Small bowel resection
10 Thyroidectomy

→ List of instruments

A Allis forceps

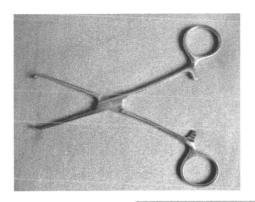

B Babcock forceps

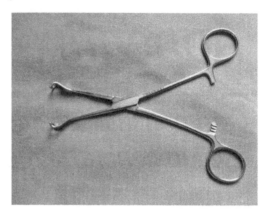

C Deaver retractor

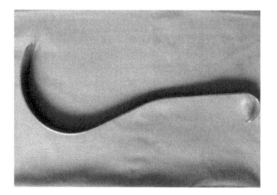

D Dyball retractor

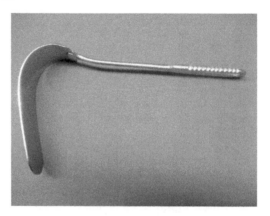

E Goligher retractor

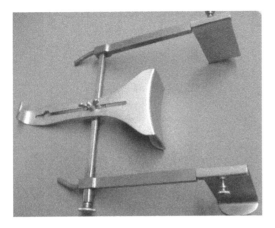

F Joll retractor

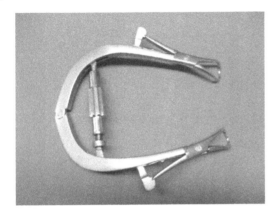

G Kocher dissector

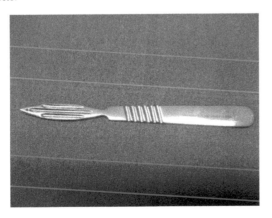

H McIndoe scissors

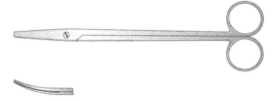

I Morris retractor

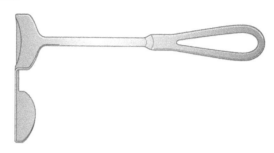

J St Mark's retractor

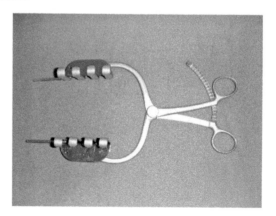

K Travers retractor

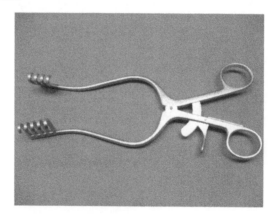

L West retractor

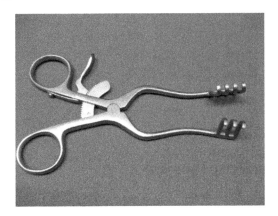

Answers to extended matching questions

1. Abdomino-perineal resection (APR) (upper end) E Goligher retractor, D Dyball retractor

This is a self-retaining three-bladed retractor used for operations on the sigmoid colon and rectum, such as upper end of APR, anterior resection or Hartmann's operation. With the patient in the Lloyd-Davies (lithotomy-Trendelenberg) position, the abdomen is opened. On opening the abdomen and performing a laparotomy, the patient is placed in the head-down position. The retractor is now inserted with only the two lateral blades to separate the wound edges. Next, the entire small bowel from the duodeno-jejunal flexure to the ileocaecal junction is packed away toward the head end with wet towels. Now the centre blade is applied to push the packs and keep them away from the site of operation. The three blades are available in different sizes to fit in with the build of the patient. The appropriate dissection is now commenced.

The Dyball retractor, which the assistant uses, is a very useful deep retractor in the latter stages of these operations to retract the urinary bladder or the uterus, or both, when dissecting in the region of the recto-vesical pouch or the pouch of Douglas.

2. Abdomino-perineal resection (lower end) J St Mark's retractor

This is a self-retaining retractor devised for the perineal end of an APR. After applying a purse-string to the anus, the stitch is left long and held in a haemostat to apply traction during dissection. An elliptical incision is made around the anus. The incision is deepened into both ischiorectal fossa. Once the incision is deep enough, the retractor is applied with the pointed ends upward to separate the ischiorectal fat, providing a good view of the anorectum that is held by the purse-string on the haemostat. As the dissection proceeds, the retractor has to be repositioned.

3. Anterior resection E Goligher retractor, D Dyball retractor

Please see number 1 above for APR.

4. Appendicectomy   B   Babcock forceps
This is an atraumatic grasping forceps used to grasp bowel. It is most commonly used in appendicectomy to grasp the appendix and deliver it out of the wound. When using this instrument, care should be taken not to perforate the inflamed appendix. It is also used to steady parts of the bowel while bringing cut edges together for anastomosis.

5. Groin dissection in varicose vein surgery   K   Travers retractor,   H   McIndoe scissors
This is a self-retaining retractor used to retract wound edges where the length of the incision is 3 to 4 cm long. For longer incisions where dissection is not too deep, two of these retractors can be used at either end of the wound. It is ideal for a groin dissection for varicose veins, inguinal or femoral hernia repairs and femoral embolectomy. It retracts skin and subcutaneous tissue and needs replacing as the incision is deepened. McIndoe scissors is the ideal dissecting instrument in these operations.

6. Laparotomy   I   Morris retractor
On making an abdominal incision, longitudinal or transverse, for a laparotomy, on opening the abdomen, the wound edges have to be retracted by the assistant. At the initial stage during exploratory laparotomy, this retractor is the ideal one to use. The lip of the retractor prevents it from slipping while the assistant pulls on it to give the surgeon a good exposure.

7. Lymph node biopsy   L   West retractor,   H   McIndoe scissors
This instrument is a smaller version of the Travers retractor. It is the ideal retractor to use when doing a lymph node biopsy under local anaesthetic, usually without an assistant. As a self-retaining retractor, it will need repositioning during the operation. The jaws should be prised open gently, because the operation is under local anaesthetic. To dissect the lymph node the McIndoe scissors is the ideal instrument to use to create as minimal trauma as possible, thus not distorting the macroscopic feature of the node.

8. Open cholecystectomy/right hemicolectomy   C   Deaver retractor   D   Dyball retractor
After entering the peritoneal cavity for one of these operations, the liver has to be retracted. This is done by the Dyball or Deaver retractor. While performing this procedure, to minimise the chances of trauma to the liver by over-enthusiastic retraction, a wet pack is often placed between the liver and the blade of the retractor.

9. Small bowel resection   A   Allis forceps,   H   McIndoe scissors
In small bowel resection, the bowel ends will need to be moved around without handling (no-touch technique). This is best done by using Allis forceps, which can also provide gentle traction. Dissection of the small bowel mesentery is an initial part of the operation. This is ideally done by McIndoe scissors.

10. Thyroidectomy   F   Joll retractor,   G   Kocher dissector,   H   McIndoe scissors
A curved collar incision is made halfway between the thyroid cartilage and suprasternal notch. After cutting through skin and platysma, the upper flap is raised up to the thyroid cartilage and lower flap down to the suprasternal notch. After mobilisation of the two flaps is complete, the Joll self-retaining thyroid retractor is inserted. This is done by first placing wet swabs over the skin edges, and then applying the two clips of the retractor to the swab-covered skin edges. The central segment of the retractor is then unscrewed to separate the skin edges to obtain full exposure.

After dealing with the middle thyroid vein/s, the superior pole is first mobilised and divided. The Kocher dissector is very useful for this manoeuvre. The dissector is used to perform blunt dissection in the upper pole and isolate the superior thyroid vessels. Once isolated, the dissector is pushed under the pedicle. A tie is then put through the eye of the dissector, which at this stage doubles as an aneurysm needle. The pedicle is thus tied three times as close to the gland as possible, so as not to damage the external laryngeal nerve. With the dissector under the tied pedicle, a fine knife is used to cut the pedicle, leaving two ties in the patient and one on the gland. Alternatively an aneurysm needle may be used to perform this step.

Dissection in this operation is ideally carried out by McIndoe scissors.

Index

Note: Reference to individual questions and their answers and given in the form of chapter number followed by question number (e.g. 56.8) with a following letter M, for extended matching questions chapter number followed by E (e. g. 8E). Topics covering a whole chapter range are given a normal page range reference without any mention of the chapter number (e.g. Abdominal pain, 519–525)